C
D
2

EDITORS

Leonard G. Gomella, MD, FACS
Steven A. Haist, MD, MS, FACP
Aimee G. Adams, PharmD

www.eDrugbook.com
www.thescutmonkey.com

New York   Chicago   San Francisco   Athens
London   Madrid   Mexico City   Milan   New Delhi
Singapore   Sydney   Toronto

Clinician's Pocket Drug Reference 2016

1 2 3 4 5 6 7 8 9 0   QLM/QLM   20 19 18 17 16 15

ISBN 978-1-25-958605-7
MHID 1-25-958605-7
ISSN 1540-6725

Notice

Medicine is an ever-changing science. As new research and clinical experience broaden our knowledge, changes in treatment and drug therapy are required. The authors and the publisher of this work have checked with sources that are believed to be reliable in their efforts to provide information that is complete and generally in accord with the standards accepted at the time of publication. However, in view of the possibility of human error or changes in medical sciences, neither the authors nor the publisher nor any other party who has been involved in the preparation or publication of this work warrants that the information contained herein is in every respect accurate or complete, and they disclaim all responsibility for any errors or omissions or for the results obtained from use of the information contained in this work. Readers are encouraged to confirm the information contained herein with other sources. For example and in particular, readers are advised to check the product information sheet included in the package of each drug they plan to administer to be certain that the information contained in this work is accurate and that changes have not been made in the recommended dose or in the contraindications for administration. This recommendation is of particular importance in connection with new or infrequently used drugs.

The book was set in Times by Cenveo® Publisher Services.
The editors were Catherine Johnson and Harriet Lebowitz.
The production supervisor was Catherine Saggese.
Project management was provided by Tanya Punj, Cenveo Publisher Services.
Quad/Graphics Leominster was printer and binder.

This book is printed on acid-free paper.

CONTENTS

Leonard G. Gomella, MD, FACS
The Bernard W. Godwin, Jr, Professor
Chairman, Department of Urology
Sidney Kimmel Medical College
Senior Director of Clinical Affairs
Sidney Kimmel Cancer Center
Thomas Jefferson University and Thomas Jefferson University Hospital
Philadelphia, Pennsylvania

Steven A. Haist, MD, MS, FACP
Clinical Professor
Department of Medicine
Drexel University College of Medicine
Philadelphia, Pennsylvania

Aimee G. Adams, PharmD
Clinical Pharmacist Specialist, Ambulatory Care
Adjunct Assistant Professor
College of Pharmacy and Department of Internal Medicine
University of Kentucky HealthCare
Lexington, Kentucky

PREFACE

We are pleased to present the 14th edition of the *Clinician's Pocket Drug Reference*. This book is based on the drug presentation style originally used in 1983 in the *Clinician's Pocket Reference*, popularly known as the "Scut Monkey Book." Our goal is to identify the most frequently used and clinically important medications, including branded, generic, OTC, and herbal products. The book now includes over 1400 generic product listings with the true number approaching 4000 entries when specific brand names are considered.

Our unique style of presentation includes key "must-know" facts of commonly used medications, essential for both the student and practicing clinician. The inclusion of common uses of medications, rather than just the official FDA-labeled indications, is based on supporting publications and community standards of care and has been reviewed by our editors and editorial board.

Encyclopedic information can be found on many websites and is occasionally needed when unique clinical situations arise. However, resources that identify the most common and essential facts are sometimes lacking. Our goal is to provide access not only to dosing but also to these clinically significant facts and key data, whether for commonly prescribed brand-name drugs, generics, or OTC products in a pocket-sized book format. Information contained within is meant for use by healthcare professionals who are already familiar with these commonly prescribed medications. For 2016, we have added over 50 new drugs, as well as hundreds of changes in other medications based on recent FDA actions and manufacturers' updates.

Versions of this book are produced in a variety of electronic or eBook formats. Visit www.eDrugbook.com for a link to some of the electronic versions currently available. Additionally, this website has several enhanced content features, such as a comprehensive listing of "look alike–sound alike" medications that can contribute to prescribing errors and other useful information related to medication prescribing.

Nursing versions of this book (*Nurses Pocket Drug Guide*) that features a section of customized nursing interventions are available. An EMS guide based on this book (*EMS Pocket Drug Guide*) with enhanced content specifically for the field provider and emergency medical practitioner is also available. Information and links for these related publications are available on the website www.eDrugbook.com.

We express special thanks to our spouses and families for their long-term support of this book and the entire Scut Monkey Project (www.thescutmonkey.com). The Scut Monkey Project, launched in 1979 at the University of Kentucky College of Medicine, is designed to provide new medical students and other health professional students with the basic tools needed when entering the world of hands-on patient care. Many other schools have adopted the concept of "students teaching students" over the years. A type of "boot camp," similar to our long-standing Scut Monkey Program course, is now offered to graduating medical students at many schools before they start their internships.

The contributions of the members of the editorial board, Harriet Lebowitz at McGraw-Hill, Tanya Punj and her colleagues at Cenveo Publisher Services, and Barbara Devine are gratefully acknowledged. As a reader, your comments and suggestions are always welcome. Improvements to this and all our books would be impossible without the interest and continual feedback of our readers. We hope this book will help you learn some of the key elements in prescribing medications and allow you to care for your patients in the best way possible.

Leonard G. Gomella, MD, FACS
Philadelphia, Pennsylvania
Leonard.Gomella@jefferson.edu

Steven A. Haist, MD, MS, FACP
Philadelphia, Pennsylvania

Aimee G. Adams, PharmD
Lexington, Kentucky

MEDICATION KEY

Medications are listed by prescribing class, and individual medications are then listed in alphabetical order by generic name. Some of the more commonly recognized trade names are listed for each medication (in parentheses after the generic name) or if available without prescription, noted as **OTC** (over-the-counter).

Generic Drug Name (Selected Common Brand Names) [Controlled Substance] BOX: Summarized/paraphrased versions of the "Black Box" precautions deemed necessary by the FDA. These are significant precautions, warnings, and contraindications concerning the individual medication. **Uses:** This includes both FDA-labeled indications bracketed by ** and other "off-label" uses of the medication. Because many medications are used to treat various conditions based on the medical literature and not listed in their package insert, we list common uses of the medication in addition to the official "labeled indications" (FDA approved) based on input from our editorial board. **Acts:** How the drug works. This information is helpful in comparing classes of drugs and understanding side effects and contraindications. *Spectrum:* Specifies activity against selected microbes for antimicrobials. **Dose:** *Adults.* Where no specific pediatric dose is given, the implication is that the drug is not commonly used or indicated in that age group. At the end of the dosing line, important dosing modifications may be noted (ie, take with food, avoid antacids, etc). *Peds.* If appropriate, dosing for children and infants is included with age ranges as needed. **W/P (Warnings and Precautions):** [Pregnancy/fetal risk categories, breast-feeding (as noted below)] Warnings and precautions concerning the use of the drug in specific settings. **CI:** Contraindications. **Disp:** Common dosing forms. **SE:** Common or significant side effects. **Notes:** Other key useful information about the drug.

CONTROLLED SUBSTANCE CLASSIFICATION

Medications under the control of the US Drug Enforcement Agency (DEA) (Schedules I–V controlled substances) are indicated by the symbol [C]. Most medications are "uncontrolled" and do not require a DEA prescriber number on the prescription. The following is a general description for the schedules of DEA-controlled substances:

Schedule (C-I) I: All non-research use forbidden (e.g., heroin, LSD, mescaline).

Schedule (C-II) II: High addictive potential; medical use accepted. No telephone call-in prescriptions; limit of one 90-day supply; no refills. Some states require special prescription form (e.g., cocaine, hydrocodone, morphine, methadone).

Schedule (C-III) III: Low to moderate risk of physical dependence, high risk of psychological dependence; prescription must be rewritten after six months or five refills (eg, acetaminophen plus codeine).

Schedule (C-IV) IV: Limited potential for dependence; prescription rules same as for schedule III (eg, benzodiazepines, propoxyphene).

Schedule (C-V) V: Very limited abuse potential; prescribing regulations often the same as for uncontrolled medications; some states have additional restrictions.

FDA FETAL RISK CATEGORIES

Category A: Adequate studies in pregnant women have not demonstrated a risk to the fetus in the first trimester of pregnancy; there is no evidence of risk in the last two trimesters.

Category B: Animal studies have not demonstrated a risk to the fetus, but no adequate studies have been done in pregnant women.

or

Animal studies have shown an adverse effect, but adequate studies in pregnant women have not demonstrated a risk to the fetus during the first trimester of pregnancy, and there is no evidence of risk in the last two trimesters.

Category C: Animal studies have shown an adverse effect on the fetus, but no adequate studies have been done in humans. The benefits from the use of the drug in pregnant women may be acceptable despite its potential risks.

or

No animal reproduction studies and no adequate studies in humans have been done.

Category D: There is evidence of human fetal risk, but the potential benefits from the use of the drug in pregnant women may be acceptable despite its potential risks.

Category X: Studies in animals or humans or adverse reaction reports, or both, have demonstrated fetal abnormalities. The risk of use in pregnant women clearly outweighs any possible benefit.

Category ?: No data available (not a formal FDA classification; included to provide complete dataset).

BREAST-FEEDING CLASSIFICATION

No formally recognized classification exists for drugs and breast-feeding. This shorthand was developed for the *Clinician's Pocket Drug Reference*. The FDA is considering creating a standard listing in the future.

+	Compatible with breast-feeding
M	Monitor patient or use with caution
±	Excreted, or likely excreted, with unknown effects or at unknown concentrations
?/–	Unknown excretion, but effects likely to be of concern
–	Contraindicated in breast-feeding
?	No data available

ABBREVIATIONS

Δ: change
Ø: none
?: possible or uncertain
✓: check, follow, or monitor
↓: decrease/decreased
↑: increase/increased
≠: not equal to; not equivalent to
÷: divided
♀: female
♂: male
μM: symbol for micromolar
5HT2A: serotonin type 2
AAP: American Academy of Pediatrics
Ab: abortion, antibody
abbrev: abbreviation
Abd: abdominal
ABG: arterial blood gas
ABMT: autologous bone marrow transplantation
abn: abnormal
ABSSSI: acute bacterial skin and skin structure infections
abx: antibiotics
ac: before meals (*ante cibum*)
ACE: angiotensin-converting enzyme
ACH: acetylcholine
ACIP: Advisory Committee on Immunization Practices, American College of International Physicians
ACLS: advanced cardiac life support
ACR: American College of Rheumatology, American College of Radiology
ACS: acute coronary syndrome, American Cancer Society, American College of Surgeons

ACT: activated coagulation time
Acts: actuation(s)
ADH: antidiuretic hormone
ADHD: attention-deficit hyperactivity disorder
ADR: adverse drug reaction
ADT: androgen deprivation therapy
AED: anti-epileptic drug
AE: adverse event
AF: atrial fibrillation
AF/A flutter: atrial fibrillation/atrial flutter
AGEP: acute generalized exanthematous pustulosis
AHA: American Heart Association
AKA: also known as
ALK: anaplastic lymphoma kinase
alk phos: alkaline phosphatase
ALL: acute lymphocytic leukemia
ALT: alanine aminotransferase
AMD: age-related macular degeneration
AMI: acute myocardial infarction
AML: acute myelogenous leukemia
amp: ample
ANA: antinuclear antibody
ANC: absolute neutrophil count
antag: antagonist
APACHE: acute physiology and chronic health evaluation
APAP: acetaminophen [*N*-acetyl-*p*-aminophenol]
aPTT: activated partial thromboplastin time
ARB: angiotensin II receptor blocker

ARDS: adult respiratory distress syndrome

ARF: acute renal failure

AS: ankylosing spondylitis, aortic stenosis

ASA: aspirin (acetylsalicylic acid)

ASAP: as soon as possible

AST: aspartate aminotransferase

AT: antithrombin

ATE: arterial thrombotic event

ATG: antithymocyte globulin

ATP: adenosine triphosphate

ATSDR: Agency for Toxic Substances and Disease Registry

attn: attention

atyp: atypical

AUB: abnormal uterine/vaginal bleeding

AUC: area under the curve

AV: atrioventricular

AVM: arteriovenous malformation

BBB: bundle branch block

BCL: B-cell lymphoma

BCP: birth control pill(s)

bid: twice daily

bili: bilirubin

BM: bone marrow, bowel movement

↓BM: bone marrow suppression, myelosuppression

BMD: bone mineral density

BMI: body mass index

BMT: bone marrow transplantation

BOO: bladder outlet obstruction

BP: blood pressure

↓BP: hypotension

↑BP: hypertension

BPH: benign prostatic hyperplasia

BPM: beats per minute

BS: blood sugar

BSA: body surface area

BUN: blood urea nitrogen

BW: body weight

Ca: calcium

CA: cancer

CABG: coronary artery bypass graft

CAD: coronary artery disease

CAP: community-acquired pneumonia

caps: capsule(s)

cardiotox: cardiotoxicity

CBC: complete blood count

CCB: calcium channel blocker

CCR5: human chemokine receptor 5 (HIV attaches to the receptor to infect CD4$^+$ T cells)

CDAD: *Clostridium* difficile–associated diarrhea

CDC: Centers for Disease Control and Prevention

CF: cystic fibrosis

CFCs: chlorofluorocarbons

CFU: colony-forming unit(s)

CGD: chronic granulomatous disease

CHD: coronary heart disease

chemo: chemotherapy

CHF: congestive heart failure

chol: cholesterol

CI: contraindicated

CIDP: chronic inflammatory polyneuropathy

CIWA: Clinical Institute Withdrawal Assessment Score (used to monitor EtOH withdrawal)

CJD: Creutzfeldt-Jakob disease

CK: creatinine kinase

CKD: chronic kidney disease

CLL: chronic lymphocytic leukemia

CLS: capillary leak syndrome

CML: chronic myelogenous leukemia

CMV: cytomegalovirus

CNS: central nervous system

combo: combination

comp: complicated

conc: concentration

cond: condition

cont: continuous
COPD: chronic obstructive pulmonary disease
COX: cyclooxygenase
CP: chest pain
CPP: central precocious puberty
CR: controlled release
CrCl: creatinine clearance
CRF: chronic renal failure
CRPC: castrate-resistant prostate cancer
CSF: cerebrospinal fluid
CTLA-4: cytotoxic T-lymphocyte antigen 4
CV: cardiovascular
CVA: cerebrovascular accident, costovertebral angle
CVH: common variable hypergammaglobulinemia
CXR: chest X-ray
CYP: cytochrome P450 enzyme
D: diarrhea
D2: Dopamine (DA) type 2
d: day
DA: dopamine
DBP: diastolic blood pressure
DBW: dosing body weight
D/C: discontinue
DDP-4: dipeptidyl peptidase-4
derm: dermatologic
D$_5$LR: 5% dextrose in lactated Ringer solution
D$_5$NS: 5% dextrose in normal saline
D$_5$W: 5% dextrose in water
DHT: dihydrotestosterone
DI: diabetes insipidus
DIC: disseminated intravascular coagulation
Disp: dispensed as; how the drug is supplied
DKA: diabetic ketoacidosis
dL: deciliter

DM: diabetes mellitus
DMARD: disease-modifying antirheumatic drug (refers to drugs in randomized trials to decrease erosions and joint space narrowing in rheumatoid arthritis; eg, methotrexate, azathioprine)
DME: diabetic macular edema
DN: diabetic nephropathy
DOPA: dihydroxyphenylalanine
DOT: directly observed therapy (used for TB treatment)
DPP-4: dipeptidyl peptidase-4
DR: delayed release; diabetic retinopathy
DRESS: drug rash with eosinophilia and systemic symptoms
d/t: due to
DTap: diphtheria toxin
DVT: deep venous thrombosis
Dz: disease
EBV: Epstein–Barr virus
EC: enteric coated
ECC: emergency cardiac care
ECG: electrocardiogram
ED: erectile dysfunction
EE: erosive esophagitis
eGFR: estimated glomerular filtration rate
EGFR: epidermal growth factor receptor
EIB: exercise-induced bronchoconstriction
ELISA: enzyme-linked immunosorbent assay
EL.U.: ELISA unit(s)
EMG: electromyelogram
EMIT: enzyme-multiplied immunoassay test
epi: epinephrine
EPS: extrapyramidal symptoms (tardive dyskinesia, tremors and

rigidity, restlessness [akathisia],
muscle contractions [dystonia],
changes in breathing and heart rate)
ER: extended release
ESA: erythropoiesis-stimulating agent
ESR: erythrocyte sedimentation rate
ESRD: end-stage renal disease
ET: endotracheal
EtOH: ethanol
extrav: extravasation
fam: family
FAP: familial adenomatous polyposis
Fe: iron
FLP: fasting lipid profile
FMF: familial Mediterranean fever
FSH: follicle-stimulating hormone
5-FU: fluorouracil
Fx: fracture
Fxn: function
g: gram(s)
GABA: gamma-aminobutyric acid
GAD: generalized anxiety disorder
GBM: glioblastoma multiforme
GC: gonorrhea
G-CSF: granulocyte colony–
stimulating factor
gen: generation
GERD: gastroesophageal reflux
disease
GF: growth factor
GFR: glomerular filtration rate
GHB: gamma-hydroxybutyrate
GI: gastrointestinal
GIST: gastrointestinal stromal tumor
GLP-1: glucagon-like peptide-1
glu: glucose
GM-CSF: granulocyte-macrophage
colony–stimulating factor
GnRH: gonadotropin-releasing
hormone
G6PD: glucose-6-phosphate
dehydrogenase

gtt: drop(s) (*gutta*)
GU: genitourinary
GVHD: graft-versus-host disease
h: hour(s)
H1N1: swine flu strain
H&P: history and physical
HA: headache
HAE: hereditary angioedema
HAP: hospital-acquired pneumonia
HBsAg: hepatitis B surface antigen
HBV: hepatitis B virus
HCL: hairy cell leukemia
HCM: hypercalcemia of malignancy
Hct: hematocrit
HCTZ: hydrochlorothiazide
HCV: hepatitis C virus
HD: hemodialysis
HDAC: histone deacetylase
HDL-C: high-density lipoprotein
cholesterol
heme: hematologic
hep: hepatitis
hepatotox: hepatotoxicity
HFA: hydrofluoroalkane chemicals
(propellant replacing CFCs in
inhalers)
HFSR: hand-foot skin reaction
Hgb: hemoglobin
HGH: human growth hormone
HHE: hypotonic–hyporesponsive
episode
Hib: *Haemophilus influenzae* type b
HIT: heparin-induced
thrombocytopenia
HITTS: heparin-induced thrombosis–
thrombocytopenia syndrome
HIV: human immunodeficiency virus
HMG-CoA: hydroxymethylglutaryl
coenzyme A
HP: high potency
HPV: human papillomavirus
HR: heart rate

↑HR: increased heart rate (tachycardia)

hs: at bedtime (*hora somni*)

HSCT: hematopoietic stem cell transplantation

HSV: herpes simplex virus

5-HT: 5-hydroxytryptamine

HTN: hypertension

Hx: history of

hypersens: hypersensitivity

IB: irritable bowel

IBD: irritable bowel disease

IBS: irritable bowel syndrome

IBW: ideal body weight

ICP: intracranial pressure

IFIS: intraoperative floppy iris syndrome

Ig: immunoglobulin

IGF: insulin-like growth factor

IHSS: idiopathic hypertrophic subaortic stenosis

IL: interleukin

IM: intramuscular

impair: impairment

in: inch(es)

Inf: infusion

inflam: inflammation

Infxn: infection

Inh: inhalation

INH: isoniazid

inhib: inhibit(s), inhibitor(s), inhibitory

Inj: injection

INR: international normalized ratio

INSTI: integrase strand transfer inhibitor

Insuff: insufficiency

Int: international

intol: intolerance

Intravag: intravaginal

IO: intraosseous

IOP: intraocular pressure

IPV: inactivated poliovirus vaccine

IR: immediate release

ISA: intrinsic sympathomimetic activity

IT: intrathecal

ITP: idiopathic thrombocytopenic purpura

Int units: international units

IUD: intrauterine device

IV: intravenous

JC virus: John Cunningham virus

JIA: juvenile idiopathic arthritis

JME: juvenile myoclonic epilepsy

JRA: juvenile rheumatoid arthritis (SJIA now preferred)

jt: joint

K: klebsiella

K^+: potassium

L&D: labor and delivery

LA: long-acting

LABA: long-acting beta$_2$-adrenergic agonist

LAIV: live attenuated influenza vaccine

LDL: low-density lipoprotein

LFT: liver function test

LH: luteinizing hormone

LHRH: luteinizing hormone–releasing hormone

Li^{+2}: lithium

liq: liquid(s)

LMW: low molecular weight

LP: lumbar puncture

LR: lactated ringers

LVD: left ventricular dysfunction

LVEF: left ventricular ejection fraction

LVSD: left ventricular systolic dysfunction

lytes: electrolytes

MAC: *Mycobacterium avium* complex

maint: maintenance dose/drug

MAO/MAOI: monoamine oxidase/ inhibitor

max: maximum
mcg: microgram(s)
mcL: microliter(s)
MCL: mantle cell lymphoma
MDD: major depressive disorder
MDI: multidose inhaler
MDS: myelodysplasia syndrome
med: medicine
MEN: multiple endocrine neoplasia
(pituitary adenoma, parathyroid
hyperplasia, pancreatic islet cell
tumors)
MEN2: multiple endocrine neoplasia
type 2 (medullary carcinoma of the
thyroid, parathyroid hyperplasia,
pheochromocytoma)
mEq: milliequivalent
met: metastatic
mg: milligram(s)
Mg^{2+}: magnesium
$MgOH_2$: magnesium hydroxide
MI: mitral insufficiency, myocardial
infarction
mill: million
min: minute(s)
mL: milliliter(s)
MMF: mycophenolate mofetil
MMR: measles, mumps, and rubella
mo: month(s)
MoAb: monoclonal antibody
mod: moderate
MRSA: methicillin-resistant
Staphylococcus aureus
MRSE: methicillin-resistant
Staphylococcus epidermidis
MS: multiple sclerosis,
musculoskeletal
ms: millisecond(s)
MSSA: methicillin-sensitive
Staphylococcus aureus
MTC: medullary thyroid cancer

mTOR: mammalian target of
rapamycin
MTT: monotetrazolium
MTX: methotrexate
MyG: myasthenia gravis
N: nausea
NA: narrow angle
NAG: narrow-angle glaucoma
NAION: nonarteritic anterior ischemic
optic neuropathy
NAPA: N-acetyl procainamide
NCI: National Cancer Institute
nephrotox: nephrotoxicity
neurotox: neurotoxicity
ng: nanogram(s)
NG: nasogastric
NHL: non-Hodgkin lymphoma
NIAON: nonischemic arterial optic
neuritis
NIDDM: non–insulin-dependent
diabetes mellitus
nl: normal
NMDA: N-methyl-D-aspartate
NMS: neuroleptic malignant syndrome
NO: nitric oxide
NPO: nothing by mouth (*nil per os*)
Nrf2: nuclear factor erythroid 2–
related factor 2
NRTI: nucleoside reverse transcriptase
inhibitor
NS: normal saline
NS5B: nonstructural protein 5B
NSAID: nonsteroidal anti-
inflammatory drug
NSCLC: non–small cell lung cancer
NSR: normal sinus rhythm
NSTEMI: non-ST elevation
myocardial infarction
NVAF: nonvalvular atrial fibrillation
N/V: nausea and vomiting
N/V/D: nausea, vomiting, and diarrhea
NYHA: New York Heart Association

OA: osteoarthritis
OAB: overactive bladder
obst: obstruction
OCD: obsessive compulsive disorder
OCP: oral contraceptive pill
OD: overdose
ODT: orally disintegrating tablets
oint: ointment
OK: recommended
ONJ: osteonecrosis of jaw
op: operative
ophthal: ophthalmic
OSAHS: obstructive sleep apnea/
    hypopnea syndrome
OTC: over-the-counter
ototox: ototoxicity
oz: ounce(s)
PA: psoriatic arthritis
PABA: para-aminobenzoic acid
    (4-aminobenzoic acid)
PARP: poly (ADP-ribose) polymerase
PAT: paroxysmal atrial tachycardia
pc: after eating (*post cibum*)
PCa: prostate cancer
PCC: prothrombin complex
    concentrate
PCI: percutaneous coronary
    intervention
PCN: penicillin
PCOS: polycystic ovary syndrome
PCP: *Pneumocystis jiroveci* (formerly
    carinii) pneumonia
PCWP: pulmonary capillary wedge
    pressure
PD-1: programmed death receptor-1
PDE: phosphodiesterase
PDE4: phosphodiesterase type 4
PDE5: phosphodiesterase type 5
PDGF: platelet-derived growth factor
PE: phenytoin equivalent, physical
    examination, pleural effusion,
    pulmonary embolus

PEA: pulseless electrical activity
PEG: polyethylene glycol
PEP: post-exposure prophylaxis
perf: perforation
periop: perioperative
PFT: pulmonary function test
pg: picogram(s)
pgp: P-glycoprotein (aka multidrug
    resistance protein [MRP])
PGE-1: prostaglandin E-1
P-gp: P-glycoprotein (membrane drug
    transporter)
PGTC: primary generalized tonic–
    clonic
Ph: Philadelphia chromosome
Pheo: pheochromocytoma
PHN: postherpetic neuralgia
photosens: photosensitivity
PI: product insert (package label)
PID: pelvic inflammatory disease
pkg: package
PKU: phenylketonuria
plt: platelet
PMDD: premenstrual dysphoric
    disorder
PML: progressive multifocal
    leukoencephalopathy
PMS: premenstrual syndrome
PNET: primitive neuroectodermal
    tumor
PO: by mouth (*per os*)
PO_4^{-3}: phosphate ion
POME: pulmonary oil microembolism
postop: post-operative
PPAR-α: peroxisome proliferator–
    activated receptor-alpha
PPD: purified protein derivative
PPI: proton pump inhibitor
PR: by rectum
preop: preoperative
PrEP: pre-exposure prophylaxis (a
    safer sex practice to reduce the risk

of sexually acquired HIV-1 in adults at high risk)

PRES: posterior reversible encephalopathy syndrome

PRG: pregnant/pregnancy

PRN: as often as needed (*pro re nata*)

PSA: prostate-specific antigen

PSVT: paroxysmal supraventricular tachycardia

pt: patient

PT: prothrombin time

PTCA: percutaneous transluminal coronary angioplasty

PTH: parathyroid hormone

PTLD: post-transplant lymphoproliferative disorder

PTSD: post-traumatic stress disorder

PTT: partial thromboplastin time

PTU: propylthiouracil

PUD: peptic ulcer disease

pulm: pulmonary

PVC: premature ventricular contraction

PVD: peripheral vascular disease

PWP: pulmonary wedge pressure

Px: prevention

pyelo: pyelonephritis

q: every (*quaque*)

q_h: every _ hours

q A.M.: every morning

qd: every day

qh: every hour

qhs: every hour of sleep (before bedtime)

qid: four times a day (*quater in die*)

q other day: every other day

q P.M.: every evening

QRS: electrocardiogram complex

QT: time from the start of QRS complex until the end of T wave on an electrocardiogram

QTc: QT interval on ECG

RA: rheumatoid arthritis

RANKL: receptor activator of nuclear factor κ-B (RANK) ligand

RAS: renin-angiotensin system

RBC: red blood cell(s) (count)

RCC: renal cell carcinoma

RDA: recommended dietary allowance

RDS: respiratory distress syndrome

rec: recommend(ed)

REMS: risk evaluation and mitigation strategy (FDA plan to help ensure that a drug's benefits outweigh its risks. As part of this plan, the company must conduct educational outreach.)

resp: respiratory

RHuAb: recombinant human antibody

RIA: radioimmune assay

RLS: restless leg syndrome

R/O, r/o: rule out

RPLS: reversible posterior leukoencephalopathy syndrome

RR: respiratory rate

RSI: rapid sequence intubation

RSV: respiratory syncytial virus

RT: reverse transcriptase

RTA: renal tubular acidosis

RVO: retinal vein occlusion

Rx: prescription/therapy

Rxn: reaction

s: second(s)

S: sign(s)

S/Sxs: signs and symptoms

SAD: social anxiety disorder, seasonal affective disorder

SAE: serious adverse event

SBE: subacute bacterial endocarditis

SBP: systolic blood pressure

SCC: squamous cell carcinoma

SCID: severe combined immunodeficiency

SCLC: small-cell lung cancer

SCr: serum creatinine

SDV: single-dose vial

SE: side effect(s)

SERM: selective estrogen receptor modulator

SGLT2: sodium-glucose co-transporter 2

SIADH: syndrome of inappropriate antidiuretic hormone

sig: significant

SIRS: systemic inflammatory response syndrome/capillary leak syndrome

SJIA: systemic juvenile idiopathic arthritis

SJS: Stevens-Johnson syndrome

SL: sublingual

SLE: systemic lupus erythematosus

SLUDGE: mnemonic for Salivation, Lacrimation, Urination, Diaphoresis, GI motility, Emesis

SMX: sulfamethoxazole

SNRI: serotonin–norepinephrine reuptake inhibitor

SOB: shortness of breath

soln: solution

sp: species

SPAG: small-particle aerosol generator

SQ: subcutaneous

SR: sustained release

SSKI: saturated solution of potassium iodide

SSNRI: selective serotonin–norepinephrine reuptake inhibitor

SSRI: selective serotonin reuptake inhibitor

SSS: sick sinus syndrome

SSSI: skin and skin structure infection

stat: immediately (*statim*)

STD: sexually transmitted disease

STEMI: ST elevation myocardial infarction

subs: substance(s)

supl: supplement

supp: suppository

susp: suspension

SVT: supraventricular tachycardia

SWFI: sterile water for injection

SWSD: shift work sleep disorder

Sx: symptom

synth: synthesis

synd: syndrome

Sz: seizure

tab: tablet

TB: tuberculosis

TBD: thyroid-binding globulin

TCA: tricyclic antidepressant

TCL: T-cell lymphoma

TE: thromboembolic event

TEN: toxic epidermal necrolysis

TFT: thyroid function test

TG: triglyceride(s)

TIA: transient ischemic attack

tid: three times a day (*ter in die*)

TIV: trivalent influenza vaccine

TKI: tyrosine kinase inhibitor

TMP: trimethoprim

TMP-SMX: trimethoprim-sulfamethoxazole

TNF: tumor necrosis factor

TOUCH: Tysabri Outreach Unified Commitment to Health

tox: toxicity

TPA: tissue plasminogen activator

TRALI: transfusion-related acute lung injury

tri: trimester

TSH: thyroid-stimulating hormone

TTP: thrombotic thrombocytopenic purpura

TTS: transdermal therapeutic system

Tx: treatment

UC: ulcerative colitis

UGT: uridine 5′ diphosphoglucuronosyl transferase
ULN: upper limits of normal
uncomp: uncomplicated
URI: upper respiratory infection
US: United States
UTI: urinary tract infection
V: vomiting
VAERS: Vaccine Adverse Events Reporting System
Vag: vaginal
VAP: ventilator-associated pneumonia
VEGF: vascular endothelial growth factor
VF: ventricular fibrillation
VIPoma: vasoactive intestinal peptide–secreting tumor
vit: vitamin
VKA: vitamin K antagonist
VLDL: very-low-density lipoprotein
VOD: venooclusive disease

vol: volume
VPA: valproic acid
VRE: vancomycin-resistant *Enterococcus*
VT: ventricular tachycardia
VTE: venous thromboembolism
w/: with
WBC: white blood cell(s) (count)
WHI: Women's Health Initiative
WHIMS: Women's Health Initiative Memory Study
w/in: within
wk: week(s)
WNL: within normal limits
w/o: without
W/P: warnings and precautions
WPW: Wolff–Parkinson–White syndrome
Wt: weight
XR: extended release
ZE: Zollinger–Ellison (syndrome)

CLASSIFICATION (Generic and common brand names)

ALLERGY

Antihistamines

Azelastine (Astelin, Astepro, Optivar)
Cetirizine (Zyrtec, Zyrtec-D, generic) [OTC]
Chlorpheniramine (Chlor-Trimeton, others) [OTC]
Clemastine fumarate (Antihist- 1, Dayhist, Tavist) [OTC]
Cyproheptadine (Periactin)
Desloratadine (Clarinex, generic)
Desloratadine/ Pseudoephedrine (Clarinex-D 12 Hour)
Diphenhydramine (Benadryl) [OTC]
Fexofenadine (Allegra, Allegra-D, generic)
Hydroxyzine (Atarax, Vistaril, generic)
Levocetirizine (Xyzal)
Loratadine (Alavert, Claritin, generic) [OTC]

Miscellaneous Antiallergy Agents

Cromolyn sodium (Intal, NasalCrom, Opticrom, others)
Montelukast (Singulair, generic)
Phenylephrine, oral (Sudafed, others) [OTC]

ANTIDOTES

Acetylcysteine (Acetadote, Mucomyst)
Amifostine (Ethyol)
Atropine, systemic (AtroPen Auto-Injector)
Atropine/pralidoxime (DuoDote Auto-Injector)
Centruroides (Scorpion) immune F(ab')$_2$ (Anascorp)
Charcoal, activated (Actidose-Aqua,
CharcoCaps, EZ Char, Kerr Insta-Char, Requa Activated Charcoal)
Deferasirox (Exjade)
Dexrazoxane (Zinecard, Totect)
Digoxin immune fab (DigiFab)
Flumazenil (Romazicon, generic)
Glucarpidase (Voraxaze)
Hydroxocobalamin (Cyanokit)
Mesna, Inf (generic), oral (Mesnex)
Methylene blue (Urolene Blue, others)
Naloxone (Evzio, generic)
Physostigmine (generic)
Potassium iodide (Iosat, Lugol's Solution, SSKI, Thyro-Block, ThyroSafe, ThyroShield) [OTC]
Succimer (Chemet)

ANTIMICROBIAL AGENTS

Antibiotics

AMINOGLYCOSIDES

Amikacin (generic)
Gentamicin, Inj (generic)

Neomycin sulfate
  (Neo-Fradin, generic)
Streptomycin (generic)
Tobramycin (generic)

Tobramycin, Inh
  (Bethkis, Kitabis Pak,
  TOBI, TOBI
  Podhaler)

CARBAPENEMS

Doripenem (Doribax)
Ertapenem (Invanz)

Imipenem/cilastatin
  (Primaxin, generic)

Meropenem (Merrem,
  generic)

CEPHALOSPORINS, FIRST-GENERATION

Cefadroxil
  (Duricef, generic)

Cefazolin (generic)

Cephalexin
  (Keflex, generic)

CEPHALOSPORINS, SECOND-GENERATION

Cefaclor (generic)
Cefotetan (generic)

Cefoxitin (Mefoxin,
  generic)
Cefprozil (generic)

Cefuroxime, oral
  (Ceftin), parenteral
  (Zinacef)

CEPHALOSPORINS, THIRD-GENERATION

Cefdinir (Omnicef)
Cefditoren (Spectracef)
Cefixime
  (Suprax, generic)

Cefotaxime (Claforan,
  generic)
Cefpodoxime (generic)
Ceftazidime (Fortaz,
  Tazicef, generic)

Ceftibuten
  (Cedax, generic)
Ceftriaxone (Rocephin,
  generic)

CEPHALOSPORIN, FOURTH-GENERATION

Cefepime (Maxipime,
  generic)

CEPHALOSPORINS, UNCLASSIFIED (FIFTH-GENERATION)

Ceftaroline (Teflaro)

Ceftolozane/tazobactam
  (Zerbaxa)

CYCLIC LIPOPEPTIDE

Daptomycin (Cubicin)

FLUOROQUINOLONES

Ciprofloxacin (Cipro, Cipro XR, generic)
Gemifloxacin (Factive)

Levofloxacin (Levaquin, generic)
Moxifloxacin (Avelox)

Ofloxacin (generic)

GLYCOPEPTIDES

Dalbavancin (Dalvance)
Oritavancin (Orbactiv)

Telavancin (Vibativ)

Vancomycin (Vancocin, generic)

GLYCYLCYCLINE

Tigecycline (Tygacil, generic)

KETOLIDE

Telithromycin (Ketek)

MACROLIDES

Azithromycin (Zithromax)
Clarithromycin (Biaxin, Biaxin XL)

Erythromycin, oral (E-Mycin, E.E.S., Ery-Tab, EryPed, generic)

OXAZOLIDINONES

Linezolid (Zyvox)

Tedizolid (Sivextro)

PENICILLINS

Amoxicillin (Amoxil, Moxatag, generic)
Amoxicillin/clavulanate potassium (Augmentin, Augmentin ES-600, Augmentin XR, generic)
Ampicillin (generic)

Ampicillin/sulbactam (Unasyn)
Dicloxacillin (generic)
Nafcillin (Nallpen, generic)
Oxacillin (generic)
Penicillin G, aqueous (potassium or sodium) (Pfizerpen, Pentids)

Penicillin G benzathine (Bicillin)
Penicillin G procaine (Wycillin, others)
Penicillin V (Pen-Vee K, Veetids, others)
Piperacillin/tazobactam (Zosyn, generic)

STREPTOGRAMIN

Quinupristin/dalfopristin (Synercid)

TETRACYCLINES

Doxycycline (Acticlate, Adoxa, Oracea, Periostat, Vibramycin, Vibra-Tabs)

Minocycline (Arestin, Dynacin, Minocin, Solodyn, generic)

Tetracycline (generic)

Miscellaneous Antibiotic Agents

Aztreonam (Azactam)

Ceftazidime/avibactam (Avycaz)

Ceftolozane/tazobactam (Zerbaxa)

Clindamycin (Cleocin, Cleocin T, others)

Fosfomycin (Monurol)

Metronidazole (Flagyl, Flagyl ER, MetroCream, MetroGel, MetroLotion)

Mupirocin (Bactroban, Bactroban Nasal)

Neomycin/bacitracin/ polymyxin B, topical (Neosporin Ointment) (*See* bacitracin/ neomycin/polymyxin B, topical [Neosporin Ointment]; bacitracin/ neomycin/polymyxin B/hydrocortisone, topical [Cortisporin])

Nitrofurantoin (Furadantin, Macrobid, Macrodantin, generic)

Retapamulin (Altabax)

Rifaximin (Xifaxan)

Trimethoprim (Primsol, generic)

Trimethoprim [TMP]/ sulfamethoxazole [SMX] [Co-Trimoxazole, TMP-SMX] (Bactrim, Bactrim DS, Septra DS, Sulfatrim, generic)

Antifungals

Amphotericin B (generic)

Amphotericin B cholesteryl (Amphotec)

Amphotericin B lipid complex (Abelcet)

Amphotericin B liposomal (AmBisome)

Anidulafungin (Eraxis)

Caspofungin (Cancidas)

Clotrimazole (Lotrimin, Mycelex, others) [OTC]

Clotrimazole/ betamethasone (Lotrisone)

Econazole (Ecoza, Spectazole, generic)

Efinaconazole (Jublia)

Fluconazole (Diflucan, generic)

Isavuconazonium sulfate (Cresemba)

Itraconazole (Onmel, Sporanox, generic)

Ketoconazole, oral (Nizoral, generic)

Ketoconazole, topical (Extina, Kuric, Nizoral A-D shampoo, Xolegel) [shampoo OTC]

Luliconazole (Luzu)

Micafungin (Mycamine)

Miconazole (Monistat 1 combination pack, Monistat 3, Monistat 7) [OTC] (Monistat-Derm)

Nystatin (Mycostatin, Nilstat, Nystop)

Oxiconazole (Oxistat)

Pentamidine (NebuPent, Pentam 300)

Posaconazole (Noxafil)

Sertaconazole (Ertaczo)

Tavaborole (Kerydin)

Terbinafine (Lamisil, Lamisil AT, generic) [OTC]

Triamcinolone/nystatin (Mycolog-II)

Voriconazole (Vfend, generic)

Antimycobacterials

Bedaquiline fumarate (Sirturo)

Dapsone, oral

Ethambutol (Myambutol, generic)

Isoniazid (INH)
Pyrazinamide (generic)
Rifabutin (Mycobutin)

Rifampin (Rifadin,
Rimactane, generic)
Rifapentine (Priftin)

Streptomycin (generic)

Antiparasitics

Benzyl alcohol (Ulesfia)
Ivermectin, oral
(Stromectol)

Ivermectin, topical
(Sklice, Soolantra)
Lindane (generic)

Spinosad (Natroba)

Antiprotozoals

Artemether/lumefantrine
(Coartem)
Atovaquone (Mepron)
Atovaquone/proguanil
(Malarone)

Hydroxychloroquine
(Plaquenil, generic)
Nitazoxanide (Alinia)
Pentamidine (NebuPent,
Pentam 300)

Tinidazole (Tindamax,
generic)

Antiretrovirals

Abacavir (Ziagen)
Atazanavir (Reyataz)
Atazanavir/cobicistat
(Evotaz)
Cobicistat (Tybost)
Darunavir (Prezista)
Darunavir/cobicistat
(Prezcobix)
Delavirdine (Rescriptor)
Didanosine [ddI] (Videx)
Dolutegravir (Tivicay)
Dolutegravir/abacavir/
lamivudine (Triumeq)
Efavirenz (Sustiva)
Efavirenz/emtricitabine/
tenofovir (Atripla)
Elvitegravir (Vitekta)

Emtricitabine (Emtriva)
Enfuvirtide (Fuzeon)
Etravirine (Intelence)
Fosamprenavir (Lexiva)
Indinavir (Crixivan)
Lamivudine (Epivir,
Epivir-HBV, 3TC
[many combo
regimens])
Lopinavir/ritonavir
(Kaletra)
Maraviroc (Selzentry)
Nelfinavir (Viracept)
Nevirapine (Viramune,
Viramune XR,
generic)
Raltegravir (Isentress)

Rilpivirine (Edurant)
Ritonavir (Norvir)
Saquinavir (Invirase)
Simeprevir (Olysio)
Stavudine (Zerit,
generic)
Tenofovir (Viread)
Tenofovir/emtricitabine
(Truvada)
Zidovudine (Retrovir,
generic)
Zidovudine/lamivudine
(Combivir, generic)

Antivirals

Acyclovir (Zovirax,
generic)
Adefovir (Hepsera)
Amantadine (Symmetrel)
Boceprevir (Victrelis)
Cidofovir (Vistide)

Famciclovir
(Famvir, generic)
Foscarnet
(Foscavir, generic)
Ganciclovir (Cytovene,
Vitrasert, generic)

Ledipasvir/sofosbuvir
(Harvoni)
Ombitasvir/paritaprevir/
ritonavir w/ dasabuvir
(Viekira Pak)
Oseltamivir (Tamiflu)

Palivizumab (Synagis)
Peginterferon alpha-2b
   [pegylated interferon]
   (PegIntron)
Penciclovir (Denavir)
Rapivab (Peramivir)

Ribavirin
   (Copegus Moderiba,
   generic)
Rimantadine
   (Flumadine, generic)
Sofosbuvir (Sovaldi)
Telaprevir (Incivek)

Telbivudine (Tyzeka)
Valacyclovir (Valtrex,
   generic)
Valganciclovir (Valcyte)
Zanamivir (Relenza)

ANTINEOPLASTIC AGENTS

Alkylating Agents

Altretamine (Hexalen)
Bendamustine (Treanda)
Busulfan (Busulfex,
   Myleran)
Carboplatin (Paraplatin)
Carmustine [BCNU]
   (BiCNU, Gliadel)
Chlorambucil (Leukeran)
Cisplatin (Platinol,
   Platinol-AQ)
Cyclophosphamide
   (Cytoxan, Neosar)

Dacarbazine
   (DTIC-Dome)
Ifosfamide (Ifex,
   generic)
Mechlorethamine
   (Mustargen)
Mechlorethamine gel
   (Valchlor)
Melphalan [L-PAM]
   (Alkeran, generic)
Oxaliplatin (Eloxatin,
   generic)

Procarbazine (Matulane)
Streptozocin (Zanosar)
Temozolomide
   (Temodar, generic)
Triethylenethio-
   phosphoramide
   (Tespa, Thioplex,
   Thiotepa, TSPA)

Antibiotics

Bleomycin sulfate
   (generic)
Dactinomycin
   (Cosmegen)

Daunorubicin
   (Cerubidine)
Doxorubicin (generic)
Epirubicin (Ellence)

Idarubicin (Idamycin,
   generic)
Mitomycin (Mitosol
   [topical], generic)

Antimetabolites

Cladribine (Leustatin)
Clofarabine (Clolar)
Cytarabine [Ara-C]
   (Cytosar-U)
Cytarabine liposome
   (DepoCyt)
Decitabine (Dacogen)
Floxuridine (generic)
Fludarabine (generic)

Fluorouracil, Inj [5-FU]
   (Adrucil, generic)
Fluorouracil, topical [5-
   FU] (Carac, Efudex,
   Fluoroplex, generic)
Gemcitabine (Gemzar,
   generic)
Mercaptopurine [6-MP]
   (Purinethol, Purixan,
   generic)

Methotrexate (Otrexup,
   Rasuvo, Rheumatrex
   Dose Pack, Trexall,
   generic)
Nelarabine (Arranon)
Omacetaxine (Synribo)
Pemetrexed (Alimta)
Pralatrexate (Folotyn)
Thioguanine (Tabloid)

Hedgehog Pathway Inhibitor
Vismodegib (Erivedge)

Hormones
Abiraterone (Zytiga)
Anastrozole (Arimidex)
Bicalutamide (Casodex)
Degarelix (Firmagon)
Enzalutamide (Xtandi)
Estramustine phosphate (Emcyt)
Exemestane (Aromasin, generic)

Flutamide (generic)
Fulvestrant (Faslodex)
Goserelin (Zoladex)
Histrelin acetate (Supprelin LA, Vantas)
Letrozole (Femara)
Leuprolide (Eligard, Lupron, Lupron

DEPOT, Lupron DEPOT-Ped, generic)
Megestrol acetate (Megace, Megace ES, generic)
Nilutamide (Nilandron)
Tamoxifen (generic)
Triptorelin (Trelstar)

Immunotherapy/Immunomodulators
BCG [Bacillus Calmette-Guérin] (TheraCys, Tice BCG)

Belimumab (Benlysta)
Interferon alpha 2b (Intron A)

Sipuleucel-T (Provenge)

Mitotic Inhibitors (Vinca Alkaloids)
Vinblastine (generic)

Vincristine [Vincristine PFS] (Marqibo, generic)

Vinorelbine (Navelbine, generic)

Monoclonal Antibodies
Ado-trastuzumab emtansine (Kadcyla)
Bevacizumab (Avastin)
Brentuximab vedotin (Adcetris)
Cetuximab (Erbitux)

Ipilimumab (Yervoy)
Nivolumab (Opdivo)
Obinutuzumab (Gazyva)
Ofatumumab (Arzerra)
Panitumumab (Vectibix)

Pembrolizumab (Keytruda)
Pertuzumab (Perjeta)
Rituximab (Rituxan)
Trastuzumab (Herceptin)

Poly (ADP-Ribose) Polymerase (PARP) Inhibitor
Olaparib (Lynparza)

Proteasome Inhibitor
Bortezomib (Velcade)

Taxanes
Cabazitaxel (Jevtana)

Docetaxel (Docefrez, Taxotere, generic)

Paclitaxel (Abraxane, Taxol, generic)

Topoisomerase Inhibitors

Etoposide [VP-16]
(Etopophos, Toposar,
Vepesid, generic)

Irinotecan
(Camptosar, generic)

Topotecan
(Hycamtin, generic)

Tyrosine Kinase Inhibitors (TKIs)

Afatinib (Gilotrif)

Axitinib (Inlyta)

Bosutinib monohydrate
(Bosulif)

Cabozanitinib
(Cometriq)

Crizotinib (Xalkori)

Dabrafenib (Tafinlar)

Dasatinib (Sprycel)

Erlotinib (Tarceva)

Everolimus (Afinitor,
Afinitor Disperz)

Gefitinib (Iressa)

Ibrutinib (Imbruvica)

Imatinib (Gleevec)

Lapatinib (Tykerb)

Lenvatinib (Lenvima)

Nilotinib (Tasigna)

Palbociclib (Ibrance)

Pazopanib (Votrient)

Ponatinib (Iclusig)

Regorafenib (Stivarga)

Ruxolitinib (Jakafi)

Sorafenib (Nexavar)

Sunitinib (Sutent)

Temsirolimus (Torisel)

Trametinib (Mekinist)

Vandetanib (Caprelsa)

Miscellaneous Antineoplastic Agents

Aldesleukin [IL-2]
(Proleukin)

Aminoglutethimide
(Cytadren)

Belinostat (Beleodaq)

Blinatumomab
(Blincyto)

Carfilzomib (Kyprolis)

Dinutuximab (Unituxin)

Eribulin (Halaven)

Hydroxyurea (Droxia,
Hydrea, generic)

Idelalisib (Zydelig)

Ixabepilone (Ixempra)

Lenalidomide (Revlimid)

Leucovorin (generic)

Mitoxantrone (generic)

Panobinostat (Farydak)

Pomalidomide
(Pomalyst)

Radium-223 dichloride
(Xofigo)

Ramucirumab (Cyramza)

Rasburicase (Elitek)

Romidepsin (Istodax)

Thalidomide (Thalomid)

Tretinoin, topical
[retinoic acid]
(Atralin, Avita,
ReFissa, Renova,
Retin-A, Retin-A
Micro)

Vemurafenib (Zelboraf)

Vorinostat (Zolinza)

Ziv-Aflibercept (Zaltrap)

CARDIOVASCULAR (CV) AGENTS

Aldosterone Antagonists

Eplerenone (Inspra)

Spironolactone
(Aldactone, generic)

Alpha$_1$-Adrenergic Blockers

Doxazosin (Cardura,
Cardura XL)

Prazosin (Minipress,
generic)

Terazosin (generic)

Angiotensin-Converting Enzyme (ACE) Inhibitors

Benazepril (Lotensin,
generic)

Captopril (Capoten,
others)

Enalapril (Enalaprilat,
Epaned Kit, Vasotec)

Fosinopril (Monopril, generic)
Lisinopril (Prinivil, Zestril)
Moexipril (Univasc, generic)

Perindopril erbumine (Aceon, generic)
Quinapril (Accupril, generic)

Ramipril (Altace, generic)
Trandolapril (Mavik, generic)

Angiotensin II Receptor Antagonists/Blockers (ARBs)

Azilsartan (Edarbi)
Candesartan (Atacand)
Eprosartan (Teveten)

Irbesartan (Avapro, generic)
Losartan (Cozaar)
Olmesartan (Benicar)

Telmisartan (Micardis, generic)
Valsartan (Diovan)

Antiarrhythmic Agents

Adenosine (Adenocard, Adenoscan)
Amiodarone (Cordarone, Nexterone, Pacerone)
Atropine, systemic (AtroPen Auto-Injector, generic)
Digoxin (Digitek, Lanoxin, Lanoxin Pediatric, generic)

Disopyramide (Norpace, Norpace CR, generic)
Dofetilide (Tikosyn)
Dronedarone (Multaq)
Esmolol (Brevibloc, generic)
Flecainide (Tambocor, generic)
Ibutilide (Corvert, generic)

Lidocaine, systemic (Xylocaine, others)
Mexiletine (generic)
Procainamide (generic)
Propafenone (Rythmol, Rythmol SR, generic)
Quinidine (generic)
Sotalol (Betapace, Sorine, Sotylize, generic)

Beta-Adrenergic Blockers

Acebutolol (Sectral)
Atenolol (Tenormin)
Betaxolol (Kerlone)
Bisoprolol (Zebeta)
Carvedilol (Coreg, Coreg CR)
Labetalol (Trandate, generic)

Metoprolol succinate (Toprol XL, generic)
Metoprolol tartrate (Lopressor, generic)
Nadolol (Corgard, generic)
Nebivolol (Bystolic)

Penbutolol (Levatol)
Pindolol (generic)
Propranolol (Hemangeol, Inderal LA, Innopran XL, generic)
Timolol (generic)

Calcium Channel Antagonists/Blockers (CCBs)

Amlodipine (Norvasc)
Clevidipine (Cleviprex)
Diltiazem (Cardizem, Cardizem CD, Cardizem LA, Cardizem SR, Cartia

XT, Dilacor XR, Dilt-XR, Taztia XT, Tiamate, Tiazac)
Felodipine (Plendil, generic)
Isradipine (Generic)

Nicardipine (Cardene, Cardene SR, generic)
Nifedipine (Adalat CC, Afedatab CR, Procardia, Procardia XL, generic)

Nimodipine (Nymalize, generic)
Nisoldipine (Sular, generic)

Verapamil (Calan, Calan SR, Isoptin SR, Verelan, Verelan PM, generic)

Centrally Acting Antihypertensive Agents

Clonidine, oral (Catapres, generic)
Clonidine, transdermal (Catapres-TTS)

Guanfacine (Intuniv, Tenex, generic)

Methyldopa (generic)

Combination Antihypertensive Agents

Aliskiren/amlodipine (Tekamlo)
Aliskiren/amlodipine/ hydrochlorothiazide (Amturnide)
Aliskiren/ hydrochlorothiazide (Tekturna HCT)
Amlodipine/olmesartan (Azor)
Amlodipine/valsartan (Exforge)

Amlodipine/valsartan/ hydrochlorothiazide (Exforge HCT)
Atenolol/chlorthalidone (Tenoretic)
Azilsartan/chlorthalidone (Edarbyclor)
Lisinopril/ hydrochlorothiazide (Prinzide, Zestoretic, generic)

Olmesartan/amlodipine/ hydrochlorothiazide (Tribenzor)
Olmesartan/ hydrochlorothiazide (Benicar HCT)
Perinodopril/amlodipine (Prestalia)
Telmisartan/amlodipine (Twynsta)

Diuretics

Acetazolamide (Diamox)
Amiloride (Midamor)
Bumetanide (Bumex)
Chlorothiazide (Diuril)
Chlorthalidone
Furosemide (Lasix, generic)
Hydrochlorothiazide (HydroDIURIL, Esidrix, others, generic)

Hydrochlorothiazide/ amiloride (Moduretic, generic)
Hydrochlorothiazide/ spironolactone (Aldactazide, generic)
Hydrochlorothiazide/ triamterene (Dyazide, Maxzide, generic)
Indapamide (Lozol, generic)

Mannitol, intravenous (Osmitrol, generic)
Metolazone (Zaroxolyn, generic)
Spironolactone (Aldactone, generic)
Torsemide (Demadex, generic)
Triamterene (Dyrenium)

Inotropic/Pressor Agents

Digoxin (Digitek, Digox, Lanoxicaps, Lanoxin)
Dobutamine (Dobutrex, generic)
Dopamine (generic)

Droxidopa (Northera)
Epinephrine (Adrenalin, Auvi-Q, EpiPen, EpiPen Jr, others)

Inamrinone [amrinone] (Inocor)
Isoproterenol (Isuprel)
Midodrine (Proamatine)

Milrinone
(Primacor, generic)
Nesiritide (Natrecor)

Norepinephrine
(Levophed)

Phenylephrine, systemic
(generic)

Lipid-Lowering Agents

Cholestyramine
(Prevalite, Questran,
Questran Light)
Colesevelam (Welchol)
Colestipol (Colestid)
Ezetimibe (Zetia)
Ezetimibe/atorvastatin
(Liptruzet)
Ezetimibe/simvastatin
(Vytorin)
Fenofibrate (Antara,
Lipofen, Lofibra,

TriCor, Triglide,
generic)
Fenofibric acid (Fibricor,
Trilipix, generic)
Gemfibrozil (Lopid,
generic)
Icosapent ethyl
(Vascepa)
Lomitapide (Juxtapid)
Mipomersen (Kynamro)
Niacin [nicotinic acid]
(Niacor, Niaspan,

Nicolar, Slo-Niacin)
[OTC forms]
Niacin/lovastatin
(Advicor)
Niacin/simvastatin
(Simcor)
Omega-3 fatty acid [fish
oil] (Epanova, Lovaza,
Omtryg)

Statins

Atorvastatin (Lipitor)
Fluvastatin
(Lescol, generic)
Lovastatin (Altoprev,
Mevacor, generic)

Pitavastatin (Livalo)
Pravastatin
(Pravachol, generic)
Rosuvastatin (Crestor)

Simvastatin
(Zocor, generic)

Statin/Antihypertensive Combination

Amlodipine/atorvastatin
(Caduet)

Vasodilators

Alprostadil
[prostaglandin E$_1$]
(Prostin VR)
Ambrisentan (Letairis)
Epoprostenol (Flolan,
Veletri, generic)
Fenoldopam (Corlopam,
generic)
Hydralazine (Apresoline,
others, generic)
Iloprost (Ventavis)

Isosorbide dinitrate
(Dilatrate-SR, Isordil,
Sorbitrate, generic)
Isosorbide mononitrate
(Imdur, Ismo,
Monoket, generic)
Minoxidil, oral (generic)
Nitroglycerin (Nitro-Bid
IV, Nitro-Bid
Ointment, Nitrodisc,
Nitrolingual,

NitroMist, Nitrostat,
Transderm-Nitro,
others)
Nitroprusside
(Nitropress)
Treprostinil, extended
release (Orenitram)
Treprostinil sodium
(Remodulin, Tyvaso)

Miscellaneous CV Agents

Aliskiren (Tekturna)

Conivaptan HCl (Vaprisol)

Macitentan (Opsumit)

Ranolazine (Ranexa)

Riociguat (Adempas)

CENTRAL NERVOUS SYSTEM (CNS) AGENTS

Alzheimer Agents

Donepezil (Aricept, generic)

Galantamine (Razadyne, Razadyne ER, generic)

Memantine (Namenda)

Memantine/donepezil (Namzaric)

Rivastigmine (Exelon, generic)

Rivastigmine, transdermal (Exelon Patch, generic)

Antianxiety Agents

Alprazolam (Niravam, Xanax X) [C-IV]

Buspirone (generic)

Chlordiazepoxide (generic) [C-IV]

Clorazepate (Tranxene T-TAB, generic) [C-IV]

Diazepam (Diastat, Valium) [C-IV]

Doxepin caps, soln (generic)

Hydroxyzine (Atarax, Vistaril, generic)

Lorazepam (Ativan, generic) [C-IV]

Meprobamate (generic) [C-IV]

Oxazepam (generic) [C-IV]

Anticonvulsants

Carbamazepine (Carbatrol, Epitol, Equetro, Tegretol XR)

Clobazam (Onfi) [C-IV]

Clonazepam (Klonopin, generic) [C-IV]

Clorazepate (Tranxene T-TAB, generic) [C-IV]

Diazepam (Diastat, Valium) [C-IV]

Eslicarbazepine (Aptiom)

Ethosuximide (Zarontin, generic)

Ezogabine (Potiga)

Fosphenytoin (Cerebyx, generic)

Gabapentin (Gralise, Neurontin, generic)

Lacosamide (Vimpat)

Lamotrigine (Lamictal)

Lamotrigine, extended release (Lamictal XR)

Levetiracetam (Elepsia XR, Keppra, Keppra XR, generic)

Lorazepam (Ativan, others) [C-IV]

Magnesium sulfate (various)

Oxcarbazepine (Oxtellar XR, Trileptal, generic)

Pentobarbital (Nembutal) [C-II]

Perampanel (Fycompa)

Phenobarbital (generic) [C-IV]

Phenytoin (Dilantin, generic)

Rufinamide (Banzel)

Tiagabine (Gabitril, generic)

Topiramate (Qudexy XR, Topamax, Topamax Sprinkle, Trokendi XR, generic)

Valproic acid (Depakene, Depakote, Stavzor, generic)

Vigabatrin (Sabril)

Zonisamide (Zonegran, generic)

Antidepressants

MONOAMINE OXIDASE INHIBITORS (MAOIs)

Phenelzine (Nardil, generic)

Selegiline, oral (Eldepryl, Zelapar, generic)

Selegiline, transdermal (Emsam)

Tranylcypromine (Parnate, generic)

SELECTIVE SEROTONIN REUPTAKE INHIBITORS (SSRIs)

Citalopram (Celexa)

Escitalopram (Lexapro, generic)

Fluoxetine (Prozac, Prozac Weekly, Sarafem, generic)

Fluvoxamine (Luvox CR, generic)

Paroxetine (Paxil, Paxil CR, Pexeva, generic)

Sertraline (Zoloft, generic)

Vortioxetine (Brintellix)

SEROTONIN–NOREPINEPHRINE REUPTAKE INHIBITORS (SNRIs)

Desvenlafaxine (Khedezla, Pristiq, generic)

Duloxetine (Cymbalta)

Levomilnacipran (Fetzima)

Milnacipran (Savella)

Venlafaxine (Effexor XR, generic)

TRICYCLIC ANTIDEPRESSANTS (TCAs)

Amitriptyline (Elavil)

Desipramine (Norpramin)

Doxepin caps, soln (generic)

Imipramine (Tofranil, generic)

Nortriptyline (Aventyl, Pamelor)

MISCELLANEOUS ANTIDEPRESSANTS

Bupropion hydrochloride (Aplenzin ER, Wellbutrin, Wellbutrin SR, Wellbutrin XL, Zyban)

Mirtazapine (Remeron, Remeron SolTab, generic)

Nefazodone (generic)

Trazodone (Oleptro, generic)

Vilazodone (Viibryd)

Antiparkinson Agents

Amantadine (Symmetrel)

Apomorphine (Apokyn)

Benztropine (Cogentin)

Bromocriptine (Parlodel)

Carbidopa/levodopa, enteral suspension (Duopa)

Carbidopa/levodopa, oral (Parcopa, Rytary, Sinemet, Sinemet SR)

Entacapone (Comtan)

Pramipexole (Mirapex, Mirapex ER, generic)

Rasagiline Mesylate (Azilect)

Rivastigmine, transdermal (Exelon Patch, generic)

Ropinirole (Requip, Requip XL, generic)

Rotigotine (Neupro)

Selegiline, oral (Eldepryl, Zelapar, generic)

Tolcapone (Tasmar)

Trihexyphenidyl (generic)

Antipsychotics

Aripiprazole (Abilify, Abilify Discmelt, Abilify Maintena Kit)

Asenapine Maleate (Saphris)

Brexpiprazole (Rexulti)

Chlorpromazine (Thorazine)

Clozapine (Clozaril, FazaClo, Versacloz)

Haloperidol (Haldol, generic)

Iloperidone (Fanapt)

Lithium carbonate, citrate (generic)

Loxapine (Adasuve)

Lurasidone (Latuda)

Olanzapine (Zyprexa, Zyprexa Zydis, generic)

Olanzapine, LA parenteral (Zyprexa Relprevv)

Paliperidone (Invega, Invega Sustenna, Invega Trinza)

Perphenazine (generic)

Pimozide (Orap)

Prochlorperazine (Compro, Procomp, generic)

Quetiapine (Seroquel, Seroquel XR, generic)

Risperidone, oral (Risperdal, Risperdal M-Tab, generic)

Risperidone, parenteral (Risperdal Consta)

Thioridazine (generic)

Thiothixene (generic)

Trifluoperazine (generic)

Ziprasidone (Geodon, generic)

Sedative Hypnotics

BENZODIAZEPINE HYPNPOTICS

Alprazolam (Xanax, Niravam) [C-IV]

Estazolam (ProSom, generic) [C-IV]

Flurazepam (Dalmane, generic) [C-IV]

Lorazepam (Ativan, others) [C-IV]

Midazolam (generic) [C-IV]

Oxazepam (generic) [C-IV]

Temazepam (Restoril, generic) [C-IV]

Triazolam (Halcion, generic) [C-IV]

NON-BENZODIAZEPINE HYPNPOTICS

Dexmedetomidine (Precedex)

Diphenhydramine (Benadryl) [OTC]

Doxepin tabs (Silenor)

Eszopiclone (Lunesta, generic) [C-IV]

Etomidate (Amidate, generic)

Pentobarbital (Nembutal, others) [C-II]

Phenobarbital (generic) [C-IV]

Propofol (Diprivan, generic)

Ramelteon (Rozerem)

Secobarbital (Seconal) [C-II]

Suvorexant (Belsomra)

Zaleplon (Sonata, generic) [C-IV]

Zolpidem (Ambien CR, Ambien IR, Edluar, Intermezzo, ZolpiMist, generic) [C-IV]

Stimulants

Armodafinil (Nuvigil)
Atomoxetine (Strattera)
Dexmethylphenidate
(Focalin, Focalin XR)
[C-II]
Dextroamphetamine
(Dexedrine, Dexedrine
Spansules, ProCentra,
Zenzedi) [C-II]

Guanfacine (Intuniv,
Tenex, generic)
Lisdexamfetamine
dimesylate (Vyvanse)
[C-II]
Methylphenidate, oral
(Concerta, Focalin,
Focalin XR, Metadate
CD, Metadate SR,

Methylin, Quillivant
XR, Ritalin, Ritalin
LA, Ritalin SR) [C-II]
Methylphenidate,
transdermal
(Daytrana) [C-II]
Modafinil (Provigil,
generic) [C-IV]

Miscellaneous CNS Agents

Alemtuzumab
(Lemtrada)
Clomipramine
(Anafranil)
Clonidine, oral, extended
release (Kapvay,
generic)
Dalfampridine (Ampyra)
Fingolimod (Gilenya)

Gabapentin enacarbil
(Horizant)
Interferon beta-1a
(Avonex, Rebif)
Meclizine (Antivert,
generic) (Dramamine,
Univert) [OTC]
Natalizumab (Tysabri)
Nimodipine (Nimotop)

Peginterferon beta-1a
(Plegridy)
Sodium oxybate/gamma
hydroxybutyrate/GHB
(Xyrem) [C-III]
Tasimelteon (Hetlioz)
Teriflunomide (Aubagio)
Tetrabenazine
(Xenazine)

DERMATOLOGIC AGENTS

Analgesic

Capsaicin (Capsin,
Zostrix, others) [OTC]

Anesthetics, Local

Dibucaine (Nupercainal,
others) [OTC]

Pramoxine (Anusol
Ointment, Proctofoam
NS, others)

Pramoxine/
hydrocortisone
(Proctofoam-HC)

Anti-Acne Agents

Adapalene (Differin)
Adapalene/benzoyl
peroxide (Epiduo Gel)
Clindamycin/benzoyl
peroxide (Benzaclin,
Onexton, generic)
Clindamycin/tretinoin
(Veltin Gel, Ziana)
Dapsone, topical
(Aczone)

Erythromycin, topical
(Akne-Mycin, Ery,
Erytha-Derm,
generic)
Erythromycin/benzoyl
peroxide
(Benzamycin)
Isotretinoin
(Amnesteem, Claravis,

Myorisan, Sotret,
Zentane, generic)
Tretinoin, topical
[retinoic acid]
(Atralin, Avita,
Refissa, Renova,
Retin-A, Retin-A
Micro)

Antibiotics

Bacitracin, topical (Baciguent)

Bacitracin/neomycin/ polymyxin B, topical (Neosporin Ointment)

Bacitracin/neomycin/ polymyxin B/ hydrocortisone, topical (Cortisporin)

Bacitracin/polymyxin B, topical (Polysporin)

Clindamycin (Cleocin, Cleocin T, others)

Gentamicin, topical (generic)

Metronidazole (Flagyl, Flagyl ER, MetroCream,

MetroGel, MetroLotion)

Minocycline (Arestin, Dynacin, Minocin, Solodyn, generic)

Mupirocin (Bactroban, Bactroban Nasal)

Silver sulfadiazine (Silvadene, Thermazene, generic)

Antifungal Agents

Ciclopirox (Cicloclan, CNL8, Loprox, Pedipirox-4 Nail Kit, Penlac)

Clotrimazole/ betamethasone (Lotrisone)

Econazole (Ecoza, Spectazole, generic)

Ketoconazole (Nizoral, generic)

Ketoconazole, topical (Extina, Nizoral A-D Shampoo, Xolegel) [shampoo OTC]

Miconazole (Monistat 1 combo pack, Monistat 3, Monistat 7) [OTC], (Monistat-Derm)

Miconazole/zinc oxide/ petrolatum (Vusion)

Naftifine (Naftin)

Nystatin (Mycostatin, Nilstat, Nystop)

Oxiconazole (Oxistat)

Terbinafine (Lamisil, Lamasil AT, generic) [OTC]

Tolnaftate (Tinactin, generic) [OTC]

Anti-Inflammatory Agents

Diclofenac, topical (Flector Patch, Pennsaid, Solaraze, Voltaren Gel)

Steroids, topical (*See* Table 3, p 336)

Antineoplastic Agent

Fluorouracil, topical [5-FU] (Carac, Efudex, Fluoroplex, generic)

Antiparasitic Agents

Lindane (generic)

Permethrin (Elimite, Nix, generic) [OTC]

Antipruritic Agent

Doxepin, topical (Prudoxin, Zonalon)

Antipsoriatic Agents

Acitretin (Soriatane)
Anthralin (Dritho,
  Zithranol,
  Zithranol-RR)

Apremilast (Otezla)
Calcipotriene (Dovonex)
Calcitriol, ointment
  (Vectical)

Secukinumab (Cosentyx)
Ustekinumab (Stelara)

Antiviral Agents

Acyclovir (Zovirax,
  generic)

Penciclovir (Denavir)

Immunomodulators

Imiquimod, cream
  (Aldara, Zyclara)
Ingenol mebutate
  (Picato)

Kunecatechins
  [sinecatechins]
  (Veregen)
Pimecrolimus (Elidel)

Tacrolimus, ointment
  (Protopic)

Keratolytic Agents

Podophyllin (Condylox,
  Condylox Gel 0.5%,
  Podocon-25)

Tazarotene (Avage,
  Fabior, Tazorac)

Neuromuscular Blocking Agents

Botulinum toxin type A
  [abobotulinumtoxin A]
  (Dysport)

Botulinum toxin type A
  [onabotulinumtoxin
  A] (Botox, Botox
  Cosmetic)

Anti-Rosacea Agent

Brimonidine topical
  (Mirvaso)

Miscellaneous Dermatologic Agents

Finasteride
  (Propecia,generic,
  Proscar generic)
Lactic acid/ammonium
  hydroxide [ammonium
  lactate] (Lac-Hydrin)
  [OTC]

Minoxidil, topical
  (Theroxidil, Rogaine,
  generic) [OTC]
Selenium sulfide (Head
  & Shoulders Clinical
  Strength Dandruff
  Shampoo, Selsun

Shampoo, Selsun Blue
  Shampoo, generic,
  others) [OTC]

DIETARY SUPPLEMENTS

Calcium acetate
(Calphron, Phos-Ex,
PhosLo)

Calcium glubionate
(Calcionate) [OTC]

Calcium salts [chloride,
gluconate, gluceptate]

Cholecalciferol [vitamin
D_3] (Delta-D, many
others)

Cyanocobalamin
[vitamin B_{12}]
(Nascobal)

Ferric carboxymaltose
(Injectafer)

Ferric gluconate
complex (Ferrlecit)

Ferrous gluconate
(Ferate, Fergon
[OTC], others)

Ferrous gluconate
complex (Ferrlecit)

Ferrous sulfate [OTC]

Ferumoxytol (Feraheme)

Folic acid, injectable,
oral (generic)

Iron dextran (Dexferrum,
INFeD)

Iron sucrose (Venofer)

Magnesium oxide
(Mag-Ox 400, others
[OTC])

Magnesium sulfate
(various)

Multivitamins, oral
[OTC] (See Table 12,
p 359)

Omega-3 fatty acid [fish
oil] (Epanova, Lovaza,
Omtryg)

Phytonadione [vitamin
K_1] (Mephyton,
generic)

Potassium supplements
(Kaochlor, Kaon,
K-Lor, Klorvess,
Micro-K, Many
others, generic) (See
Table 6, p 351)

Pyridoxine [vitamin B_6]
(generic)

Sodium bicarbonate
[$NaHCO_3$] (generic)

Sucroferric
Oxyhydroxide
(Velphoro)

Thiamine [vitamin B_1]
(generic)

EAR (OTIC) AGENTS

Acetic acid/aluminum
acetate, otic
(Domeboro Otic)
[OTC]

Benzocaine/antipyrine
(Aurodex, generic)

Ciprofloxacin, otic
(Cetraxal)

Ciprofloxacin/
dexamethasone, otic
(Ciprodex)

Ciprofloxacin/
hydrocortisone, otic
(Cipro HC Otic)

Finafloxacin otic (Xtoro
Otic)

Neomycin/colistin/
hydrocortisone

(Cortisporin-TC
Otic Drops)

Neomycin/colistin/
hydrocortisone/
thonzonium
(Cortisporin-TC Otic
Suspension)

Ofloxacin, otic (Floxin
Otic, Floxin Otic
Singles)

ENDOCRINE SYSTEM AGENTS

Antidiabetic Agents

ALPHA-GLUCOSIDASE INHIBITORS

Acarbose (Precose)   Miglitol (Glyset)

BIGUANIDES

Metformin (Fortmet, Glucophage, Glucophage XR, Glumetza, Riomet, generic)

COMBINATION ANTIDIABETIC AGENTS

Alogliptin/metformin (Kazano)
Alogliptin/pioglitazone (Oseni)
Canagliflozin/metformin (Invokamet)
Dapagliflozin/metformin (Xigduo XR)
Empagliflozin/linagliptin (Glyxambi)

Glyburide/metformin (Glucovance, generic)
Linagliptin/metformin (Jentadueto)
Pioglitazone/metformin (ACTOplus Met, ACTOplus MET XR, generic)
Repaglinide/metformin (PrandiMet)

Saxagliptin/metformin (Kombiglyze XR)
Sitagliptin/metformin (Janumet, Janumet XR)
Sitagliptin/simvastatin (Juvisync)

DIPEPTIDYL PEPTIDASE-4 (DPP-4) INHIBITORS

Alogliptin (Nesina)
Linagliptin (Tradjenta)

Saxagliptin (Onglyza)
Sitagliptin (Januvia)

GLUCAGON-LIKE PEPTIDE-1 (GLP-1) RECEPTOR AGONISTS

Albiglutide (Tanzeum)
Dulaglutide (Trulicity)
Exenatide (Byetta)

Exenatide ER (Bydureon, Bydureon Pen)

Liraglutide, recombinant (Saxenda, Victoza)

INSULINS

Insulin, human inhalation powder (Afrezza)

Insulin, injectable (*See* Table 4, p 338)

MEGLITINIDES

Nateglinide (Starlix, generic)

Repaglinide (Prandin)

SODIUM-GLUCOSE CO-TRANSPORTER 2 (SGLT2) INHIBITORS

Canagliflozin (Invokana)
Dapagliflozin (Farxiga)

Empagliflozin (Jardiance)

SULFONYLUREAS

Chlorpropamide (generic)
Glimepiride (Amaryl, generic)

Glimepiride/pioglitazone (Duetact)

Glipizide (Glucotrol, Glucotrol XL, generic)

Glyburide (DiaBeta, Glynase, generic)

Tolazamide (generic)

Tolbutamide (generic)

THIAZOLIDINEDIONES

Pioglitazone (Actos, generic)

Rosiglitazone (Avandia)

MISCELLANEOUS ANTIDIABETIC AGENTS

Bromocriptine mesylate (Cycloset)

Hormone and Synthetic Substitutes

Calcitonin (Fortical, Miacalcin)

Calcitriol [vitamin D₃ analog] (Calcijex, Rocaltrol)

Cortisone, systemic, topical (*See* Table 2, p 335, and Table 3, p 336)

Desmopressin (DDAVP, Stimate)

Dexamethasone, systemic, topical (Decadron)

Fludrocortisone acetate (Florinef, generic)

Glucagon, recombinant (GlucaGen)

Hydrocortisone, systemic, topical (Cortef, Solu-Cortef, generic)

Methylprednisolone (A-Methapred, Depo-Medrol, Medrol, Medrol Dosepak, Solu-Medrol, generic) [*See* Steroids, p 287, and Table 2, p 335]

Prednisolone (Flo-Pred, Omnipred, Orapred, Pediapred, generic) (*See* Steroids, p 287, and Table 2, p 335)

Prednisone (generic) (*See* Steroids, p 287, and Table 2, p 335)

Testosterone, implant (Testopel) [C-III]

Testosterone, nasal gel (Natesto) [C-III]

Testosterone, topical (Androderm, AndroGel 1%, AndroGel 1.62%, Axiron, Fortesta, Striant, Testim, Vogelxo, generic) [C-III]

Testosterone undecanoate, Inj (Aveed) [C-III]

Vasopressin [Antidiuretic hormone, ADH] (Vasostrict, generic)

Hypercalcemia/Osteoporosis Agents

Alendronate (Binosto, Fosamax, Fosamax Plus D, generic)

Denosumab (Prolia, Xgeva)

Etidronate disodium (Didronel, generic)

Gallium nitrate (Ganite)

Ibandronate (Boniva, generic)

Pamidronate (generic)

Raloxifene (Evista)

Risedronate (Actonel, Actonel w/ Calcium, generic)

Risedronate, delayed release (Atelvia)

Teriparatide (Forteo)

Zoledronic acid (Reclast, Zometa, generic)

Obesity

Bupropion/naltrexone (Contrave)
Liraglutide, recombinant (Saxenda, Victoza)

Lorcaserin (Belviq)
Orlistat (Alli [OTC], Xenical)

Phentermine (Adipex-P, Suprenza, generic)
Phentermine/topiramate (Qsymia) [C-IV]

Thyroid/Antithyroid

Levothyroxine (Levoxyl, Synthroid, others)
Liothyronine [T₃] (Cytomel, Triostat)

Methimazole (Tapazole, generic)
Potassium iodide (Iosat, Lugol's Solution, SSKI, Thyro-Block,

ThyroSafe, ThyroShield) [OTC]
Propylthiouracil (generic)

Miscellaneous Endocrine System Agents

Cinacalcet (Sensipar)
Demeclocycline (Declomycin)
Diazoxide (Proglycem)
Mifepristone (Korlym, Mifeprex)

Parathyroid hormone (Natpara)
Pasireotide (Signifor)
Somatropin (Genotropin, Nutropin AQ,

Omnitrope, Saizen, Serostim, Zorbtive)
Tesamorelin (Egrifta)

EYE (OPHTHALMIC) AGENTS

Glaucoma Agents

Acetazolamide (Diamox)
Apraclonidine (Iopidine)
Betaxolol, ophthalmic (Betoptic)
Brimonidine, ophthalmic (Alphagan P)
Brimonidine/timolol (Combigan)
Brinzolamide (Azopt)

Brinzolamide/ brimonidine (Simbrinza)
Carteolol, ophthalmic (generic)
Dipivefrin (Propine)
Dorzolamide (Trusopt)
Dorzolamide/timolol (Cosopt)

Echothiophate iodide, ophthalmic (Phospholine Iodide)
Latanoprost (Xalatan)
Levobunolol (AK-Beta, Betagan)
Tafluprost (Zioptan)
Timolol, ophthalmic (Betimol, Istalol, Timoptic, Timoptic XE, generic)

Ophthalmic Antibiotics

Azithromycin, ophthalmic, 1% (AzaSite)
Bacitracin, ophthalmic (AK-Tracin Ophthalmic)

Bacitracin/neomycin/ polymyxin B, ophthalmic (Neo-Polycin, Neosporin Ophthalmic)

Bacitracin/neomycin/ polymyxin B/ hydrocortisone, ophthalmic (Neo-Polycin HC Cortisporin Ophthalmic)

Bacitracin/polymyxin B, ophthalmic (AK-Poly-Bac Ophthalmic, Polysporin Ophthalmic)

Besifloxacin (Besivance)

Ciprofloxacin, ophthalmic (Ciloxan)

Erythromycin, ophthalmic (Ilotycin, Romycin)

Gentamicin, ophthalmic (Garamycin, Genoptic, Gentak, generic)

Gentamicin/ prednisolone, ophthalmic (Pred-G Ophthalmic)

Levofloxacin, ophthalmic (Iquix, Quixin)

Moxifloxacin, ophthalmic (Moxeza, Vigamox)

Neomycin/ dexamethasone (AK-Neo-Dex Ophthalmic, NeoDecadron Ophthalmic)

Neomycin/polymyxin B/ dexamethasone, ophthalmic (Maxitrol)

Neomycin/polymyxin B/ hydrocortisone (Cortisporin Ophthalmic)

Neomycin/polymyxin B/ prednisolone (Poly-Pred Ophthalmic)

Ofloxacin, ophthalmic (Ocuflox)

Sulfacetamide, ophthalmic (Bleph-10, Cetamide, Sodium Sulamyd)

Sulfacetamide/ prednisolone, ophthalmic (Blephamide, others)

Tobramycin, ophthalmic (Tobradex ST, Tobrex, generic)

Tobramycin/ dexamethasone, ophthalmic (TobraDex)

Miscellaneous Ophthalmic Agents

Aflibercept (Eylea)

Alcaftadine, ophthalmic (Lastacaft)

Artificial tears (Tears Naturale) [OTC]

Atropine, ophthalmic (Isopto Atropine, generic)

Bepotastine besilate (Bepreve)

Bromfenac (Bromday, Prolensa)

Cidofovir (Vistide)

Cromolyn sodium (Intal, NasalCrom, Opticrom, others)

Cyclopentolate, ophthalmic (Cyclate, Cyclogyl)

Cyclopentolate/ phenylephrine (Cyclomydril)

Cyclosporine, ophthalmic (Restasis)

Dexamethasone, ophthalmic (AK-Dex Ophthalmic, Decadron Ophthalmic, Maxidex)

Dexamethasone, ophthalmic implant (Ozurdex)

Diclofenac, ophthalmic (Voltaren Ophthalmic)

Emedastine (Emadine)

Epinastine (Elestat)

Ganciclovir, ophthalmic gel (Zirgan)

Ketorolac, ophthalmic (Acular, Acular LS, Acular PF, Acuvail)

Ketotifen (Alaway, Claritin Eye, Zaditor, Zyrtec Itchy Eye) [OTC]

Lodoxamide (Alomide)

Loteprednol (Alrex, Lotemax)

Naphazoline (Albalon, Naphcon, generic)

Naphazoline/ pheniramine (Naphcon A, Visine A, generic)

Nepafenac (Nevanac)

Olopatadine, ophthalmic (Pataday, Patanol, Pazeo)

Pemirolast (Alamast)
Phenylephrine,
    ophthalmic
    (AK-Dilate,
    Neo-Synephrine
    Ophthalmic, Zincfrin
    [OTC])

Ranibizumab (Lucentis)
Rimexolone (Vexol
    Ophthalmic)
Trifluridine, ophthalmic
    (Viroptic)

GASTROINTESTINAL (GI) AGENTS

Antacids

Alginic acid/aluminum
    hydroxide/magnesium
    trisilicate (Gaviscon)
    [OTC]
Aluminum hydroxide
    (AlternaGEL,
    Amphojel,
    Dermagran) [OTC]
Aluminum hydroxide/
    alginic acid/
    magnesium carbonate
    (Gaviscon Extra

Strength Liquid)
    [OTC]
Aluminum hydroxide/
    magnesium hydroxide
    (Maalox, Mylanta
    Ultimate Strength)
    [OTC]
Aluminum hydroxide/
    magnesium hydroxide/
    simethicone (Maalox
    Plus, Mylanta,
    Mylanta II) [OTC]

Aluminum hydroxide/
    magnesium trisilicate
    (Gaviscon Regular
    Strength) [OTC]
Calcium carbonate
    (Alka-Mints, Tums)
    [OTC]
Magaldrate/simethicone
    (Riopan Plus) [OTC]

Antidiarrheals

Bismuth subsalicylate
    (Pepto-Bismol) [OTC]
Diphenoxylate/atropine
    (Lomotil, Lonox)
    [C-V]
Lactobacillus (Lactinex
    Granules) [OTC]

Loperamide (Diamode,
    Imodium) [OTC]
Octreotide (Sandostatin,
    Sandostatin LAR,
    generic)

Paregoric [camphorated
    tincture of opium]
    [C-III]
Rifaximin (Xifaxan,)

Antiemetics

Aprepitant (Emend)
Chlorpromazine
    (Thorazine)
Dimenhydrinate
    (Dramamine, others)
    [OTC]
Dolasetron (Anzemet)
Dronabinol (Marinol)
    [C-III]

Droperidol (Inapsine)
Fosaprepitant (Emend
    for Injection)
Granisetron, oral,
    transdermal (Sancuso,
    generic)
Meclizine (Antivert,
    Bonine, Dramamine
    [OTC], Univert,
    generic)

Metoclopramide
    (Metozolv ODT,
    Reglan, generic))
Nabilone (Cesamet)
    [C-II]
Netupitant/Palonosetron
    (Akynzeo)
Ondansetron (Zofran,
    Zofran ODT, generic)

Ondansetron, oral
   soluble film (Zuplenz)
Palonosetron (Aloxi)
Prochlorperazine
   (Compazine)

Promethazine
   (Promethegan,
   generic)

Scopolamine,
   transdermal
   (Transderm Scop)
Trimethobenzamide
   (Tigan, generic)

Antiulcer Agents

Bismuth subcitrate/
   metronidazole/
   tetracycline (Pylera)
Cimetidine (Tagamet,
   Tagamet HB 200
   [OTC], generic)
Dexlansoprazole
   (Dexilant)
Esomeprazole
   magnesium, sodium,
   strontium (Nexium,
   Nexium IV, Nexium
   24HR [OTC], generic)

Famotidine (Pepcid,
   Pepcid AC, generic)
   [OTC]
Lansoprazole (Prevacid,
   Prevacid 24HR
   [OTC])
Nizatidine (Axid, Axid
   AR [OTC], generic)
Omeprazole (Prilosec,
   Prilosec [OTC],
   generic)
Omeprazole/sodium
   bicarbonate (Zegerid,
   Zegerid [OTC])

Omeprazole/sodium
   bicarbonate/
   magnesium hydroxide
   (Zegerid w/
   Magnesium
   Hydroxide)
Pantoprazole (Protonix,
   generic)
Rabeprazole (AcipHex,
   generic)
Ranitidine (Zantac,
   Zantac EFFERDose
   [OTC], generic)
Sucralfate (Carafate,
   generic)

Cathartics/Laxatives

Bisacodyl (Dulcolax)
   [OTC]
Citric acid/magnesium
   oxide/sodium
   picosulfate (Prepopik)
Docusate calcium
   (Surfak)
Docusate potassium
   (Dialose)
Docusate sodium
   (Colace, DOSS)
Glycerin suppository
Lactulose (Constulose,
   Enulose, Generlac,
   others)

Magnesium citrate
   (Citroma, others)
   [OTC]
Magnesium hydroxide
   (Milk of Magnesia)
   [OTC]
Magnesium oxide
   (Mag-Ox, Maox, Uro-
   Mag, Others) [OTC]
Mineral oil, oral [OTC],
   Mineral oil enema
   (Fleet Mineral Oil)
   [OTC]Mineral oil
   enema (Fleet Mineral
   Oil) [OTC]

Polyethylene glycol
   [PEG] 3350
   (MiraLAX) [OTC]
Polyethylene glycol
   [PEG]–electrolyte
   solution [PEG-ES]
   (CoLyte, GoLYTELY)
Psyllium (Konsyl,
   Metamucil, generic)
   [OTC]
Sodium phosphate
   (OsmoPrep, Visicol)
Sorbitol (generic)

Enzyme

Pancrelipase (Creon,
Panakare Plus,
Pancreaze, Pertzye,
Ultresa, Voikace,
Zenpep, generic)

Miscellaneous GI Agents

Alosetron (Lotronex)
Alvimopan (Entereg)
Balsalazide (Colazal,
Giazo, generic)
Budesonide, oral
(Entocort EC, Uceris)
Budesonide, rectal foam
(Uceris foam)
Certolizumab pegol
(Cimzia)
Crofelemer (Fulyzaq)
Dexpanthenol (generic)
Dibucaine (Nupercainal,
others [OTC])
Dicyclomine (Bentyl)
Fidaxomicin (Dificid)
Hydrocortisone, rectal
(Anusol-HC
Suppository,
Cortifoam Rectal,
Proctocort, others,
generic)
Hyoscyamine (Anaspaz,
Cystospaz, Levsin,
others, generic)
Hyoscyamine/atropine/
scopolamine/

phenobarbital
(Donnatal, others,
generic)
Infliximab (Remicade)
Linaclotide (Linzess)
Lubiprostone (Amitiza)
Mesalamine (Apriso,
Asacol, Asacol HD,
Canasa, Lialda,
Pentasa, Rowasa,
generic)
Methylnaltrexone
bromide (Relistor)
Metoclopramide (Clopra,
Octamide, Reglan)
Mineral oil/pramoxine
HCl/zinc oxide (Tucks
Ointment) [OTC]
Misoprostol (Cytotec,
generic)
Naloxegol (Movantik)
Natalizumab (Tysabri)
Neomycin (Neo-Fradin,
generic)
Olsalazine (Dipentum)
Oxandrolone (Oxandrin,
generic) [C-III]

Pramoxine (Anusol
Ointment, Proctofoam
NS, others)
Pramoxine/
hydrocortisone
(Enzone,
Proctofoam-HC)
Propantheline (Pro-
Banthine, generic)
Simethicone (generic)
[OTC]
Starch, topical, rectal
(Tucks Suppositories)
[OTC]
Sulfasalazine
(Azulfidine,
Azulfidine EN,
generic)
Teduglutide [rDNA
origin] (Gattex)
Vedolizumab (Entyvio)
Witch hazel (Tucks Pads,
others) [OTC]

HEMATOLOGIC AGENTS

Anticoagulants

Antithrombin, pooled
(Thrombate III),
recombinant (ATryn)

Apixaban (Eliquis)
Argatroban (generic)
Bivalirudin (Angiomax)

Dabigatran (Pradaxa)
Dalteparin (Fragmin)
Desirudin (Iprivask)

Enoxaparin (Lovenox)

Fondaparinux (Arixtra, generic)

Heparin (generic)

Lepirudin (Refludan)

Protamine (generic)

Rivaroxaban (Xarelto)

Savaysa (Edoxaban)

Warfarin (Coumadin, Jantoven, generic)

Antiplatelet Agents

Abciximab (ReoPro)

Aspirin (Bayer, Ecotrin, St. Joseph's, generic) [OTC]

Cilostazol (Pletal)

Clopidogrel (Plavix, generic)

Dipyridamole (Persantine)

Dipyridamole/aspirin (Aggrenox)

Eptifibatide (Integrilin)

Prasugrel (Effient)

Ticagrelor (Brilinta)

Tirofiban (Aggrastat)

Vorapaxar (Zontivity)

Antithrombotic Agents

Alteplase, recombinant [tPA] (Activase)

Reteplase (Retavase)

Streptokinase (generic)

Tenecteplase (TNKase)

Hematopoietic Agents

Darbepoetin alfa (Aranesp)

Eltrombopag (Promacta)

Epoetin alfa [erythropoietin, EPO] (Epogen, Procrit)

Filgrastim [G-CSF] (Granix, Neupogen, Zarxio)

Oprelvekin (Neumega)

Pegfilgrastim (Neulasta)

Plerixafor (Mozobil)

Romiplostim (Nplate)

Sargramostim [GM-CSF] (Leukine)

Volume Expanders

Albumin (Albuked, Albuminar 20, Albuminar 25, AlbuRx 25, Albutein, Buminate, Human

Albumin Grifols, Kedbumin, Plasbumin

Dextran 40 (Gentran 40, Rheomacrodex)

Hetastarch (Hespan)

Plasma protein fraction (Plasmanate)

Miscellaneous Hematologic Agents

Aminocaproic acid (Amicar)

Antihemophilic factor (Recomb), porcine sequence (Obizur)

Antihemophilic factor, recombinant (Advate, Eloctate, Hexilate FS,

Kogenate FS, Novoeight, Recombinate, Xyntha)

Antihemophilic factor VIII (Hemofil M, Monoclate-P)

Deferiprone (Ferriprox)

Desmopressin (DDAVP, Stimate)

Pentoxifylline (Trental, generic)

Prothrombin complex concentrate, human (Kcentra)

IMMUNE SYSTEM AGENTS

Immunomodulators

Dimethyl fumarate
(Tecfidera)
Icatibant (Firazyr)
Interferon alpha (Intron
A, Roferon-A)
Interferon alphacon-1
(Infergen)
Interferon beta-1a
(Avonex, Rebif)
Interferon beta-1b
(Betaseron, Extavia)

Interferon gamma-1b
(Actimmune)
Peginterferon alpha-2a
[pegylated interferon]
(Pegasys)
Peginterferon alpha-2b
[pegylated interferon]
(PegIntron)
Short ragweed pollen
allergen extract
(Ragwitek)

Sweet vernal, orchard,
perennial rye, Timothy
and Kentucky blue
grass mixed pollens
allergenic extract
(Oralair)
Timothy grass pollen
allergen extract tablet
for sublingual use
(Grastek)

Disease-Modifying Antirheumatic Drugs (DMARDs)

Abatacept (Orencia)
Adalimumab (Humira)
Anakinra (Kineret)
Apremilast (Otezla)
Certolizumab pegol
(Cimzia)
Etanercept (Enbrel)

Golimumab (Simponi,
Simponi Aria)
Infliximab (Remicade)
Leflunomide (Arava)
Methotrexate (Otrexup,
Rasuvo, Rheumatrex

Dose Pack, Trexall,
generic)
Tocilizumab (Actemra)
Tofacitinib (Xeljanz)

Immunosuppressive Agents

Azathioprine (Azasan,
Imuran)
Basiliximab (Simulect)
Belatacept (Nulojix)
Cyclosporine (Gengraf,
Neoral, Sandimmune)
Daclizumab (Zenapax)
Everolimus (Zortress)
Lymphocyte immune
globulin

[antithymocyte
globulin, ATG]
(Atgam)
Mycophenolate mofetil
(CellCept, generic)
Mycophenolic acid
(Myfortic, generic)
Sirolimus [rapamycin]
(Rapamune)

Steroids, systemic (*See*
Table 2, p 335)
Tacrolimus, extended
release (Astragraf XL)
Tacrolimus, immediate
release (Prograf,
generic)

MUSCULOSKELETAL AGENTS

Antigout Agents

Allopurinol (Aloprim,
Lopurin, Zyloprim)
Colchicine (Colcrys,
Mitigare, generic)

Febuxostat (Uloric)
Pegloticase (Krystexxa)
Probenecid (Probalan,
generic)

Muscle Relaxants

Baclofen (Gablofen, Lioresal Intrathecal)
Carisoprodol (Soma)
Chlorzoxazone (Parafon Forte DSC, others)
Cyclobenzaprine (Flexeril)

Cyclobenzaprine, ER(Amrix)
Dantrolene (Dantrium, Revonto, Ryanodex, generic)
Diazepam (Diastat rectal gel, Valium) [C-IV]

Metaxalone (Skelaxin)
Methocarbamol (Robaxin, generic)
Orphenadrine (Norflex, generic)

Neuromuscular Blockers

Atracurium (Tracrium)
Botulinum toxin type A [incobotulinumtoxin A] (Xeomin)
Botulinum toxin type A [onabotulinumtoxin

A] (Botox, Botox Cosmetic)
Botulinum toxin type B [rimabotulinumtoxin B] (Myobloc)
Pancuronium (generic)

Rocuronium (Zemuron, generic)
Succinylcholine (Anectine, Quelicin, generic)
Vecuronium (generic)

Miscellaneous Musculoskeletal Agents

Edrophonium (Enlon)

Tizanidine (Zanaflex, generic)

OB/GYN AGENTS

Contraceptives

Copper IUD (ParaGard T 380A)
Ethinyl estradiol/ norelgestromin patch (Ortho Evra, Xulane)
Etonogestrel, implant (Implanon)

Etonogestrel/ethinyl estradiol, vaginal insert (NuvaRing)
Levonorgestrel intrauterine device (IUD) (Liletta, Mirena)

Medroxyprogesterone (Depo-Provera, Depo-Sub Q Provera, Provera, generic)
Oral contraceptives (*See* Table 5, p 341)

Emergency Contraceptives

Levonorgestrel (Next Choice, Plan B One-Step [OTC], generic [OTC])

Ulipristal acetate (Ella)

Estrogen Supplementation

ESTROGEN ONLY

Esterified estrogens (Menest)
Estradiol, gel (Divigel)

Estradiol, metered gel (Elestrin, Estrogel)

Estradiol, oral (Delestrogen, Estrace, Femtrace, others)

Estradiol, spray
(Evamist)
Estradiol, transdermal
(Alora, Climara,
Estraderm, Minivelle,
Vivelle Dot)

Estradiol, vaginal
(Estring, Femring,
Vagifem)
Estrogen, conjugated
(Premarin)

Estrogen, conjugated
synthetic (Enjuvia)

COMBINATION ESTROGEN/PROGESTIN

Estradiol/levonorgestrel,
transdermal
(Climara Pro)

Estradiol/norethindrone
(Activella, Lopreeza,
Mimvey, Mimvey Lo,
generic)

Estrogen, conjugated/
medroxyprogesterone
(Premphase, Prempro)

COMBINATION ESTROGEN/ESTROGEN ANTAGONIST

Conjugated estrogens/
bazedoxifene
(Duavee)

Vaginal Preparations

Amino-Cerv pH 5.5
Cream
Miconazole (Monistat 1
combination pack,
Monistat 3, Monistat 7)

[OTC]
(Monistat-Derm)
Nystatin (Mycostatin,
Nilstat, Nystop)

Terconazole (Terazol 3,
Terazol 7, Zazole,
generic)
Tioconazole (Vagistat-1,
generic [OTC])

Miscellaneous OB/GYN Agents

Clomiphene (generic)
Dinoprostone (Cervidil
Insert, Prepidil Gel,
Prostin E2)
Doxylamine/pyridoxine
(Diclegis)
Leuprolide (Eligard,
Lupron, Lupron
DEPOT, Lupron
DEPOT-Ped, generic)
Leuprolide acetate/
norethindrone acetate
kit (Lupaneta Pack)

Magnesium sulfate
(various)
Medroxyprogesterone
(Depo-Provera, Depo-
Sub Q Provera,
Provera, generic)
Methylergonovine
(Methergine)
Mifepristone (Korlym,
Mifeprex)
Nafarelin, metered spray
(Synarel)
Ospemifene (Osphena)

Oxytocin (Pitocin,
generic)
Paroxetine (Brisdelle)
Terbutaline (generic)
Tranexamic acid
(Cyklokapron,
Lysteda, generic)

PAIN MEDICATIONS

Antimigraine Agents

Acetaminophen/
butalbital, w/ and w/o
caffeine (Fioricet w/
Codeine, generic)
[C-III]

Almotriptan (Axert)

Aspirin/butalbital/
caffeine compound
(Fiorinal) [C-III]

Aspirin/butalbital/
caffeine/codeine
(Fiorinal w/ Codeine)

Eletriptan (Relpax)

Frovatriptan (Frova)

Naratriptan (Amerge,
generic)

Rizatriptan (Maxalt,
Maxalt-MLT, generic)

Sumatriptan (Alsuma,
Imitrex, Imitrex Nasal
Spray, Imitrex
Statdose, Sumavel
DosePro, generic)

Sumatriptan needleless
system (Sumavel
DosePro)

Sumatriptan/naproxen
sodium (Treximet)

Zolmitriptan (Zomig,
Zomig Nasal, Zomig
ZMT)

Local/Topical (*See also* Table 1, p 334)

Benzocaine (Americaine,
Hurricane, Lanacane,
others [OTC])

Benzocaine/antipyrine
(Aurodex)

Bupivacaine (Marcaine)

Capsaicin (Capsin,
Zostrix, others) [OTC]

Cocaine [C-II]

Dibucaine (Nupercainal,
others [OTC])

Lidocaine, lidocaine/
epinephrine
(Anestacon Topical,
Xylocaine, Xylocaine
MPF, Xylocaine
Viscous, others)

Lidocaine/prilocaine
(EMLA, ORAQIX)

Lidocaine/tetracaine,
transdermal patch
(Synera), cream
(Pliaglis)

Mepivacaine
(Carbocaine)

Pramoxine (Anusol
Ointment, Proctofoam
NS, others)

Procaine (Novocaine)

Narcotic Analgesics

Acetaminophen/codeine
(Tylenol 2, 3, 4)
[C-III, C-IV]

Alfentanil (Alfenta)
[C-II]

Buprenorphine, oral,
sublingual (Buprenex,
generic) [C-III]

Buprenorphine, systemic
(Buprenex, generic)
[C-III]

Buprenorphine,
transdermal (Butrans)
[C-III]

Buprenorphine/naloxone
(Bunavail, Suboxone,
Zubsolv) [C-III]

Butorphanol (Stadol)
[C-IV]

Codeine [C-II]

Fentanyl (Sublimaze,
generic) [C-II]

Fentanyl, transdermal
(Duragesic, generic)
[C-II]

Fentanyl, transmucosal
(Abstral, Actiq,
Fentora, Lazanda,

Onsolis, generic)
[C-II]

Hydrocodone, extended
release (Hysingla ER,
Zohydro) [C-II]

Hydrocodone/
acetaminophen
(Hycet, Lorcet,
Vicodin, others) [C-II]

Hydrocodone/ibuprofen
(Vicoprofen, generic)
[C-II]

Hydromorphone (Dilaudid, generic) [C-II]

Hydromorphone, extended release (Exalgo) [C-II]

Levorphanol (Levo-Dromoran) [C-II]

Meperidine (Demerol, Meperitab, generic) [C-II]

Methadone (Dolophine, Methadose, generic) [C-II]

Morphine (Astramorph/PF, Duramorph, Infumorph, Kadian SR, MS Contin, Oramorph SR, Roxanol) [C-II]

Morphine/naltrexone (Embeda) [C-II]

Nalbuphine (generic)

Oxycodone (OxyContin, Roxicodone, generic) [C-II]

Oxycodone/acetaminophen (Percocet, Primlev, Tylox) [C-II]

Oxycodone/acetaminophen,

extended release (Xartemis XR) [C-II]

Oxycodone/aspirin (Percodan) [C-II]

Oxycodone/ibuprofen (Combunox) [C-II]

Oxycodone/naloxone (Targiniq ER) [C II]

Oxymorphone (Opana, Opana ER) [C-II]

Pentazocine (Talwin) [C-IV]

Tapentadol (Nucynta) [C-II]

Nonnarcotic Analgesics

Acetaminophen, Inj (Ofirmev)

Acetaminophen, oral [N-acetyl-p-aminophenol, APAP] (Tylenol, others, generic) [OTC]

Acetaminophen/butalbital, w/ and w/o caffeine (Algesic LQ, Bupap, Esgic, Fioricet, Margesic, Zebutal, generic) [C-III]

Aspirin (Bayer, Ecotrin, St. Joseph's) [OTC]

Tramadol (ConZip, Ultram, Ultram ER, generic) [C-IV]

Tramadol/acetaminophen (Ultracet) [C-IV]

Nonsteroidal Anti-inflammatory Agents (NSAIDs)

Celecoxib (Celebrex, generic)

Diclofenac, Inj (Dyloject)

Diclofenac, oral (Cataflam, Voltaren, Voltaren-XR, Zorvolex)

Diclofenac, topical (Flector Patch, Pennsaid, Solaraze, Voltaren Gel)

Diclofenac/misoprostol (Arthrotec 50, Arthrotec 75)

Diflunisal (Dolobid)

Etodolac

Fenoprofen (Nalfon, generic)

Flurbiprofen (Ansaid, Ocufen, generic)

Ibuprofen, oral (Advil, Motrin, Motrin IB, Rufen, others, generic) [OTC]

Ibuprofen, parenteral (Caldolor)

Indomethacin (Indocin, Tivorbex, generic)

Ketoprofen (generic)

Ketorolac (Toradol, generic)

Ketorolac, nasal (Sprix)

Meloxicam (Mobic, generic)

Nabumetone (Relafen, generic)

Naproxen (Aleve [OTC], Anaprox, Anaprox DS, EC-Naprosyn, Naprelan, Naprosyn, generic)

Naproxen/esomeprazole (Vimovo)

Oxaprozin (Daypro, generic)
Piroxicam (Feldene, generic)

Sulindac (Clinoril, generic)
Tolmetin (generic)

Miscellaneous Pain Medications

Amitriptyline (Elavil)
Clonidine, epidural (Duraclon)

Imipramine (Tofranil, generic)
Pregabalin (Lyrica, generic)

Ziconotide (Prialt)

RESPIRATORY AGENTS

Antitussives, Decongestants, and Expectorants

Acetylcysteine (Acetadote, Mucomyst)
Benzonatate (Tessalon, Zonatuss)
Codeine [C-II]
Dextromethorphan (Benylin DM, Delsym, Mediquell, PediaCare 1, others) [OTC]
Guaifenesin (Robitussin, others, generic) [OTC]
Guaifenesin/codeine (Robafen AC, others, generic) [C-V]

Guaifenesin/ dextromethorphan (various) [OTC]
Hydrocodone/ chlorpheniramine (Vituz), hydrocodone/ chlorpheniramine/ pseudoephedrine (generic) [C-II]
Hydrocodone/ guaifenesin (Obredon) [C-II]
Hydrocodone/ homatropine (Hycodan, Hydromet,

Tussigon, others, generic) [C-II]
Hydrocodone/ pseudoephedrine (Detussin, Histussin-D, others, generic) [C-II]
Potassium iodide (Iosat, Lugol's Solution, SSKI, Thyro-Block, ThyroSafe, ThyroShield) [OTC]
Pseudoephedrine (many mono and combo brands) [OTC]

Bronchodilators

Aclidinium bxanaxromide
Albuterol (ProAir HFA, ProAir RespiClick, Proventil HFA, Ventolin HFA)
Albuterol/ipratropium (Combivent Respimat, DuoNeb)
Aminophylline (generic)
Arformoterol (Brovana)

Ephedrine (generic)
Epinephrine (Adrenalin, Auvi-Q, EpiPen, EpiPen Jr, others)
Formoterol fumarate (Foradil, Perforomist)
Indacaterol (Arcapta Neohaler)
Isoproterenol (Isuprel)
Levalbuterol (Xopenex, Xopenex HFA)

Metaproterenol (generic)
Pirbuterol (Maxair, generic)
Salmeterol (Serevent, Serevent Diskus)
Terbutaline (Brethine, Bricanyl)
Theophylline (Elixophylline, Theo-24, Theolair, Uniphyl, generic)

Respiratory Inhalants

Acetylcysteine (Acetadote, Mucomyst)

Aztreonam, Inh (Cayston)

Beclomethasone (QVAR)

Beclomethasone, nasal (Beconase AQ, Qnasl)

Budesonide, Inh (Pulmicort Flexhaler, Respules, Turbuhaler, generic)

Budesonide, nasal (Rhinocort Aqua, generic)

Budesonide/formoterol (Symbicort)

Ciclesonide, Inh (Alvesco)

Ciclesonide, nasal (Omnaris, Zettona)

Cromolyn sodium (Intal, NasalCrom, Opticrom, others)

Dornase alfa (DNase, Pulmozyme)

Fluticasone furoate (Arnuity Ellipta)

Fluticasone furoate, nasal (Veramyst)

Fluticasone furoate/ vilanterol trifenatate (Breo Ellipta)

Fluticasone propionate, Inh (Flovent Diskus, Flovent HFA)

Fluticasone propionate, nasal (Flonase, generic) [OTC]

Fluticasone propionate/ salmeterol xinafoate (Advair Diskus, Advair HFA)

Formoterol fumarate (Foradil Aerolizer, Perforomist)

Ipratropium (Atrovent HFA, Atrovent Nasal, generic)

Mannitol, Inh (Aridol)

Mometasone, Inh (Asmanex, Asmanex HFA)

Mometasone, nasal (Nasonex)

Mometasone/formoterol (Dulera)

Olodaterol (Striverdi Respimat)

Olopatadine, nasal (Patanase)

Phenylephrine, nasal (Neo-Synephrine Nasal) [OTC]

Tiotropium (Spiriva HandiHaler, Spiriva Respimat)

Tobramycin, Inh (Bethkis, Kitabis Pak, TOBI, TOBI Podhaler)

Umeclidinium (Incruse Ellipta)

Umeclidinium/vilanterol (Anoro Ellipta)

Surfactants

Beractant (Survanta)

Calfactant (Infasurf)

Lucinactant (Surfaxin)

Miscellaneous Respiratory Agents

Alpha-1 proteinase inhibitor (Aralast NP, Glassia, Prolastin C, Zemaira)

Montelukast (Singulair, generic)

Nintedanib (Ofev)

Omalizumab (Xolair)

Pirfenidone (Esbriet)

Roflumilast (Daliresp)

Sildenafil (Revatio, Viagra)

Tadalafil (Adcirca)

Zafirlukast (Accolate, generic)

Zileuton (Zyflo, Zyflo CR)

UROGENITAL SYSTEM AGENTS

Benign Prostatic Hyperplasia (BPH) Agents

Alfuzosin (Uroxatral)

Doxazosin (Cardura, Cardura XL)

Dutasteride (Avodart)

Dutasteride/tamsulosin (Jalyn)

Finasteride (Propecia, Proscar [generic])

Silodosin (Rapaflo)

Tamsulosin (Flomax, generic)

Terazosin (generic)

Bladder Agents

Belladonna/opium, suppositories (generic) [C-II]

Bethanechol (Urecholine, generic)

Darifenacin (Enablex)

Fesoterodine (Toviaz)

Flavoxate (generic)

Hyoscyamine (Anaspaz, Cystospaz, Levsin, others, generic)

Hyoscyamine/atropine/ scopolamine/

phenobarbital (Donnatal, others, generic)

Methenamine hippurate (Hiprex), methenamine mandelate (Urex, Uroquid-Acid No.2)

Mirabegron (Myrbetriq)

Oxybutynin (Ditropan, Ditropan XL, generic)

Oxybutynin, topical (Gelnique)

Oxybutynin transdermal system (Oxytrol)

Phenazopyridine (Azo-Standard, Pyridium, Urogesic, many others) [OTC]

Solifenacin (VESIcare)

Tolterodine (Detrol, Detrol LA, generic)

Trospium (generic)

Erectile Dysfunction Agents

Alprostadil, intracavernosal (Caverject, Edex)

Alprostadil, urethral suppository (Muse)

Avanafil (Stendra)

Sildenafil (Revatio, Viagra)

Tadalafil (Cialis)

Vardenafil (Levitra, Stayxn, generic)

Yohimbine (Yocon, Yohimex)

Urolithiasis Agents

Potassium citrate (Urocit-K, generic)

Sodium citrate/citric acid (Bicitra, Oracit)

Miscellaneous Urogenital System Agents

Ammonium aluminum sulfate (Alum) [OTC]

BCG [Bacillus Calmette-Guérin] (TheraCys, Tice BCG)

Dimethyl sulfoxide [DMSO] (Rimso-50)

Methenamine/phenyl salicylate/methylene blue/benzoic acid/

hyoscyamine (Hyophen)

Neomycin/polymyxin bladder irrigant (Neosporin GU Irrigant)

Nitrofurantoin
(Furadantin, Macrobid,
Macrodantin, generic)

Pentosan polysulfate
sodium (Elmiron)

Trimethoprim
(Proloprim, Trimpex)

VACCINES/SERUMS/TOXOIDS

Cytomegalovirus
immune globulin
[CMV-IG IV]
(CytoGam)
Diphtheria/tetanus
toxoids [DT] (generic
only) (Ages < 7 y)
Diphtheria/tetanus
toxoids [Td]
(Decavac, Tenivac)
(Ages > 7 y)
Diphtheria/tetanus
toxoids/acellular
pertussis, adsorbed
[DTaP] (Ages < 7 y)
(Daptacel, Infanrix,
Tripedia)
Diphtheria/tetanus
toxoids/acellular
pertussis, adsorbed
[Tdap] (Ages > 10–11 y)
(Boosters: Adacel,
Boostrix)
Diphtheria/tetanus
toxoids/acellular
pertussis, adsorbed/
hepatitis B
(recombinant)/ IPV,
combined (Pediarix)
Diphtheria/tetanus
toxoids/acellular
pertussis, adsorbed/
IPV (Kinrix,
Quadracel)
Diphtheria/tetanus
toxoids/acellular
pertussis, adsorbed/

IPV/Haemophilus b
conjugate vaccine,
combined (Pentacel)
Haemophilus B
conjugate vaccine
(ActHIB, Hiberix,
HibTITER,
PedvaxHIB, others)
Hepatitis A vaccine
(Havrix, Vaqta)
Hepatitis A (inactivated)/
hepatitis B
(recombinant) vaccine
(Twinrix)
Hepatitis B immune
globulin (H-BIG,
HepaGam B,
HyperHep B,
Nabi-HB)
Hepatitis B vaccine
(Engerix-B,
Recombivax HB)
Human papillomavirus
recombinant vaccine
(Cervarix [Types 16,
18], Gardasil [Types
6, 11, 16, 18],
Gardasil 9)
Immune globulin g,
human, IV [IVIG]
(Bivigam, others)
Immune globulin g,
human, SQ
(Hizentra,Vivaglobin,
others)
Influenza vaccine,
inactivated,

quadrivalent (IIV₄)
(Fluarix Quadrivalent,
Fluzone Quadrivalent)
Influenza vaccine,
inactivated, trivalent
(IIV₃) (Afluria,
Fluarix, Flucelvax,
FluLaval, Fluvirin,
Fluzone, Fluzone
High Dose, Fluzone
Intradermal)
Influenza vaccine, live
attenuated,
quadrivalent (LAIV₄)
(FluMist)
Influenza vaccine,
recombinant, trivalent
(RIV₃) (FluBlok)
Measles/mumps/rubella
vaccine, live [MMR]
(M-M-R II)
Measles/mumps/rubella/
varicella virus
vaccine, live [MMRV]
(ProQuad)
Meningococcal
conjugate vaccine
[quadrivalent, MCV₄]
(Menactra, Menveo)
Meningococcal group B
vaccine (Bexsero,
Trumenba)
Meningococcal groups C
and Y/Haemophilus b
tetanus toxoid
conjugate vaccine
(Menhibrix)

Meningococcal polysaccharide vaccine [MPSV4] (Menomune A/C/Y/W-135)

Pneumococcal 13-valent conjugate vaccine (Prevnar 13)

Pneumococcal vaccine, polyvalent (Pneumovax 23)

Rotavirus vaccine, live, oral, monovalent (Rotarix)

Rotavirus vaccine, live, oral, pentavalent (RotaTeq)

Smallpox vaccine (ACAM2000)

Tetanus immune globulin (HyperTET S/D, generic)

Tetanus toxoid [TT] (generic)

Varicella virus vaccine (Varivax)

Varicella zoster immune globulin (VarZIG)

Zoster vaccine, live (Zostavax)

WOUND CARE

Becaplermin (Regranex Gel)

Silver nitrate (generic)

MISCELLANEOUS THERAPEUTIC AGENTS

Acamprosate (Campral)

Alglucosidase alfa (Lumizyme, Myozyme)

C1 esterase inhibitor, human (Berinert, Cinryze)

Dextrose 50%/25%

Ecallantide (Kalbitor)

Eculizumab (Soliris)

Ferric citrate (Auryxia)

Flibanserin (ADDYI)

Ivacaftor (Kalydeco)

Ketamine (Ketalar, generic) [C-III]

Lanthanum carbonate (Fosrenol)

Mecasermin (Increlex)

Megestrol acetate (Megace, Megace-ES, generic)

Methylene blue (Urolene Blue, others)

Naltrexone (ReVia, Vivitrol, generic)

Nicotine, gum (Nicorette, others) [OTC]

Nicotine, nasal spray (Nicotrol NS)

Nicotine, transdermal (Habitrol, NicoDerm CQ [OTC], others)

Palifermin (Kepivance)

Potassium iodide (Iosat, Lugol's Solution,

SSKI, Thyro-Block, ThyroSafe, ThyroShield) [OTC]

Tolvaptan (Samsca)

Sevelamer carbonate (Renvela)

Sevelamer hydrochloride (Renagel)

Sodium polystyrene sulfonate (Kayexalate, Kionex, generic)

Talc [sterile talc powder] (Sclerosol, generic)

Taliglucerase alfa (Elelyso)

Varenicline (Chantix)

NATURAL AND HERBAL AGENTS

Black cohosh

Chamomile

Cranberry (Vaccinium macrocarpon)

Dong quai (Angelica polymorpha, sinensis)

Echinacea (Echinacea purpurea)

Evening primrose oil

Feverfew (Tanacetum parthenium)

Fish oil supplements (omega-3 polyunsaturated fatty acid)

Garlic (Allium sativum)

Ginger (*Zingiber officinale*)
Ginkgo biloba
Ginseng
Glucosamine sulfate (chitosamine) and chondroitin sulfate
Kava kava (kava kava root extract, *Piper methysticum*)

Melatonin
Milk thistle (*Silybum marianum*)
Red yeast rice
Resveratrol
Saw palmetto (*Serenoa repens*)
St. John's wort (*Hypericum perforatum*)

Valerian (*Valeriana officinalis*)
Yohimbine (*Pausinystalia yohimbe*) (Yocon, Yohimex)

GENERIC AND SELECTED BRAND DRUG DATA

These listings do not include all the information needed to use these medications safely and effectively. These are highly summarized listings of key prescribing information. See full prescribing label information for further detailed information that may be necessary.

Abacavir (Ziagen) BOX: Allergy (fever, rash, fatigue, GI, resp) reported; stop drug immediately & do not rechallenge; lactic acidosis & hepatomegaly/steatosis reported Uses: *HIV Infxn in combo w/ other antiretrovirals* Acts: NRTI Dose: *Adults.* 300 mg PO bid or 600 mg PO daily *Peds.* 8 mg/kg bid 16–20 mg/kg daily (stable CD4, undetect VRL) 300 mg bid max W/P: [C, –] CDC rec: HIV-infected mothers not breast-feed (transmission risk) Disp: Tabs 300 mg; soln 20 mg/mL CI: Mod–severe hepatic impair hypersens SE: See Box, ↑ LFTs, fat redistribution, N/V, HA, chills Notes: Many drug interactions; HLA-B*5701 ↑ risk for fatal hypersens Rxn, genetic screen before use

Abatacept (Orencia) Uses: *Mod–severe RAs, juvenile idiopathic arthritis* Acts: Selective costimulation modulator, ↓ T-cell activation Dose: *Adults.* Initial 500 mg (< 60 kg), 750 mg (60–100 kg); 1 g (> 100 kg) IV over 30 min; repeat at 2 and 4 wk, then q4wk; SQ regimen: after IV dose, 125 mg SQ w/in 24 h of Inf, then 125 SQ weekly *Peds 6–17 y.* 10 mg/kg (< 75 kg), 750 mg (75–100 kg), IV over 30 min; repeat at 2 and 4 wk then q4wk (> 100 kg, adult dose) W/P: [C; ?/–] w/ TNF blockers, anakinra; COPD; Hx predisposition to Infxn; w/ immunosuppressants CI: w/ Live vaccines w/in 3 mo of D/C abatacept Disp: IV 250 mg/vial; SQ 125 mg/mL refilled syringe SE: HA, URI, N, nasopharyngitis, Infxn, malignancy, Inf Rxns/hypersens (dizziness, HA, HTN), COPD exacerbations, cough, dyspnea Notes: Screen for TB before use

Abciximab (ReoPro) Uses: *Prevent acute ischemic comps in PCP*, MI* Acts: ↓ Plt aggregation (glycoprotein IIb/IIIa inhib) Dose: *ECC 2010.* ACS w/ immediate PCI: 0.25 mg/kg IV bolus 10–60 min before PCI, then 0.125 mcg/kg/min max 10 mcg/min IV for 12 h; w/ heparin. ACS w/ planned PCI w/in 24 h: 0.25 mg/kg IV bolus, then 10 mcg/min IV over 18–24 h concluding 1 h post-PCI; *PCI:* 0.25 mg/kg bolus 10–60 min pre-PTCA, then 0.125 mcg/kg/min (max = 10 mcg/min) cont Inf for 12 h W/P: [C, ?/–] CI: Active/recent (w/in 6 wk) internal hemorrhage, CVA w/in 2 y or CVA w/ sig neuro deficit, bleeding diathesis or PO anticoagulants w/in 7 d (unless PT < 1.2 × control), ↓ plt (< 100,000 cells/mcL), recent trauma or major surgery (w/in 6 wk), CNS tumor, AVM, aneurysm, severe uncontrolled HTN, vasculitis, dextran use w/ PTCA, murine protein allergy, w/ other glycoprotein IIb/IIIa inhib Disp: Inj 2 mg/mL SE: Back pain, ↓ BP, CP, allergic Rxns, bleeding, ↓ plt Notes: Use w/ heparin/ASA

Abiraterone (Zytiga) **Uses:** *Castrate-resistant metastatic PCa* **Acts:** CYP17 inhibitor; ↓ testosterone precursors **Dose:** 1000 mg PO qd w/ 5 mg prednisone bid; w/o food 2 h ac and 1 h pc; ↓ w/ hepatic impair **W/P:** [X, N/A] w/ Severe CHF, monitor for adrenocortical Insuff/excess, w/ CYP2D6 substrate/CYP3A4 inhib or inducers **CI:** PRG **Disp:** Tabs 250 mg **SE:** ↑ LFTs, jt swell, ↑ TG, ↓ K^+, ↓ PO_4^{-3} edema, muscle pain, hot flush, D, UTI, cough,↑ BP, ↑ URI, urinary frequency, dyspepsia **Notes:** ✓ LFTs, K^+; CYP17 inhib may ↑ mineralocorticoid SEs; prednisone ↓ ACTH limiting SEs

Acamprosate (Campral) **Uses:** *Maintain abstinence from EtOH* **Acts:** ↓ Glutamatergic transmission; ↓ NMDA receptors; related to GABA **Dose:** 666 mg PO tid; CrCl 30–50 mL/min: 333 mg PO tid **W/P:** [C; ?/–] Not advisable to father children; use barrier contraceptive and one additional form by partner **CI:** CrCl < 30 mL/min **Disp:** Tabs 333 mg **EC SE:** N/D, depression, anxiety, insomnia **Notes:** Does not eliminate EtOH withdrawal Sx; continue even if relapse occurs

Acarbose (Precose) **Uses:** *Type 2 DM* **Acts:** α-Glucosidase inhib; delays carbohydrate digestion to ↓ glu **Dose:** 25–100 mg PO tid w/ 1st bite each meal; 50 mg tid (< 60 kg); 100 mg tid (> 60 kg); usual maint 50–100 mg PO tid **W/P:** [B, ?] w/ Scr > 2 mg/dL; can affect digoxin levels **CI:** IBD, colonic ulceration, partial intestinal obst; cirrhosis **Disp:** Tabs 25, 50, 100 mg **SE:** Abd pain, D, flatulence, ↑ LFTs, hypersens Rxn **Notes:** OK w/ sulfonylureas; ✓ LFTs q3mo for 1st y; use simple sugars to correct glucose

Acebutolol (Sectral) **Uses:** *HTN, arrhythmias* chronic stable angina **Acts:** Blocks β-adrenergic receptors, β₁, & ISA **Dose:** *HTN:* 400–800 mg/d 2 + doses *Arrhythmia:* 400–1200 mg/d 2 + doses; ↓ 50% w/ CrCl < 50 mL/min, elderly; max 800 mg/d ↓ 75% w/ CrCl < 25 mL/min; max 400 mg/d **W/P:** [B, + M] Can exacerbate ischemic heart Dz, do not D/C abruptly **CI:** 2nd-/3rd-degree heart block, cardiac failure, cardiogenic shock **Disp:** Caps 200, 400 mg **SE:** Fatigue, HA, dizziness, ↓ HR

Acetaminophen, Inj (Ofirmev) **BOX:** Avoid dosing errors (accidental overdose/death). Acetaminophen associated w/acute liver failure; most injury d/t dose above recommended max daily limits, and more than one acetaminophen-containing product **Uses:** *Mild–mod pain, fever* **Acts:** Nonnarcotic analgesic; CNS synth of prostaglandins & hypothalamic heat-regulating center **Dose:** *Adults & Peds > 50 kg:* 1000 mg q6h or 650 mg q4h IV; 4000 mg max/d. *< 50 kg:* 15 mg/kg q6h or 12.5 mg/kg q4h, 75 mg/kg/d max *Peds ≥ 2–12 y.* 15 mg/kg q6h or 12.5 mg/kg q4h IV, 75 mg/kg/d max. Min. interval of 4 h **W/P:** [C, +] Excess dose can cause hepatic injury; caution w/ liver Dz, alcoholism, malnutrition, hypovolemia, CrCl < 30 g/min **CI:** Hypersens to components, severe/active liver Dz **Disp:** IV 1000 mg (10 mg/mL) **SE:** N/V, HA, insomnia (adults); N/V, constipation, pruritus, agitation, atelectasis (peds) **Notes:** Min. dosing interval 4 h; infuse over 15 min. No anti-inflammatory or plt-inhibiting action

Acetaminophen, Oral [N-acetyl-p-aminophenol, APAP] Tylenol, Others, Generic) [OTC] **BOX:** May cause acute liver failure; associated w/ doses > 4000 mg/d & taking APAP in > 1 product **Uses:** *Mild–mod pain, HA, fever* **Acts:** Nonnarcotic analgesic; ↓ CNS synth of prostaglandins & hypothalamic heat-regulating center **Dose:** *Adults.* 325–650 mg PO or PR q4–6h or 1000 mg PO 3–4 x/d; max 3 g/d; 4 g/d if HCP supervision < *50 kg:* 15 mg/kg IV q6h or 12.5 mg/kg IV q4h; max 75 mg/kg/d; ≥ *50 kg:* 650 mg IV q4h or 1000 mg IV q6h; max 4 g/d *Peds.* < *12 y.* 10–15 mg/kg/dose PO or PR q4–6h; max 5 doses/24 h. Administer q6h if CrCl 10–50 mL/min & q8h if CrCl < 10 mL/min *IV:* 15 mg/kg IV q6h or 12.5 mg/kg IV q4h; max 75mg/kg/d **W/P:** [C, +] w/ Hepatic/renal impair in elderly & w/ EtOH use (> 3 drinks/d); w/ > 4 g/d; EtOH liver Dz, G6PD deficiency; w/ warfarin; serious skin Rxns (SJS, TEN, AGEP) **CI:** Hypersens **Disp:** Tabs dissolving 80, 160 mg; tabs 325, 500, 650 mg; chew tabs 80, 160 mg; gel caps 500 mg; liq 160 mg/5 mL, 500 mg/15 mL; drops 80 mg/0.8 mL; supp 80, 120, 325, 650 mg; Inj 10 mg/mL **SE:** hepatox; OD hepatox at 10 g; 15 g can be lethal; Rx w/N-acetylcysteine **Notes:** No anti-inflammatory or plt-inhib action; avoid EtOH; combo products w/ > 325 mg APAP/dosage unit removed from market 2014 by FDA, ↓ dose also ↓ risk of APAP overdose. FDA advisory has rec ↓ in max dose to 3000 mg/d

Acetaminophen/Butalbital, w/ and w/o Caffeine (Alagesic LQ, Bupap, Esgic, Fioricet, Margesic, Zebutal, Generic) [C-III] BOX: APAP hepatotox (acute liver failure, liver transplant, death) reported. Often d/t APAP > 4000 mg/d or more than one APAP product **Uses:** *Tension HA* **Acts:** Nonnarcotic analgesic w/ barbiturate **Dose:** 1–2 tabs or caps (or 15–30 mL) PO q4–6h PRN; max 6 tabs/caps or 90 mL/d; max 4 g/d APAP from all sources; ↓ w/ renal/hepatic impair **W/P:** [C, ?/–] Alcoholic liver Dz, G6PD deficiency; serious skin Rxn **CI:** Hypersens **Disp:** Tabs butalbital/APAP 50/300 mg (*Bupap*), 50/325 mg; caps butalbital/APAP/caffeine 50/300/40 mg (*Fioricet*), 50/325/40 mg (*Esgic, Margesic, Zebutal*); liq butalbital/APAP/caffeine 50/325/40 mg/15 mL (*Alagesic LQ*); tabs butalbital/APAP/caffeine 50/325/40 mg **SE:** Drowsiness, dizziness, "hangover," N/V **Notes:** Butalbital habit forming; gradual taper to D/C; avoid EtOH (≥ 3 drinks/d, ↑ hepatotox risk)

Acetaminophen/Butalbital/Caffeine, w/ and w/o Codeine (Fioricet w/ Codeine, Generic) [C-III] BOX: APAP hepatotox (acute liver failure, transplant, death) reported. Often d/t APAP > 4000 mg/d or more than one APAP product; death d/t rapid metabolism of codeine to morphine; resp depression/death in children w/ codeine after tonsillectomy/adenoidectomy w/ evidence of ultra-rapid metabolizers of codeine d/t CYP2D6 polymorphism **Uses:** *Tension HA* **Acts:** Narcotic analgesic w/ barbiturate **Dose:** 1–2 caps PO q4h PRN; max 6 caps/d; max 4 g/d APAP from all sources; ↓ w/ renal/hepatic impair **W/P:** [C, ?/–] Alcoholic liver Dz, G6PD deficiency; serious skin Rxn **CI:** Component hypersens **Disp:** Caps butalbital/APAP/caffeine/codeine 50/300/40/30 mg **SE:** Drowsiness, dizziness, "hangover," N/V **Notes:** Butalbital habit forming; gradual taper to D/C; avoid EtOH (≥ 3 drinks/d, ↑ risk of hepatotox)

Acetaminophen/Codeine (Tylenol 2, 3, and 4) [C-III, C-V] BOX: Acetaminophen hepatotox (acute liver failure, liver transplant, death) reported. Often d/t acetaminophen > 4000 mg/day or more than one acetaminophen product. Death d/t ultra-rapid metabolism of codeine to morphine; resp depression/death reported in children who received codeine after tonsillectomy/adenoidectomy w/ evidence of an ultra-rapid metabolizers of codeine due to a CYP2D6 polymorphism **Uses:** *Mild–mod pain (No. 2–3); mod–severe pain (No. 4)* **Acts:** Combined APAP & narcotic analgesic **Dose: Adults.** 1–2 tabs q4–6h PRN or 30–60 mg/codeine q4–6h based on codeine content (max dose APAP = 4 g/d) **Peds.** APAP 10–15 mg/kg/dose; codeine 0.5–1 mg/kg dose q4–6h (guide: 3–6 y, 5 mL/dose; 7–12 y, 10 mL/dose) (max 2.6 g/d if < 12 y); ↓ in renal/hepatic impair **W/P:** [C, ?] Alcoholic liver Dz; G6PD deficiency **CI:** Hypersens **Disp:** Tabs 300 mg APAP + codeine (No. 2 = 15 mg, No. 3 = 30 mg, No. 4 = 60 mg); susp (C-V) APAP 120 mg + codeine 12 mg/5 mL **SE:** Drowsiness, dizziness, N/V **Notes:** See Acetaminophen note p 40

Acetazolamide (Diamox) **Uses:** *Diuresis, drug and CHF edema, glaucoma, prevent high-altitude sickness, refractory epilepsy*, metabolic alkalosis, resp stimulant in COPD **Acts:** Carbonic anhydrase inhib; ↓ renal excretion of hydrogen & ↑ renal excretion of Na^+, K^+, HCO_3^-, & H_2O **Dose: Adults.** Diuretic: 250–375 mg IV or PO q24h Glaucoma: 250–1000 mg PO q24h in ÷ doses Epilepsy: 8–30 mg/kg/d PO in ÷ doses Altitude sickness: Prevention: 125 mg BID; 250 BID if >100 kg (per CDC) start 24 h before & 48–72 h after highest ascent Treatment: 250 mg PO BID Metabolic alkalosis: 500 mg IV × 1 Resp stimulant: 25 mg bid **Peds.** Epilepsy: 8–30 mg/kg/24 h PO in ÷ doses; max 1 g/d Diuretic: 5 mg/kg/24 h PO or IV Alkalinization of urine: 5 mg/kg/dose PO bid-tid Glaucoma: 8–30 mg/kg/24 h PO in 3 ÷ doses; max 1 g/d; ↓ dose w/ CrCl 10–50 mL/min; avoid if CrCl < 10 mL/min **W/P:** [C, +/–] **CI:** Renal/hepatic/adrenal failure, sulfa allergy, hyperchloremic acidosis **Disp:** Tabs 125, 250 mg; ER caps 500 mg; Inj 500 mg/vial, powder for recons **SE:** Malaise, metallic taste, drowsiness, photosens, hyperglycemia **Notes:** Follow Na^+ & K^+; watch for metabolic acidosis; ✓ CBC & plts; SR forms not for pediatrics

Acetic Acid/Aluminum Acetate, Otic (Domeboro Otic) [OTC] **Uses:** *Otitis externa* **Acts:** Anti-infective **Dose:** 4–6 gtt in ear(s) q2–3h **W/P:** [C, ?] **CI:** Perforated tympanic membranes **Disp:** 2% otic soln **SE:** Local irritation

Acetylcysteine (Acetadote, Mucomyst) **Uses:** *Mucolytic, antidote to APAP hepatotox/OD*, adjuvant Rx chronic bronchopulmonary Dzs & CF* prevent contrast-induced renal dysfunction **Acts:** Splits mucoprotein disulfide linkages; restores glutathione in APAP OD to protect liver **Dose: Adults & Peds.** Nebulizer: 3–5 mL of 20% soln diluted w/ equal vol of H_2O or NS tid-qid Antidote: PO or NG: 140 mg/kg load, then 70 mg/kg q4h × 17 doses (dilute 1:3 in carbonated beverage or OJ), repeat if emesis w/in 1 h of dosing Acetadote: 150 mg/kg IV over 60 min, then 50 mg/kg over 4 h, then 100 mg/kg over 16 h Prevent renal dysfunction: 600–1200 mg PO bid × 2 d **W/P:** [B, ?] **Disp:** Soln, Inh and oral, 20%;

Acetadote IV soln 20% **SE:** Bronchospasm (Inh), N/V, drowsiness, anaphylactoid Rxns w/ IV **Notes:** Activated charcoal adsorbs PO acetylcysteine for APAP ingestion; start Rx for APAP OD w/in 6–8 h

Acitretin (Soriatane) **BOX:** Not to be used by females who are PRG or who intend to become PRG during/for 3 y following drug D/C; no EtOH during/2 mo following D/C; no blood donation for 3 y following D/C; hepatotoxic **Uses:** *Severe psoriasis*; other keratinization Dz (lichen planus, etc) **Acts:** Retinoid-like activity **Dose:** 25–50 mg/d PO, w/ main meal; **W/P:** [X, ?/–] Renal/hepatic impair; in women of reproductive potential **CI:** See Box; ↑ serum lipids; w/ MTX or tetracyclines; w/ chronic ↑ lipids, severe renal/hepatic impair **Disp:** Caps 10, 17.5, 25 mg **SE:** Hyperesthesia, cheilitis, skin peeling, alopecia, pruritus, rash, arthralgia, GI upset, photosens, thrombocytosis, ↑ triglycerides, ↑ Na^+, K^+, PO_4^{-2} **Notes:** ✓ LFTs/lytes/lipids; response takes up to 2–3 mo; informed consent & FDA guide for each Rx required; due to teratogenicity Do Your P.A.R.T. educational program for pt and HCP (www.soriatane.com/fdo/do_your_part.pdf)

Aclidinium Bromide (Tudorza Pressair) **Uses:** *Bronchospasm w/ COPD* **Acts:** LA anticholinergic, blocks ACH receptors **Dose:** 400 mcg/inhal, 1 inhal bid **W/P:** [C, ?] w/ Atropine hypersens, NAG, BPH, or MG; avoid w/ milk allergy **CI:** None **Disp:** Inhal powder, 30/60 doses **SE:** HA, D, nasopharyngitis, cough **Notes:** Not for acute exacerbation; lactose in powder, avoid w/ milk allergy; OK w/ renal impair

Acyclovir (Zovirax, generic) **Uses:** *Herpes simplex* (HSV) (genital/mucocutaneous, encephalitis, keratitis), *Varicella zoster* (Chickenpox), *Herpes zoster* (shingles) Infxns* **Acts:** ↓ viral DNA synth **Dose:** *Adults.* Dose on IBW if obese (> 125% IBW) PO: *Initial genital HSV:* 200 mg PO q4h while awake (5 caps/d) × 7–10 d or 400 mg PO tid × 7–10 d *Intermittent HSV Rx:* As initial, except Rx × 5 d, or 800 mg PO bid, at prodrome *Chronic HSV suppression:* 400 mg PO bid *Topical: Initial herpes genitalis:* Apply q3h (6×/d) for 7 d *HSV encephalitis:* 10 mg/kg IV q8h × 10 d *Herpes zoster:* 800 mg PO 5×/d for 7–10 d or *IV* 10 mg/kg/dose IV q8h × 7 d *Peds. Genital HSV: 3 mo–12 y:* 40–80 mg/kg/d ÷ 3–4 doses (max 1 g); ≥ *12 y:* 200 mg 5×/d or 400 mg 3×/d × 5–10 d; IV 5 mg/kg/dose q8h × 5–7 d *HSV encephalitis: 3 mo–12 y:* 60 mg/kg/d IV ÷ q8h × 14–21 d; > *12 y:* 30 mg/kg/d IV ÷ q8h × 14–21 d *Chickenpox:* ≥ *2 y:* 20 mg/kg/dose PO qid × 5 d *Shingles:* < *12 y:* 30 mg/kg/d PO or 1500 mg/m²/d IV ÷ q8h × 7–10 d; ↓ w/ CrCl < 50 mL/min **W/P:** [B, +] **CI:** Component hypersens **Disp:** Caps 200 mg; tabs 400/800 mg; susp 200 mg/5 mL; oint 5%; Inj 50mg/mL **SE:** Dizziness, lethargy, malaise, confusion, rash, IV site inflam; transient ↑ Cr/BUN **Notes:** PO better than topical for herpes genitalis

Adalimumab (Humira) **BOX:** Cases of TB have been observed; ✓ TB skin test prior to use; hep B reactivation possible, invasive fungal, and other opportunistic Infxns reported; lymphoma/other CA possible in children/adolescents **Uses:** *Mod–severe RA w/ an inadequate response to one or more DMARDs, PA, JIA, plaque psoriasis, AS, Crohn Dz, ulcerative colitis Crohns Dz in adults & peds* **Acts:** TNF-α inhib **Dose:** *RA, PA, AS:* 40 mg SQ q other wk; may ↑ 40 mg qwk if not on MTX. JIA 15–30 kg 20 mg q other wk *Crohn Dz/ ulcerative colitis:* 160 mg d 1, 80 mg 2 wk later, then 2 wk later start maint 40 mg q other wk **W/P:** [B, ?/–] See Box; do not use w/ live vaccines **CI:** None **Disp:** Prefilled 0.4 mL (20 mg) & 0.8 mL (40 mg) syringe **SE:** Inj site Rxns, HA, rash, ↑ CHF, anaphylaxis, pancytopenia (aplastic anemia) devastating Dz, new-onset psoriasis **Notes:** Refrigerate prefilled syringe, rotate Inj sites, OK w/ other DMARDs

Adapalene (Differin) **Uses:** *Acne vulgaris* **Acts:** Retinoid-like, modulates cell differentiation/keratinization/inflam **Dose:** *Adults & Peds > 12 y.* Apply 1×/d to clean/dry skin QHS **W/P:** [C, ?/–] products w/ sulfur/resorcinol/salicylic acid ↑ irritation **CI:** Component hypersens **Disp:** Topical lotion, gel, cream 0.1%; gel 0.3% **SE:** Skin redness, dryness, burning, stinging, scaling, itching, sunburn **Notes:** Avoid exposure to sunlight/sunlamps; wear sunscreen

Adapalene/Benzoyl Peroxide (Epiduo Gel) **Uses:** *Acne vulgaris* **Acts:** Retinoid-like, modulates cell differentiation, keratinization, and inflam w/ antibacterial **Dose:** *Adults & Peds > 12 y.* Apply 1 × daily to clean/dry skin **W/P:** [C, ?/–] Bleaching effects, photosens **CI:** Component hypersens **Disp:** Topical gel: adapalene 0.1% and benzoyl peroxide 2.5% (45g) **SE:** Local irritation, dryness **Notes:** Vit A may ↑ SE

Adefovir (Hepsera) **BOX:** Acute exacerbations of hep B seen after D/C Rx (monitor LFTs); nephrotox w/ underlying renal impair w/ chronic use (monitor renal Fxn); HIV resistance/untreated may emerge; lactic acidosis & severe hepatomegaly w/ steatosis reported **Uses:** *Chronic active hep B* **Acts:** Nucleotide analog **Dose:** CrCl > 50 mL/min: 10 mg PO daily; CrCl 20–49 mL/min: 10 mg PO q48h; CrCl 10–19 mL/min: 10 mg PO q72h; HD: 10 mg PO q7d postdialysis **W/P:** [C, ?/–] **Disp:** Tabs 10 mg **SE:** Asthenia, HA, D, hematuria Abd pain; see Box **Notes:** ✓ HIV status before use

Adenosine (Adenocard, Adenoscan) **Uses:** *Adenocard* *PSVT*; including w/ WPW; *Adenoscan* (pharmacologic stress testing) **Acts:** Class IV antiarrhythmic; slows AV node conduction **Dose:** *Stress test.* 140 mcg/kg/min × 6 min cont Inf *Adults. ECC 2010.* 6-mg rapid IV push, then 20-mL NS bolus. Elevate extremity; repeat 12 mg in 1–2 min PRN; ↓ to 3 mg if pt receiving carbamazepine or dipyridamole *Peds. ECC 2010. Symptomatic SVT:* 0.1 mg/kg rapid IV/IO push (max dose 6 mg); can follow w/ 0.2 mg/kg rapid IV/IO push (max dose 12 mg); follow each dose w/ ≥ 5 mL NS flush **W/P:** [C, ?] Hx bronchospasm **CI:** 2nd-/3rd-degree AV block or SSS (w/o pacemaker); Afib/flutter w/ WPW, V tachycardia, recent MI or CNS bleed, asthma **Disp:** Inj 3 mg/mL **SE:** Facial flushing, HA, dyspnea, chest pressure, ↓ BP, pro-arrhythmic **Notes:** Doses > 12 mg not OK; can cause momentary asystole w/ use; caffeine, theophylline antagonize effects

Ado-trastuzumab emtansine (Kadcyla) **BOX:** Do not substitute for trastuzumab; hepatotox (liver failure & death) reported (monitor LFTs/bili prior to & w/ each dose); cardiac tox: may ↓ LVEF (✓ LVEF prior to/ during Tx); embryo-fetal tox **Uses:** *Tx of HER2-positive, met breast CA previously treated w/ trastu-zumab and/or taxane* **Acts:** HER2-targeted Ab/microtubule inhibitor conjugate **Dose:** 3.6 mg/kg IV inf q3 wk until progression or tox; do not use dextrose 5% soln; see label for tox dosage mods **W/P:** [D, –] interruption of Tx, ↓ dose, or D/C may be necessary due to ADRs (see SE); avoid w/ strong CYP3A4 inhib **CI:** None **Disp:** Lyoph powder 100, 160 mg/vial **SE:** See Abs, fatigue, N/V/D, constipation, HA, ↑ LFTs, ↓ plts, ↓ WBC, musculoskeletal pain, Inf-related Rxns, hypersens Rxns, neurotox, pulmonary tox, pyrexia **Notes:** Monitor for tox; counsel on PRG prevention/planning (MotHER Pregnancy Registry)

Afatinib (Gilotrif) **Uses:** *Tx NSCLC w/ EGFR exon 19 del or exon 21 (L858R) subs* **Acts:** TKI **Dose:** 40 mg PO 1×/d; 1 h ac or 2 h pc; see label for tox dosage modifications **W/P:** [D, –] embryo-fetal tox; severe D, interstitial lung Dz, hepatotox, keratitis, bullous & exfoliative skin disorders; interruption of Tx, ↓ dose, or Tx D/C may be necessary due to ADRs; w/ P-gp inhibitors/inducers (adjust dose) **CI:** None **Disp:** Tabs 20, 30, 40 mg **SE:** V/D, rash/dermatitis acne-iform, pruritus, stomatitis, paronychia, dry skin, ↓ appetite, ↓ Wt, conjunctivitis, epistaxis, rhinorrhea, dyspnea, fatigue, ↓ LVEF, pyrexia, cystitis

Aflibercept (Eylea) **Uses:** *Neovascular (wet) AMD; macular edema follow-ing RVO; DME; DR in pt w/DME* **Acts:** Binds VGEF-A & placental growth fac-tor; ↑ neovascularization & vascular permeability **Dose:** 2 mg (0.05 mL) intravitreal Inj; AMD q4wk × 3 mo, then q8wk; RVO q4wk; DME q4wk × 5, then q8wk; DR q4wk × 5, then q8wk **W/P:** [C, ?] May cause endophthalmitis/retinal detachment **CI:** Ocular or periocular Infxn, active intraocular inflam, hypersens **Disp:** Inj kit 3-mL vial to deliver 0.05 mL of 40 mg/mL **SE:** Blurred vision, eye pain, conjuncti-val hemorrhage, cataract, IOP, vitreous detachment, floaters, arterial thrombosis **Notes:** Intravitreal Inj only w/ 30-gauge × 1/2-in needle

Albiglutide (Tanzeum) **BOX:** Risk of thyroid tumors/carcinoma **Uses:** *Type 2 DM; adjunct to ↓ calories/↑ exercise* **Acts:** Human GLP-1 agonist; ↑ insu-lin secretion; ↓ gastric emptying **Dose:** 30 mg SQ q1wk; may ↑ to 50 mg PRN; any time w/o regard to food **W/P:** [C/–] Not rec 1st line w/poor control on diet/exercise; not w/ type 1 DM/DKA/severe GI Dz; not an insulin substitute; ↓ blood sugar w/ insulin secretagogue (eg, sulfonylurea) or insulin; D/C w/ serious hypersens Rxn, pancreatitis; thyroid tumors in animals w/ GLP-1; caution w/renal impair **CI:** Hx thyroid CA, multiple MEN2 **Disp:** Singe-dose pen Inj 30, 50 mg **SE:** Hypoglycemia, N/D, Inj site Rxn, URI, AF, ↑ GGT, GERD, influenza, arthralgia, back pain, cough, pneumonia **Notes:** ↓ absorption of PO meds; SQ Inj into upper arm/thigh/abdomen

Albumin (Albuked, Albuminar 20, Albuminar 25, AlbuRx 25, Albutein, Buminate, Human Albumin Grifols, Kedbumin, Plasbumin) **Uses:** *Based on specific product label; plasma vol expansion for shock (eg, burns, trauma, surgery, infections)*; ovarian hyperstimulation synd, CABG support, hypoalbuminemia/hypoproteinemia **Acts:** Intravascular oncotic pressure **Dose:** *Adults.* Initial 25 g IV, then based on response; 250 g/48 h max

Peds. 0.5–1 g/kg/dose; max 6 g/kg/d **W/P:** [C, ?] Severe anemia; cardiac, renal, or hepatic Insuff d/t protein load & hypervolemia; avoid 25% in preterm infants; products from human plasma may contain infectious agents (viruses, prions, etc) **CI:** CHF, severe anemia **Disp:** Vials 20/50/100 mL 20%, 25% **SE:** Chills, fever, CHF, tachycardia, ↓ BP, hypervolemia **Notes:** Contains 130–160 mEq Na⁺/L; may cause pulm edema; max Inf rates: 25% vial: 2–3 mL/min; See also Plasma Protein Fraction (Albumin 5% Solution)

Albuterol (ProAir HFA, ProAir Respiclick, Proventil HFA, Ventolin HFA)
Uses: *Asthma, COPD, prevent exercise-induced bronchospasm* **Acts:** β-adrenergic sympathomimetic bronchodilator; relaxes bronchial smooth muscle **Dose:** *Adults.* Inhaler: 2 Inh q4–6h PRN; q4–6h *PO*: 2–4 mg PO tid-qid *Nebulizer*: 1.25–5 mg (0.25–1 mL of 0.5% soln in 2–3 mL of NS) q4–8h PRN *Prevent exercise-induced asthma*: 2 puffs 5–30 min prior to activity *Peds > 4 yr.* Inhaler: 2 Inh q4–6h *PO*: 0.1–0.2 mg/kg/dose PO; max 2–4 mg PO tid *Nebulizer*: 0.63–5 mg in 2–3 mL of NS q4–8h PRN **W/P:** [C, ?] **Disp:** Tabs 2, 4 mg; XR tabs 4, 8 mg; syrup 2 mg/5 mL; 90 mcg/dose metered-dose inhaler (typically 200 acts/canister); *RespiClick* (breath-actuated) inhaler; soln for nebulizer 0.63, 1.25, 2.5/3 mL; 2.5 mg/0.5 mL **SE:** Palpitations, tachycardia, nervousness, GI upset

Albuterol/Ipratropium (Combivent Respimat, DuoNeb)
Uses: *COPD* **Acts:** β-adrenergic bronchodilator w/ quaternary anticholinergic **Dose:** 2 Inh qid; nebulizer 3 mL q6h; max 3 mL q4h **W/P:** [C, ?] **CI:** Peanut/soybean allergy **Disp:** MDI 18 mcg ipratropium/90 mcg albuterol/puff, 60/120 metered actuations; nebulization soln (*DuoNeb*) ipratropium 0.5 mg/albuterol 2.5 mg/3 mL **SE:** Palpitations, tachycardia, nervousness, GI upset, dizziness, blurred vision **Notes:** *Respimat* no longer contains CFCs

Alcaftadine, Ophthalmic (Lastacaft)
Uses: *Allergic conjunctivitis* **Acts:** Histamine H₁-receptor antag **Dose:** 1 gtt in eye(s) daily **W/P:** [B, ?] **CI:** Hypersens **Disp:** Ophth soln 0.25% **SE:** Eye irritation **Notes:** Remove contacts before use

Aldesleukin [IL-2] (Proleukin)
BOX: Restrict to pts w/ nl cardiac/pulmonary Fxns as defined by formal testing. Caution w/ Hx of cardiac/pulmonary Dz. Administer in hospital setting w/ physician experienced w/ anticancer agents. Assoc w/ CLS characterized by ↓ BP and organ perfusion w/ potential for cardiac/resp tox, GI bleed/infarction, renal insufficiency, edema, and mental status changes. Increased risk of sepsis and bacterial endocarditis. Treat bacterial Infxn before use. Pts w/ central lines are at ↑ risk for Infxn. Prophylaxis w/ oxacillin, nafcillin, ciprofloxacin, or vancomycin may reduce staphylococcal Infxn. Hold w/ mod–severe severe lethargy or somnolence; continued use may result in coma **Uses:** *Met RCC & melanoma* **Acts:** Acts via IL-2 receptor; many immunomodulatory effects **Dose:** 600,000 Int units/kg q8h × max 14 doses d 1–5 and d 15–19 of 28-d cycle (FDA-dose/schedule for RCC); other schedules (eg, "high dose") 720,000 Int units/kg IV q8h up to 12 doses, repeat 10–15 d later) **W/P:** [C, ?/ –] **CI:** Organ allografts; abn thallium stress test or PFT **Disp:** Powder for recons 22 × 10⁶

Int units, when reconstituted 18 mill Int units/mL = 1.1 mg/mL **SE:** Flu-like synd (malaise, fever, chills), N/V/D, ↑ bili; capillary leak synd; ↓ BP, tachycardia, pulm & periph edema, fluid retention, & Wt gain; renal & mild heme tox (↓ Hgb, plt, WBC), eosinophilia; cardiac tox (ischemia, atrial arrhythmias); neurotox (CNS depression, somnolence, delirium, rare coma); pruritic rashes, urticaria, & erythroderma common

Alemtuzumab (Lemtrada) BOX: Serious/fatal autoimmune Dz (↓ plt and antiglomerular basement membrane Dz); ✓ CBC w/ diff, Cr, & UA periodically × 48 mo after last dose; life-threatening Inf Rxn, administer in appropriate facility; monitor × 2 h post-Inf; ↑ risk of malignancy; baseline/annual skin exams; REMS **Uses:** *Relapsing MS* **Acts:** CD52 cytolytic MoAb **Dose:** 1st course: 12 mg/d IV Inf × 5 d (60 mg total); 2nd course: 12 mg/d IV Inf × 3 d 12 mo after 1st course (36 mg total); infuse over 4 h; premedicate w/ steroids (1000 mg methylprednisolone or equivalent) × 1st 3 d of Tx; have HSV antiviral Px d 1 of Tx & × 2 mo after end of Tx or until CD4 count is > 200 cells/mm³ **W/P:** [C, -] Do not give live vaccines; avoid w/ active Infxn **CI:** HIV **Disp:** Inj soln 12 mg/1.2 mL **SE:** N/V/D, Abd pain, rash, pruritus, uticaria, HA, fatigue, insomnia, URI, UTI, nasopharyngitis, HSV, fungal Infxn, sinusitis, dizziness, flushing, pyrexia, paresthesia, oropharyngeal/extremity/back pain, arthralgia, thyroid disorder **Notes:** ✓ TFT baseline & q3mo until 48 mo after last Inf; ✓ CBC qmo until 48 mo after last Inf; *Lemtrada* REMS program 1-855-676-6326; *Campath* for CLL available only through *Campath* Distribution Program.

Alendronate (Binosto, Fosamax, Fosamax Plus D, Generic) Uses: *Rx & prevent osteoporosis male & postmenopausal female, Rx steroid-induced osteoporosis, Paget Dz* **Acts:** ↓ Nl & abn bone resorption; ↓ osteoclast Act **Dose:** *Postmenopausal & male osteoporosis:* Rx: 70 mg tab or soln/wk or 10 mg tab qd or 70 mg alendronate/2800 or 5600 Int units vit D₃ *Prevent postmenopausal osteoporosis:* Rx: 35 mg tab/wk or 5 mg tab qd *Steroid-induced osteoporosis:* Rx: 5 mg tab qd except postmenopausal not on estrogen: one 10 mg tab qd *Paget's disease of bone:* Rx: 40 mg/d × 6 mo; if low fracture risk consider D/C after 3–5 y of use **W/P:** [C, ?] Not OK if CrCl < 35 mL/min, w/ NSAID use **CI:** Esophageal anomalies, inability to sit/stand upright for 30 min, ↓ Ca²⁺ **Disp:** Tabs 5, 10, 35, 40, 70 mg, *Fosamax plus D:* Alendronate 70 mg w/ cholecalciferol (vit D₃) 2800 or 5600 Int units; Binosto 70 mg effervescent tab **SE:** Abd pain, acid regurgitation, constipation, D/N, dyspepsia, musculoskeletal pain, jaw osteonecrosis (w/ dental procedures, chemo) **Notes:** Take 1st thing in AM w/ H₂O (8 oz) > 30 min before 1st food/beverage of d; do not lie down for 30 min after. Use Ca²⁺ & vit D supl w/ regular tab; may ↑ atypical subtrochanteric femur fractures; avoid taking with antacids (↓ absorption)

Alfentanil (Alfenta) [C-II] Uses: *Adjunct in maint of anesthesia; analgesia* **Acts:** Short-acting narcotic analgesic **Dose:** *Adults & Peds > 12 y. Assisted ventilation:* Induction 8–20 mcg/kg; maint 3–5 mcg/kg q5–20min or 0.5 to 1 mcg/kg/min; total 8–40 mcg/kg *Controlled ventilation:* Induction 20–50 mcg/kg; maint 5–15 mcg/kg q5–20min; total 75 mcg/kg max *Continuous Inf* (↓ response to intubation/incision):

Induction 50–75 mcg/kg; maint 0.5–3 mcg/kg/min; total based on procedure duration *Induction:* 130–245 mcg/kg; maint 0.5–1.5 mcg/kg/min or general anesthetic; total based on procedure duration (Note: At these doses, truncal rigidity expected; use muscle relaxant); administer over 3 min and ↓ inhal agents 30–50% 1st h *Monitored anesthesia care (MAC):* Induction 3–8 mcg/kg; maint: 3–5 mcg/kg q5–20min or 0.25–1 mcg/kg/min; total 3–40 mcg/kg **W/P:** [C, –] ↑ ICP, resp depression **Disp:** Inj 500 mcg/mL **SE:** ↓ HR, ↓ BP arrhythmias, peripheral vasodilation, ↑ ICP, drowsiness, resp depression, N/V/constipation, ADH release

Alfuzosin (Uroxatral) **Uses:** *Symptomatic BPH* **Acts:** α-Blocker **Dose:** 10 mg PO daily immediately after the same meal **W/P:** [B, ?/–]w/ any Hx ↓ BP; use w/ PDE5 inhibitors may ↓ BP; may ↑ QTc interval; IFIS during cataract surgery **CI:** w/ CYP3A4 inhib; mod–severe hepatic impair; protease inhibitors for HIV **Disp:** Tabs 10 mg ER **SE:** Postural ↓ BP, dizziness, HA, fatigue **Notes:** Do not cut or crush

Alginic Acid/Aluminum Hydroxide/Magnesium Trisilicate (Gaviscon) [OTC] **Uses:** *Heartburn* **Acts:** Protective layer blocks gastric acid **Dose:** Chew 2–4 tabs or 15–30 mL PO qid followed by H_2O **W/P:** [C, ?] Avoid w/ renal impair or Na$^+$-restricted diet **Disp:** Chew tabs, susp **SE:** D, constipation **Notes:** Avoid w/in 2 h of other meds; chew tab to actuate

Alglucosidase Alfa (Lumizyme, Myozyme) **BOX:** Life-threatening anaphylactic Rxns seen w/ Inf; medical support measures should be immediately available; caution w/ ↓ CV/resp Fxn **Uses:** *Rx Pompe DZ* **Acts:** Recombinant acid α-glucosidase; degrades glycogen in lysosomes **Dose:** *Peds 1 mo–3.5 y.* 20 mg/kg IV q2wk over 4 h (see PI) **W/P:** [B, ?/–] Illness at time of Inf may ↑ Inf Rxns **Disp:** Powder 50 mg/vial limited distribution **SE:** Hypersens, fever, rash, D, V, gastroenteritis, pneumonia, URI, cough, resp distress/failure, Infxns, cardiac arrhythmia, ↑/↓ HR, flushing, anemia, pain, constipation

Aliskiren (Tekturna) **BOX:** May cause injury and death to a developing fetus; D/C immediately when PRG detected **Uses:** *HTN* **Acts:** 1st direct renin inhib **Dose:** 150–300 mg/d PO **W/P:** [D, ?/–]; Avoid w/ CrCl < 30 mL/min; ketoconazole and other CYP3A4 inhib may ↑ aliskiren levels **CI:** Anuria, sulfur sensitivity **Disp:** Tabs 150, 300 mg **SE:** D, Abd pain, dyspepsia, GERD, cough, ↑ K$^+$, angioedema, ↓ BP, dizziness, ↑ BUN, ↑ SCr

Aliskiren/Amplopidine (Tekamlo) **BOX:** May cause fetal injury & death; D/C immediately when PRG detected **Uses:** *HTN* **Acts:** Renin inhib w/ dihydropyridine CCB **Dose:** 150/5 mg PO 1×/d; max 300/10 mg/d); max effect in 2 wk **W/P:** [D, ?/–] do not use w/ cyclosporine/itraconazole avoid CrCl < 30 mL/min **Disp:** Tabs (aliskiren mg/amlodipine mg) 150/5, 150/10, 300/5, 300/10 **SE:** ↓ BP, ↑ K$^+$, angioedema, peripheral edema, D, dizziness, angina, MI, ↑ SCr, ↑ BUN

Aliskiren/Amlodipine/Hydrochlorothiazide (Amturnide) **BOX:** May cause fetal injury & death; D/C immediately when PRG detected **Uses:** *HTN* **Acts:** Renin inhib, dihydropyridine CCB, & thiazide diuretic **Dose:** Titrate q2wk PRN to 300/10/25 mg PO max/d **W/P:** [D, ?/–] Avoid w/ CrCl < 30 mL/min;

do not use w/ cyclosporine/itraconazole; ↓ BP in salt/volume depleted pts; HCTZ may exacerbate/activate SLE; D/C if myopia or NAG **CI:** Anuria, sulfonamide allergy **Disp:** Tabs (aliskiren mg/amlodipine mg/HCTZ mg) 150/5/12.5, 300/5/12.5, 300/5/25, 300/10/12.5, 300/10/25 **SE:** ↓ BP, ↑ K⁺, hyperuricemia, angioedema, peripheral edema, D, HA, dizziness, angina, MI, nasopharyngitis

Aliskiren/Hydrochlorothiazide (Tekturna HCT) BOX: May cause injury and death to a developing fetus; D/C immediately when PRG detected **Uses:** *HTN* **Acts:** Renin inhib w/ thiazide diuretic **Dose:** 150 mg/12.5 mg PO qd; may ↑ after 2–4 wk up to *max* 300 mg/25 mg **W/P:** [D, –] Avoid w/ CrCl ≤ 30 mL/min; avoid w/ CYP3A4 inhib (Li, ketoconazole, etc) may ↑ aliskiren levels; ↓ BP in salt/volume depleted pts sulfonamide allergy HCTZ may exacerbate/activate SLE **Disp:** Tabs (aliskiren mg/HCTZ mg) 150/12.5, 150/25, 300/12.5, 300/25 **SE:** Dizziness, influenza, D, cough, vertigo, asthenia, arthralgia, angioedema, ↑ BUN

Allopurinol (Aloprim, Lopurin, Zyloprim) **Uses:** *Gout, hyperuricemia of malignancy, uric acid urolithiasis* **Acts:** Xanthine oxidase inhib; ↓ uric acid production **Dose:** *Adults.* *PO:* Initial 100 mg/d; usual 300 mg/d; max 800 mg/d; ÷ dose if > 300 mg/d; ↑ 100 mg/d q–5wk for uric acid < 5 mg/dL (per ACR guidelines) *IV:* 200–400 mg/m²/d (max 600 mg/24 h); (after meal w/ plenty of fluid) *Peds.* Only for hyperuricemia of malignancy if < 10 y: 10 mg/kg/d PO (max 800 mg) or 50–100 mg/m² q8h (max 300 mg/m²/d); 200–400 mg/m²/d IV (max 600 mg) ↓ in renal impair **W/P:** [C, M] **Disp:** Tabs 100, 300 mg; Inj 500 mg/30 mL (Aloprim) **SE:** Rash, N/V, renal impair, angioedema **Notes:** Aggravates acute gout; begin after acute attack resolves; IV dose of 6 mg/mL final conc as single daily Inf or ÷ 6-, 8-, or 12-h intervals

Almotriptan (Axert) **Uses:** *Rx acute migraine* **Acts:** Vascular serotonin receptor agonist **Dose:** *Adults & Peds 12–17 y.* *PO:* 6.25–12.5 mg PO, repeat in 2 h PRN; (max 25 mg/24 h); w/ hepatic/renal impair, w/ potent CYP3A4 6.25-mg single dose (max 12.5 mg/d) **W/P:** [C, ?/–] **CI:** Angina, ischemic heart Dz, coronary artery vasospasm, hemiplegic or basilar migraine, uncontrolled HTN, ergot use, w/ sulfonamide allergy MAOI use w/in 14 d **Disp:** Tabs 6.25, 12.5 mg **SE:** N, somnolence, paresthesias, HA, dry mouth, weakness, numbness, coronary vasospasm, HTN

Alogliptin (Nesina) **Uses:** *Mono/combo type 2 DM* **Acts:** DDP-4 inhib, ↑ insulin synth/release **Dose:** 25 mg/d PO; if CrCl 30–60 mL/min 12.5 mg/d; CrCl < 30 mL/min 6.25 mg/d **W/P:** [B, M] 0.2% pancreatitis risk, hepatic failure, hypersens Rxn **CI:** Hypersens **Disp:** Tabs 6.25, 12.5, 25 mg **SE:** Hypoglycemia, HA, nasopharyngitis, URI, severe arthralgia

Alogliptin/Metformin (Kazano) BOX: Lactic acidosis w/ metformin accumulation; ↑ risk w/ sepsis, vol depletion, CHF, renal/hepatic impair, excess alcohol; w/ lactic acidosis suspected D/C and hospitalize **Uses:** *Combo type 2 DM* **Acts:** DDP-4 inhib; ↑ insulin synth/release w/ biguanide; ↓ hepatic glu prod & absorption; ↑ insulin sens **Dose:** Max daily 25 mg alogliptin, 2000 mg metformin **W/P:** [B, M] may cause lactic acidosis, pancreatitis, hepatic failure, hypersens Rxn, vit

B_{12} def **CI:** hx of hypersens, renal impair (♀ SCr ≥ 1.4 mg/dL or ♂ ≥ 1.5 mg/dL), metabolic acidosis **Disp:** Tabs (alogliptin mg/metformin mg): 12.5/500, 12.5/1000 **SE:** ↓ glu, HA, nasopharyngitis, D, ↑ BP, back pain, URI **Notes:** Warn against excessive EtOH intake, may ↑ metformin lactate effect; temp D/C w/ surgery or w/ iodinated contrast studies

Alogliptin/Pioglitazone (Oseni)
BOX: May cause/worsen CHF **Uses:** *Combo type 2 DM* **Acts:** DDP-4 inhibitor, ↑ insulin synth/release w/ thiazolidin-edione; ↑ insulin sens **Dose:** 25 mg alogliptin/15 mg pioglitazone or 25 mg/30 mg/d; NYHA Class I/II, start 25 mg/15 mg **W/P:** [C, –] w/bladder Ca **CI:** CHF NYHA Class III/IV, Hx of hypersens **Disp:** Tabs (alogliptin mg/pioglitazone mg): 25/15, 25/30, 25/45, 12.5/15, 12.5/30, 12.5/45 **SE:** Back pain, nasopharyngitis, URI **Notes:** 25 mg/15 mg max w/ strong CYP2C8 inhib; may ↑ bladder CA risk

Alosetron (Lotronex)
BOX: Serious GI SEs, some fatal, including ischemic colitis reported. Prescribed only through participation in the prescribing program **Uses:** *Severe D/predominant IBS in women who fail conventional Rx* **Acts:** Selective 5-HT$_3$ receptor anta **Dose:** 0.5 mg PO bid; ↑ to 1 mg bid max after 4 wk; D/C after 8 wk not controlled **W/P:** [B, ?/–] **CI:** Hx chronic/severe constipation, GI obst, strictures, toxic megacolon, GI perforation, adhesions, ischemic/UC, Crohn Dz, diver-ticulitis, thrombophlebitis, hypercoagulability **Disp:** Tabs 0.5, 1 mg **SE:** Constipation, Abd pain, N, fatigue, HA **Notes:** D/C immediately if constipation or Sxs of ischemic colitis develop; informed consent prior to use

Alpha-1 Proteinase Inhibitor (Aralast NP, Glassia, Prolastin C, Zemaira)
Uses: *α_1-Antitrypsin deficiency* **Acts:** Replace human α_1-protease inhib **Dose:** 60 mg/kg IV 1×/wk **W/P:** [C, ?] **CI:** Selective IgA deficiencies w/ IgA antibodies **Disp:** Inj 500, 1000 mg powder; 1000 mg soln vial for Inj **SE:** HA, CP, edema, MS discomfort, fever, dizziness, flu-like Sxs, allergic Rxns, ↑ AST/ALT

Alprazolam (Niravam, Xanax XR) [C-IV]
Uses: *Anxiety & panic disor-ders, anxiety w/ depression* **Acts:** Benzodiazepine; antianxiety agent **Dose:** *Anxiety:* Initial, 0.25–0.5 mg tid; ↑ to 4 mg/d max ÷ doses *Panic:* Initial, 0.5 mg tid; may gradually ↑ to response; ↓ in elderly, debilitated, & hepatic impair **W/P:** [D, –] **CI:** NAG, concomitant itra-/ketoconazole **Disp:** Tabs 0.25, 0.5, 1, 2 mg; *Xanax XR* 0.5, 1, 2, 3 mg; *Niravam* (ODTs) 0.25, 0.5, 1, 2 mg; soln 1 mg/mL **SE:** Drowsi-ness, fatigue, irritability, memory impair, sexual dysfunction, paradoxical Rxns **Notes:** Avoid abrupt D/C after prolonged use

Alprostadil [Prostaglandin E$_1$] (Prostin VR)
BOX: Apnea in up to 12% of neonates, especially < 2 kg at birth **Uses:** *Conditions where ductus arteriosus flow must be maintained*, sustain pulm/systemic circulation until OR (eg, pulm atre-sia/stenosis, transposition) **Acts:** Vasodilator (ductus arteriosus very sensitive), plt inhib **Dose:** 0.05–0.1 mcg/kg/min IV; ↓ to response **ECC 2010:** *Maintain ductus patency:* 0.01–0.4 mcg/kg/min **W/P:** [X, –] **CI:** Neonatal resp distress synd **Disp:** Inj 500 mcg/mL **SE:** Cutaneous vasodilation, Sz-like activity, jitteriness, ↑ temp, ↓ K$^+$, thrombocytopenia, ↓ BP; may cause apnea **Notes:** Keep intubation kit at bedside

Alprostadil, Intracavernosal (Caverject, Edex) Uses: *ED* Acts: Relaxes smooth muscles, dilates cavernosal arteries, ↑ lacunar spaces w/ blood entrapment Dose: 2.5–60 mcg intracavernosal; titrate in office for erection suitable for intercourse, but not > 1 h; max 1 dose/24 h or 3×/wk W/P: [X, –] CI: ↑ risk of priapism (eg, sickle cell); penile deformities/implants; men in whom sexual activity inadvisable Disp: *Caverject:* 5-, 10-, 20-, 40-mcg powder for Inj vials ± diluent syringes 10-, 20-, 40-mcg amp *Caverject Impulse:* Self-contained syringe (29 gauge) 10 & 20 mcg *Edex:* 10-, 20-, 40-mcg cartridges SE: Local pain w/ Inj Notes: Counsel about priapism, penile fibrosis, & hematoma risks, titrate dose in office

Alprostadil, Urethral Suppository (Muse) Uses: *ED* Acts: Urethral absorption; vasodilator, relaxes smooth muscle of corpus cavernosa Dose: 125–250 mcg PRN to achieve erection (max 2 systems/24 h) duration 30–60 min W/P: [X, –] CI: ↑ Priapism risk (especially sickle cell, myeloma, leukemia); penile deformities/implants; men in whom sex inadvisable Disp: 125, 250, 500, 1000 mcg w/ transurethral system SE: ↓ BP, dizziness, syncope, penile/testicular pain, urethral burning/bleeding, priapism Notes: Titrate dose in office

Alteplase, Recombinant [tPA] (Activase) Uses: *AMI, PE, acute ischemic stroke, & CV cath occlusion* Acts: Thrombolytic; binds fibrin in thrombus, initiates fibrinolysis Dose: *ECC 2010. STEMI:* 15-mg bolus; then 0.75 mg/kg over 30 min (50 mg max); then 0.50 mg/kg over next 60 min (35 mg max; max total dose 100 mg) *Acute ischemic stroke:* 0.9 mg/kg IV (max 90 mg) over 1 h, give 10% of total dose over 1 min; remaining 90% over 1 h (dose before 3–4.5-h window) *PE:* 100 mg over 2 h (submassive PE: can administer 10-mg bolus, then 90 mg over 2 h) *Cath occlusion:* < 30 kg 110% lumen vol max 2 mg/2 mL; > 30 kg 2 mg/2 mL W/P: [C, ?] CI: Active internal bleeding; uncontrolled HTN (SBP > 185 mm Hg, DBP > 110 mm Hg); recent (w/in 3 mo) CVA, GI bleed, trauma; intracranial or intraspinal surgery or Dzs (AVM/aneurysm/subarachnoid hemorrhage/neoplasm); prolonged cardiac massage; suspected aortic dissection, w/ anticoagulants or INR > 1.7, heparin w/in 48 h, plts < 100,000, Sz at the time of stroke, significant closed head/facial trauma Disp: Powder for Inj 2, 50, 100 mg SE: Bleeding, bruising (eg, venipuncture sites), ↓ BP Notes: Give heparin to prevent reocclusion; in AMI, doses of > 150 mg associated w/ intracranial bleeding

Altretamine (Hexalen) BOX: BM suppression, neurotox common, should be administered by experienced chemo MD Uses: *Palliative Rx persistent or recurrent ovarian CA* Acts: Unknown; ? cytotoxic/alkylating agent; ↓ nucleotide incorporation Dose: 260 mg/m²/d in 4 ÷ doses for 14–21 d of a 28-d Rx cycle; after meals and hs W/P: [D, ?/–] CI: Preexisting BM depression or neurologic tox Disp: Gel caps 50 mg SE: N/V/D, cramps; neurotox (neuropathy, CNS depression); myelosuppression, anemia, ↓ PLT, ↓ WBC Notes: ✓ CBC, routine neurologic exams

Aluminum Hydroxide (AlternaGEL, Amphojel, Dermagran) [OTC] Uses: *Heartburn, upset or sour stomach, or acid indigestion*; supl to Rx of ↑PO₄²⁻; *minor cuts, burns (Dermagran)* Acts: Neutralizes gastric acid; binds

PO_4^{2-} **Dose:** *Adults.* 10–30 mL or 300–1200 mg PO q4–6h **Peds.** 5–15 mL PO q4–6h or 50–150 mg/kg/24 h PO ÷ q4–6h (hyperphosphatemia) **W/P:** [C, ?] **Disp:** Tabs 300, 600 mg; susp 320, 600 mg/5 mL; oint 0.275% (*Dermagran*) **SE:** Constipation **Notes:** OK w/ renal failure; topical ointment for cuts/burns; not preferred for hyperphosphatemia

Aluminum Hydroxide/Alginic Acid/Magnesium Carbonate (Gaviscon Extra Strength Liquid) [OTC] **Uses:** *Heartburn, acid indigestion* **Acts:** Neutralizes gastric acid **Dose:** 15–30 mL PO pc & hs; 2–4 chew tabs up to qid **W/P:** [C, ?] ↑ Mg^{2+}, avoid in renal impair **Disp:** Liq w/ AlOH 95 mg/Mg carbonate 358 mg/15 mL; Extra Strength liq AlOH 254 mg/Mg carbonate 237 mg/15 mL; chew tabs AlOH 160 mg/Mg carbonate 105 mg **SE:** Constipation, D **Notes:** Qid doses best pc & hs; may ↓ absorption of some drugs, take 2–3 h apart to ↓ effect

Aluminum Hydroxide/Magnesium Hydroxide (Maalox, Mylanta Ultimate Strength) [OTC] **Uses:** *Hyperacidity* (peptic ulcer, hiatal hernia, etc) **Acts:** Neutralizes gastric acid **Dose:** 10–20 mL or 1–2 tabs PO qid or PRN **W/P:** [C, ?] **Disp:** Chew tabs, susp **SE:** May ↑ Mg^{2+} w/ renal Insuff, constipation, D **Notes:** Doses qid best pc & hs

Aluminum Hydroxide/Magnesium Hydroxide & Simethicone (Maalox Plus, Mylanta, Mylanta II) [OTC] **Uses:** *Hyperacidity w/ bloating* **Acts:** Neutralizes gastric acid & defoaming **Dose:** *Adults.* 10–20 mL or 1–2 tabs PO qid or PRN, avoid in renal impair **W/P:** [C, ?] **Disp:** Tabs, susp, liq **SE:** ↑ Mg^{2+} in renal Insuff, D, constipation **Notes:** Mylanta II contains twice Al & Mg hydroxide of Mylanta; may affect absorption of some drugs

Aluminum Hydroxide/Magnesium Trisilicate (Gaviscon Regular Strength) [OTC] **Uses:** *Relief of heartburn, upset or sour stomach, acid indigestion* **Acts:** Neutralizes gastric acid **Dose:** Chew 1–2 tabs qid; avoid in renal impair **W/P:** [C, ?] **CI:** Mg^{2+} sensitivity **Disp:** AlOH 80 mg/Mg trisilicate 20 mg/tab **SE:** ↑ Mg^{2+} in renal Insuff, constipation, D **Notes:** May affect absorption of some drugs

Alvimopan (Entereg) **BOX:** For short-term hospital use only (max 15 doses); ↑ risk MI vs placebo **Uses:** *↑↓ Time to GI recovery w/ bowel resection and primary anastomosis* **Acts:** Opioid (µ) receptor antag; selectively binds GI receptors, antagonizes effects of opioids on GI motility/secretion **Dose:** 12 mg 30 min–5 h preop PO, then 12 mg bid up to 7 d; max 15 doses **W/P:** [B, ?/–] Not rec in complete bowel obstruction surgery, hepatic/renal impair **CI:** Therapeutic opioids > 7 d consecutive prior **Disp:** Caps 12 mg **SE:** ↓ K^+, dyspepsia, urinary retention, anemia, back pain **Notes:** Hospitals must be registered to use

Amantadine (Symmetrel) **Uses:** *Rx/prophylaxis influenza A (no longer recommended d/t resistance), Parkinsonism, & drug-induced EPS* **Acts:** Prevents infectious viral nucleic acid release into host cell; releases DA and blocks reuptake of DA in presynaptic nerves **Dose:** *Adults. Influenza A:* 200 mg/d PO or 100 mg PO bid w/in 48 h of Sx until 24–48 h post-Sx *EPS:* 100 mg PO bid (up to 300 mg/d ÷ doses) *Parkinsonism:* 100 mg PO daily-bid (up to 400 mg/d) *Peds 1–9 y.* 4.4–8.8 mg/kg/24 h to 150 mg/24 h max ÷ doses daily-bid *10–12 y. Per CDC 2011:* > 10 y, < 40 kg 5 mg/kg/d ÷ 2 doses; > 10 y, > 40 kg 100 mg bid ↓ in renal impair **W/P:** [C, ?/–] **Disp:** Caps 100 mg; tabs 100 mg; soln 50 mg/5 mL **SE:** Orthostatic ↓ BP, edema, insomnia, depression, irritability, hallucinations, dream abnormalities, N/D, dry mouth **Notes:** Not for influenza use in US d/t resistance, including H1N1

Ambrisentan (Letairis) BOX: CI in PRG; ✓ monthly PRG tests; limited access program **Uses:** *Pulm arterial HTN* **Acts:** Endothelin receptor antag **Dose:** 5 mg PO/d, max 10 mg/d; not OK w/ hepatic impair **W/P:** [X, –] Do not use > 5 mg/d w/ Cyclosporine, strong CYP3A or 2C19 inhib, inducers of P-glycoprotein, CYPs and UGTs **CI:** PRG **Disp:** Tabs 5, 10 mg **SE:** Edema, ↓ Hct/Hgb nasal congestion, sinusitis, dyspnea, flushing, constipation, HA, palpitations, hepatotoxic **Notes:** Available only through the Letairis Education and Access Program (LEAP); D/C AST/ALT > 5× ULN or bili > 2× ULN or S/Sx of liver dysfunction; childbearing females must use 2 methods of contraception

Amifostine (Ethyol) **Uses:** *Xerostomia prophylaxis during RT (head, neck, etc) where parotid is in radiation field; ↓ renal tox w/ repeated cisplatin* **Acts:** Prodrug, dephosphorylated to active thiol metabolite, free radical scavenger binds cisplatin metabolites **Dose:** Chemo prevent: 910 mg/m²/d 15-min IV Inf 30 min pre-chemo; *Xerostomia Px:* 200 mg/m² over 2 min 1×/d 15 min pre-rad **W/P:** [C, ?/–] **Disp:** 500-mg vials powder, reconstitute in NS **SE:** Transient ↓ BP (> 60%), N/V, flushing w/ hot or cold chills, dizziness, ↓ Ca²⁺, somnolence, sneezing, serious skin Infxn **Notes:** Does not ↓ effectiveness of cyclophosphamide + cisplatin chemotherapy; off label 500 mg SQ before RT

Amikacin (Generic) BOX: May cause nephrotoxicity, neuromuscular blockade, & respiratory paralysis **Uses:** *Serious gram(–) bacterial Infxns* & mycobacteria **Acts:** Aminoglycoside; ↓ protein synth **Spectrum:** Good gram(–) bacterial coverage: *Pseudomonas* & *Mycobacterium* sp **Dose:** *Adults & Peds. Conventional:* Use DBW = IBW + 0.4 (actual body weight – IBW) for normal renal Fxn: 15 mg/kg/d ÷ 2–3 equal doses; *Extended interval dosing:* 1×/d; 15–20 mg/kg q24h, follow levels 4 and 12 h; ↑ interval for renal impair; max 1.5 g/d *Peds: Neonates < 1200 g, 0–4 wk:* 7.5 mg/kg/dose q18h–24h *Age < 7 d, 1200–2000 g:* 7.5 mg/kg/dose q12h *> 2000 g:* 7.5–10 mg/kg/dose q12h *Age > 7 d, 1200–2000 g:* 7.5–10 mg/kg/dose q8–12h *> 2000 g:* 7.5–10 mg/kg/dose q8h **W/P:** [O, +/–] Avoid w/ diuretics **Disp:** Inj 500 mg/2 mL; 1 g/4 mL **SE:** Renal impairment, oto **Notes:** May be effective in gram(–) resistance to gentamicin & tobramycin; follow Cr; Levels: *Peak:* 30 min after Inf *Trough:* < 0.5 h before next dose *Therapeutic: Peak* 20–30 mcg/mL (varies by lab), *Trough:* < 8 mcg/mL *Half-life:* 2 h

Amiloride (Midamor) BOX: ↑ K⁺ esp renal Dz, DM, elderly **Uses:** *HTN, CHF, & thiazide or loop diuretic induced ↓ K⁺* **Acts:** K⁺-sparing diuretic; interferes w/ Na⁺/Na⁺ exchange in distal tubule & collecting duct **Dose:** *Adults.* 5–10 mg PO daily (max 20 mg/d); max 20 mg/d; ↓ w/ renal impair **Peds.** 0.4–0.625 mg/kg/d; max 20 mg/d; ↓ w/ renal impair **W/P:** [B, ?] avoid CrCl < 10 mL/min **CI:** ↑ K⁺, acute or chronic renal Dz, diabetic neuropathy, w/ other K+-sparing diuretics **Disp:** Tabs 5 mg **SE:** ↑ K+; HA, dizziness, dehydration, impotence **Notes:** ✓ K+

Aminocaproic Acid (Amicar) Uses: *Excessive bleeding from systemic hyperfibrinolysis & urinary fibrinolysis* **Acts:** ↓ Fibrinolysis; inhibits TPA, inhibits conversion of plasminogen to plasmin **Dose: Adults.** 4–5 g IV or PO (1st h), then 1 g/h IV or 1.25 g/h PO × 8 h or until bleeding controlled; 30 g/d max **Peds.** 100 mg/kg IV (1st h), then 1 g/m²/h; max 18 g/m²/d; ↓ w/ renal Insuff **W/P:** [C, ?] Not for upper urinary tract bleeding **CI:** DIC **Disp:** Tabs 500, 1000 mg, syrup 1.25 g/5 mL; Inj 250 mg/mL **SE:** ↓ BP, ↓ HR, dizziness, HA, fatigue, rash, GI disturbance, skeletal muscle weakness, ↓ plt Fxn **Notes:** Administer × 8 h or until bleeding controlled

Aminophylline (Generic) Uses: *Asthma, COPD*, & bronchospasm **Acts:** Relaxes smooth muscle (bronchi, pulm vessels); stimulates diaphragm **Dose: Adults.** *Acute asthma.* Load 5.7 mg/kg IV, then 0.38–0.51 mg/kg/h (900 mg/d max); titrate to levels *Chronic asthma.* 380 mg/d PO ÷ q6–8h; maint ↑ 760 mg/d **Peds.** Load 5.7 mg/kg/dose IV; *1 ≤ 9 y:* 1.01 mg/kg/h; *9 ≤ 12 y:* 0.89 mg/kg/h; w/ hepatic Insuff & w/ some drugs (macrolide & quinolone antib, cimetidine, propranolol) **W/P:** [C, +] Uncontrolled arrhythmias, HTN, Sz disorder, hyperthyroidism, peptic ulcers **Disp:** Tabs 100 mg, Inj 25 mg/mL **SE:** N/V, irritability, tachycardia, ventricular arrhythmias, Szs **Notes:** Individualize dosage *Level:* 10–20 mcg/mL, toxic > 20 mcg/mL; aminophylline 85% theophylline; erratic rectal absorption

Amiodarone (Cordarone, Nexterone, Pacerone) **BOX:** Liver tox, exacerbation of arrhythmias and lung damage reported Uses: *Recurrent VF or unstable VT*, supraventricular arrhythmias, AF **Acts:** Class III antiarrhythmic inhibits alpha/beta adrenergic system (Table 9, p 355) **Dose: Adults.** *Ventricular arrhythmias:* IV: 15 mg/min × 10 min, then 1 mg/min × 6 h, maint 0.5-mg/min cont Inf typically × 18 h, then Δ to PO or *PO:* Load: 800–1600 mg/d PO × 1–3 wk; goal 8–10 g total *Maint:* 600–800 mg/d PO for 1 mo, then 200–400 mg/d *Supraventricular arrhythmias: IV:* 300 mg IV over 1 h, then 20 mg/kg for 24 h, then 600 mg PO daily for 1 wk, maint 100–400 mg daily or *PO:* Load 600–800 mg/d PO for 1–4 wk; goal 6–8 g total *Maint:* ↓ to 100–400 mg daily *ECC 2010. VF/VT cardiac arrest refractory to CPR, shock and pressor:* 300 mg IV/IO push; can give additional 150 mg IV/IO once *Life-threatening arrhythmias:* Max dose: 2.2 g IV/24 h; rapid Inf: 150 mg IV over 1st 10 min (15 mg/min); can repeat 150 mg IV q10min PRN; slow Inf: 360 mg IV over 60 min (1 mg/min) *Maint:* 540 mg IV over 18 h (0.5 mg/min) **Peds.** 10–15 mg/kg/24 h ÷ q12h PO for 7–10 d, then 5 mg/kg/24 h ÷ q12h or daily (infants require ↑ loading) *ECC 2010. Pulseless VT/Refractory VF:* 5 mg/kg IV/IO bolus, repeat PRN to 15 mg/kg (2.2 g in adolescents)/24 h; max single dose 300 mg; *Perfusing SVT/Ventricular arrhythmias:* 5 mg/kg IV/IO load over 20–60 min; repeat PRN to 15 mg/kg (2.2 g in adolescents)/24h **W/P:** [D, –] May require ↓ digoxin/warfarin dose, ↓ w/ liver Insuff; many drug interactions **CI:** Sinus node dysfunction, 2nd-/3rd-degree AV block, sinus brady (w/o pacemaker), iodine sensitivity **Disp:** Tabs 100, 200, 400 mg; Inj 50 mg/mL; Premixed

Inf 150, 360 mg SE: Pulm fibrosis, exacerbation of arrhythmias, ↑ QT interval; CHF, hypo-/hyperthyroidism, ↑ LFTs, liver failure, ↓ BP/ ↓ HR (Inf related) dizziness, HA, corneal microdeposits, optic neuropathy/neuritis, peripheral neuropathy, photosens; blue skin Notes: IV conc > 2.0 mg/mL central line only Levels: *Trough:* just before next dose *Therapeutic:* 0.5–2.5 mcg/mL *Toxic:* > 2.5 mcg/mL *Half-life:* 40–55 d (↓ peds)

Amitriptyline (Elavil) BOX: Antidepressants may ↑ suicide risk; consider risks/benefits of use. Monitor pts closely Uses: *Depression (not bipolar depression)*, peripheral neuropathy, chronic pain, tension HAs, migraine HA prophylaxis PTSD* Acts: TCA; ↓ reuptake of serotonin & norepinephrine by presynaptic neurons Dose: *Adults. Initial:* 25–150 mg PO hs; may ↑ to 300 mg hs *Peds.* Not OK < 12 y unless for chronic pain *Initial:* 0.1 mg/kg PO hs, ↑ over 2–3 wk to 0.5–2 mg/kg PO hs; taper to D/C W/P: CV Dz, Szs [D,+/–] NAG, hepatic impair CI: w/ MAOIs or w/in 14 d of use, during AMI recovery Disp: Tabs 10, 25, 50, 75, 100, 150 mg; Inj 10 mg/mL SE: Strong anticholinergic SEs; OD may be fatal; urine retention, sedation, ECG changes BM suppression, orthostatic ↓ BP, photosens Notes: Levels: *Therapeutic:* 100–250 mg/mL *Toxic:* > 500 ng/mL; levels may not correlate w/ effect

Amlodipine (Norvasc) Uses: *HTN, stable or unstable angina* Acts: CCB; relaxes coronary vascular smooth muscle Dose: 2.5–10 mg/d PO; ↓ w/ hepatic impair W/P: [C, ?] Disp: Tabs 2.5, 5, 10 mg SE: Edema, HA, palpitations, flushing, dizziness Notes: Take w/o regard to meals

Amlodipine/Atorvastatin (Caduet) Uses: *HTN, chronic stable/vasospastic angina, control cholesterol & triglycerides* Acts: CCB & HMG-CoA reductase inhib Dose: Amlodipine 2.5–10 mg w/ atorvastatin 10–80 mg PO daily W/P: [X, –] CI: Active liver Dz, ↑ LFTs Disp: Tabs amlodipine/atorvastatin: 2.5/10, 2.5/20, 2.5/40, 5/10, 5/20, 5/40, 5/80, 10/10, 10/20, 10/40, 10/80 mg SE: Edema, HA, palpitations, flushing, myopathy, arthralgia, myalgia, GI upset, liver failure Notes: ✓ LFTs; instruct pt to report muscle pain/weakness

Amlodipine/Olmesartan (Azor) BOX: Use of renin-angiotensin agents in PRG can cause injury and death to fetus, D/C immediately when PRG detected Uses: *Hypertension* Acts: CCB w/ angiotensin II receptor blocker Dose: Initial 5 mg/20 mg, max 10 mg/40 mg qd W/P: [D, –] w/ K⁺ supl or K⁺-sparing diuretics, renal impair, RAS, severe CAD, AS CI: PRG Disp: Tabs amlodipine/olmesartan 5 mg/20 mg, 10/20, 5/40, 10/40 SE: Edema, vertigo, dizziness, ↓ BP

Amlodipine/Valsartan (Exforge) BOX: Use of renin-angiotensin agents in PRG can cause fetal injury and death, D/C immediately when PRG detected Uses: *HTN* Acts: CCB w/ angiotensin II receptor blocker Dose: Initial 5 mg/160 mg, may ↑ after 1–2 wk, max 10 mg/320 mg qd, start elderly at 1/2 initial dose W/P: [D /–] w/ K⁺ supl or K⁺-sparing diuretics, renal impair, RAS, severe CAD CI: PRG, Disp: Tabs amlodipine/valsartan 5/160, 10/160, 5/320, 10 mg/320 mg SE: Edema, vertigo, nasopharyngitis, URI, dizziness, ↓ BP

Amlodipine/Valsartan/Hydrochlorothiazide (Exforge HCT) BOX: Use of renin-angiotensin agents in PRG can cause fetal injury and death. D/C immediately when PRG detected Uses: *Hypertension (not initial Rx)* Acts: CCB, angiotensin II receptor blocker, & thiazide diuretic Dose: 5–10/160–320/12.5–25 mg 1 tab 1 × d; may ↑ dose after 2 wk; max dose 10/320/25 mg W/P: [D, –] w/ Severe hepatic or renal impair CI: Anuria, sulfonamide allergy Disp: Tabs amlodipine/valsartan/HCTZ: 5/160/12.5, 10/160/12.5, 5/160/25, 10/160/25, 10/320/25 mg SE: edema, dizziness, HA, fatigue, ↑/↓ K⁺ ↑ BUN, ↑ SCr, nasopharyngitis, dyspepsia, N, back pain, muscle spasm, ↓ BP

Ammonium Aluminum Sulfate [Alum] [OTC] Uses: *Hemorrhagic cystitis when saline bladder irrigation fails* Acts: Astringent Dose: 1–2% soln w/ constant NS bladder irrigation W/P: [+/–] Disp: Powder for recons SE: Encephalopathy possible; ✓ aluminum levels, especially w/ renal Insuff; can precipitate & occlude catheters Notes: Safe w/o anesthesia & w/ vesicoureteral reflux

Amoxicillin (Amoxil, Moxatag, Generic) Uses: *Ear, nose, & throat, lower resp, skin, urinary tract Infxns from susceptible gram(+) bacteria*, endocarditis prophylaxis, *H. pylori* eradication w/ other agents (gastric ulcers) Acts: β-Lactam antibiotic; ↓ cell wall synth Spectrum: Gram(+) (*Streptococcus* sp, *Enterococcus* sp); some gram(–) (*H. influenzae, E. coli, N. gonorrhoeae, H. pylori,* & *P. mirabilis*) Dose: Adults. 250–500 mg PO tid or 500–875 mg bid ER 775 mg 1 × d Peds. 25–100 mg/kg/24 h PO ÷ q8h, ↓ in renal impair W/P: [B, +] Disp: Caps 250, 500 mg; chew tabs 125, 200, 250, 400 mg; susp, 125, 200, 250 mg/mL & 400 mg/5 mL; tabs 500, 875 mg; tab ER 775 mg SE: D; rash Notes: Cross-hypersens w/ PCN; many *E. coli* strains resistant; chew tabs contain phenylalanine

Amoxicillin/Clavulanic Potassium (Augmentin, Augmentin ES 600, Augmentin XR, Generic) Uses: *Ear, lower resp, sinus, urinary tract, skin Infxns caused by β-lactamase–producing H. influenzae, S. aureus, & E. coli* Acts: β-Lactam antibiotic w/ β-lactamase inhib Spectrum: Gram(+) same as amoxicillin alone, MSSA; gram(–) as w/ amoxicillin alone, β-lactamase–producing *H. influenzae, Klebsiella* sp, *M. catarrhalis* Dose: Adults. 250–500 mg PO q8h or 875 mg q12h; XR 2000 mg PO q12h Peds. 20–40 mg/kg/d as amoxicillin PO ÷ q8h or 45–90 mg/kg/d ÷ q12h; ↓ in renal impair; take w/ food W/P: [B, enters breast milk] Disp: Supplied (amoxicillin/clavulanic): Tabs 250/125, 500/125, 875/125 mg; chew tabs 125/31.25, 200/28.5, 250/62.5, 400/57 mg/mg; susp 125/31.25, 250/62.5, 200/28.5, 400/57 mg/5 mL; susp ES 600/42.9 mg/5 mL; XR tab 1000/62.5 mg/mg SE: Abd discomfort, N/V/D, allergic Rxn, vaginitis Notes: Do not substitute two 250-mg tabs for one 500-mg tab (possible OD of clavulanic acid); max clavulanic acid 125 mg/dose

Amphotericin B (Generic) BOX: Primarily used for life-threatening fungal Infxn; max dose 1.5 mg/kg; OD can cause cardiopulmonary arrest Uses: *Severe, systemic fungal Infxns; oral & cutaneous candidiasis* **Acts:** Binds ergosterol in the fungal membrane to alter permeability **Dose:** *Adults & Peds.* 0.25–1.5 mg/kg/24 h IV over 2–6 h (25–50 mg/d or q other day). Total varies w/ indication ↑ PR, N/V **W/P:** [B, ?] **Disp:** Powder (Inj) 50 mg/vial **SE:** ↓ K⁺/Mg²⁺ from renal wasting; anaphylaxis, HA, fever, chills, nephrotox, ↑ BP, anemia, rigors **Notes:** ✓ Cr/LFTs/K⁺/Mg²⁺; ↓ in renal impair; pretreatment w/ APAP & diphenhydramine ± hydrocortisone, ↓ SE; meperidine administration may control Inf rigors

Amphotericin B Cholesteryl (Amphotec) **Uses:** *Aspergillosis if intolerant/refractory to conventional amphotericin B*, systemic candidiasis **Acts:** Binds ergosterol in fungal membrane, alters permeability **Dose:** *Adults & Peds.* 3–4 mg/kg/d; 1 mg/kg/h Inf, 7.5 mg/kg/d max; ↓ w/ renal Insuff **W/P:** [B, ?] **Disp:** Powder for Inj 50, 100 mg/vial **SE:** Anaphylaxis; fever, chills, HA, ↓ PLT, N/V, ↑ HR, ↓ K⁺, ↓ Mg²⁺, nephrotox, ↓ BP, infusion Rxns, anemia **Notes:** Do not use in-line filter; ✓ LFTs/lytes

Amphotericin B Lipid Complex (Abelcet) **Uses:** *Refractory invasive fungal Infxn in pts intolerant to conventional amphotericin B* **Acts:** Binds ergosterol in fungal membrane, alters permeability **Dose:** *Adults & Peds.* 2.5–5 mg/kg/d IV × 1 daily **W/P:** [B, ?] **Disp:** Inj 5 mg/mL **SE:** Anaphylaxis; fever, chills, HA, ↓ K⁺, ↑ SCr ↓ Mg²⁺, nephrotox, ↓ BP, anemia **Notes:** Filter w/ 5-micron needle; do not mix in electrolyte containing solns; if Inf > 2 h, manually mix bag

Amphotericin B Liposomal (AmBisome) **Uses:** *Refractory invasive fungal Infxn w/ intolerance to conventional amphotericin B; cryptococcal meningitis in HIV; empiric for febrile neutropenia; visceral leishmaniasis* **Acts:** Binds ergosterol in fungal membrane, alters membrane permeability **Dose:** *Adults & Peds.* 3–6 mg/kg/d, Inf 60–120 min; varies by indication; ↓ in renal Insuff **W/P:** [B, ?] **Disp:** Powder Inj 50 mg **SE:** Anaphylaxis, fever, chills, HA, ↓ K⁺, ↓ Mg²⁺ peripheral edema, insomnia, rash, ↑ LFTs, nephrotox, ↓ BP, anemia **Notes:** Do not use < 1-micron filter

Ampicillin (Generic) **Uses:** *Resp, GU, or GI tract Infxns, meningitis d/t gram(−) & (+) bacteria, SBE prophylaxis* **Acts:** β-Lactam antibiotic; ↓ cell wall synth **Spectrum:** Gram(+) (*Streptococcus* sp, *Staphylococcus* sp, *Listeria*); gram(−) (*Klebsiella* sp, *E. coli, H. influenzae, P. mirabilis, Shigella* sp, *Salmonella* sp) **Dose:** *Adults.* 1000 mg–2 g IM or IV q4–6h or 250–500 mg PO q6h; varies by indication *Peds Neonates < 7 d.* 50 mg/kg/24 h IV ÷ q8h *Term infants.* 75–150 mg/kg/24 h ÷ q6–8h IV or PO *Children > 1 mo.* 200 mg/kg/24 h ÷ q6h IM or IV; 50–100 mg/kg/24 h ÷ q6h PO up to 250 mg/dose *Meningitis:* 200–400 mg/kg/24 h; ↓ w/ renal impair; take on empty stomach **W/P:** [B, M] Cross-hypersens w/ PCN **Disp:** Caps 250, 500 mg; susp 125 mg/5 mL, 250 mg/5 mL; powder (Inj) 125, 250, 500 mg, 1, 2, 10 g/vial **SE:** D, rash, allergic Rxn **Notes:** Many *E. coli* resistant

Ampicillin/Sulbactam (Unasyn) **Uses:** *Gynecologic, intra-Abd, skin Infxns d/t β-lactamase–producing S. aureus, Enterococcus, H. influenzae, P. mirabilis, & Bacteroides sp* **Acts:** β-Lactam antibiotic & β-lactamase inhib **Spectrum:** Gram(+) & (−)

as for amp alone; also *Enterobacter, Acinetobacter, Bacteroides* **Dose:** *Adults.* 1.5–3 g IM or IV q6h *Peds.* 100–400 mg ampicillin/kg/d (150–300 mg Unasyn) q6h; ↓ w/ renal Insuff **W/P:** [B, M] **Disp:** Powder for Inj 1.5, 3 g/vial, 15 g bulk package **SE:** Allergic Rxns, rash, D, Inj site pain **Notes:** A 2:1 ratio ampicillin:sulbactam

Anakinra (Kineret) Uses: *Reduce S/Sxs of mod–severe active RA, failed 1 or more DMARDs* **Acts:** Human IL-1 receptor antag **Dose:** 100 mg SQ daily; w/ CrCl < 30 mL/min, q other day **W/P:** [B, ?] Only > 1% y avoid in active Inf **CI:** *E. coli*-derived protein allergy **Disp:** 100-mg prefilled syringes; 100 mg (0.67 mL/vial) **SE:** ↓ WBC, especially w/ TNF-blockers, Inj site Rxn (may last up to 28 d), Infxn, N/D, Abd pain, flu-like sx, HA **Notes:** ✓ immunization up to date prior to starting Rx

Anastrozole (Arimidex) Uses: *Breast CA: postmenopausal w/ metastatic breast CA, adjuvant Rx postmenopausal early hormone-receptor(+) breast CA* **Acts:** Selective nonsteroidal aromatase inhib, ↓ circulatory estradiol **Dose:** 1 mg/d **W/P:** [X, ?/–] **CI:** PRG **Disp:** Tabs 1 mg **SE:** May ↑ cholesterol; N/V/D, HTN, flushing, ↑ bone/tumor pain, HA, somnolence, mood disturbance, depression, rash, fatigue, weakness **Notes:** No effect on adrenal steroids or aldosterone

Anidulafungin (Eraxis) Uses: *Candidemia, esophageal candidiasis, other *Candida* Infxn (peritonitis, intra-Abd abscess)* **Acts:** Echinocandin; ↓ cell wall synth *Spectrum: C. albicans, C. glabrata, C. parapsilosis, C. tropicalis* **Dose:** Candidemia, others: 200 mg IV × 1, then 100 mg IV daily [Tx ≥ 14 d after last (+)culture]; *Esophageal candidiasis:* 100 mg IV × 1, then 50 mg IV daily (Tx > 14 d and 7 d after resolution of Sx); 1.1 mg/min max Inf rate **W/P:** [B, ?/–] **CI:** Echinocandin hypersens **Disp:** Powder 50, 100 mg/vial **SE:** Histamine-mediated Inf Rxns (urticaria, flushing, ↓ BP, dyspnea, etc), fever, N/V/D, ↓ K⁺, HA, ↑ LFTs, hep, worsening hepatic failure **Notes:** ↓ Inf rate to < 1.1 mg/min w/ Inf Rxns

Anthralin (Dritho, Zithranol, Zithranol-RR) Uses: *Psoriasis* **Acts:** Keratolytic **Dose:** Apply daily **W/P:** [C, ?] **CI:** Acutely inflamed psoriatic eruptions, erythroderma **Disp:** Cream, 0.5, 1, 1.2%; shampoo **SE:** Irritation; hair/fingernails/skin discoloration, erythema

Antihemophilic Factor (Recomb), Porcine Sequence (Obizur) Uses: *Tx bleeding episodes in adults w/ acquired hemophilia A* **Acts:** Replaces factor VIII; ↑ clotting **Dose:** Start 200 U/kg IV, titrate q4–12h to keep factor VIII 50–100% of nl w/ minor/mod bleeding; 100–200% of nl w/major bleeding; ↓ to 50–100% after bleeding resolves **W/P:** [C, ?] Hypersens rxns, inhib antibodies **CI:** Component hypersens (hamster protein) **Disp:** 500 U/vial **SE:** development of inhibs to porcine factor VIII **Notes:** ✓ factor VIII activity via 1-stage clotting assay 30 min & 3 h after initial dose, then 30 min after subsequent doses; ✓ Nijmegen Bethesda inhib assay if concern for inhib antibody development

Antihemophilic Factor [AHF, Factor VIII] (Hemofil M, Monoclate-P) Uses: *Classic hemophilia A* **Acts:** Provides factor VIII needed to convert prothrombin to thrombin **Dose:** *Adults & Peds.* 1 AHF unit/kg ↑ factor VIII level by 2 Int units/dL; units required = (Wt in kg) factor VIII ↑ as % nl) × (0.5); minor hemorrhage = 20–40% nl; mod hemorrhage/minor surgery = 30–50% nl; major surgery, life-threatening hemorrhage = 80–100% nl **W/P:** [C, ?] **Disp:** ✓ each vial for units contained, powder for recons **SE:** Rash, fever, HA, chills, N/V **Notes:** Determine ø nl factor VIII before dosing

Antihemophilic Factor, Recombinant (Advate, Eloctate, Hexilate FS, Kogenate FS, Novoeight, Recombinate, Xyntha) Uses: *Control/prevent bleeding & surgical prophylaxis in hemophilia A* **Acts:** ↑ Levels of factor VIII **Dose:** Units required = Wt (kg) × desired factor VIII rise (Int units/dL or % of nl) × 0.5 (Int units/kg per Int units/dL); frequency/duration determined by type of bleed (see PI) **W/P:** [C, ?/–] Severe hypersens Rxn possible **CI:** None **Disp:** ✓ each vial for units contained, powder for recons **SE:** HA, fever, N/V/D, weakness, allergic Rxn **Notes:** Monitor for the development of factor VIII neutralizing antibodies; Eloctate ↑ half-life (20 vs 12 h)

Antithrombin, Recombinant (Atryn), Pooled (Thrombate III) Uses: *Prevent periop/peripartum thromboembolic events w/ hereditary AT deficiency* **Acts:** Inhibs thrombin and factor Xa **Dose:** *Adults.* Based on pre-Rx AT level, BW (kg), and drug monitoring; see PI. Goal AT levels 0.8–1.2 Int units/mL **W/P:** [C, +/–] Hypersens Rxns; ↑ effect of heparin/LMWH; *Thrombate* infectious disease risk **CI:** *Atryn:* Hypersens to goat/goat milk proteins; *Thrombate* Ø **Disp:** *Atryn:* powder 1750 Int units/vial; *Thrombate:* 500 Int units/vial **SE:** Bleeding, Inf site Rxns, dizziness, chest discomfort, N, dysgeusia, chills, pain (cramps), dyspnea **Notes:** ✓ aPTT and antifactor Xa; monitor for bleeding or thrombosis; *Thrombate* from pooled human plasma

Antithymocyte Globulin (See Lymphocyte Immune Globulin, p 201) **Apixaban (Eliquis)** **BOX:** ↑ Risk of spinal/epidural hematoma w/ paralysis & ↑ thrombotic events w/ D/C in afib pts; monitor closely Uses: *Prevent CVA/TE in nonvalvular afib and hip/knee replacement surgery; Rx DVT and PE* **Acts:** Factor Xa inhib **Dose:** *CVA & thrombosis w/ NVAF:* 5 mg PO bid; *DVT/PE Px after hip/knee surgery:* Start 2.5 mg PO bid 12–24 h postop (hip 35 d, knee 12 d); *Rx DVT/PE:* 10 mg PO bid × 7 d, then 5 mg PO bid; ↓ *DVT/PE recurrence:* 2.5 mg PO bid after at least 6 mo of DVT/PE Rx; ↓ dose if > 80 y/< 60 kg, Cr > 1.5 mg/dL; 2.5 mg PO bid; 2.5 mg w/ strong dual inhib of CYP3A4 and P-glycoprotein; if on 2.5 mg do **NOT** use w/ strong dual inhib of CYP3A4 and P-glycoprotein **W/P:** [B, –] Do not use w/ prosthetic valves **CI:** Pathological bleeding & apixaban hypersens **Disp:** Tabs 2.5, 5 mg **SE:** Bleeding **Notes:** If missed dose, do **NOT** double next dose; no antidote to reverse; anticoagulant effect can last 24 h after dose

Apomorphine (Apokyn) Uses: *Acute, intermittent hypomobility ("off") episodes of Parkinson Dz* **Acts:** Dopamine agonist **Dose:** 0.2 mL SQ supervised test dose; if BP OK, initial 0.2 mL (2 mg) SQ during "off" periods; only 1 dose per "off" period; titrate dose; 0.6 mL (6 mg) max single doses; use w/ antiemetic; ↓ in renal impair **W/P:** [C, ?] Avoid EtOH; antihypertensives, vasodilators, cardio-/cerebrovascular Dz, hepatic impair **CI:** IV administration, w/ 5-HT antags, sulfite/comp allergy **Disp:** Inj 10 mg/mL, 3-mL pen cartridges **SE:** Emesis, syncope, ↑ QT, orthostatic ↓ BP, somnolence, ischemia, Inj site Rxn, edema, N/V, hallucination abuse potential, dyskinesia, fibrotic conditions, priapism, CP/angina, yawning, rhinorrhea **Notes:** Daytime somnolence may limit activities; trimethobenzamide 300 mg tid PO or other non–5-HT₃ antag antiemetic given 3 d prior to & up to 2 mo following initiation

Apraclonidine (Lopidine) **Uses:** *Control postop intraocular HTN* **Acts:** α₂-Adrenergic agonist **Dose:** 1–2 gtt of 0.5% tid; 1 gtt of 1% before and after surgical procedure **W/P:** [C, ?] **CI:** w/in 14 d of or w/ MAOI **Disp:** 0.5, 1% soln **SE:** Ocular irritation, lethargy, xerostomia, blurred vision

Apremilast (Otezla) **Uses:** *Psoriatic arthritis, pts w/ mod/severe plaque psoriasis who are candidates for photo- or systemic therapy* **Acts:** PDE4 inhib **Dose:** 10 mg PO qam × 1, then 10 mg bid × 1, then 10 mg PO qam/20 mg PO qpm × 1, then 20 mg PO bid × 1, then 20 mg PO qam/30 mg PO qpm, then 30 mg PO bid **W/P:** [C, ?/–] ↑ depression/suicidal ideation; ↓ Wt **CI:** Ø **Disp:** Tabs 10, 20, 30 mg **SE:** *Arthritis:* N/D, HA; *Psoriasis:* N/D, HA, URI **Notes:** ↓ Dose w/ CrCl< 30

Aprepitant, Oral (Emend) **Uses:** *Prevents N/V associated w/ emetogenic CA chemotherapy (eg, cisplatin) (use in combo w/ other antiemetics)*, postop N/V* **Acts:** Substance P/neurokinin 1 (NK₁) receptor antag **Dose:** 125 mg PO day 1, 1 h before chemotherapy, then 80 mg PO qam d 2 & 3; postop N/V: 40 mg w/in 3 h of induction **W/P:** [B, ?/–]; substrate & mod CYP3A4 inhib; CYP2C9 inducer (Table 10, p 356); ↓ Effect OCP and warfarin **CI:** Use w/ pimozide or cisapride **Disp:** Caps 40, 80, 125 mg **SE:** Fatigue, asthenia, hiccups **Notes:** See also Fosaprepitant, Inj (Emend)

Arformoterol (Brovana) **BOX:** Long-acting β₂-adrenergic agonists may increase the risk of asthma-related death. Use only for pts not adequately controlled on other asthma-controller meds; safety + efficacy in asthma not established **Uses:** *Maint in COPD* **Acts:** Selective LA β₂-adrenergic agonist **Dose:** 15 mcg bid nebulization **W/P:** [C, ?] **CI:** Hypersens **Disp:** Soln 15 mcg/2 mL **SE:** Pain, back pain, CP, D, sinusitis, nervousness, palpitations, allergic Rxn, peripheral edema, rash, leg cramps **Notes:** Not for acute bronchospasm. Refrigerate, use immediately after opening

Argatroban (Generic) **Uses:** *Prevent/Tx thrombosis in HIT, PCI in pts w/ HIT risk* **Acts:** Anticoagulant, direct thrombin inhib **Dose:** 2 mcg/kg/min IV; adjust until aPTT 1.5–3 × baseline not to exceed 100 s; 10 mcg/kg/min max; ↓ w/ hepatic impair **W/P:** [B, ?] Avoid PO anticoagulants unless transitioning to oral, ↑ bleeding risk; avoid use w/ thrombolytics in critically ill pts **CI:** Overt overt bleeding **Disp:** Inj 100 mg/mL; Premixed Inf 50, 125 mg **SE:** AF, cardiac arrest, cerebrovascular disorder, ↓ BP, VT, N/V/D, sepsis, cough, renal tox, ↓ Hgb

Notes: Steady state in 1–3 h; ✓ aPTT w/ Inf start and after each dose change; use care when transitioning to oral anticoagulants (see PI)

Aripiprazole (Abilify, Abilify Discmelt, Abilify Maintena Kit) BOX: Increased mortality in elderly w/ dementia-related psychosis; ↑ suicidal thinking in children, adolescents, and young adults w/ MDD Uses: *Schizophrenia adults and peds 13–17 y, mania or mixed episodes associated w/ bipolar disorder, MDD in adults, agitation w/ schizophrenia* Acts: DA & serotonin antag Dose: *Adults. Schizophrenia:* 10–15 mg PO/d; may repeat ≥ 2 h *Acute agitation:* 9.75 mg/1.3 mL IM *Bipolar:* 15 mg/d; *MDD adjunct* w/ other antidepressants initial 2 mg/d *Peds. Schizophrenia:* **13–17 y:** Start 2 mg/d, usual 10 mg/d; max 30 mg/d for all adult and peds uses; ↓ dose w/ CYP3A4/CYP2D6 inhib (Table 10, p 356); ↑ dose w/ CYP3A4 inducer W/P: [C, –] w/ Low WBC, CV Dz, irritability in 16–17 y; possible autistic disorder assn Disp: Tabs 2, 5, 10, 15, 20, 30 mg; *Discmelt* (disintegrating tabs 10, 15 mg), soln 1 mg/mL, Inj 9.75 mg/1.3 mL; Maintena kit 300, 400 mg vial w/ Inj supl SE: Neuroleptic malignant synd, tardive dyskinesia, orthostatic ↓ BP, cognitive & motor impair, ↑ glu, leukopenia, neutropenia, and agranulocytosis Notes: Discmelt contains phenylalanine; monitor CBC

Armodafinil (Nuvigil) Uses: *Narcolepsy, SWSD, and OSAHS* Acts: ?; binds DA receptor, ↓ DA reuptake Dose: *OSAHS/narcolepsy:* 150–250 mg PO daily in A.M. *SWSD:* 150 mg PO qd 1 h prior to start of shift; ↓ w/ hepatic impair; monitor for interactions w/ substrates CYP3A4/5, CYP7C19 W/P: [C, ?] CI: Hypersens to modafinil/armodafinil Disp: Tabs 50, 150, 200, 250 mg SE: HA, N, dizziness, insomnia, xerostomia, rash, including SJS, angioedema, anaphylactoid Rxns, multiorgan hypersens Rxns

Artemether/Lumefantrine (Coartem) Uses: *Acute, uncomplicated malaria (P. falciparum)* Acts: Antiprotozoal/Antimalarial Dose: *Adults > 16 y. 25–< 35 kg:* 3 tabs h 0 & 8 day 1, then 3 tabs bid d 2 & 3 (18 tabs/course) *≥ 35 kg:* 4 tabs h 0 & 8 d 1, then 4 tabs bid d 2 & 3 (24 tabs/course) *Peds 2 mo–< 16 y. 5–15 kg:* 1 tab h 0 & 8 d 1, then 1 tab bid d 2 & 3 (6 tabs/course) *15–25 kg:* 2 tabs h 0 & 8 d 1, then 2 tabs bid d 2 & 3 (12 tabs/course) *> 25 kg:* See adult dose W/P: [C, ?] ↑ QT, hepatic/renal impair, CYP3A4 inhib/substrate/inducers, CYP2D6 substrates CI: Component hypersens Disp: Tabs artemether 20 mg/lumefantrine 120 mg SE: Palp, HA, dizziness, chills, sleep disturb, fatigue, anorexia, N/V/D, Abd pain, weakness, arthralgia, myalgia, cough, splenomegaly, fever, anemia, hepatomegaly, ↑ AST, ↑ QT Notes: Not rec w/ other agents that ↑ QT

Artificial Tears (Tears Naturale) [OTC] Uses: *Dry eyes* Acts: Ocular lubricant Dose: 1–2 gtt PRN Disp: OTC soln SE: Mild stinging, temp blurred vision

Asenapine Maleate (Saphris) BOX: ↑Mortality in elderly w/ dementia-related psychosis Uses: *Schizophrenia; manic/mixed bipolar disorder* Acts: DA/serotonin antag Dose: *Adults. Schizophrenia:* 5 mg SL twice daily; max 20 mg/d *Bipolar disorder:* 5–10 mg twice daily *Peds 10–17 y.* 2.5 mg SL bid, after 3 d to 5 mg bid, then to 5–10 mg bid after 3 more d PRN (peds pts have ↑ dystonia if escalation not followed) **W/P:** [C, ?/–] **Disp:** SL tabs 2.5, 5, 10 mg **SE:** Dizziness, insomnia, ↑ TG, edema, ↑/↓ BP, somnolence, akathisia, oral hypoesthesia, EPS, ↑ Wt, ↑ glu, ↑ QT interval, hyperprolactinemia, ↓ WBC, NMS, severe allergic Rxns **Notes:** Do not swallow/crush/chew tab; avoid eating/drinking 10 min after dose

Aspirin (Bayer, Ecotrin, St. Joseph's, Generic) [OTC] Uses: *CABG, PTCA, carotid endarterectomy, ischemic stroke, TIA, ACS/MI, arthritis, pain, HA, fever, inflammation, ↓ pre-eclampsia in ♀ at risk*, Kawasaki Dz **Acts:** Prostaglandin inhib by COX-2 inhib **Dose:** *Adults.* Pain, fever: 325–650 mg q4–6h PO or PR (4 g/d max) *Plt inhib:* 81–325 mg PO daily; *Prevent MI:* 81 (preferred)–325 mg PO daily; *Pre-eclampsia:* 81 mg/d *ECC 2010. ACS:* 160–325 mg nonenteric coated PO ASAP (chewing preferred at ACS onset) *Peds. Antipyretic:* 10–15 mg/kg/dose PO or PR q4–6h; *Kawasaki Dz:* 80–100 mg/kg/d ÷ q6h, 3–5 mg/kg/d after fever resolves for at least 48 h or total 14 d; for all uses 4 g/d max; avoid w/ CrCl < 10 mL/min, severe liver Dz **W/P:** [C, M] linked to Reye synd; avoid w/ viral illness in peds < 16 y **CI:** Allergy to ASA, chickenpox/flu Sxs, synd of nasal polyps, angioedema, & bronchospasm to NSAIDs, bleeding disorder **Disp:** Tabs 325, 500 mg; chew tabs 81 mg; EC tabs 81, 162, 325, 500 mg, effervescent tabs 500 mg; supp 300, 600 mg; caplets 81, 375, 500 mg **SE:** GI upset, erosion, & bleeding **Notes:** D/C 1 wk preop; avoid/limit EtOH; Salicylate levels: *Therapeutic:* 100–250 mcg/mL *Toxic:* > 300 mcg/mL

Aspirin/Butalbital/Caffeine Compound (Fiorinal) [C-III] Uses: *Tension HA*, pain **Acts:** Barbiturate w/ analgesic **Dose:** 1–2 PO q4h PRN, max 6 tabs/d; dose in renal/hepatic Dz **W/P:** [C (D w/ prolonged use or high doses at term)] **CI:** ASA allergy, GI ulceration, bleeding disorder, porphyria, synd of nasal polyps, angioedema, & bronchospasm to NSAIDs **Disp:** Caps/tabs ASA 325 mg/ butalbital 50 mg/caffeine 40 mg **SE:** Drowsiness, dizziness, GI upset, ulceration, bleeding, light-headedness heartburn, confusion, HA **Notes:** Butalbital habit-forming; D/C 1 wk prior to surgery, avoid/limit EtOH

Aspirin/Butalbital/Caffeine/Codeine (Fiorinal w/ Codeine) [C-III] Uses: *Complex tension HA* **Acts:** Sedative and narcotic analgesic **Dose:** 1–2 tabs/caps PO q4h PRN max 6/d **W/P:** [C, –] **CI:** Allergy to ASA and codeine; synd of nasal polyps, angioedema, & bronchospasm to NSAIDs, bleeding diathesis, peptic ulcer or sig GI lesions, porphyria **Disp:** Caps contain 325 mg ASA, 40 mg caffeine, 50 mg butalbital, 30 mg codeine **SE:** Drowsiness, dizziness, GI upset, ulceration, bleeding **Notes:** D/C 1 wk prior to surgery, avoid/limit EtOH

Atazanavir (Reyataz) Uses: *HIV-1 Infxn* **Acts:** Protease inhib **Dose:** Antiretroviral naïve 300 mg PO daily w/ ritonavir 100 mg or 400 mg PO daily; experienced pts 300 mg w/ ritonavir 100 mg; when given w/ efavirenz 600 mg, administer atazanavir 400 mg + ritonavir 100 mg once/d; separate doses from didanosine; ↓ w/ hepatic impair **W/P:** CDC rec: HIV-infected mothers not breast-feed [B, –]; ↑ levels of statins sildenafil, antiarrhythmics, warfarin, cyclosporine, TCAs; ↓ w/ St. John's wort, PPIs H₂-receptor antags; do not use w/ salmeterol, colchicine (w/ renal/hepatic failure); adjust dose w/ bosentan, tadalafil for

PAH **CI:** w/ Midazolam, triazolam, ergots, pimozide, simvastatin, lovastatin, cisapride, etravirine, indinavir, irinotecan, rifampin, alpha 1-adrenoreceptor antag (alfuzosin), PDE5 inhib (e.g., sildenafil) **Disp:** Caps 100, 150, 200, 300 mg; powder 50 mg **SE:** HA, N/V/D, Bilirubin, rash, Abd pain, DM, photosens, ↑ PR interval **Notes:** Administer w/ food; may have less adverse effect on cholesterol; if given w/ H₂ blocker, separate by 10 h H₂; if given w/ proton pump inhib, separate by 12 h; concurrent use not OK in experienced pts

Atazanavir/Cobicistat (Evotaz) Uses: *HIV* **Acts:** HIV-1 protease inhib w/ CYP3A inhib **Dose:** 1 tab PO qd w/ food **W/P:** [B, HIV mothers should not breast-feed] ↑ PR; rash; renal failure w/ tenofovir; w/ tenofovir, ✓ urine glu, protein, CrCl, PO₄⁻³; do not use w/ tenofovir if CrCl < 70 mL/min or w/ other nephrotoxic meds; gallstones; kidney stones; pts w/ hep B/C risk for hepatic decomp; do **NOT** use w/ ritonavir or other antiretroviral drugs requiring CYP3A inhib (eg, other protease inhibs or elvitegravir); indirect bili may ↑ **CI:** Component hypersens; use w/ certain meds alters concentration and associated w/ life-threatening complications or ↓ effect **Disp:** Tabs 300 mg atazanavir/150 mg cobicistat **SE:** N, jaundice, icterus **Notes:** ✓ LFTs in pts w/ hep B/C

Atenolol (Tenormin) **BOX:** Avoid abrupt withdrawl (esp CAD pts), gradual taper to ↓, acute ↑ HR, HTN +/– ischemia Uses: *HTN*, angina, post-MI* **Acts:** selective β-adrenergic receptor blocker **Dose:** *HTN & angina:* 25–100 mg/d PO *ECC 2010. AMI:* 5 mg IV over 5 min; in 10 min, 5 mg slow IV; if tolerated in 10 min, start 50 mg PO, titrate; ↓ in renal impair **W/P:** [D, M] DM, bronchospasm; abrupt D/C can exacerbate angina & ↑ MI risk **CI:** ↑ HR, cardiogenic shock, cardiac failure, 2nd-/3rd-degree AV block, sinus node dysfunction, pulm edema **Disp:** Tabs 25, 50, 100 mg **SE:** ↓ HR, ↓ BP, 2nd-/3rd-degree AV block, dizziness, fatigue

Atenolol/Chlorthalidone (Tenoretic) Uses: *HTN* **Acts:** β-Adrenergic blockade w/ diuretic **Dose:** 50–100 mg/d PO based on atenolol; ↓ dose w/ CrCl < 35 mL/min **W/P:** [D, ?/–] DM, bronchospasm **CI:** See Atenolol (Tenormin); anuria, sulfonamide, cross-sensitivity **Disp:** Atenolol 50 mg/chlorthalidone 25 mg, atenolol 100 mg/chlorthalidone 25 mg **SE:** ↓ HR, ↓ BP, 2nd-/3rd-degree AV block, dizziness, fatigue, ↓ K⁺, photosens

Atomoxetine (Strattera) **BOX:** ↑ Frequency of suicidal thinking; monitor closely, especially in peds pts. Uses: *ADHD* **Acts:** Selective norepinephrine reuptake inhib **Dose:** *Adults & Peds > 70 kg.* 40 mg PO/d, after 3 d minimum, ↑ to 80–100 mg ÷ daily-bid *Peds < 70 kg.* 0.5 mg/kg × 3 d, then ↑ 1.2 mg/kg daily or bid (max 1.4 mg/kg or 100 mg); ↓ dose w/ hepatic Insuff or in combo w/ CYP2D6 inhibs (Table 10, p 356) **W/P:** [C, ?/–] w/ known structural cardiac anomalies, cardiac Hx hepatox **CI:** NAG, w/in 2 wk of D/C an MAOI **Disp:** Caps 10, 18, 25, 40, 60, 80, 100 mg **SE:** HA, insomnia, dry mouth, Abd pain, N/V, anorexia ↑ BP, tachycardia, Wt loss, somnolence, sexual dysfunction, jaundice, ↑ LFTs **Notes:** AHA rec: All children receiving stimulants for ADHD receive CV assessment before Rx initiated; D/C immediately w/ jaundice

Atorvastatin (Lipitor) Uses: *Dyslipidemia, primary prevention CV Dz Acts: HMG-CoA reductase inhib Dose: Initial 10–20 mg/d, may ↑ to 80 mg/d W/P: [X, –] CI: Active liver Dz, unexplained ↑ LFTs Disp: Tabs 10, 20, 40, 80 mg SE: Myopathy, HA, arthralgia, myalgia, GI upset, CP, edema, insomnia, dizziness, liver failure Notes: Monitor LFTs, instruct pt to report unusual muscle pain or weakness

Atovaquone (Mepron) Uses: *Rx & prevention PCP*; *Toxoplasma gondii* encephalitis, babesiosis (w/ azithromycin) Acts: ↓ Nucleic acid & ATP synth Dose: *Rx*: 750 mg PO bid for 21 d *Prevention*: 1500 mg PO once/d (w/ meals) W/P: [C, ?] Disp: Susp 750 mg/5 mL SE: Fever, HA, anxiety, insomnia, rash, N/V, cough, pruritus, weakness

Atovaquone/Proguanil (Malarone) Uses: *Prevention or Rx *P. falciparum* malaria* Acts: Antimalarial Dose: *Adults. Prevention*: 1 tab PO 1–2 d before, during, & 7 d after leaving endemic region *Rx*: 4 tabs PO single dose daily × 3 d *Peds.* See PI W/P: [C, ?/–] CI: Prophylactic use when CrCl < 30 mL/min Disp: Tabs atovaquone 250 mg/proguanil 100 mg; peds 62.5/25 mg SE: HA, fever, myalgia, Abd pain dizziness, weakness N/V, ↑ LFTs

Atracurium (Tracrium) Uses: *Anesthesia adjunct to facilitate ET intubation, facilitate ventilation in ICU pts* Acts: Nondepolarizing neuromuscular blocker Dose: *Adults & Peds > 2 y.* 0.4–0.5 mg/kg IV bolus, then 0.08–0.1 mg/kg q20–45min PRN; ICU: 0.4–0.5 mg/kg/min titrated W/P: [C, ?] Disp: Inj 10 mg/mL SE: Flushing Notes: Pt must be intubated & on controlled ventilation; use adequate amounts of sedation & analgesia

Atropine, Ophthalmic (Isopto Atropine, Generic) Uses: *Mydriasis, cycloplegia, uveitis* Acts: Antimuscarinic; cycloplegic, dilates pupils Dose: *Refraction*: 1–2 gtt 1 h before *Uveitis*: 1–2 gtt daily-qid CI: NAG, adhesions between iris and lens Disp: 1% ophthal soln, 1% oint SE: Local irritation, burning, blurred vision, light sensitivity Notes: Compress lacrimal sac 2–3 min after instillation; effects can last 1–2 wk

Atropine, Systemic (AtroPen Auto-Injector) Uses: *Organophosphate (insecticide) and acetylcholinesterase (nerve gas) inhib antidote* Acts: Antimuscarinic; blocks ACH at parasympathetic sites Dose: *Adults & Peds > 90 lbs/> 10 y.* 2 mg (green) *Peds 40–90 lb/4–10 y.* 1 mg (dark red) *15–40 lb/6 mo–4 y.* 0.5 mg (blue) *Infants < 15 lb/< 6 mo.* 0.25 mg (yellow); inject into outer thigh (through clothing OK); general limit to 3 doses q10min W/P: B/[C, +] CI: Ø Disp: *Auto-injector*: color–coded 0.25, 0.5, 1, 2 mg/dose SE: Flushing, mydriasis, tachycardia, dry mouth/nose, blurred vision, urinary retention, constipation, psychosis, Inj site pain Notes: SLUDGE (Sx of organophosphate poisoning); *Auto-injector* limited distribution; for use in nerve agent/insecticide poisoning only; primary protection to agents is protective garments/masks Notes: See also Atropine, Systemic (Generic)

Atropine, Systemic (Generic) Uses: *Preanesthetic; symptomatic ↓ HR & asystole, AV block, organophosphate (insecticide) and acetylcholinesterase (nerve gas) inhib antidote; cycloplegic* **Acts:** Antimuscarinic; blocks ACH at parasympathetic sites; cycloplegic **Dose: Adults. ECC 2010.** *Asystole/PEA:* Asystole/PEA use no longer recommended *Bradycardia:* 0.5 mg IV q3–5min PRN; max 3 mg or 0.04 mg/kg *Preanesthetic:* 0.4–0.6 mg IM/IV *Poisoning:* 1–6 mg IV bolus, repeat q3–5min PRN to reverse effects (ATSDR 2011) **Peds. ECC 2010.** *Symptomatic bradycardia:* 0.02 mg/kg IV/IO (min dose 0.1 mg, max single dose 0.5 mg); repeat PRN × 1; max total dose 1 mg or 0.04 mg/kg child, 3 mg adolescent **W/P:** B/[C, +] **CI:** NAG, adhesions between iris and lens, pyloric stenosis, BPH **Disp:** Inj 0.05, 0.1, 0.4, 1 mg/mL **SE:** Flushing, mydriasis, tachycardia, dry mouth/nose, blurred vision, urinary retention, constipation, psychosis **Notes:** See also Atropine, Systemic (AtroPen Auto-Injector)

Atropine/Pralidoxime (DuoDote Auto-Injector) **Uses:** *Nerve agent (tabun, sarin, others); organophosphate insecticide poisoning* **Acts:** Atropine blocks effects of excess ACH; pralidoxime reactivates acetylcholinesterase inactivated by poisoning **Dose:** 1 Inj midlateral thigh; 10–15 min for effect; w/ severe Sx, give 2 additional Inj; if alert/oriented no more doses **W/P:** [C, ?] **Disp:** Autoinjector 2.1 mg atropine/600 mg pralidoxime **SE:** Dry mouth, blurred vision, dry eyes, photophobia, confusion, HA, tachycardia, ↑ BP, flushing, urinary retention, constipation, Abd pain, N/V, emesis **Notes:** See "SLUDGE" under atropine, systemic (AtroPen Auto-Injector); limited distribution; for use by personnel w/ appropriate training; wear protective garments; do not rely solely on med; evacuation and decontamination ASAP

Avanafil (Stendra) **Uses:** *ED* **Acts:** ↓ PDE5 (responsible for cGMP breakdown); ↑ cGMP activity to relax smooth muscles to ↑ flow to corpus cavernosum **Dose:** *(men only)* 100 mg PO 30 min before sex activity, no more than 1×d; ↑/↓ dose 50–200 mg based on effect; do not use w/ strong CYP3A4 inhib; use 50 mg w/ mod CYP3A4 inhib; w/ or w/o food **W/P:** [C, ?] Priapism risk; hypotension w/ BP meds or substantial alcohol; seek immediate attention w/ hearing loss or acute vision loss (may be NAION); w/ CYP3A4 inhib (eg, ketoconazole, ritonavir, erythromycin) ↑ effects; do not use w/ severe renal/hepatic impair CI: w/nitrates or guanylate cyclase stim (eg, riociguat) **Disp:** Tabs 50, 100, 200 mg **SE:** HA, flushing, nasal congestion, nasopharyngitis back pain **Notes:** More rapid onset than sildenafil (15–30 min)

Axitinib (Inlyta) **Uses:** *Advanced RCC* **Acts:** TKI inhib **Dose:** 5 mg PO q12h; if tolerated > 2 wk, ↑ to 7 mg q12h, then 10 mg q12h; w/ or w/o food; swallow whole; ↓ dose by ½ w/ mod hepatic impair; avoid w/ or ↓ dose by ½ if used w/ strong CYP3A4/5 inhib; for ADR ↓ to 2–3 mg bid **W/P:** [D, ?] w/ brain mets, recent GI bleed **Disp:** Tabs 1, 5 mg **SE:** N/V/D/C, HTN, fatigue, asthenia, ↓ appetite, ↓ Wt, ↑ LFTs, hand-foot synd, venous/arterial thrombosis; hemorrhage, ↓ thyroid, GI perf/fistula, proteinuria, hypertensive crisis, impaired wound healing, reversible posterior leukoencephalopathy synd **Notes:** Hold 24 h prior to surgery

Azathioprine (Imuran, Azasan, Imuran) **BOX:** May ↑ neoplasia w/ chronic use; mutagenic and hematologic tox possible **Uses:** *Adjunct to prevent renal transplant rejection, RA*, SLE, Crohn Dz, UC **Acts:** Immunosuppressive; antagonizes purine metabolism **Dose:** *Adults. Crohn and UC:* Start 50 mg/d, ↑ 25 mg/d q1–2wk, target dose 2–3 mg/kg/d *Adults & Peds. Renal transplant:* 3–5 mg/kg/d IV/PO single daily dose, then 1–3 mg/kg/d maint *RA:* 1 mg/kg/d once daily or ÷ bid × 6–8 wk, ↑ 0.5 mg/kg/d q4wk to 2.5 mg/kg/d; ↓ w/ renal Insuff **W/P:** [D, ?/–] **CI:** PRG **Disp:** Tabs 50, 75, 100 mg; **SE:** GI intolerance, fever, chills, leukopenia, ↑ LFTs, bilirubin, ↑ risk Infxns, thrombocytopenia **Notes:** Handle Inj w/ cytotoxic precautions; interaction w/ allopurinol; do not administer live vaccines on drug; ✓ CBC and LFTs; dose per local transplant protocol, usually start 1–3 d pretransplant

Azelastine (Astelin, Astepro, Optivar) **Uses:** *Allergic rhinitis (rhinorrhea, sneezing, nasal pruritus), vasomotor rhinitis; allergic conjunctivitis (Optivar)* **Acts:** Histamine H₁-receptor antag **Dose:** *Adults & Peds > 12 y. Nasal:* 1–2 sprays/nostril bid *Ophth:* 1 gtt in each affected eye bid *Peds > 5 y.* 1 spray/nostril bid (0.1%) *Peds 5–11 y.* 1 spray/nostril bid (01.% or 0.15%) **W/P:** [C, ?/–] **CI:** Component sens **Disp:** Nasal 137 mcg/spray; nasal soln 01%, 0.15%; ophthal soln 0.05% **SE:** Somnolence, bitter taste, HA, colds Sx (rhinitis, cough)

Azilsartan (Edarbi) **BOX:** Use in 2nd/3rd trimester can cause fetal injury and death; D/C when PRG detected **Uses:** *HTN* **Acts:** ARB **Dose:** 80 mg PO 1 × d; consider 40 mg PO 1 × d if on high dose diuretic **W/P:** [D, ?] correct vol/salt depletion before **Disp:** Tabs 40, 80 mg **SE:** D, ↓ BP, N, asthenia, fatigue, dizziness, cough

Azilsartan/Chlorthalidone (Edarbyclor) **BOX:** Use in 2nd/3rd trimester can cause fetal injury and death; D/C when PRG detected **Uses:** *HTN* **Acts:** ARB w/ thiazide diuretic **Dose:** 40/12.5 mg–40/25 mg PO 1 × d **W/P:** [D, ?] Correct vol/salt depletion prior to use; use w/ lithium, NSAIDs **CI:** Anuria **Disp:** Tabs (azilsartan/chlorthalidone) 40/12.5, 40/25 mg **SE:** N/D, ↓ BP, asthenia, fatigue, dizziness, cough, ↓ K⁺, hyperuricemia, photosens, ↑ glucose

Azithromycin (Zithromax) **Uses:** *Community-acquired pneumonia, pharyngitis, otitis media, skin Infxns, nongonococcal (chlamydial) urethritis, chancroid & PID; Rx & prevention of MAC in HIV* **Acts:** Macrolide antibiotic; bacteriostatic; ↓ protein synth **Spectrum:** *Chlamydia, H. ducreyi, H. influenzae, Legionella, M. catarrhalis, M. pneumoniae, M. hominis, N. gonorrhoeae, S. aureus, S. agalactiae, S. pneumoniae, S. pyogenes* **Dose:** *Adults. Resp tract Infxns:* PO: Caps 500 mg d 1, then 250 mg/d PO × 4 d *Sinusitis:* 500 mg/d PO × 3 d *IV:* 500 mg × 2 d, then 500 mg PO × 7–10 d *Nongonococcal urethritis:* 1 g PO × 1 d *Gonorrhea, uncomplicated:* 2 g PO × 1 *Prevent MAC:* 1200 mg PO once/wk *Peds. Otitis media:* 10 mg/kg PO d 1, then 5 mg/kg/d d 2–5 *Pharyngitis* (≥ 2 y): 12 mg/kg/d PO × 5 d; take susp on empty stomach; tabs OK w/ or w/o food; ↓ w/ CrCl < 10 mL/ mg **W/P:** [B, +] May ↑ QTc w/ arrhythmias **Disp:** Tabs 250, 500, 600 mg; Z-Pack (5-d, 250 mg); Tri-Pack (500-mg tabs × 3); susp 2 g; single-dose packet (Zmax) ER susp (2 g); susp 100, 200 mg/5 mL; Inj powder 500 mg; **SE:** GI upset, metallic taste **Notes:** ER susp on empty stomach; GC monotherapy may be associated w/ resistance; consider 1 g w/ 250 mg ceftriaxone IM × 1

Azithromycin, Ophthalmic, 1% (AzaSite) Uses: *Bacterial conjunctivitis* **Acts:** Bacteriostatic **Dose:** *Adults & Peds ≥ 1 y.* 1 gtt bid, q8–12 h apart × 2 d, then 1 gtt qd × 5 d **W/P:** [↑ B, ?] **CI:** Ø **Disp:** 1% in 2.5-mL bottle **SE:** Irritation, burning, stinging, contact dermatitis, corneal erosion, dry eye, dysgeusia, nasal congestion, sinusitis, ocular discharge, keratitis

Aztreonam (Azactam) Uses: *Aerobic gram(−) UTIs, lower resp, intra-Abd, skin, gynecologic Infxns & septicemia* **Acts:** Monobactam: ↓ Cell wall synth **Spectrum:** Gram(−) (*Pseudomonas, E. coli, Klebsiella, H. influenzae, Serratia, Proteus, Enterobacter, Citrobacter*) **Dose:** *Adults.* 1–2 g IV/IM q6–12h *UTI:* 500 mg–1 g IV q8–12h *Meningitis:* 2 g IV q6–8h *Peds.* 90–120 mg/kg/d ÷ q6–8h; ↓ in renal impair **W/P:** [B, +] **Disp:** Inj (soln), 1 g, 2 g/50 mL Inj powder for recons 1 g, 2 g **SE:** N/V/D, rash, pain at Inj site **Notes:** No gram(+) or anaerobic activity; OK in PCN-allergic pts

Aztreonam, Inh (Cayston) Uses: *Improve resp Sx in CF pts w/ P. aeruginosa* **Acts:** Monobactam: ↓ cell wall synth **Dose:** *Adults & Peds ≥ 7 y.* One dose tid × 28 d (space doses q4h) **W/P:** [B, +] w/ Beta-lactam allergy **CI:** Allergy to aztreonam **Disp:** 75 mg reconstituted to 84 mL **SE:** Allergic Rxn, bronchospasm, cough, nasal congestion, wheezing, pharyngolaryngeal pain, V, Abd pain, chest discomfort, pyrexia, rash **Notes:** Use immediately after reconstitution, use only w/ Altera Nebulizer System; bronchodilator prior to use

Bacitracin/Neomycin/Polymyxin B, Ophthalmic (Neo-Polycin Neosporin Ophthalmic); Bacitracin/Neomycin/Polymyxin B/Hydrocortisone, Ophthalmic (Neo-Polycin HC Cortisporin Ophthalmic); Bacitracin/Polymyxin B, Ophthalmic (AK-Poly-Bac Ophthalmic, Polysporin Ophthalmic) Uses: *Steroid-responsive inflam ocular conds* **Acts:** Topical antibiotic w/ anti-inflam **Dose:** Apply q3–4h into conjunctival sac **W/P:** [C, ?] **CI:** Viral, mycobacterial, fungal eye Infxn **Disp:** See Bacitracin, Topical

Bacitracin, Topical (Baciguent); Bacitracin/Neomycin/Polymyxin B, Topical (Neosporin Ointment); Bacitracin/Neomycin/Polymyxin B/Hydrocortisone, Topical (Cortisporin); Bacitracin/Polymyxin B, Topical (Polysporin) Uses: *Prevent/Rx of *minor skin Infxns* **Acts:** Topical antibiotic w/ added components (anti-inflam & analgesic) **Dose:** Apply sparingly bid-qid **W/P:** [C, ?] Not for deep wounds, punctures, or animal bites **Disp:** Bacitracin 500 units/g oint; bacitracin 400 units/neomycin 3.5 mg/polymyxin B 5000 units/g oint; bacitracin 400 units/neomycin 3.5 mg/polymyxin B 5000 units/hydrocortisone 10 mg/g oint; Bacitracin 500 units/neomycin 3.5 mg/polymyxin B 5000 units/lidocaine 40 mg/g oint bacitracin 500 units/polymyxin B sulfate 10,000 units/g oint & powder; **Notes:** Ophthal, systemic, & irrigation forms available, not generally used d/t potential tox

Baclofen (Gablofen, Lioresal Intrathecal) **BOX:** Abrupt D/C, especially IT use can lead to organ failure, rhabdomyolysis, and death Uses: *Spasticity d/t severe chronic disorders (eg, MS, amyotrophic lateral sclerosis, or spinal cord lesions)*, trigeminal neuralgia, intractable hiccups **Acts:** Centrally acting skeletal muscle relaxant; ↓ transmission of monosynaptic & polysynaptic cord reflexes **Dose:** *Adults.* Initial, 5 mg PO tid; ↑ q3d by 5 mg to effect; max 80 mg/d *IT:* Via implantable pump (see PI) *Peds 2–7 y.* 20–30 mg ÷ q8h (max 60 mg) *> 8 y:* Max 120 mg/d *IT:* Via implantable pump (see PI); ↓ in renal impair; take w/ food or milk **W/P:** [C, +] Epilepsy, neuropsychological disturbances; **Disp:** Tabs 10, 20 mg; IT Inj 50, 500, 1000, 2000 mcg/mL; 2% cream **SE:** Dizziness, drowsiness, insomnia, rash, fatigue, ataxia, weakness, ↓ BP

Balsalazide (Colazal, Giazo, Generic) **Uses:** *UC* **Acts:** 5-ASA derivative, anti-inflammatory **Dose:** 2.25 g (3 caps) tid × 8–12 wk; *Giazo* 1.1-g tabs bid up to 8 wk **W/P:** [B, ?/–] Severe renal failure **CI:** Mesalamine or salicylate hypersens **Disp:** Caps 750 mg **SE:** Dizziness, HA, N, Abd pain, agranulocytosis, renal impair, allergic Rxns **Notes:** Daily dose of 6.75 g = 2.4 g mesalamine, UC exacerbation upon initiation of Rx

Basiliximab (Simulect) **BOX:** Use only under the supervision of a physician experienced in immunosuppression Rx in an appropriate facility **Uses:** *Prevent acute transplant rejection* **Acts:** IL-2 receptor antag **Dose:** *Adults & Peds > 35 kg.* 20 mg IV 2 h before transplant, then 20 mg IV 4 d posttransplant. *Peds < 35 kg.* 10 mg 2 h prior to transplant; same dose IV 4 d posttransplant **W/P:** [B, ?/–] **CI:** Hypersens to murine proteins **Disp:** Inj powder 10, 20 mg **SE:** Edema, ↓ BP, HTN, HA, dizziness, fever, pain, Infxn, GI effects, electrolyte disturbances **Notes:** A murine/human MoAB

BCG [Bacillus Calmette-Guérin] (TheraCys, Tice BCG) **BOX:** Contains live, attenuated mycobacteria; transmission risk; handle as biohazard; nosocomial & disseminated Infxns reported in immunosuppressed **Uses:** *Bladder CA (superficial)*, TB prophylaxis: Routine US adult BCG immunization not recommended. Children who are PPD(–) and continually exposed to untreated/ineffectively treated adults or whose TB strain is INH/rifampin resistant. Healthcare workers in high-risk environments **Acts:** Attenuated live BCG culture, immunomodulator **Dose:** *Bladder CA:* 1 vial prepared & instilled in bladder for 2 h. Repeat once/wk × 6 wk; then 1 Tx at 3, 6, 12, 18, & 24 mo after **W/P:** [C, ?] Asthma w/ TB immunization **CI:** Immunosuppression, PRG, steroid use, febrile illness, UTI, gross hematuria, w/ traumatic catheterization **Disp:** Powder 81 mg (*TheraCys*), 50 mg (*Tice BCG*) **SE:** Intravesical: Hematuria, urinary frequency, dysuria, bacterial UTI, rare BCG sepsis malaise, fever, chills, pain, N/V, anorexia, anemia **Notes:** PPD is not CI in BCG vaccinated persons; intravesical use, dispose/void in toilet w/ chlorine bleach

Becaplermin (Regranex Gel) **BOX:** Increased mortality d/t malignancy reported; use w/ caution in known malignancy **Uses:** Local wound care adjunct w/ *diabetic foot ulcers* **Acts:** Recombinant PDGF, enhances granulation tissue **Dose:** *Adults. Based on lesion:* Calculate the length of gel, measure the greatest length of ulcer by the greatest width; tube size and measured result determine the formula used in the calculation. Recalculate q1–2wk based on change in lesion size. *15-g tube:* [length × width] × 0.6 = length of gel (in inches) or for *2-g tube:* [length × width] × 1.3 = length of gel (in inches) **Peds.** See PI **W/P:** [C, ?] **CI:** Neoplasmatic site **Disp:** 0.01% gel in 2-, 15-g tubes **SE:** Rash **Notes:** Use w/ good wound care; wound must be vascularized; reassess after 10 wk if ulcer not ↓ by 30% or not healed by 20 wk

Beclomethasone (QVAR) Uses: Chronic *asthma* Acts: Inhaled corticosteroid Dose: **Adults & Peds 5–11 y.** 40–160 mcg 1–4 Inhs bid; initial 40–80 mcg Inh bid if on bronchodilators alone; 40–160 mcg bid w/ other inhaled steroids; 320 mcg bid max; taper to lowest effective dose bid; rinse mouth/throat after **W/P:** [C, ?] **CI:** Acute asthma **Disp:** PO metered-dose inhaler; 40, 80 mcg/Inh **SE:** HA, cough, hoarseness, oral candidiasis **Notes:** Not effective for acute asthma; effect in 1–2 d or as long as 2 wk; rinse mouth after use

Beclomethasone Nasal (Beconase AQ, Qnasl) Uses: *Allergic rhinitis, nasal polyps (*Beconase AQ*); allergic rhinitis (*Qnasl*)* Acts: Inh steroid Dose: **Adults & Peds >12 y.** *Beconase AQ:* 1–2 sprays/nostril bid **Peds 6–12 y.** *Beconase AQ:* 1 spray/nostril qd, may ↑ to 2 sprays to control Sx, then ↓ **Peds 4–6 y.** *Qnasl:* 1 spray/nostril qd **W/P:** [C, ?] **Disp:** Nasal metered-dose inhaler: *Beconase AQ* 42 mcg/spray; *Qnasl* 40 mcg/spray **SE:** Local irritation, burning, epistaxis **Notes:** Effect in days to 2 wk

Bedaquiline Fumarate (Sirturo) BOX: ↑ QT can occur and may be additive w/ other QT-prolonging drugs; ↑ risk of death vs placebo, only use when an effective TB regimen cannot be provided Uses: *Tx of MDR TB* Acts: Diarylquinoline antimycobacterial Dose: 400 mg/d × 2 wk, then 200 mg 3 ×/wk for 22 wk **W/P:** [B, –] ↑ QT, ✓ ECG frequently; D/C if ventricular arrhythmias or QTc > 500 ms; hepatic Rxn, ✓ LFTs, D/C w/ AST/ALT > 8× ULN, T bili > 2× ULN or LFTs persist > 2 wk; w/ renal failure **CI:** w/ drugs that ↑ QTc **Disp:** Tabs 100 mg **SE:** HA, N, arthralgias, hemoptysis, CP **Notes:** Frequent ✓ ECG; ✓ LFTs; avoid use of potent CYP3A4 inducers; avoid w/in < 14 d use of CYP3A4 inhib

Belatacept (Nulojix) BOX: May ↑ risk of posttransplant PTLD mostly CNS; ↑ risk of Infxn; for use by physicians experienced in immunosuppressive therapy; ↑ risk of malignancies; not for liver transplant Uses: *Prevention rejection in EBV-positive kidney transplant recipients* Acts: T-cell costimulation blocker Dose: D 1 (transplant day, preop) & d 5 10 mg/kg; end of wk 2, wk 4, wk 8, wk 12 after transplant 10 mg/kg; Maint: End of wk 16 after transplant 4 wk 5 mg/kg **W/P:** [C, –] w/ CYP3A4 inhib/inducers, other anticoagulants or plt inhib **CI:** EBV seronegative or unknown EBV status **Disp:** 250 mg Inj **SE:** anemia, N/V/D, UTI, edema, constipation, ↑ BP, pyrexia, graft dysfunction, cough, HA, ↑/↓ K+, ↓ WBC **Notes:** REMS; use in combo w/ basiliximab, mycophenolate mofetil (MMF), & steroids; PML w/ excess dedicated dosing

Belimumab (Benlysta) Uses: *SLE* Acts: B-lymphocyte inhib Dose: 10 mg/kg IV q2wk × 3 doses, then q4wk; Inf over 1 h; premed against Inf &

hypersens Rxns **W/P:** [C, ?/–] Hx active or chronic Infxns; possible ↑ mortality **CI:** Live vaccines, hypersens **Disp:** Inj powder 120, 400 mg/vial **SE:** N/D, bronchitis, nasopharyngitis, pharyngitis, insomnia, extremity pain, pyrexia, depression, migraine, serious/fatal, hypersens, anaphylaxis **Notes:** Not for severe active lupus nephritis or CNS lupus or w/ other biologics or IV cyclophosphamide

Belinostat (Beleodaq) Uses: *Relapsed/refractory TCL* **Acts:** histone deacetylase inhib **Dose:** 1000 mg/m^2 over 30 min qd d 1–5 of a 21-d cycle **W/P:** [D, –] ↓ plts/WBC/RBC; serious Infxn; hepatotox; tumor lysis synd; embryo-fetal tox **Disp:** Powder, single vial, 500 mg **SE:** N/V, fatigue, fever, anemia **Notes:** D/C or ↓ dose 25% w/ AE's; ✓ CBC, LFTs; modify dose w/toxicity; ✓ tumor lysis

Belladonna/Opium, Suppositories (Generic) [C-II] Uses: *Mod–severe pain associated w/ bladder spasms* **Acts:** Antispasmodic, analgesic **Dose:** 1 supp PR 1–2/d (up to 4 doses/d) **W/P:** [C, ?] **CI:** Glaucoma, resp depression, severe renal or hepatic dz, convulsive disorder, acute alcoholism **Disp:** 30 mg opium/16.2 mg belladonna extract; 60 mg opium/16.2 mg belladonna extract **SE:** Anticholinergic (eg, sedation, urinary retention, constipation)

Benazepril (Lotensin, Generic) BOX: PRG avoid use Uses: *HTN* **Acts:** ACE inhib **Dose:** 10–80 mg PO qd or bid; follow BP 2–6 h postdose; target in CHF 20–40 mg **W/P:** [D, –] **CI:** Angioedema **Disp:** Tabs 5, 10, 20, 40 mg **SE:** Symptomatic ↓ BP w/ diuretics; dizziness, HA, ↑ K$^+$, nonproductive cough, ↑ SCr

Bendamustine (Treanda) Uses: *CLL, B-cell NHL* **Acts:** Mechlorethamine derivative; alkylating agent **Dose:** 100 mg/m^2 IV over 30 min on d 1 & 2 of 28-d cycle, up to 6 cycles (w/ tox see PI for dose changes) *NHL:* 120 mg/m^2 IV over 30 min d 1 & 2 of 21-d cycle, up to 8 cycles; do not use w/ CrCl < 40 mL/min, severe hepatic impair **W/P:** [D, ?/–] Do not use w/ CrCl < 40 mL/min, severe hepatic impair **CI:** Hypersens to bendamustine or mannitol **Disp:** Inj powder, 25 mg, 100 mg **SE:** Pyrexia, N/V, dry mouth, fatigue, cough, stomatitis, rash, myelosuppression, Infxn, Inf Rxns & anaphylaxis, tumor lysis synd, skin Rxns, extravasation **Notes:** Consider use of allopurinol to prevent tumor lysis synd

Benzocaine (Americaine, Hurricane Lanacane, Others) [OTC] BOX: Do not use for infant teething Uses: *Topical anesthetic, lubricant on ET tubes, catheters, etc; pain relief in external otitis, cerumen removal, skin conditions, sunburn, insect bites, mouth and gum irritation, hemorrhoids* **Acts:** Topical local anesthetic **Dose:** *Adults & Peds > 1 y.* *Anesthetic lubricant:* Apply evenly to tube/instrument; other uses per manufacturer instructions **W/P:** [C, –] Do not use on broken skin; see provider if condition does not respond; avoid in infants and those w/ pulmonary Dzs **Disp:** Many site-specific OTC forms creams, gels, liquids, sprays, 2–20% **SE:** Itching, irritation, burning, edema, erythema, pruritus, rash, stinging, tenderness, urticaria; methemoglobinemia (infants or in COPD) **Notes:** Use minimum amount to obtain effect; risk of methemoglobinemia S/SXs: HA, lightheadedness, SOB, anxiety, fatigue, pale, gray or blue colored skin, and tachycardia

Benzocaine/Antipyrine (Aurodex, Generic) Uses: *Analgesia in severe otitis media* Acts: Anesthetic w/ local decongestant Dose: Fill ear & insert a moist cotton plug; repeat 1–2 h PRN W/P: [C, ?] CI: w/ Perforated eardrum Disp: Soln 5.4% antipyrine, 1.4% benzocaine SE: Local irritation, methemoglobinemia, ear discharge

Benzonatate (Tessalon, Zonatuss) Uses: Symptomatic relief of *nonproductive cough* Acts: Anesthetizes the stretch receptors in the resp passages Dose: *Adults & Peds > 10 y.* 100 mg PO tid (max 600 mg/d) W/P: [C, ?] Disp: Caps 100, 150, 200 mg SE: Sedation, dizziness, GI upset Notes: Do not chew or puncture the caps; deaths reported in peds < 10 y w/ ingestion

Benztropine (Cogentin) Uses: *Parkinsonism & drug-induced extrapyramidal disorders* Acts: Anticholinergic & antihistaminic effects Dose: *Adults. Parkinsonism:* initial 0.5–1 mg PO/IM/IV qhs, ↑ q 5–6 d PRN by 0.5 mg, usual dose 1–2 mg/d, 6 mg/d max *Extrapyramidal:* 1–4 mg PO/IV/IM qd-bid. *Peds > 3 y.* 0.02–0.05 mg/kg/dose 1–2/d W/P: [C, ?] w/ Urinary Sxs, NAG, hot environments, CNS or mental disorders, other phenothiazines or TCA (IV: < 3 y pyloric/duodenal obstruction, myasthenia gravis Disp: Tabs 0.5, 1, 2 mg; Inj 1 mg/mL SE: Anticholinergic (tachycardia, ileus, N/V, etc), anhidrosis, heat stroke

Benzyl Alcohol (Ulesfia) Uses: *Head lice* Acts: Pediculicide Dose: *Adults & Peds.* Apply vol for hair length to dry hair; saturate the scalp; leave on 10 min; rinse w/ water; repeat in 7 d; *Hair length 0–2 in:* 4–6 oz; *2–4 in:* 6–8 oz; *4–8 in:* 8–12 oz; *8–16 in:* 12–24 oz; *16–22 in:* 24–32 oz; *> 22 in:* 32–48 oz W/P: [B, ?] Avoid eyes CI: Ø Disp: 5% lotion 4-, 8-oz bottles SE: Pruritus, erythema, irritation (local, eyes) Notes: Use fine-tooth/nit comb to remove nits and dead lice; no ovocidal activity.

Bepotastine Besilate (Bepreve) Uses: *Allergic conjunctivitis* Acts: H_1-receptor antag Dose: 1 gtt into affected eye(s) twice daily W/P: [C, ?/–] Do not use while wearing contacts Disp: Soln 1.5% SE: Mild taste, eye irritation, HA, nasopharyngitis

Beractant (Survanta) Uses: *Prevention & Rx RDS in premature infants* Acts: Replaces pulm surfactant Dose: 4 mL/kg via ET tube; repeat q6h PRN; max 4 doses Disp: Susp 25 mg of phospholipid/mL SE: Transient ↓ HR, desaturation, apnea

Besifloxacin (Besivance) Uses: *Bacterial conjunctivitis* Acts: Inhib DNA gyrase & topoisomerase IV Dose: *Adults & Peds > 1 y.* 1 gtt into eye(s) tid 4–12 h apart × 7 d W/P: [C, ?] Remove contacts during Tx CI: Ø Disp: 0.6% susp SE: HA, redness, blurred vision, irritation

Betaxolol (Kerlone) Uses: *HTN* Acts: Competitively blocks β-adrenergic receptors, $β_1$ Dose: 5–20 mg/d W/P: [C, ?/–] CI: Sinus ↓ HR, AV conduction abnormalities, uncompensated cardiac failure Disp: Tabs 10, 20 mg SE: Dizziness, HA, ↓ HR, edema, CHF, fatigue, lethargy

Betaxolol, Ophthalmic (Betoptic) Uses: Open-angle glaucoma Acts: Competitively blocks β_1-adrenergic receptors Dose: 1–2 gtt bid W/P: [C, ?/–] Disp: Soln 0.5%; susp 0.25% SE: Local irritation, photophobia

Bethanechol (Urecholine, Generic) Uses: *Acute postop/postpartum nonobstructive urinary retention; neurogenic bladder w/ retention* Acts: Stimulates cholinergic smooth muscle in bladder & GI tract Dose: *Adults.* Initial 5–10 mg PO, then repeat qh until response or 50 mg, typical 10–50 mg tid-qid, 200 mg/d max tid-qid. *Peds.* 0.3–0.6 mg/kg/24 h PO ÷ tid-qid; take on empty stomach W/P: [C, –] CI: BOO, PUD, epilepsy, hyperthyroidism, ↓ HR, COPD, AV conduction defects, Parkinsonism, ↓ BP, vasomotor instability Disp: Tabs 5, 10, 25, 50 mg SE: Abd cramps, D, salivation, ↓ BP

Bevacizumab (Avastin) BOX: Associated w/ GI perforation, wound dehiscence, & fatal hemoptysis Uses: *Met colorectal CA w/5-FU, NSCLC w/ paclitaxel and carboplatin; glioblastoma; metastatic RCC w/ IFN-alpha, cervical & ovarian Ca w/ paclitaxel and platinum or topotecan* Acts: Vascular endothelial GF inhib Dose: *Colon:* 5 mg/kg or 10 mg/kg IV q14d *NSCLC:* 15 mg/kg q21d; 1st dose over 90 min; 2nd over 60 min, 3rd over 30 min if tolerated *RCC:* 10 mg/kg IV q2wk w/ IFN-α W/P: [C, –] Do not use w/in 28 d of surgery if time for separation of drug & anticipated surgical procedures is unknown; D/C w/ serious adverse CI: Ø Disp: 100 mg/4 mL, 400 mg/16 mL vials SE: Wound dehiscence, GI perforation, tracheoesophageal fistula, arterial thrombosis, hemoptysis, hemorrhage, HTN, proteinuria, CHF, Inf Rxns, D, leukopenia Notes: Monitor for ↑ BP & proteinuria

Bicalutamide (Casodex) Uses: *Advanced PCa w/ GnRH agonists (eg, leuprolide, goserelin)* Acts: Nonsteroidal antiandrogen Dose: 50 mg/d W/P: [X, ?] CI: Women Disp: Caps 50 mg SE: Hot flashes, ↓ loss of libido, impotence, edema, pain, D/N/V, gynecomastia, ↑ LFTs

Bicarbonate (See Sodium Bicarbonate, p 284)

Bisacodyl (Dulcolax) [OTC] Uses: *Constipation; preop bowel prep* Acts: Stimulates peristalsis Dose: *Adults.* 5–15 mg PO or 10 mg PR PRN; up to 30 mg when complete evacuation needed. *Peds < 2 y.* 5 mg PR PRN *> 2 y.* 5 mg PO or 10 mg PR PRN (do not chew tabs or give w/in 1 h of antacids or milk) W/P: [C, ?] CI: Abd pain or obstruction, N/V Disp: EC tabs 5, 10 mg; supp 10 mg; enema soln 10 mg/30 mL SE: Abd cramps, proctitis, & inflammation w/ supps

Bismuth Subcitrate/Metronidazole/Tetracycline (Pylera) Uses: *H. pylori Infxn w/ omeprazole* Acts: Eradicates *H. pylori,* see agents Dose: 3 caps qid w/ omeprazole 20 mg bid for × 10 d W/P: [D, –] CI: PRG, peds < 8 y (tetracycline during tooth development causes teeth discoloration), w/ renal/hepatic impair, component hypersens Disp: Caps w/ 140 mg bismuth subcitrate potassium, 125 mg metronidazole, & 125 mg tetracycline hydrochloride SE: Stool abnormality, N, anorexia, D, dyspepsia, Abd pain, HA, flu-like synd, taste perversion, vaginitis, dizziness; see SE for each component Notes: Metronidazole carcinogenic in animals

Bismuth Subsalicylate (Pepto-Bismol) [OTC] Uses: Indigestion, N, & *D*; combo for Rx of *H. pylori* Infxn* Acts: Antisecretory & anti-inflam Dose: *Adults.* 2 tabs or 30 mL PO PRN (max 8 doses/24 h) *Peds.* (For all max 8 doses/24 h) *3–6 y:* 1/3 tab or 5 mL PO PRN *6–9 y:* 2/3 tab or 10 mL PO PRN *9–12 y:* 1 tab or 15 mL PO PRN W/P: [C, D (3rd tri), −] Avoid w/ renal failure; Hx severe GI bleed; influenza or chickenpox (↑ risk of Reye synd) CI: Hx severe GI bleeding or coagulopathy, ASA allergy Disp: Chew tabs, caplets 262 mg; liq 262, 525 mg/15 mL; susp 262 mg/15 mL SE: May turn tongue & stools black

Bisoprolol (Zebeta) Uses: *HTN* Acts: Competitively blocks β_1-adrenergic receptors Dose: 2.5–10 mg/d (max dose 20 mg) ↓ w/ renal impair W/P: [C, ?/−] CI: Sinus bradycardia, AV conduction abnormalities, uncompensated cardiac failure Disp: Tabs 5, 10 mg SE: Fatigue, lethargy, HA, ↓ HR, edema, CHF Notes: Not dialyzed

Bivalirudin (Angiomax) Uses: *Anticoagulant w/ ASA in unstable angina undergoing PTCA, PCI, or in pts undergoing PCI w/ or at risk for HIT/HITTS* Acts: Anticoagulant, thrombin inhib Dose: 0.75 mg/kg IV bolus, then 1.75 mg/kg/h for duration of procedure and up to 4 h postprocedure; ✓ ACT 5 min after bolus, may repeat 0.3 mg/kg bolus if necessary (give w/ aspirin ASA 300–325 mg/d; start pre-PTCA) W/P: [B, ?] CI: Major bleeding Disp: Powder 250 mg for Inj W/P: ↓ BP, bleeding, back pain, N, HA

Bleomycin Sulfate (Generic) BOX: Idiopathic Rxn (↓ BP, fever, chills, wheezing) in lymphoma pts; pulm fibrosis; should be administered by chemo-experienced physician Uses: *Testis CA; Hodgkin Dz & NHLs; cutaneous lymphomas; squamous cell CA (head & neck, larynx, cervix, skin, penis); malignant pleural effusion sclerosing agent* Acts: Induces DNA breakage (scission) Dose: (per protocols); ↓ w/ renal impair W/P: [D, ?] CI: w/ Hypersens, idiosyncratic Rxn Disp: Powder (Inj) 15, 30 units SE: Hyperpigmentation & allergy (rash to anaphylaxis); fever in 50%; lung tox (idiosyncratic & dose related); pneumonitis w/ fibrosis; Raynaud phenomenon, N/V Notes: Test dose 1 unit, especially in lymphoma pts; lung tox w/ total dose > 400 units or single dose > 30 units; avoid high FiO_2 in general anesthesia to ↑ tox

Blinatumomab (Blincyto) BOX: Cytokine release synd, may be life-threatening; neurologic tox may be fatal Uses: *Philadelphia chromosome (−) relapsed or refractory B-cell precursor ALL* Acts: Bispecific CD19 directed CD3 T-cell engager Dose: > 45 kg, cycle 1, 9 mcg/d, d 1–7, then 28 mcg/d, d 8–28; subsequent cycles 28 mcg/d; 4 wk cont Inf, 2 wk Tx free; hospitalize first 9 d of 1st cycle and first 2 d of 2nd cycle; premed w/ dexamethasone 20 mg IV 1 h prior to 1st dose each cycle and between d 7 and 8 w/ ↑ dose or when restarting if Inf off > 4 h; IV bag infused over 24 or 48 h W/P: [C, −] Infxn; ↓ ability to drive/use machines (refrain from driving/hazardous activities); strict prep & administration Disp: Single-use vial, 35 mcg powder SE: HA, N, fever, edema, tremor, rash, constipation, ↓ WBC, febrile neutropenia, ↓ K^+

Boceprevir (Victrelis) Uses: *Chronic hep C, genotype 1, w/ compensated liver Dz, including naïve to Tx or failed Tx w/ peginterferon and ribavirin* Acts: Hep C antiviral Dose: After 4 wk of peginterferon and ribavirin, then 800 mg tid w/ food for 44 wk w/ peginterferon and ribavirin; must be used w/ peginterferon and ribavirin W/P: [B, X w/ peginterferon and ribavirin, –] (X because must be used w/ peginterferon and ribavirin, class B by itself) CI: All CIs to peginterferon and ribavirin; men if PRG female partner; drugs highly dependent on CYP3A4/5, including alfuzosin, sildenafil, tadalafil, lovastatin, simvastatin, ergotamines, cisapride, triazolam, midazolam, rifampin, St. John's wort, phenytoin, carbamazepine, phenobarbital, drosperinone; strong CYP3A4/5 Disp: Caps 200 mg SE: Anemia, ↓ WBCs, neutrophils, fatigue, insomnia, HA, anorexia, N/V/D, dysgeusia, alopecia Notes: (NS3/4A protease inhib); ✓ HCV-RNA levels wk 4, 8, 12, 24, end of Tx; ✓ WBC w/ diff at wk 4, 8, 12

Bortezomib (Velcade) Uses: *Rx multiple myeloma or mantel cell lymphoma w/ one failed previous Rx* Acts: Proteasome inhib Dose: (per protocol or PI); ↓ dose w/ heme tox, neuropathy W/P: [D, ?/–] w/ Drugs CYP450 metabolized (Table 10, p 356) Disp: 3.5 mg vial Inj powder SE: Asthenia, GI upset, anorexia, dyspnea, HA, orthostatic ↓ BP, edema, insomnia, dizziness, rash, pyrexia, arthralgia, neuropathy

Bosutinib Monohydrate (Bosulif) Uses: *Ph¹ CML intol/resist to prior therapy* Acts: TKI Dose: 500 mg/d, ↑ dose to 600 mg/d by wk 8 w/ incomplete response, or by wk 12 w/ cytogenetic incomplete response and no grade 3/greater adverse Rxn; w/ hepatic impair 200 mg/d W/P: [D, –] GI toxicity; ↓ BM, ✓ CBC/LFTs qmo; fluid retention; hold/↓ dose or D/C w/ tox CI: Hypersens Disp: Tabs 100, 500 mg SE: N/V/D, Abd pain, fever, rash, fatigue, anemia, ↓ plts Notes: Avoid w/ mod/strong CYP3A inhib & inducers; avoid use of PPIs

Botulinum Toxin Type A [abobotulinumtoxin A] (Dysport) BOX: Effects may spread beyond Tx area leading to swallowing and breathing difficulties (may be fatal); Sxs may occur hours to weeks after Inj Uses: *Cervical dystonia (adults), glabellar lines (cosmetic)* Acts: Neurotoxin, ↓ ACH release from nerve endings, ↓ neuromuscular transmission Dose: *Cervical dystonia:* 500 units IM ÷ dose units into muscles; retreat no less than 12–16 wk PRN dose range 250–100 units based on response. *Glabellar lines:* 50 units ÷ in 10 units/Inj into muscles, do not administer at intervals < q3mo; repeat no less than q3mo W/P: [C, ?] Sedentary pt to resume activity slowly after Inj; aminoglycosides and nondepolarizing muscle blockers may ↑↑ effects; do not exceed dosing CI: Hypersens to components (cow milk), Infxn at Inj site Disp: 300, 500 units, Inj SE: Anaphylaxis, erythema multiforme, dysphagia, dyspnea, syncope, HA, NAG, Inj site pain Notes: Botulinum toxin products not interchangeable

Botulinum Toxin Type A [incobotulinumtoxin A] (Xeomin) BOX: Effects may spread beyond Tx area leading to swallowing and breathing difficulties (may be fatal); Sxs may occur hours to weeks after Inj Uses: *Cervical dystonia (adults), glabellar lines* Acts: Neurotoxin, ↓ ACH release from nerve endings, ↓

neuromuscular transmission **Dose:** *Cervical dystonia:* 120 units IM ÷ dose into muscles *Glabellar lines:* 4 units into each of the 5 sites (total = 20 units); do not administer at intervals < q3mo **W/P:** [C, ?] Sedentary pts to resume activity slowly after Inj; aminoglycosides and nondepolarizing muscle blockers may ↑↑ effects; do not exceed dosing **CI:** Hypersens to components (cow milk), Infxn at Inj site **Disp:** 50, 100 units, Inj SE: Dysphagia, neck/musculoskeletal pain, muscle weakness, Inj site pain **Notes:** Botulinum toxin products not interchangeable

Botulinum Toxin Type A [onabotulinumtoxin A] (Botox, Botox Cosmetic)
BOX: Effects may spread beyond Tx area leading to swallowing and breathing difficulties (may be fatal); Sxs may occur hours to weeks after Inj **Uses:** *Glabellar lines (cosmetic) < 65 y, blepharospasm, cervical dystonia, axillary hyperhidrosis, strabismus, chronic migraine, upper limb spasticity, incontinence in OAB due to neurologic Dz* **Acts:** Neurotoxin, ↓ ACH release from nerve endings; denervates sweat glands/muscles **Dose:** (See PI for site injection details) *Glabellar lines (cosmetic):* 0.1 mL IM × 5 sites q3–4mo *Blepharospasm:* 1.25–2.5 units IM/site q3mo; max 200 units/30 d total *Cervical dystonia:* 198–300 units IM ÷ < 100 units into muscles *Hyperhidrosis:* 50 units intradermal/each axilla *Strabismus:* 1.25–2.5 units IM/site q3mo; inject eye muscles w/ EMG guidance *Chronic migraine:* 155 units total, 0.1 mL (5 unit) Inj ÷ into 7 head/neck muscles *Upper limb spasticity:* Dose based on Hx; use EMG guidance *OAB:* Inj via cytoscope 20 Inj 0.5 mL (100 units/10 mL) 1 cm apart, repeat minimum 12 wks later **W/P:** [C, ?] w/ Neurologic Dz; do not exceed rec doses; sedentary pts to resume activity slowly after Inj; aminoglycosides and nondepolarizing muscle blockers may ↑↑ effects; do not exceed dosing **CI:** Hypersens to components, Infxn at Inj site **Disp:** Inj powder, single-use vial (dilute w/ NS); *(Botox cosmetic)* 50, 100 units; *(Botox)* 100, 200 unit vials; store 2–8°C **SE:** Anaphylaxis, erythema multiforme, dysphagia, dyspnea, syncope, HA, NAG, Inj site pain **Notes:** Botulinum toxin products not interchangeable; do not exceed total dose of 360 units q12–16wk

Botulinum Toxin Type B [rimabotulinumtoxin B] (Myobloc)
BOX: Effects may spread beyond Tx area leading to swallowing and breathing difficulties (may be fatal); Sxs may occur hours to weeks after Inj **Uses:** *Cervical dystonia (adults)* **Acts:** Neurotoxin, ↓ ACH release from nerve endings, ↓ neuromuscular transmission **Dose:** *Cervical dystonia:* 2500–5000 units IM ÷ dose units into muscles; lower dose if näive **W/P:** [C, ?] Sedentary pts to resume activity slowly after Inj; aminoglycosides and nondepolarizing muscle blockers may ↑↑ effects; do not exceed dosing **CI:** Hypersens to components, Infxn at Inj site **Disp:** Inj 5000 units/mL **SE:** Anaphylaxis, erythema multiforme, dysphagia, dyspnea, syncope, HA, NAG, Inj site pain **Notes:** Effect 12–16 wk w/ 5000–10,000 units; botulinum toxin products not interchangeable

Brentuximab Vedotin (Adcetris)
BOX: JC virus Infxn leading to PML and death may occur **Uses:** *Hodgkin lymphoma, systemic anaplastic large cell lymphoma* **Acts:** CD30-directed antibody-drug conjugate **Dose:** 1.8 mg/kg IV over

30 min q3wk; max 16 cycles; pts > 100 kg, dose based on Wt of 100 kg; ↓ dose w/ periph neuropathy & neutropenia (see label) **W/P:** [D, ?/–] w/ Strong CYP3A4 inhib/inducers **CI:** w/ Bleomycin **Disp:** Inj (powder) 50 mg/vial **SE:** Periph neuropathy, ↓ WBC/Hgb/plt, N/V/D, HA, dizziness, pain, arthralgia, myalgia, insomnia, anxiety, alopecia, night sweats, URI, fatigue, pyrexia, rash, cough, dyspnea, Inf Rxns, tumor lysis synd, PML, SJS, pulmonary tox

Brexpiprazole (Rexulti) **BOX:** Increased mortality in elderly w/ dementia-related psychosis; ↑ suicidal thinking in children, adolescents, and young adults w/ MDD **Uses:** *Schizophrenia & as add-on to antidepressant for MDD* **Acts:** D2 dopamine partial agonist **Dose:** 2–4 mg/d PO **W/P:** [C, –] See Box **CI:** Component hypersens **Disp:** Tabs 1, 2, 4 mg **SE:** Wt gain, restlessness

Brimonidine, Ophthalmic (Alphagan P) **Uses:** *Open-angle glaucoma, ocular HTN* **Acts:** α₂-Adrenergic agonist **Dose:** 1 gtt in eye(s) tid (wait 15 min to insert contacts) **W/P:** [B, ?] **CI:** MAOI Rx **Disp:** 0.15, 0.1, 0.2% soln **SE:** Local irritation, HA, fatigue

Brimonidine, Topical (Mirvaso) **Uses:** *Tx of rosacea* **Acts:** α₂-adrenergic agonist **Dose:** Apply pea-size quantity to forehead, chin, nose, & cheeks qd **W/P:** [B, ?/–] w/ Hx depression, orthostatic ↓ BP, severe CV Dz, cerebral or coronary insuff, scleroderma, thromboangiitis obliterans, Sjögren synd, Raynaud phenomenon (may potentiate vascular insufficiency) **Disp:** Gel 0.33% **CI:** Ø **SE:** Flushing, erythema, skin burning sensation, contact dermatitis, acne, HA, nasopharyngitis, ↑ IOP **Notes:** Do not apply to eyes/lips

Brimonidine/Timolol (Combigan) **Uses:** *↓ IOP in glaucoma or ocular HTN* **Acts:** Selective α₂-adrenergic agonist and nonselective β-adrenergic antag **Dose:** *Adults & Peds ≥ 2 y.* 1 gtt bid **W/P:** [C, –] **CI:** Asthma, severe COPD, sinus bradycardia, 2nd-/3rd-degree AV block, CHF cardiac failure, cardiogenic shock, component hypersens **Disp:** Soln (2 mg/mL brimonidine, 5 mg/mL timolol) 5, 10, 15 mL **SE:** Allergic conjunctivitis, conjunctival folliculosis, conjunctival hyperemia, eye pruritus, ocular burning & stinging **Notes:** Instill other ophthal products 5 min apart

Brinzolamide (Azopt) **Uses:** *Open-angle glaucoma, ocular HTN* **Acts:** Carbonic anhydrase inhib **Dose:** 1 gtt in eye(s) tid **W/P:** [C, ?/–] **CI:** Sulfonamide allergy **Disp:** 1% susp **SE:** Blurred vision, dry eyes, blepharitis, taste disturbance, HA

Brinzolamide/Brimonidine (Simbrinza) **Uses:** *↓ IOP in open-angle glaucoma or ocular HTN* **Acts:** Carbonic anhydrase inhib and α₂-adrenergic agonist **Dose:** 1 gtt in eye(s) tid **W/P:** [C, ?/–] sulfonamide hypersens Rxn (brinzolamide); corneal endothelium cell loss; not rec if CrCl < 30 ml/min **CI:** Component hypersens **Disp:** Ophthal susp (brinzolamide/brimonidine) 10/2 mg/mL **SE:** Eye irritation/allergy, blurred vision, dysgeusia, dry mouth, HA, fatigue **Notes:** Shake well before use; remove contacts during admin, reinsert after 15 min; separate other topical eye meds by 5 min

Bromfenac (Bromday, Prolensa) Uses: *Inflam & ocular pain post-cataract surgery* Acts: NSAID Dose: 1 gtt in eye(s) 1 d prior & 14 d post-surgery W/P: [C, ?/–] Sulfite hypersens; may delay healing, keratitis, ↑ bleeding time CI: Ø Disp: Ophthal soln Bromday 0.09%, Prolensa 0.07% SE: Eye pain, blurred vision, photophobia, anterior chamber inflam, foreign body sensation Notes: Shake well before use; remove contacts during admin, reinsert after 10 min; separate other topical eye meds by 5 min

Bromocriptine (Parlodel) Uses: *Parkinson Dz, hyperprolactinemia, acromegaly, pituitary tumors* Acts: Agonist to striatal DA receptors; ↓ prolactin secretion Dose: *Initial;* 1.25 mg PO bid; titrate to effect, w/ food W/P: [B, –] CI: uncontrolled HTN, PRG, severe CAD or CVS Dz Disp: Tabs 2.5 mg; caps 5 mg SE: ↓ BP, Raynaud phenomenon, dizziness, N, GI upset, hallucinations

Bromocriptine Mesylate (Cycloset) Uses: *Improve glycemic control in adults w/ type 2 DM* Acts: Dopamine receptor agonist; ? DM mechanism Dose: *Initial:* 0.8 mg PO daily, ↑ weekly by 1 tab; usual dose 1.6–4.8 mg 1×/d; w/in 2 h after waking w/ food W/P: [B, –] May cause orthostatic ↓ BP, psychotic disorders; not for type 1 DM or DKA; w/ strong inducers/inhib of CYP3A4, avoid w/ dopamine antags/receptor agonist CI: Hypersens to ergots drugs, w/ syncopal migraine, nursing mothers Disp: Tabs 0.8 mg SE: N/V, fatigue, HA, dizziness, somnolence

Budesonide, Inh (Pulmicort Flexhaler, Respules, Turbuhaler, Generic) Uses: *Maint prophylaxis asthma* Acts: Steroid Dose: *Adults.* Dose based on previous Rx. *Bronchodilators alone:* 0.25 mg BID *Inh steroids:* 0.25–0.5 mg bid *Oral steroids:* 0.5 mg bid *Pulmicort Flexhaler:* 1–2 Inh bid *Peds 6–17 y. Pulmicort Flexhaler:* 1–2 Inh bid *Respules:* 0.25–0.5 mg qd or bid (rinse mouth after use) W/P: [B, ?/–] CI: w/ Acute asthma Disp: *Turbuhaler:* 200 mcg/Inh; *Flexhaler:* 90, 180 mcg/Inh; *Respules:* 0.25, 0.5, 1 mg/2 mL susp (administered by jet nebulizer) SE: HA, N, cough, hoarseness, *Candida* Infxn, epistaxis

Budesonide, Nasal (Rhinocort Aqua, Generic) Uses: *Seasonal/perennial allergic rhinitis* Acts: Steroid Dose: *Adults & Peds > 6 y. Rhinocort Aqua:* 1 spray/nostril/d W/P: [B. ?/–] Systemic effects of steroid use (impaired wound healing, immunosuppression, hypersens, etc) CI: w/ Acute asthma Disp: 32 mcg/spray SE: epistaxis, pharyngitis, bronchospasm, coughing, nasal irritation, *Candida* Infxn, nasal perforation

Budesonide, Oral (Entocort EC, Uceris) Uses: *Mild–mod Crohn Dz* Acts: Steroid, anti-inflam Dose: *Adults. Entocort:* Initial: 9 mg PO qam to 8 wk max; maint 6 mg PO qam; taper by 3 mo *Uceris:* 9 mg PO qam × 8 wk CI: Hypersens W/P: [C, ?/–] hypercorticism, adrenal suppression DM, glaucoma, cataracts, HTN, CHF Disp: *Entocort:* Caps 3 mg; *Uceris:* Tabs 9 mg ER SE: HA, N, ↑ Wt, mood change, immunosuppression Notes: Do not cut/crush/chew; taper to D/C; avoid grapefruit juice

Budesonide, Rectal Foam (Uceris Foam) Uses: *Mild–mod Crohn Dz* Acts: Steroid, anti-inflam Dose: *Adults.* Initial: 9 mg PO qam to 8 wk max; maint

6 mg PO qam; taper by 3 mo **CI:** Hypersens **W/P:** [C, ?/–] DM, glaucoma, cataracts, HTN, CHF **Disp:** Caps 3 mg ER **SE:** HA, N, ↑ Wt, mood change, *Candida* Infxn, epistaxis **Notes:** Do not cut/crush/chew; taper to D/C; avoid grapefruit juice

Budesonide/Formoterol (Symbicort) **BOX:** Long-acting β₂-adrenergic agonists may ↑ risk of asthma-related death. Use only for pts not adequately controlled on other meds **Uses:** *Rx of asthma, maint in COPD (chronic bronchitis and emphysema)* **Acts:** Steroid w/ LA β₂-adrenergic agonist **Dose:** *Adults & Peds > 12 y.* 2 Inh bid (use lowest effective dose), 640/18 mcg/d max **CI:** [C, ?/–] **CI:** Status asthmaticus/acute asthma **Disp:** Inh (budesonide/formoterol): 80/4.5 mcg, 160/4.5 mcg **SE:** HA, GI discomfort, nasopharyngitis, palpitations, tremor, nervousness, URI, paradoxical bronchospasm, hypokalemia, cataracts, glaucoma **Notes:** Not for acute bronchospasm; not for transferring pt from chronic systemic steroids; rinse & spit w/ water after each dose

Bumetanide (Bumex) **BOX:** Potent diuretic, may result in profound fluid & electrolyte loss **Uses:** *Edema from CHF, hepatic cirrhosis, & renal Dz* **Acts:** Loop diuretic; ↓ reabsorption of Na⁺ & Cl⁻, in ascending loop of Henle & the distal tubule **Dose:** *Adults.* 0.5–2 mg/d PO; 0.5–1 mg IV/IM q8–24h (max 10 mg/d). *Peds.* 0.015–0.1 mg/kg PO q6–24h (max 10 mg/d) **W/P:** [C, ?/–] **CI:** Anuria, hepatic coma, severe electrolyte depletion **Disp:** Tabs 0.5, 1, 2 mg; Inj 0.25 mg/mL **SE:** ↓ K⁺, ↓ Na⁺, ↑ Cr, ↑ uric acid, dizziness, ototox **Notes:** Monitor fluid & lytes; 1 mg Bumex ≈ 40 mg Lasix

Bupivacaine (Marcaine) **BOX:** Avoid 0.75% for OB anethesia d/t reports of cardiac arrest and death **Uses:** *Local, regional, & spinal anesthesia, obstetrical procedures*, local & regional analgesia **Acts:** Local anesthetic **Dose:** *Adults & Peds.* Dose dependent on procedure (tissue vascularity, depth of anesthesia, etc) (See Table 1, p 334) **W/P:** [C, –] Severe bleeding, ↓ BP, shock & arrhythmias, local Infxns at site, septicemia **CI:** Obstetrical paracervical block anesthesia **Disp:** Inj 0.25, 0.5, 0.75% **SE:** ↓ BP, ↓ HR, dizziness, anxiety

Buprenorphine, Oral, Sublingual (Buprenex, Generic) [C-III] **Uses:** *Opioid dependence* **Acts:** Opiate agonist-antag **Dose:** Daily dosing: Adjust ↑/↓ 2–4 mg to maint suppression of withdrawal; maint 2–24 mg/d typical **W/P:** [C, –] **Disp:** Tabs, SL: 2, 8 mg **SE:** Sedation, ↓ BP, resp depression **Notes:** Requires special registration and unique identifier; for opioid dependence buprenorphine/naloxone combo preferred

Buprenorphine, Systemic (Buprenex, Generic) [C-III] **Uses:** *Mod-severe pain* **Acts:** Opiate agonist-antag **Dose:** 0.3–0.6 mg IM or slow IV push q6h PRN **W/P:** [C, ↓] **Disp:** 0.3 mg/mL **SE:** Sedation, ↓ BP, resp depression **Notes:** Withdrawal if opioid dependent

Buprenorphine, Transdermal (Butrans) [C-III] **BOX:** Limit use to severe around-the-clock chronic pain; assess for opioid abuse/addiction before use; 20 mcg/h max due to ↑ QTc; avoid heat on patch, may result in OD **Uses:** *Mod-severe chronic pain requiring around-the-clock opioid analgesic* **Acts:** Partial opioid agonist **Dose:** Wear patch × 7/d; if opioid naïve, start 5 mcg/h; see PI for conversion from opioid; wait 72 h before Δ dose; wait 3 wk before using same application site **W/P:** [C, −] **CI:** Resp depression, severe asthma, ileus, component hypersens, short-term opioid need, postop/mild/intermittent pain **Disp:** Transdermal patch 5, 7.5, 10, 15, 20 mcg/h **SE:** N/V, HA, site Rxns, pruritus, dizziness, constipation, somnolence, dry mouth **Notes:** Taper to D/C; not for PRN use

Buprenorphine/Naloxone (Bunavail, Suboxone, Zubsolv) [C-III] Uses: *Maint opioid withdrawal* **Acts:** Opioid agonist-antag + opioid antag **Dose:** Usual: *Suboxone:* 4–24 mg/d SL; ↑/↓ by 2/0.5 mg or 4/1 mg to effect *Zubsolv:* 11.4 mg/2.8 mg buprenorphine/naloxone *Bunavail:* Apply to buccal mucosa qd, titrate **W/P:** [C, +/−] **CI:** Hypersens **Disp:** *Suboxone:* SL film buprenorphine/naloxone: 2/0.5, 8/2 mg; *Bunavail:* buccal film (mg buprenorphine/mg naloxone) 2.1/0.3, 4.2/0.7, 6.3/1; *Zubsolv:* SL tabs (mg buprenorphine/mg naloxone) 1.4/0.36, 5.7/1.4, 8.6/2.1, 11.4/2.9 **SE:** Oral hypoparesthesia, HA, V, pain, constipation, diaphoresis **Notes:** Not for analgesia; limited distribution under the Drug Addiction Treatment Act

Bupropion HCl (Aplenzin ER, Wellbutrin, Wellbutrin SR, Wellbutrin XL, Zyban) **BOX:** All pts being treated w/ bupropion for smoking cessation Tx should be observed for neuropsychiatric S/Sxs (hostility, agitation, depressed mood, and suicide-related events); most during/after *Zyban*; Sxs may persist following D/C; closely monitor for worsening depression or emergence of suicidality, increased suicidal behavior in young adults **Uses:** *Depression, smoking cessation adjunct*, ADHD **Acts:** Weak inhib of neuronal uptake of serotonin & norepinephrine; ↓ neuronal DA reuptake **Dose:** *Depression:* 100–450 mg/d ÷ bid-tid; SR 150–200 mg bid; XL 150–450 mg daily *Smoking cessation (Zyban, Wellbutrin XR):* 150 mg/d × 3 d, then 150 mg bid × 8–12 wk, last dose before 6 P.M.; ↓ dose w/ renal/hepatic impair **W/P:** [C, ?/−] **CI:** Sz disorder, Hx anorexia nervosa or bulimia, MAOI w/in 14 d; abrupt D/C of EtOH or sedatives; inhibitors/inducers of CYP2B6 (See Table 10, p 356) **Disp:** Tabs 75, 100 mg; SR tabs 100, 150, 200 mg; XL tabs 150, 300 mg; *Zyban* tabs 150 mg; *Aplenzin XR* tabs: 175, 348, 522 mg **SE:** Xerostomia, dizziness, Szs, agitation, insomnia, HA, tachycardia, ↓ Wt **Notes:** Avoid EtOH & other CNS depressants, SR & XR do not cut/chew/crush, may ↑ adverse events including Szs not for peds use

Bupropion/Naltrexone (Contrave) **BOX:** ↑ Risk suicidal thinking/behavior in children, adolescents, & young adults taking antidepressants; monitor for suicidal thoughts/actions **Uses:** *Adjunct to reduced-calorie diet and exercise for chronic Wt management for BMI > 30 or 27 w/ at least one comorbid cond* **Acts:** Aminoketone antidepressant w/ opioid antag **Dose:** wk 1, 1 tab qam; wk 2, 1 tab qam & qpm; wk 3, 2 tabs qam, 1 tab qpm; wk 4 & beyond, 2 tabs qam, 2 tabs qpm **W/P:** [X, −] Suicidal behavior/ideation; Sz risk; ↑ BP, ↑ HR; hepatotox; NAG; ↓ glu w/ Wt loss & antidiabetic meds **CI:** Uncontrolled ↑ BP; Sz disorder; anorexia nervosa, bulimia; abrupt D/C of EtOH, benzodiazepines, barbiturates, or antiepileptics; other bupropion products; chronic opioid use; w/in 14 d of MAOI **Disp:** Tabs 90 mg bupropion/8 mg naltrexone **SE:** HA, N/V/D, constipation, insomnia, dizziness, dry mouth **Notes:** Many bupropion interactions; false + urine test for amphetamines

Buspirone (Generic) Uses: *Generalized anxiety disorder* **Acts:** Antianxiety; antag CNS serotonin and DA receptors **Dose:** Initial: 7.5 mg PO bid; ↑ by 5 mg q2–3d to effect; usual 20–30 mg/d; max 60 mg/d **CI:** Hypersens **W/P:** [B, ?/–] Avoid w/ severe hepatic/renal Insuff w/ MAOI **Disp:** Tabs 5, 7.5, 10, 15, 30 mg **SE:** Drowsiness, dizziness, HA, N, EPS, serotonin synd, hostility, depression **Notes:** No abuse potential or physical/psychological dependence

Busulfan (Busulfex, Myleran) **BOX:** Can cause severe bone marrow suppression, should be administered by an experienced physician Uses: *CML*, preparative regimens for allogeneic & ABMT in high doses **Acts:** Alkylating agent **Dose:** (per protocol) **W/P:** [D, ?] **Disp:** Tabs 2 mg, Inj 60 mg/10 mL **SE:** Bone marrow suppression, ↑ BP, pulm fibrosis, N (w/ high dose), gynecomastia, adrenal Insuff, skin hyperpigmentation, ↑ HR, rash, weakness, Sz

Butorphanol (Stadol) [C-IV] Uses: *Anesthesia adjunct, pain & migraine HA* **Acts:** Opiate agonist-antag w/ central analgesic actions **Dose:** 0.5–2 mg IV or 1–4 mg IM q3–4h PRN *Migraine:* 1 spray in 1 nostril, repeat × 1 60–90 min, then q3–4h; ↓ in renal impair **W/P:** [C, +] **Disp:** Inj 1, 2 mg/mL; nasal 1 mg/spray (10 mg/mL) **SE:** Drowsiness, dizziness, nasal congestion **Notes:** May induce withdrawal in opioid dependency

C1 Esterase Inhibitor, Human (Berinert, Cinryze) Uses: *Berinert: Rx acute Abd or facial attacks of HAE*, *Cinryze: Prophylaxis of HAE* **Acts:** ↓ complement system by ↓ factor XIIa and kallikrein activation **Dose:** *Adults & Adolescents. Berinert:* 20 units/kg IV × 1; *Cinryze:* 1000 units IV q3–4d **W/P:** [C, ?/–] Hypersens Rxns, monitor for thrombotic events, may contain infectious agents **CI:** Hypersens Rxns to C1 esterase inhib preparations **Disp:** 500 units/vial **SE:** HA, Abd pain, N/V/D, muscle spasms, pain, subsequent HAE attack, anaphylaxis, thromboembolism

Cabazitaxel (Jevtana) **BOX:** Neutropenic deaths reported; ✓ CBC, CI w/ ANC ≤ 1500 cells/mm³; severe hypersens (rash/erythema, ↓ BP, bronchospasm) may occur, D/C drug & Tx; CI w/ Hx of hypersens to cabazitaxel or others formulated w/ polysorbate 80 Uses: *Hormone-refractory metastatic PCa after taxotere* **Acts:** Microtubule inhib **Dose:** 25 mg/m² IV Inf (over 1 h) q3wk w/ prednisone 10 mg PO daily; premed w/ antihistamine, corticosteroid, H₂ antag; do not use w/ bili ≥ ULN, AST/ALT ≥ 1.5 × ULN **W/P:** [D, ?/–] w/ CYP3A inhib/inducers **CI:** See Box **Disp:** 40 mg/mL Inj **SE:** ↓ WBC, ↓ Hgb, ↓ plt, sepsis, N/V/D, constipation, Abd/back/jt pain, dysgeusia, fatigue, hematuria, neuropathy, anorexia, cough, dyspnea, alopecia, pyrexia, hypersens Rxn, renal failure **Notes:** Monitor closely pts > 65 y

Cabozanitinib (Cometriq) **BOX:** GI perf/fistulas, severe and sometimes fatal hemorrhage (3%), including GI bleeding/hemoptysis Uses: *Metastatic medullary thyroid CA* **Acts:** Multi TKI **Dose:** 140 mg/d, take on an empty stomach **W/P:** [D, –] D/C w/ arterial thromboembolic events; dehiscence; ↑ BP, ONJ; palmar-plantar erythrodysesthesia synd; proteinuria; reversible posterior leukoencephalopathy **CI:** w/ Severe bleeding **Disp:** Caps 20, 80 mg counted blister pack **SE:** N/V Abd pain, constipation, stomatitis, oral pain, dysgeusia, fatigue, ↓ Wt, anorexia, ↑ BP, ↑ AST/ALT, ↑ alk phos, ↑ bili, ↓ Ca, ↓ PO_4, ↓ plts, ↓ lymphocytes, ↓ neutrophils **Notes:** A CYP3A4 subs, w/ strong CYP3A4 induc ↓ cabozantinib exposure, w/ strong CYP3A4 inhib ↑ cabozantinib exposure; ✓ for hemorrhage

Calcipotriene (Dovonex) **Uses:** *Plaque psoriasis* **Acts:** Synthetic vitamin D_3 analog **Dose:** Apply bid **W/P:** [C, ?] **CI:** ↑ Ca^{2+}; vit D tox; do not apply to face **Disp:** Cream; foam oint; soln 0.005% **SE:** Skin irritation, dermatitis

Calcitonin (Fortical, Miacalcin) **Uses:** *Miacalcin:* *Paget Dz, emergent Rx hypercalcemia, postmenopausal osteoporosis*; *Fortical:* *Postmenopausal osteoporosis* **Acts:** Polypeptide hormone (salmon derived), inhibits osteoclasts **Dose:** *Paget Dz:* 100 units/d IM/SQ initial, 50 units/d or 50–100 units q1–3d maint *Hypercalcemia:* 4 units/kg IM/SQ q12h; ↑ to 8 units/kg q12h, max q6h *Osteoporosis:* 100 units/d IM/SQ; intranasal 200 units = 1 nasal spray/d; alternate nostrils **W/P:** [C, ?] **Disp:** *Fortical, Miacalcin* nasal spray 200 Int units/activation; Inj, *Miacalcin* 200 units/mL (2 mL) **SE:** Facial flushing, N, Inj site edema, nasal irritation, polyuria, may ↑ granular casts in urine **Notes:** For nasal spray alternate nostrils daily; ensure adequate calcium and vit D intake; *Fortical* is rDNA derived from salmon

Calcitriol [Vitamin D_3 Analog] (Calcijex, Rocaltrol) **Uses:** *Predialysis reduction of ↑ PTH levels to treat bone Dz; ↑ Ca^{2+} on dialysis* **Acts:** 1,25-Dihydroxycholecalci-ferol (vit D analog); ↑ Ca^{2+} and phosphorus absorption; ↑ bone mineralization **Dose:** *Adults. Renal failure:* 0.25 mcg/d PO, ↑ 0.25 mcg/d q4–8wk up to 0.5–1.0 mcg qd PRN; 0.5–4 mcg 3×/wk IV, ↑ PRN *Hypoparathyroidism:* 0.5–2 mcg/qd. *Peds. Renal failure:* 15 ng/kg/d, ↑ PRN; maint 30–60 ng/kg/d *Hypoparathyroidism:* < 5 y: 0.25–0.75 mcg/d > 6 y: 0.5–2 mcg/d **W/P:** [C, ?] ↑ Mg^{2+} possible w/ antacids **CI:** ↑ Ca^{2+}; vit D tox **Disp:** Inj 1 mcg/mL (in 1 mL); caps 0.25, 0.5 mcg; soln 1 mcg/mL **SE:** ↑ Ca^{2+} possible **Notes:** ✓ To keep Ca^{2+} WNL; use nonaluminum phosphate binders and low-phosphate diet to control serum phosphate

Calcitriol, Ointment (Vectical) **Uses:** *Mild–moderate plaque psoriasis* **Acts:** Vit D_3 analog **Dose:** Apply to area bid; max 200 mg/wk **W/P:** [C, ?/–] Avoid excess sunlight **CI:** Ø **Disp:** Oint 3 mcg/g (5-, 100-g tube) **SE:** Hypercalcemia, hypercalciuria, nephrolithiasis, worsening psoriasis, pruritus, skin discomfort

Calcium Acetate (Calphron, Phos-Ex, PhosLo) **Uses:** *ESRD-associated hyperphosphatemia* **Acts:** Ca^{2+} supl w/o aluminum to ↓ PO_4^- absorption **Dose:** 2–4 tabs PO w/ meals, usual 2001–2668 mg PO w/ meals **W/P:** [C, +] **CI:** ↑ Ca^{2+} renal calculi **Disp:** Gel-Cap 667 mg **SE:** Can ↑ Ca^{2+}, hypophosphatemia, constipation **Notes:** Monitor Ca^{2+}

Calcium Carbonate (Alka-Mints, Tums) [OTC] Uses: *Hyperacidity associated w/ peptic ulcer Dz, hiatal hernia, etc* Acts: Neutralizes gastric acid Dose: 500 mg–2 g PO PRN, 7 g/d max; ↓ w/ renal impair W/P: [C, ?] CI: ↑ CA, ↓ phos, renal calculi, suspected digoxin tox Disp: Chew tabs 350, 420, 500, 550, 750, 850 mg; susp SE: ↑ Ca²⁺, ↓ PO⁴⁻, constipation

Calcium Glubionate (Calcionate) [OTC] Uses: *Rx & prevent calcium deficiency* Acts: Ca²⁺ supl Dose: Adults. 1000–1200 mg/d ÷ doses Peds. 200–1300 mg/d W/P: [C, ?] Disp: OTC syrup 1.8 g/5 mL = elemental Ca²⁺ 115 mg/5 mL SE: ↑ Ca²⁺, ↓ PO⁴⁻, constipation

Calcium Salts (Chloride, Gluconate, Gluceptate) Uses: *Ca²⁺ replacement*, VF, Ca²⁺ blocker tox (CCB), *severe ↑ Mg²⁺ tetany*, *hyperphosphatemia in ESRD* Acts: Ca²⁺ supl/replacement Dose: Adults. Replacement: 1–2 g/d PO Tetany: 1 g CaCl over 10–30 min; repeat in 6 h PRN; ECC 2010. Hyperkalemia/ hypermagnesemia/CCB OD: 500–1000 mg (5–10 mL of 10% soln) IV; repeat PRN; comparable dose of 10% calcium gluconate is 15–30 mL Peds. Tetany: 10 mg/kg CaCl over 5–10 min; repeat in 6–8 h or use Inf (200 mg/kg/d max); ECC 2010. Hypocalcemia/hyperkalemia/hypermagnesemia/CCB OD: Calcium chloride or gluconate 20 mg/kg (0.2 mL/kg) slow IV/IO, repeat PRN; central venous route preferred Adults & Peds. ↓ Ca²⁺ d/t citrated blood Inf: 0.45 mEq Ca/100 mL citrated blood Inf (↓ in renal impair) W/P: [C, ?] CI: ↑ Ca²⁺, suspected digoxin tox Disp: CaCl Inj 10% = 100 mg/mL = Ca 27.2 mg/mL = 10-mL amp; Ca gluconate Inj 10% = 100 mg/mL = Ca 9 mg/mL; tabs 500 = 45-mg Ca, 650 mg = 58.5 mg Ca, 975 mg = 87.75 mg Ca, 1 g = 90 mg Ca; Ca gluceptate Inj 220 mg/mL = 18 mg/mL Ca SE: ↓ HR, cardiac arrhythmias, ↑ Ca²⁺, constipation Notes: CaCl 270 mg (13.6 mEq) elemental Ca/g & calcium gluconate 90 mg (4.5 mEq) Ca/g. RDA for Ca intake: Adults. 1000 mg/d; > 50 y: 1200 mg/d Peds < 6 mo. 200 mg/d; 6 mo–1 y: 260 mg/d; 1–3 y: 700 mg/d; 4–8 y: 1000 mg/d; 10–18 y: 1300 mg/d

Calfactant (Infasurf) Uses: *Prevention & Rx of RSD in infants* Acts: Exogenous pulm surfactant Dose: 3 mL/kg instilled into lungs. Can repeat 3 total doses given 12 h apart W/P: [?, ?] Disp: Intratracheal susp 35 mg/mL SE: Monitor for cyanosis, airway obst, ↓ HR during administration

Canagliflozin (Invokana) Uses: *Type 2 DM* Acts: SGLT2 inhib Dose: Start 100 mg/d; ↑ to 300 mg PRN w/ GFR > 60 mL/min W/P: [C, –] ↓ BP from ↓ vol from glucosuria; ↑ K⁺; ↑ Cr; ✓renal Fxn; genital mycotic Infxns; hypoglycemia lower risk than insulin & sulfonylureas; hypersens CI: Hypersens reaction, severe renal impairment (GFR < 45 mL/min) Disp: Tabs 100, 300 mg SE: UTI, genital mycotic Infxns (3–15%) less likely to occur in circumcised males, polyuria, ↑ K⁺, ↑ PO₄⁻³, ↑ Mg²⁺, ↑ creat, ↑ LDL-chol Notes: 1st in class w/ FDA approval; may ↑ CV morbidity in first 30 d of Tx; CrCl 45–60 mL/min 100 mg/d max, do NOT use w/ CrCl < 45 mL/min; Wt loss likely; do not use w/ severe liver Dz; ↑ adverse events in geriatric population; metabolized by UDP-glucuronosyltransferase 1A9 & 2B4, concomitant rifampin, phenytoin, or ritonavir use reduces exposure, may need to ↑ dose; may need to ↓ digoxin dose

Canagliflozin/Metformin (Invokamet) **BOX:** Lactic acidosis d/t metformin; risk w/renal impair, sepsis, dehydration, excess EtOH, hepatic impair, CHF. Sx include malaise, myalgia, resp distress, abd distress, low pH, ↑ anion gap, ↑ lactate; if acidosis suspected, D/C and hospitalize **Uses:** *Adjunct to diet/exercise w/type 2 DM; not for type 1 DM or DKA* **Acts:** SGLT2 inhibitor (↓urinary glu excretion) w/a biguanide **Dose:** Individualize; take bid w/meals, ↑ dose slowly to ↓GI effects; ↓ w/ renal impair; max/d: metformin 2000 mg, canagliflozin 300 mg; w/ eGFR 45-60 limit canagliflozin to 50 mg bid; ✓ Cr, do not start if >1.5 (♂) or 1.4 (♀) **W/P:** [C, –] monitor/correct volume, especially in elderly; ✓ Cr, K, CBC (may ↓ B₁₂), dig levels; temp D/C with IV contrast or surgery w/↓ PO intake; ↓insulin or insulin secretagogue to limit hypoglycemia risk **CI:** Hypersens, severe renal impair, dialysis, ESRD, acidosis, DKA **Disp:** Tabs (mg canagliflozin/mg metformin) 50/500, 50/1000, 150/500, 150/1000 **SE:** *Canagliflozin:* genital mycotic infections, UTI, ↑ urination; *metformin* N/V/D, flatulence, asthenia, indigestion, Abd pain, H/A

Candesartan (Atacand) **BOX:** w/ PRG D/C immediately **Uses:** *HTN, CHF* **Acts:** Angiotensin II receptor antag **Dose:** 4–32 mg/d (usual 16 mg/d); CHF target = 32 mg/d **W/P:** [C(1st tri), D (2nd tri), ?/–] w/ renal Dz **CI:** Component hypersens **Disp:** Tabs 4, 8, 16, 32 mg **SE:** Dizziness, HA, flushing, angioedema, ↑ K⁺, ↑ Cr

Capsaicin (Capsin, Zostrix, Others) [OTC] **Uses:** Pain d/t *postherpetic neuralgia*, *arthritis, diabetic neuropathy*, *minor pain of muscles & joints* **Acts:** Topical analgesic **Dose:** Apply tid-qid **W/P:** [B, ?] **Disp:** OTC creams; gel; lotions; roll-ons **SE:** Local irritation, neurotox, cough **Notes:** Wk to onset of action

Captopril (Capoten, Others) **Uses:** *HTN, CHF, MI*, LVD, diabetic nephropathy **Acts:** ACE inhib **Dose:** *Adults. HTN:* Initial, 25 mg PO bid-tid; ↑ to maint q1–2wk by 25-mg increments/dose (max 450 mg/d) to effect. *CHF:* Initial, 6.25–12.5 mg PO tid; titrate PRN; CHF target = 50 mg tid *LVD:* 50 mg PO tid *DN:* 25 mg PO tid *Peds Infants.* 0.15–0.3 mg/kg/dose PO ÷ 1–4 doses *Children.* Initial, 0.3–0.5 mg/kg/dose PO; ↑ to 6 mg/kg/d max in 2–4 ÷ doses; 1 h ac; ↓ dose renal impair **W/P:** [D, –] **CI:** Hx angioedema **Disp:** Tabs 12.5, 25, 50, 100 mg **SE:** Rash, proteinuria, cough, ↑ K⁺

Carbamazepine (Carbatrol, Epitol, Equetro, Tegretol XR) **BOX:** Aplastic anemia & agranulocytosis have been reported w/ carbamazepine; pts w/ Asian ancestry should be tested to determine potential for skin Rxns **Uses:** *Epilepsy, trigeminal neuralgia, acute mania w/ bipolar disorder (Equetro)* EtOH withdrawal **Acts:** Anticonvulsant **Dose:** *Adults. Initial:* 200 mg PO bid or 100 mg 4 ×/d as susp; ↑ by 200 mg/d; usual 800–1200 mg/d ÷ doses *Acute mania (Equetro):* 400 mg/d, ÷ bid, adjust by 200 mg/d to response 1600 mg/d max *Peds < 6 y.* 10–20 mg/kg ÷ bid-tid or qid (susp) *6–12 y. Initial:* 200 mg/d bid (tab) or qid (susp), ↑ 100 mg/d, usual: 400–800 mg/d, max 1000 mg/d; ↓ in renal impair; take w/ food **W/P:** [D, M]

CI: w/in 14 d, w/ nefazodone, MAOI use, Hx BM suppression **Disp:** Tabs 200 mg; chew tabs 100 mg; XR tabs 100, 200, 400 mg; *Equetro* Caps ER 100, 200, 300 mg; susp 100 mg/5 mL **SE:** Drowsiness, dizziness, blurred vision, N/V, rash, SJS/toxic epidermal necrolysis (TEN), ↓ Na⁺, leukopenia, agranulocytosis **Notes:** Monitor CBC & levels: *Trough:* Just before next dose; *Therapeutic: Peak:* 8–12 mcg/mL (monotherapy), 4–8 mcg/mL (polytherapy); *Toxic Trough:* > 15 mcg/mL; *Half-life:* 15–20 h; generic products not interchangeable, many drug interactions, induces its own metabolism, administer susp in 3–4 ÷ doses daily; skin tox (SJS/TEN) ↑ w/ HLA-B*1502 allele

Carbidopa/Levodopa, Enteral Susp (Duopa) **Uses:** *Rx motor fluctuations in advanced Parkinson Dz* **Acts:** Carbidopa (amino acid decarboxylation inhibitor) & levodopa (aromatic amino acid) ↑ CNS DA levels **Dose:** IV over 16 h; max 2000 mg levodopa/d (1 cassette); complex doing schema, see PI; convert pts from all forms of levodopa to oral IR carbidopa–levodopa tabs (1:4 ratio) **W/P:** [C, ?] PEG tube–related complications, daytime sleepiness, ✓ ↓ BP, hallucinations/psychosis, depression/suicidality, avoid sudden D/C to ↓ risk of hyperpyrexia/confusion, may cause dyskinesia, ✓ peripheral neuropathy **CI:** MAOI use (w/in 14 d) **Disp:** 4.63 mg carbidopa/20 mg levodopa/mL **SE:** PEG complications, N, depression, edema, ↑ BP, URI, oropharyngeal pain, atelectasis, incision site erythema **Notes:** requires PEG-J tube w/inner jejunal, see PI for rec tubes

Carbidopa/Levodopa, Oral (Parcopa, Rytary, Sinemet, Sinemet SR) **Uses:** *Parkinson Dz* **Acts:** ↑ CNS DA levels **Dose:** 25/100 mg tid, ↑ as needed (max 200/2000 mg/d) *Rytary:* (levodopa-naïve) 23.75/ 95 mg PO tid × 3 d; d 4 ↑ to 36.25/145 mg tid, ↑ PRN to 97.5/390 mg tid max/d; if converting from another product see PI **W/P:** [C, ?] **CI:** NAG, suspicious skin lesion (may activate melanoma), melanoma, MAOI use (w/in 14 d) **Disp:** Tabs (mg carbidopa/mg levodopa) 10/100, 25/100, 25/250; tabs SR (mg carbidopa/mg levodopa) 25/100, 50/200; ODT 10/100, 25/100, 25/250; *Rytary:* caps (mg carbidopa/mg levodopa) 23.75/95, 36.25/145,48.75/195, 61.25/245 **SE:** Psychological disturbances, orthostatic ↓ BP, dyskinesias, cardiac arrhythmias **Notes:** Do not crush/chew SR, can sprinkle on applesauce

Carboplatin (Paraplatin) **BOX:** Administration only by physician experienced in CA chemotherapy; ↓ PLT, anemia, ↑ Infxn; BM suppression possible; anaphylaxis and V may occur **Uses:** *Ovarian*, lung, head & neck, testicular, urothelial, & brain CA, NHL & allogeneic & ABMT in high doses **Acts:** DNA cross-linker; forms DNA-platinum adducts **Dose:** Per protocols based on target (Calvert formula: mg = AUC × [25 + calculated GFR]); adjust based on plt count, CrCl, & BSA (Egorin formula); up to 1500 mg/m² used in ABMT setting (per protocols) **W/P:** [D, ?] Severe hepatic tox **CI:** Severe BM suppression, excessive bleeding **Disp:** Inj 50-, 150-, 450-, 650-mg vial (10 mg/mL) **SE:** Pain, ↓ Na⁺/Mg²⁺/Ca²⁺/K⁺, anaphylaxis, ↓ BM, N/V/D, nephrotox, hematuria, neurotox, ↑ LFTs **Notes:** Physiologic dosing based on Calvert or Egorin formula allows ↑ doses w/ ↓ tox

Carfilzomib (Kyprolis) Uses: *Multiple myeloma w/ > 2 prior therapies and prog w/in 60 d* **Acts:** Proteasome inhib **Dose:** 20 mg/m²/d, if tolerated ↑ to 27 mg/m²/d; IV over 2–10 min; cycle = 2 consecutive d/wk × 3 wk, then 12-d rest; hydrate before and after admin, premedicate w/ dexamethasone 1st cycle, dose escalation, or if infusion reactions **W/P:** [D, –] CHF, cardiac ischemia; pulm HTN, dyspnea; tumor lysis synd; ↓ plts, ✓ plts; hepatic toxicity, ✓ LFTs **CI:** Ø **Disp:** Vial, 60 mg powder **SE:** N/D fever, fatigue, dyspnea, ARF, anemia, ↓ plts, ↓ lymphocytes, ↑ LFTs, peripheral neuropathy

Carisoprodol (Soma) Uses: *Acute (limit 2–3 wk) painful musculoskeletal conditions* **Acts:** Centrally acting muscle relaxant **Dose:** 250–350 mg PO tid-qid **W/P:** [C, M] Tolerance may result; w/ renal/hepatic impair, w/ CYP219 poor metabolizers **CI:** Allergy to meprobamate; acute intermittent porphyria **Disp:** Tabs 250, 350 mg **SE:** CNS depression, drowsiness, dizziness, HA, tachycardia, weakness, rare Sz **Notes:** Avoid EtOH & other CNS depressants; avoid abrupt D/C; available in combo w/ ASA or codeine

Carmustine [BCNU] (BiCNU, Gliadel) BOX: BM suppression, dose-related pulm tox possible; administer under direct supervision of experienced physician Uses: *Primary or adjunct brain tumors, multiple myeloma, Hodgkin and non-Hodgkin lymphomas*, induction for autologous stem cell or BMT (off label) surgery & RT adjunct high-grade glioma and recurrent glioblastoma (Gliadel implant) **Acts:** Alkylating agent; nitrosourea forms DNA cross-links to inhibit DNA **Dose:** 150–200 mg/m² q6–8wk single or ÷ dose daily Inj over 2 d; 20–65 mg/m² q4–6wk; 300–600 mg/m² in BMT (per protocols); up to 8 implants in CNS op site; ↓ w/ hepatic & renal impair **W/P:** [D, ?/–] ↓ WBC, RBC, plt counts, renal/hepatic impair **CI:** ↓ BM, PRG **Disp:** Inj 100 mg/vial; Gliadel wafer 7.7 mg **SE:** Inf Rxn, ↓ BP, N/V, ↓ WBC & plt, phlebitis, facial flushing, hepatic/renal dysfunction, pulm fibrosis (may occur years after), optic neuroretinitis; heme tox may persist 4–6 wk after dose **Notes:** Do not give course more frequently than q6wk (cumulative tox); ✓ baseline PFTs, monitor pulm status

Carteolol Ophthalmic (Generic) Uses: *↑ IOP pressure, chronic open-angle glaucoma* **Acts:** Blocks β-adrenergic receptors (β₁, β₂), mild ISA **Dose:** Ophthal 1 gtt in eye(s) bid **W/P:** [C, ?/–] Cardiac failure, asthma **CI:** Sinus bradycardia; heart block > 1st degree; bronchospasm **Disp:** Ophthal soln 1 % **SE:** Conjunctival hyperemia, anisocoria, keratitis, eye pain **Notes:** Oral forms no longer available in US

Carvedilol (Coreg, Coreg CR) Uses: *HTN, mild–severe CHF, LVD post-MI* **Acts:** Blocks adrenergic receptors, β₁, β₂, α₁ **Dose:** HTN: 6.25–12.5 mg bid or CR 20–80 mg PO daily. CHF: 3.125–50 mg bid; 50 mg max if > 85 kg; 25 mg max if < 85 kg; w/ food to minimize orthostatic ↓ BP **W/P:** [C, ?/–] asthma, DM **CI:** Decompensated CHF, 2nd-/3rd-degree heart block, SSS, severe ↓ HR w/o pacemaker, acute asthma, severe hepatic impair **Disp:** Tabs 3.125, 6.25, 12.5, 25 mg; CR tabs 10, 20, 40, 80 mg **SE:** Dizziness, fatigue, hyperglycemia, may mask/potentiate hypoglycemia, ↓ HR, edema, hypercholesterolemia **Notes:** Do not D/C abruptly; ↑ digoxin levels

Caspofungin (Cancidas) **Uses:** *Invasive aspergillosis refractory/intolerant to standard Rx, candidemia & other candida Inf*, empiric Rx in febrile neutropenia w/ presumed fungal Infxn **Acts:** Echinocandin; ↓ fungal cell wall synth; highest activity in regions of active cell growth **Dose:** 70 mg IV load d 1, 50 mg/d IV; slow Inf over 1 h; ↓ in hepatic impair **W/P:** [C, ?/–] Do not use w/ cyclosporine **CI:** Allergy to any component **Disp:** Inj 50, 70 mg powder for recons **SE:** Fever, HA, N/V, thrombophlebitis at site, ↑ LFTs ↓ BP, edema, ↑ HR, rash, ↓ K, D, Inf Rxn **Notes:** Monitor during Inf; limited experience beyond 2 wk of Rx

Cefaclor (Generic) **Uses:** *Bacterial Infxns of the upper & lower resp tract, skin, bone, urinary tract* **Acts:** 2nd-gen cephalosporin; ↓ cell wall synth. *Spectrum:* More gram(–) activity than 1st-gen cephalosporins; effective against gram(+) (*Streptococcus* sp, *S. aureus*); good gram(–) against *H. influenzae, E. coli, Klebsiella, Proteus* **Dose:** *Adults.* 250–500 mg PO q8h; 375, 500 mg ER q12h. *Peds.* 20–40 mg/kg/d PO ÷ 8–12 h; ↓ renal impair **W/P:** [B, M] **CI:** Cephalosporin/PCN allergy **Disp:** Caps 250, 500 mg; tabs ER 500 mg; susp 125, 250, 375 mg/5 mL **SE:** N/D, rash, eosinophilia, ↑ LFTs, HA, rhinitis, vaginitis

Cefadroxil (Duricef, Generic) **Uses:** *Infxns skin, bone, upper & lower resp tract, urinary tract* **Acts:** 1st-gen cephalosporin; ↓ cell wall synth. *Spectrum:* Good gram(+) (group A β-hemolytic *Streptococcus, Staphylococcus*); gram(–) (*E. coli, Proteus, Klebsiella*) **Dose:** *Adults.* 1–2 g/d PO, 2 ÷ doses *Peds.* 30 mg/kg/d ÷ bid; ↓ in renal impair **W/P:** [B, M] **CI:** Cephalosporin/PCN allergy **Disp:** Caps 500 mg; tabs 1 g; susp, 250, 500 mg/5 mL **SE:** N/V/D, rash, eosinophilia, ↑ LFTs

Cefazolin (Generic) **Uses:** *Infxns of skin, bone, upper & lower resp tract, urinary tract* **Acts:** 1st-gen cephalosporin; β-lactam ↓ cell wall synth. *Spectrum:* Good gram(+) bacilli & cocci (*Streptococcus, Staphylococcus* [except *Enterococcus*]); some gram(–) (*E. coli, Proteus, Klebsiella*) **Dose:** *Adults.* 1–2 g IV q8h *Peds.* 25–100 mg/kg/d IV ÷ q6–8h; ↓ in renal impair **W/P:** [B, M] **CI:** Cephalosporin/PCN allergy **Disp:** Inj, powder, soln **SE:** D, rash, eosinophilia, ↑ LFTs, Inj site pain **Notes:** Widely used for surgical prophylaxis

Cefdinir (Omnicef) **Uses:** *Infxns of the resp tract, skin, and skin structure* **Acts:** 3rd-gen cephalosporin; ↓ cell wall synth *Spectrum:* Many gram(+) & (–) organisms; more active than cefaclor & cephalexin against *Streptococcus, Staphylococcus*; some anaerobes **Dose:** *Adults.* 300 mg PO bid or 600 mg/d PO *Peds.* 7 mg/kg PO bid or 14 mg/kg/d PO; ↓ in renal impair **W/P:** [B, M] w/ PCN-sensitive pts **CI:** Hypersens to cephalosporins **Disp:** Caps 300 mg; susp 125, 250 mg/5 mL **SE:** Anaphylaxis, D, rare pseudomembranous colitis, HA

Cefditoren (Spectracef) **Uses:** *Acute exacerbations of chronic bronchitis, pharyngitis, tonsillitis; skin Infxns* **Acts:** 3rd-gen cephalosporin; ↓ cell wall synth. *Spectrum:* Good gram(+) (*Streptococcus & Staphylococcus*); gram(–) (*H. influenzae & M. catarrhalis*) **Dose:** *Adults & Peds > 12 y. Skin Infxn, pharyngitis, tonsillitis:*

200 mg PO bid × 10 d *Chronic bronchitis:* 400 mg PO bid × 10 d; avoid antacids w/in 2 h; take w/ meals; ↓ in renal impair **W/P:** [B, ?] Renal/hepatic impair **CI:** Cephalosporin/PCN allergy, milk protein, or carnitine deficiency **Disp:** Tabs 200, 400 mg **SE:** HA, N/V/D, colitis, nephrotox, hepatic dysfunction, SJS, toxic epidermal necrolysis, allergic Rxns **Notes:** Causes renal excretion of carnitine; tabs contain milk protein

Cefepime (Maxipime, Generic) Uses: *Comp/uncomp UTI, pneumonia, empiric febrile neutropenia, skin/soft-tissue Infxns, comp intra-Abd Infxns* **Acts:** 4th-gen cephalosporin; ↓ cell wall synth. *Spectrum:* Gram(+) *S. pneumoniae, S. aureus,* gram(−) *K. pneumoniae, E. coli, P. aeruginosa,* & *Enterobacter* sp **Dose:** *Adults.* 1–2 g IV q8–12h. *Peds.* 50 mg/kg q8h for febrile neutropenia; 50 mg/kg bid for skin/soft-tissue Infxns; ↓ in renal impair **W/P:** [B, +] Sz risk w/ CrCl < 60 mL/min; adjust dose w/ renal Insuff **CI:** Cephalosporin/PCN allergy **Disp:** Inj 500 mg, 1, 2 g **SE:** Rash, pruritus, N/V/D, fever, HA, (+) Coombs test w/o hemolysis **Notes:** Can give IM or IV; concern over ↑ death rates not confirmed by FDA

Cefixime (Suprax, Generic) Uses: *Resp tract, skin, bone, & urinary tract Infxns* **Acts:** 3rd-gen cephalosporin; ↓ cell wall synth. *Spectrum: S. pneumoniae, S. pyogenes, H. influenzae,* & *enterobacteria* **Dose:** *Adults.* 400 mg PO ÷ daily-bid. *Peds.* 8 mg/kg/d PO ÷ daily-bid; ↓ w/ renal impair **W/P:** [B, ?] **CI:** Cephalosporin/PCN allergy **Disp:** Tabs 400 mg; chew tabs 100, 200 mg; susp 100, 200 mg/5 mL **SE:** N/V/D, flatulence, & Abd pain **Notes:** ✓Renal & hepatic Fxn; use susp for otitis media

Cefotaxime (Claforan, Generic) Uses: *Infxns of lower resp tract, skin, bone & jt, urinary tract, meningitis, sepsis, PID, GC* **Acts:** 3rd-gen cephalosporin; ↓ cell wall synth. *Spectrum:* Most gram(−) (not *Pseudomonas*), some gram(+) cocci *S. pneumoniae, S. aureus* (penicillinase/nonpenicillinase producing), *H. influenzae* (including ampicillin-resistant), not *Enterococcus*; many PCN-resistant pneumococci **Dose:** *Adults. Uncomplicated Infxn:* 1 g IV/IM q12h; *Mod-severe Infxn:* 1–2 g IV/IM q8–12 h; *Severe/septicemia:* 2 g IV/IM q4–8h; *GC urethritis, cervicitis, rectal in female:* 0.5 g IM × 1; *Rectal GC in men:* 1 g IM × 1 *Peds.* 50–200 mg/kg/d IV ÷ q6–8h; ↓ w/ renal/hepatic impair **W/P:** [B, +] Arrhythmia w/ rapid Inj; w/ colitis **CI:** Cephalosporin/PCN allergy **Disp:** Powder for Inj 500 mg, 1, 2, 10 g; premixed Inf 20, 40 mg/mL **SE:** D, rash, pruritus, colitis, eosinophilia, ↑ transaminases

Cefotetan (Generic) Uses: *Infxns of the upper & lower resp tract, skin, bone, urinary tract, Abd, & gynecologic system* **Acts:** 2nd-gen cephalosporin; ↓ cell wall synth *Spectrum:* Less active against gram(+) anaerobes including *B. fragilis;* gram(−), including *E. coli, Klebsiella,* & *Proteus* **Dose:** 1–3 g IV q12h. *Peds.* 20–40 mg/kg/dose IV ÷ q12h (6 g/d max) ↓ w/ renal impair **W/P:** [B, +] May ↑ bleeding risk; w/ Hx of PCN allergies; w/ other nephrotoxic drugs **CI:** Cephalosporin/PCN allergy **Disp:** Powder for Inj 1, 2, 10 g **SE:** D, rash, eosinophilia, ↑ transaminases, hypoprothrombinemia, & bleeding (d/t MTT side chain) **Notes:** May interfere w/ warfarin

Cefoxitin (Mefoxin, Generic) Uses: *Infxns of the upper & lower resp tract, skin, bone, urinary tract, Abd, & gynecologic system* Acts: 2nd-gen cephalosporin; ↓ cell wall synth. *Spectrum:* Good gram(−) against enteric bacilli (i.e., *E. coli, Klebsiella,* & *Proteus*); anaerobic: *B. fragilis* Dose: *Adults.* 1–2 g IV q6–8h. *Peds.* 80–160 mg/kg/d ÷ q4–6h (12 g/d max); ↓ w/ renal impair W/P: [B, M] CI: Cephalosporin/PCN allergy Disp: Powder for Inj 1, 2, 10 g SE: D, rash, eosinophilia, ↑ transaminases

Cefpodoxime (Generic) Uses: *Rx resp, skin, & urinary tract Infxns* Acts: 3rd-gen cephalosporin; ↓ cell wall synth. *Spectrum: S. pneumoniae* or non–β-lactamase–producing *H. influenzae;* acute uncomplicated *N. gonorrhoeae;* some uncomplicated gram(−) (*E. coli, Klebsiella, Proteus*) Dose: *Adults.* 100–400 mg PO q12h *Peds.* 10 mg/kg/d PO ÷ bid; ↓ in renal impair; w/ food W/P: [B, M] CI: Cephalosporin/PCN allergy Disp: Tabs 100, 200 mg; susp 50, 100 mg/5 mL SE: D, rash, HA, eosinophilia, ↑ transaminases Notes: Drug interactions w/ agents that ↑ gastric pH

Cefprozil (Generic) Uses: *Rx resp tract, skin, & urinary tract Infxns* Acts: 2nd-gen cephalosporin; ↓ cell wall synth. *Spectrum:* Active against MSSA, *Streptococcus,* & gram(−) bacilli (*E. coli, Klebsiella, P. mirabilis, H. influenzae,* Moraxella) Dose: *Adults.* 250–500 mg PO daily-bid *Peds.* 7.5–15 mg/kg/d PO ÷ bid; ↓ in renal impair W/P: [B, M] CI: Cephalosporin/PCN allergy Disp: Tabs 250, 500 mg; susp 125, 250 mg/5 mL SE: D, dizziness, rash, eosinophilia, ↑ transaminases Notes: Use higher doses for otitis & pneumonia

Ceftaroline (Teflaro) Uses: *Tx skin/skin structure Infxn & CAP* Acts: Unclassified ("5th-gen") cephalosporin; ↓ cell wall synthesis; *Spectrum:* Gram(+) *Staph aureus* (MSSA/MRSA), *Strep pyogenes, Strep agalactiae, Strep pneumoniae;* Gram(−) *E. coli, K. pneumoniae, K. oxytoca, H. influenzae* Dose: 600 mg IV q12h; CrCl 30–50 mL/min: 400 mg IV q12h CrCl 15–29 mL/min: 300 mg IV q12h; CrCl < 15 mL/min: 200 mg IV q12h; Inf over 1 h W/P: [B, ?/−] monitor for *C. difficile*-associated D CI: Cephalsporin sensitivity Disp: Inj 600 mg SE: Hypersens Rxn, D/N, rash, constipation, ↓ K⁺, phlebitis, ↑ LFTs

Ceftazidime (Fortaz, Tazicef, Generic) Uses: *Rx resp tract, skin, bone, urinary tract Infxns, meningitis, & septicemia* Acts: 3rd-gen cephalosporin; ↓ cell wall synth. *Spectrum: P. aeruginosa* sp, good gram(−) activity Dose: *Adults.* 500–2 g IV/IM q8–12h *Peds.* 30–50 mg/kg/dose IV q8h, 6g/d max; ↓ renal impair W/P: [B, +] PCN sensitivity CI: Cephalosporin/PCN allergy Disp: Powder for Inj 500 mg; 1, 2, 6 g SE: D, rash, eosinophilia, ↑ transaminases Notes: Use only for proven or strongly suspected Infxn to ↓ development of drug resistance

Ceftazidime/Avibactam (Avycaz) Uses: *Complicated intra-Abd Infxn w/ metronidazole; complicated UTI* Acts: β-lactam antibiotic/β-lactamase inhib Dose: *Adults.* 2.5 g w/ CrCl > 50 mL/min; CKD adjust (see PI) W/P: [B, M] Anaphylaxis, serious skin Rxn, *C.difficile* Infxn, Sz w/ renal impair, ↓ efficacy w /CrCl

30-50 mL/min, ✓ CrCl qd **CI:** Component hypersens **Disp:** Single vial, 2 g ceftazidime/0.5 g avibactam **SE:** N/V, constipation, anxiety **Notes:** Inf over 2 h

Ceftibuten (Cedax, Generic) Uses: *Rx resp tract, skin, urinary tract Infxns, & otitis media* **Acts:** 3rd-gen cephalosporin; ↓ cell wall synth. *Spectrum: H. influenzae & M. catarrhalis*; weak against *S. pneumoniae* **Dose: Adults.** 400 mg/d PO **Peds.** 9 mg/kg/d PO; ↓ in renal impair; take on empty stomach (susp) **W/P:** [B, +/−] **CI:** Cephalosporin/PCN allergy **Disp:** Caps 400 mg; susp 90 mg/5 mL **SE:** D, rash, eosinophilia, ↑ transaminases

Ceftolozane/Tazobactam (Zerbaxa) Uses: *Complicated intra-Abd Infxn/UTI* **Acts:** Unclassified ("5th-gen") cephalosporin, ↓ cell wall synth (C); ↓ bacterial β-lactamases (T) *Spectrum: Enterobacter cloacae, E. coli, K. oxytoca, K. pneumoniae, P. mirabilis, P. aeruginosa, B. fragilis, Streptococcus anginosus/constellatus/salivarius* **Dose:** Intra-Abd Infxn: 1.5 g q8h × 4–14 d IV w/ metronidazole 500 mg IV q8h; UTI: 1.5 g q8h IV × 7 d; adjust w/ ↓ renal fxn **W/P:** [B, ?] ↓ Efficacy w/ CrCl 30–50 mL/min; monitor CrCl **CI:** Cephalosporin/PCN/tazobactam allergy; allergy **Disp:** 1.5-g powder vials: 1 g ceftolozane/0.5 g tazobactam **SE:** HA, N/D, fever **Notes:** Combo product; dose expressed as g of combo

Ceftriaxone (Rocephin, Generic) **BOX:** Avoid in hyperbilirubinemic neonates or co-infusion w/ calcium-containing products Uses: *Resp tract (pneumonia); skin, bone, Abd, & urinary tract Infxns; septicemia; GC; PID; perioperative* **Acts:** 3rd-gen cephalosporin; ↓ cell wall synth. *Spectrum:* Mod gram(+); excellent β-lactamase producers **Dose: Adults.** 1–2 g IV/IM q12–24h **Peds.** 50–100 mg/kg/d IV/IM ÷ q12–24h **W/P:** [B, +] **CI:** Cephalosporin allergy; hyperbilirubinemic neonates **Disp:** Powder for Inj 250 mg, 500 mg, 1, 2, 10 g; premixed 20, 40 mg/mL **SE:** D, rash, ↑ WBC, thrombocytosis, eosinophilia, ↑ LFTs

Cefuroxime, Oral (Ceftin), Parenteral (Zinacef) Uses: *Upper & lower resp tract, skin, bone, urinary tract, Abd, gynecologic Infxns* **Acts:** 2nd-gen cephalosporin; ↓ cell wall synth. *Spectrum:* Staphylococci, group B streptococci, *H. influenzae, E. coli, Enterobacter, Salmonella, & Klebsiella* **Dose: Adults.** 750 mg–1.5 g IV q8h or 250–500 mg PO bid **Peds.** 75–150 mg/kg/d IV ÷ q8h or 20–30 mg/kg/d PO ÷ bid; ↓ w/ renal impair; take PO w/ food **W/P:** [B, +] **CI:** Cephalosporin/PCN allergy **Disp:** Tabs 250, 500 mg; susp 125, 250 mg/5 mL; powder for Inj 750 mg, 1.5, 7.5 g **SE:** D, rash, eosinophilia, ↑ LFTs **Notes:** Cefuroxime film-coated tabs & susp not bioequivalent; do not substitute on a mg/mg basis; IV crosses blood–brain barrier

Celecoxib (Celebrex, Generic) **BOX:** ↑ Risk of serious CV thrombotic events, MI, & stroke; can be fatal: ↑ risk of serious GI adverse events including bleeding, ulceration, & perforation of the stomach or intestines; can be fatal Uses: *OA, RA, ankylosing spondylitis, acute pain, primary dysmenorrhea, preventive in FAP* **Acts:** NSAID; ↓ COX-2 pathway **Dose: Adults.** 100–200 mg/d or bid; *FAP:* 400 mg PO bid **Peds > 2 y.** 10–25 kg 50 mg PO bid; >25 kg 100 mg PO bid; ↓ w/ hepatic impair; take w/ food/milk **W/P:** [C/D (3rd tri), ?] w/ Renal impair; ↑ risk of MI/CVA **CI:** Sulfonamide allergy, perioperative CABG **Disp:** Caps 50, 100, 200, 400 mg **SE:** See Box; GI upset, HTN, edema, renal failure, HA **Notes:** Watch for Sxs of GI bleeding; no effect on plt/bleeding time; can affect drugs metabolized by P450 pathway

Centruroides (Scorpion) Immune F(ab')₂ (Anascorp) Uses: *Antivenom for scorpion envenomation w/ symptoms* **Acts:** IgG, bind/neutralize *Centruroides sculpturatus* toxin **Dose: *Adults & Peds.*** 3 vials, recons w/ 5 mL NS, combine all 3, dilute to 50 mL, Inf IV over 10 min; additional 1 vial q 30–60 min PRN Sx **W/P:** [C, M] Hypersens, especially w/ Hx equine protein Rxn **CI:** Ø **Disp:** Vial **SE:** Fever, N/V, pruritus, rash, myalgias, serum sickness **Notes:** Use only w/ important Sx (loss of muscle control, abn eye movements, slurred speech, resp distress, salivation, V); may contain infectious agents

Cephalexin (Keflex, Generic) Uses: *Skin, bone, upper/lower resp tract (streptococcal pharyngitis), otitis media, uncomp cystitis Infxns* **Acts:** 1st-gen cephalosporin; ↓ cell wall synth. *Spectrum: Streptococcus* (including β-hemolytic), *Staphylococcus, E. coli, Proteus, & Klebsiella* **Dose: *Adults & Peds > 15 y.*** 250–1000 mg PO qid; Rx cystitis 7–14 d (4 g/d max). *Peds < 15 y.* 25–100 mg/kg/d PO ÷ bid-qid; ↓ in renal impair; w/ or w/o food **W/P:** [B, +] **CI:** Cephalosporin/PCN allergy **Disp:** Caps 250, 500 mg; susp 125, 250 mg; susp 125, 250 mg/5 mL **SE:** D, rash, eosinophilia, gastritis, dyspepsia, ↑ LFTs, *C. difficile* colitis, vaginitis

Certolizumab Pegol (Cimzia) BOX: Serious Infxns (bacterial, fungal, TB, opportunistic) possible; D/C w/ severe Infxn/sepsis, test and monitor for TB w/ Tx; lymphoma/other CA possible in children/adolescents **Uses:** *Crohn Dz w/ inadequate response to conventional Tx; mod–severe RA* **Acts:** TNF-α blocker **Dose:** *Crohn:* Initial: 400 mg SQ, repeat 2 & 4 wk after; maint: 400 mg SQ q4wk. *RA:* Initial: 400 mg SQ, repeat 2 & 4 wk after; maint: 200 mg SQ q other wk or 400 mg SQ q4wk **W/P:** [B, ?] Infxn, TB, autoimmune Dz, demyelinating CNS Dz, hep B reactivation **CI:** Ø **Disp:** Inj powder for reconstitution 200 mg; Inj soln 200 mg/mL (1 mL) **SE:** HA, N, URI, serious Infxns, TB, opportunistic Infxns, malignancies, demyelinating Dz, CHF, pancytopenia, lupus-like synd, new-onset psoriasis **Notes:** 400-mg dose: 2 Inj of 200 mg each; monitor for Infxn; do not give live/attenuated vaccines during Rx; avoid use w/ anakinra

Cetirizine (Zyrtec, Zyrtec D, Generic) [OTC] Uses: *Allergic rhinitis & other allergic Sxs, including urticaria* **Acts:** Nonsedating antihistamine; *Zyrtec D* contains decongestant **Dose: *Adults & Peds > 6 y.*** 5–10 mg/d; *Zyrtec D* 5/120 mg PO bid whole *Peds 6–11 mo.* 2.5 mg daily *12 mo–5 y.* 2.5 mg daily-bid; ↓ to qd in renal/hepatic impair **W/P:** [C, ?/–] w/ HTN, BPH, rare CNS stimulation, DM, heart Dz **CI:** Allergy to cetirizine, hydroxyzine **Disp:** Tabs 5, 10 mg; chew tabs 5, 10 mg; syrup 5 mg/5 mL; *Zyrtec D:* Tabs 5/120 mg (cetirizine/pseudoephedrine) **SE:** HA, drowsiness, xerostomia **Notes:** Can cause sedation; swallow ER tabs whole

Cetuximab (Erbitux) **BOX:** Severe Inf Rxns, including rapid onset of airway obst (bronchospasm, stridor, hoarseness), urticaria, & ↓ BP; permanent D/C required; ↑ risk sudden death and cardiopulmonary arrest **Uses:** *EGFR + metastatic colorectal CA w/ or w/o irinotecan, unresectable head/neck small-cell carcinoma w/ RT; monotherapy in metastatic head/neck CA* **Acts:** Human/mouse recombinant MoAb; binds EGFR, ↓ tumor cell growth **Dose:** (per protocol) Load 400 mg/m² IV over 2 h; 250 mg/m² given over 1 h weekly **W/P:** [C, –] **Disp:** Inj 100 mg/50 mL, 200 mg/100 mL **SE:** Acneiform rash, asthenia/malaise, N/V/D, Abd pain, alopecia, Inf Rxn, derm tox, interstitial lung Dz, fever, sepsis, dehydration, kidney failure, PE **Notes:** Assess tumor for EGFR before Rx; pretreatment w/ diphenhydramine; w/ mild SE ↓ Inf rate by 50%; limit sun exposure

Charcoal, Activated (Actidose-Aqua, CharcoCaps, EZ Char, Kerr Insta-Char, Requa Activated Charcoal) **Uses:** *Emergency poisoning by most drugs & chemicals (see CI)* **Acts:** Adsorbent detoxicant **Dose:** Give w/ 70% sorbitol (2 mL/kg); repeated use of sorbitol not OK **Adults.** *Acute intoxication:* 25–100 g/dose. *GI dialysis:* 20–50 g q6h for 1–2 d **Peds 1–12 y.** *Acute intoxication:* 1–2 g/kg/dose **W/P:** [C, ?] May cause V (hazardous w/ petroleum & caustic ingestions); do not mix w/ dairy **CI:** Not effective for cyanide, mineral acids, caustic alkalis, organic solvents, iron, EtOH, methanol poisoning, Li; do not use sorbitol in pts w/ fructose intolerance, intestinal obst, nonintact GI tracts **Disp:** Powder, liq, caps, tabs **SE:** Some liq dosage forms in sorbitol base (a cathartic); V/D, black stools, constipation **Notes:** Charcoal w/ sorbitol not OK in children < 1 y; monitor for ↓ K⁺ & Mg²⁺; protect airway in lethargic/comatose pts

Chlorambucil (Leukeran) **BOX:** Myelosuppressive, carcinogenic, teratogenic, associated w/ infertility **Uses:** *CLL, Hodgkin Dz*, Waldenström macroglobulinemia **Acts:** Alkylating agent (nitrogen mustard) **Dose:** (per protocol) 0.1–0.2 mg/kg/d for 3–6 wk or 0.4 mg/kg/dose q2wk; ↓ w/ renal impair **W/P:** [D, ?] Sz disorder & BM suppression; affects human fertility **CI:** Previous resistance; alkylating agent allergy; w/ live vaccines **Disp:** Tabs 2 mg **SE:** ↓ BM, CNS stimulation, N/V, drug fever, rash, secondary leukemias, alveolar dysplasia, pulm fibrosis, hepatotoxic **Notes:** Monitor LFTs, CBC, plts, serum uric acid; ↓ dose if pt has received radiation

Chlordiazepoxide (Generic) [C-IV] **Uses:** *Anxiety, tension, EtOH withdrawal*, & preop apprehension **Acts:** Benzodiazepine; antianxiety agent **Dose:** **Adults.** *Mild anxiety:* 5–10 mg PO tid-qid or PRN. *Severe anxiety:* 25–50 mg PO q6–8h or PRN **Peds > 6 y.** 5 mg PO q6–8h; ↓ in renal impair, elderly **W/P:** [D, ?] Resp depression, CNS impair, Hx of drug dependence; avoid in hepatic impair **CI:** Preexisting CNS depression, NAG **Disp:** Caps 5, 10, 25 mg **SE:** Drowsiness, CP, rash, fatigue, memory impair, xerostomia, Wt gain **Notes:** Erratic IM absorption

Chlorothiazide (Diuril) **Uses:** *HTN, edema* **Acts:** Thiazide diuretic **Dose:** **Adults.** 500 mg–1 g PO daily-bid; 500–1000 mg/d IV (for edema only) **Peds > 6 mo.** 10–20 mg/kg/24 h PO ÷ bid; 4 mg/kg ÷ daily bio IV; OK w/ food **W/P:** [C, +]

CI: Sens to thiazides/sulfonamides, anuria **Disp:** Tabs 250, 500 mg; susp 250 mg/5 mL; Inj 500 mg/vial **SE:** ↓ K+, Na+, dizziness, hyperglycemia, hyperuricemia, hyperlipidemia, photosens **Notes:** Do not use IM/SQ; take early in the day to avoid nocturia; use sunblock; monitor lytes

Chlorpheniramine (Chlor-Trimeton, Others) [OTC] **BOX:** OTC meds w/ chlorpheniramine should not be used in peds < 2 y **Uses:** *Allergic rhinitis*, common cold **Acts:** Antihistamine **Dose:** *Adults & Peds > 12 y.* 4 mg PO q4–6h or 8–12 mg PO bid of SR 24 mg/d max *Peds.* *2–5 y:* 1 mg q4–6h, max 6 mg/24 h; *6–11 y.* 2mg q4–6h, max 12 mg/24hr; > *12 y* adult dosing **W/P:** [C, ?/–] BOO; NAG; hepatic Insuff **CI:** Allergy **Disp:** Tabs 4 mg; SR tabs 12 mg **SE:** Anticholinergic SE & sedation common, postural ↓ BP, QT changes, extrapyramidal Rxns, photosens **Notes:** Do not cut/crush/chew ER forms; deaths in pts < 2 y associated w/ cough and cold meds [*MMWR* 2007;56(1):1–4]

Chlorpromazine (Thorazine) **Uses:** *Psychotic disorders, N/V*, apprehension, intractable hiccups **Acts:** Phenothiazine antipsychotic; antiemetic **Dose:** *Adults.* *Psychosis:* 30–800 mg/d in 1–4 ÷ doses, start low dose, ↑ PRN; typical 200–600 mg/d; 1–2 g/d may be needed in some cases. *Severe Sxs:* 25 mg IM/IV initial; may repeat in 1–4 h, then 25–50 mg PO or PR tid. *Hiccups:* 25–50 mg PO tid-qid. *Peds > 6 mo.* *Psychosis & N/V:* 0.5–1 mg/kg/dose PO q4–6h or IM/IV q6–8h **W/P:** [C, ?/–] Safety in children < 6 mo not established; Szs, avoid w/ hepatic impair, BM suppression **CI:** Sensitivity w/ phenothiazines; NAG **Disp:** Tabs 10, 25, 50, 100, 200 mg; Inj 25 mg/mL **SE:** Extrapyramidal SE & sedation; α-adrenergic blocking properties; ↓ BP; ↑ QT interval **Notes:** Do not D/C abruptly

Chlorpropamide (Diabinese, Generic) **Uses:** *Type 2 DM* **Acts:** Sulfonylurea; ↑ pancreatic insulin release; ↑ peripheral insulin sensitivity; ↓ hepatic glucose output **Dose:** 100–500 mg/d; w/ food, ↓ hepatic impair **W/P:** [C, ?/–] CrCl < 50 mL/min; ↓ in hepatic impair **CI:** Cross-sens w/ sulfonamides **Disp:** Tabs 100, 250 mg **SE:** HA, dizziness, rash, photosens, hypoglycemia, SIADH **Notes:** Avoid EtOH (disulfiram-like Rxn)

Chlorthalidone **Uses:** *HTN* **Acts:** Thiazide diuretic **Dose:** *Adults.* 25–100 mg PO daily *Peds.* (Not approved) 0.3–2 mg/kg/dose PO 3×/wk or 1–2 mg/kg/d PO; ↓ in renal impair; OK w/ food, milk **W/P:** [B, +] **CI:** Cross-sens w/ thiazides or sulfonamides; anuria **Disp:** Tabs 25, 50, 100 mg **SE:** ↓ K+, dizziness, photosens, ↑ glucose, hyperuricemia, sexual dysfunction

Chlorzoxazone (Parafon Forte DSC, Others) **Uses:** *Adjunct to rest & physical therapy Rx to relieve discomfort associated w/ acute, painful musculoskeletal conditions* **Acts:** Centrally acting skeletal muscle relaxant **Dose:** *Adults.* 500–750 mg PO tid–qid. *Peds.* 20 mg/kg/d in 3–4 ÷ doses **W/P:** [C, ?] Avoid EtOH & CNS depressants **CI:** Severe liver Dz **Disp:** Tabs 250, 375, 500, 750 mg **SE:** Drowsiness, tachycardia, dizziness, hepatotox, angioedema

Cholecalciferol [Vitamin D₃] (Delta D, Many Others) **Uses:** *Dietary supl to Rx vit D deficiency* **Acts:** ↑ intestinal Ca^{2+} absorption **Dose:** Institute of

Medicine RDA. *Adults ≤ 70 y. & Peds >1 y.* 600 Int units *Adults > 71 y.* 800 IU **PRG/lactating** ♀. 600 Int units; *Peds 0–12 mo.* 400 Int units. Severe deficiency may require higher dosing of 50,000 Int units qwk × 8 wk, then 1500–200 Int units daily PO **W/P:** [A (D doses above the RDA), +] **CI:** ↑ Ca²⁺, hypervitaminosis, allergy **Disp:** Tabs 400, 1000 Int units **SE:** Vit D tox (renal failure, HTN, psychosis) **Notes:** 1 mg cholecalciferol = 40,000 Int units vit D activity

Cholestyramine (Prevalite, Questran, Questran Light) Uses: *Hypercholesterolemia; hyperlipidemia, pruritus associated w/ partial biliary obst; D associated w/ excess fecal bile acids* pseudomembranous colitis, dig tox, hyperoxaluria **Acts:** Binds intestinal bile acids, forms insoluble complexes **Dose: Adults.** Titrate: 4 g/d-bid, ↑ to max 24 g/d ÷ 1–6 doses/d *Peds.* 240 mg/kg/d in 2–3 ÷ doses, max 8 g/d **W/P:** [C, ?] Constipation, phenylketonuria, may interfere w/ other drug absorption; consider supl w/ fat-soluble vits **CI:** Complete biliary or bowel obst; w/ mycophenolate hyperlipoproteinemia types III, IV, V **Disp:** (*Prevalite*) w/ aspartame: 4 g resin/5.5 g powder; (*Questran*) 4 g cholestyramine resin/9 g powder; (*Questran Light*) 4 g resin/5 g powder **SE:** Constipation, Abd pain, bloating, HA, rash, vit K deficiency **Notes:** OD may cause GI obst; mix 4 g in 2–6 oz of noncarbonated beverage; take other meds 1–2 h before or 6 h after; ✓ lipids

Ciclesonide, Inh (Alvesco) Uses: *Asthma maint* **Acts:** Inh steroid **Dose: Adults & Peds > 12 y. On bronchodilators alone:** 80 mcg bid (320 mcg/d max) *Inhaled corticosteroids:* 80 mcg bid (640 mcg/d max) *On oral corticosteroids:* 320 mcg bid (640 mcg/d max) **W/P:** [C, ?] **CI:** Status asthmaticus or other acute episodes of asthma, hypersens **Disp:** Inh 80, 160 mcg/actuation (60 doses) **SE:** HA, nasopharyngitis, sinusitis, pharyngolaryngeal pain, URI, arthralgia, nasal congestion **Notes:** Oral *Candida* risk, rinse mouth and spit after, taper systemic steroids slowly when transferring to ciclesonide, monitor growth in peds, counsel on use of device, clean mouthpiece weekly

Ciclesonide, Nasal (Omnaris, Zettona) Uses: *Allergic rhinitis* **Acts:** Nasal corticosteroid **Dose: Adults & Peds > 12 y. Omnaris** 2 sprays (max 200 mcg/d) *Zettona* 1 spray each nostril 1 ×/d (max 74 mcg/d) **W/P:** [C, ?/–] w/ ketoconazole; monitor peds for growth ↓ **CI:** Component allergy **Disp:** Intranasal spray, *Omnaris* 50 mcg/spray (120 doses); *Zettona* 37 mcg/spray (60 doses) **SE:** Adrenal suppression, delayed nasal wound healing, URI, HA, ear pain, epistaxis, ↑ risk viral Dz (eg, chickenpox), delayed growth in children

Ciclopirox (Ciclodan, CNL8, Loprox, Pedipirox-4 Nail Kit, Penlac) Uses: *Tinea pedis, tinea cruris, tinea corporis, cutaneous candidiasis, tinea versicolor, tinea rubrum; onychomycosis w/o lunula involvement* **Acts:** Antifungal antibiotic; cellular depletion of essential substrates &/or ions **Dose: Adults & Peds > 10 y.** Massage into affected area bid. *Onychomycosis:* Apply to nails daily, w/ removal q7d **W/P:** [B, ?] **CI:** Component sens **Disp:** Cream 0.77%, gel 0.77%, topical susp 0.77%, shampoo 1%, nail lacquer 8% **SE:** Pruritus, local irritation, burning **Notes:** D/C w/ irritation; avoid dressings; gel best for athlete's foot; for onychomycosis, re-evaluate if no response after 4 wk

Cidofovir (Vistide)   BOX: Renal impair is the major tox; neutropenia possible, ✓ CBC before dose; follow administration instructions; possible carcinogenic, teratogenic **Uses:** *CMV retinitis w/ HIV* **Acts:** Selective inhib viral DNA synth **Dose:** *Rx:* 5 mg/kg IV over 1 h once/wk × 2 wk w/ probenecid *Maint:* 5 mg/kg IV once/2 wk w/ probenecid (2 g PO 3 h prior to cidofovir, then 1 g PO at 2 h & 8 h after cidofovir); ↓ w/ renal impair **W/P:** [C, –] SCr > 1.5 mg/dL or CrCl < 55 mL/min or urine protein ≥ 100 mg/dL; w/ other nephrotoxic drugs **CI:** Probenecid/sulfa allergy **Disp:** Inj 75 mg/mL **SE:** Renal tox, chills, fever, HA, N/V/D, ↓ plt, ↓ WBC **Notes:** Hydrate w/ NS prior to each Inf

Cilostazol (Pletal)   BOX: PDE III inhib have ↓ survival w/ class III/IV heart failure **Uses:** *↓ Sxs of intermittent claudication* **Acts:** Phosphodiesterase III inhib; ↑ cAMP in plts & blood vessels; vasodilation & inhibit plt aggregation **Dose:** 100 mg PO bid, 1/2 h before or 2 h after breakfast & dinner **W/P:** [C, ?] ↓ dose w/ drugs that inhibit CYP3A4 & CYP2C19 (Table 10, p 356) **CI:** CHF, hemostatic disorders, active bleeding **Disp:** Tabs 50, 100 mg **SE:** HA, palpitation, D

Cimetidine (Tagamet, Tagamet HB 200, Generic [OTC]) Uses: *Duodenal ulcer; ulcer prophylaxis in hypersecretory states (eg, trauma, burns); GERD* **Acts:** H₂-receptor antagonist **Dose:** *Adults. Active ulcer:* 400 mg PO bid or 800 mg hs *Maint:* 400 mg PO hs *GERD:* 300–600 mg PO q6h; maint 800 mg PO hs *Peds Infants.* 10–20 mg/kg/24 h PO *Children.* 20–40 mg/kg/24 h PO ÷ q6h; ↓ w/ renal Insuff & in elderly **W/P:** [B, +] Many drug interactions (P450 system); do not use w/ clopidogrel (↓ effect) **CI:** Component sens **Disp:** Tabs 200 (OTC), 300, 400, 800 mg; liq 300 mg/5 mL **SE:** Dizziness, HA, agitation, ↓ plt, gynecomastia **Notes:** 1 h before or 2 h after antacids; avoid EtOH

Cinacalcet (Sensipar)   Uses: *Secondary hyperparathyroidism in CRF; primary hyperparathyroidism;* ↑ Ca²⁺ in parathyroid carcinoma* **Acts:** ↓ PTH by ↑ calcium-sensing receptor sensitivity **Dose:** *Secondary hyperparathyroidism:* 30 mg PO daily *Parathyroid carcinoma & primary hyperparathyroidism:* 30 mg PO bid; for all indications titrate q2–4wk based on calcium & PTH levels; swallow whole; take w/ food **W/P:** [C, ?/–] Monitor for ↓ CA²⁺; w/ Szs, adjust w/ CYP3A4 inhib (Table 10, p 356) **Disp:** Tabs 30, 60, 90 mg **SE:** N/V/D, myalgia, dizziness, ↓ Ca²⁺ **Notes:** Monitor Ca²⁺, PO₄²⁻, PTH

Ciprofloxacin (Cipro, Cipro XR, Generic)   BOX: ↑ risk of tendonitis and tendon rupture; ↑ risk w/ age > 60, transplant pts **Uses:** *Rx lower resp tract, sinuses, skin & skin structure, bone/joints, complex intra-Abd Infxn (w/ metronidazole); typhoid, infectious D, uncomp GC, anal anthrax, UTI including prostatitis* **Acts:** Quinolone antibiotic; ↓ DNA gyrase *Spectrum:* Broad gram(+) & (–) aerobics; little *Streptococcus;* good *Pseudomonas, E. coli, B. fragilis, P. mirabilis, K. pneumoniae, C. jejuni,* or *Shigella* **Dose:** 250–750 mg PO q12h; XR 500–1000 mg PO q24h; or 200–400 mg IV q12h; ↓ in renal impair **W/P:** [C, ?/–] Children < 18 y; avoid in MG

CI: Component sens; w/ tizanidine **Disp:** Tabs 100, 250, 500, 750 mg; tabs XR 500, 1000 mg; susp 5 g, 10 g/100 mL; Inj 200, 400 mg; premixed piggyback 200, 400 mg/100 mL **SE:** Restlessness, N/V/D, rash, ruptured tendons, ↑ LFTs, peripheral neuropathy, mania, delirium **Notes:** Avoid antacids; reduce/restrict caffeine intake; interactions w/ theophylline, caffeine, sucralfate, warfarin, antacids; most tendon problems in Achilles, rare shoulder and hand

Ciprofloxacin, Ophthalmic (Ciloxan) **Uses:** *Rx & prevention of ocular Infxns (conjunctivitis, blepharitis, corneal abrasions)* **Acts:** Quinolone antibiotic; ↓ DNA gyrase **Dose:** 1–2 gtt in eye(s) q2h while awake for 2 d, then 1–2 gtt q4h while awake for 5 d; oint 1/2-in ribbon in eye tid × 2 d, then bid × 5 d **W/P:** [C, ?/–] **CI:** Component sens **Disp:** Soln 3.5 mg/mL; oint 0.3%, 3.5 g **SE:** Local irritation

Ciprofloxacin, Otic (Cetraxal) **Uses:** *Otitis externa* **Acts:** Quinolone antibiotic; ↓ DNA gyrase. *Spectrum: P. aeruginosa, S. aureus* **Dose:** *Adults & Peds > 1 y.* 0.25 mL in ear(s) q 12 h × 7 d **W/P:** [C, ?/–] **CI:** Component sens **Disp:** Soln 0.2% **SE:** Hypersens Rxn, ear pruritus/pain, HA, fungal superinfection

Ciprofloxacin/Dexamethasone, Otic (Ciprodex Otic) **Uses:** *Otitis externa, otitis media peds* **Acts:** Quinolone antibiotic; ↓ DNA gyrase; w/ steroid **Dose:** *Adults.* 4 gtt in ear(s) bid × 7 d *Peds > 6 mo.* 4 gtt in ear(s) bid for 7 d **W/P:** [C, ?/–] **CI:** Viral ear Infxns **Disp:** Susp ciprofloxacin 0.3% & dexamethasone 1% **SE:** Ear discomfort Notes: OK w/ tympanostomy tubes

Ciprofloxacin/Hydrocortisone, Otic (Cipro HC Otic) **Uses:** *Otitis externa* **Acts:** Quinolone antibiotic; ↓ DNA gyrase; w/ steroid **Dose:** *Adults & Peds > 1 y.* 3 gtt in ear(s) bid × 7 d **W/P:** [C, ?/–] **CI:** Perforated tympanic membrane, viral Infxns of the external canal **Disp:** Susp ciprofloxacin 0.2% & hydrocortisone 1% **SE:** HA, pruritus

Cisplatin (Platinol, Platinol AQ) **BOX:** Anaphylactic-like Rxn, ototox, cumulative renal tox; doses > 100 mg/m² q3–4wk rarely used, do not confuse w/ carboplatin **Uses:** *Testicular, bladder, ovarian Ca's*, SCLC, NSCLC, breast, head & neck, & penile CAs; osteosarcoma; peds brain tumors **Acts:** DNA-binding; denatures double helix; intrastrand cross-linking **Dose:** 10–20 mg/m²/d for 5 d q3wk; 50–120 mg/m² q3–4wk (per CA-specific protocols); ↓ w/ renal impair **W/P:** [D, –] Cumulative renal tox may be severe; ↓ BM, hearing impair, preexisting renal Insuff **CI:** w/ Anthrax or live vaccines; platinum-containing compound allergy; w/ cidofovir **Disp:** Inj 1 mg/mL **SE:** Allergic Rxns, N/V, nephrotox (↑ w/ administration of other nephrotox drugs; minimize w/ NS Inf & mannitol diuresis), high-frequency hearing loss in 30%, peripheral "stocking glove"-type neuropathy, cardiotox (ST, T-wave changes), ↓ Mg²⁺, mild ↓ BM, hepatotox; renal impair dose-related & cumulative **Notes:** Give taxanes before platinum derivatives; ✓ Mg²⁺, lytes before & w/in 48 h after cisplatin

Citalopram (Celexa) **BOX:** Closely monitor for worsening depression or emergence of suicidality, particularly in pts < 24 y; not for peds **Uses:** *Depression* **Acts:** SSRI **Dose:** Initial 20 mg/d, may ↑ to 40 mg/d max dose; ↓ 20 mg/d max > 60 y, w/ cimetidine, or hepatic/renal Insuff **W/P:** [C, +/–] Hx of mania, Szs & pts at risk for suicide; ↑ risk serotonin synd (p 13) w/ triptans, linezolid, lithium, tramadol, St. John's wort; use w/ other SSRIs, SNRIs, or tryptophan not rec **CI:** MAOI or w/in 14 d of MAOI use **Disp:** Tabs 10, 20, 40 mg; soln 10 mg/5 mL **SE:** Somnolence, insomnia, anxiety, xerostomia, N, diaphoresis, sexual dysfunction; may ↑ Qt interval and cause arrhythmias; ↓ Na⁺/SIADH

Citric Acid/Magnesium Oxide/Sodium Picosulfate (Prepopik)
Uses: *Colonoscopy colon prep* **Acts:** Stimulant/osmotic laxative **Dose:** Powder recons w/ 5 oz cold water; *"Split Dose":* 1st dose night before and 2nd dose morning of procedure; OR *"Day Before":* 1st dose afternoon/early evening day before and 2nd dose later evening (ie, 4–6 P.M., then 10 P.M.–12 A.M.); clear liquids after dose **W/P:** [B, ?] Fluid/electrolyte abnormalities, arrhythmias, seizures; ↑ risk in renal Insuff or w/ nephrotox drugs; mucosal ulcerations; aspiration risk **CI:** CrCl < 30 mL/min; GI perf/obstr/ileus/gastric retention/toxic colitis/megacolon **Disp:** Packets, 16.1 g powder (15 mg sodium picosulfate, 3.5 g mag oxide, 12 g anhyd citric acid) w/ dosing cup **SE:** N/V/D, HA, Abd pain, cramping, bloating **Notes:** Meds taken 1 h w/in dose might not be absorbed

Cladribine (Leustatin) **BOX:** Dose-dependent reversible myelosuppression; neurotox, nephrotox, administer by physician w/ experience in chemotherapy regimens **Uses:** *HCL, CLL, NHLs, progressive MS* **Acts:** Induces DNA strand breakage; interferes w/ DNA repair/synth; purine nucleoside analog **Dose:** 0.09–0.1 mg/kg/d cont IV Inf for 1–7 d (per protocols); ↓ w/ renal impair **W/P:** [D, ?/–] Causes neutropenia & Infxn **CI:** Component sens **Disp:** Inj 1 mg/mL **SE:** ↓ BM, T lymphocyte ↓ may be prolonged (26–34 wk), fever in 46%, tumor lysis synd, Infxns (especially lung & IV sites), rash (50%), HA, fatigue, N/V **Notes:** Consider prophylactic allopurinol; monitor CBC

Clarithromycin (Biaxin, Biaxin XL) **Uses:** *Upper/lower resp tract, skin/ skin structure Infxns, H. pylori Infxns, & Infxns caused by nontuberculosis (atypical) Mycobacterium; prevention of MAC Infxns in HIV Infxn* **Acts:** Macrolide antibiotic, ↓ protein synth. **Spectrum:** *H. influenzae, M. catarrhalis, S. pneumoniae, M. pneumoniae, & H. pylori* **Dose:** *Adults.* 250–500 mg PO bid or 1000 mg (2 × 500 mg XL tab)/d *Mycobacterium:* 500 mg PO bid *Peds > 6 mo.* 7.5 mg/kg/dose PO bid; ↓ w/ renal impair **W/P:** [C, ?] Antibiotic-associated colitis; rare ↑ QT & ventricular arrhythmias; not rec w/ PDE5 inhib **CI:** Macrolide allergy; w/ Hx jaundice w/ Biaxin; w/ cisapride, pimozide, astemizole, terfenadine, ergotamines; w/ colchicine & renal impair; w/ statins; w/ ↑ QT or ventricular arrhythmias **Disp:** Tabs 250, 500 mg; susp 125, 250 mg/5 mL; 500 mg XL tab **SE:** ↑ QT interval, causes metallic taste, N/D, Abd pain, HA, rash **Notes:** Multiple drug interactions, ↑ theophylline & carbamazepine levels; do not refrigerate susp

Clemastine Fumarate (Antihist-1, Dayhist, Tavist) [OTC] **Uses:** *Allergic rhinitis & Sxs of urticaria* **Acts:** Antihistamine **Dose:** *Adults & Peds > 12 y.* 1.34 mg bid–2.68 mg tid; max 8.04 mg/d *Peds 6–12 y.* 0.67–1.34 mg bid (max 4.02/d) *< 6 y.* 0.335–0.67 mg/d ÷ into 2–3 doses (max 1.34 mg/d) **W/P:** [B, M] BOO;

do not take w/ MAOI **CI:** NAG **Disp:** Tabs 1.34, 2.68 mg; syrup 0.67 mg/5 mL **SE:** Drowsiness, dyscoordination, epigastric distress, urinary retention **Notes:** Avoid EtOH

Clevidipine (Cleviprex) **Uses:** *HTN when PO not available/desirable* **Acts:** Dihydropyridine CCB, potent arterial vasodilator **Dose:** 1–2 mg/h IV, then maint 4–6 mg/h; 21 mg/h max **W/P:** [C, ?] ↓ BP, syncope, rebound HTN, reflex tachycardia, CHF **CI:** Hypersens: component or formulation (soy, egg products); impaired lipid metabolism; severe aortic stenosis **Disp:** Inj 0.5 mg/mL (50 mL, 100 mL) **SE:** AF, fever, insomnia, N/V, HA, renal impair

Clindamycin (Cleocin, Cleocin-T, Others) **BOX:** Pseudomembranous colitis may range from mild to lifethreatening **Uses:** *Rx aerobic & anaerobic Infxns; topical for severe acne & Vag Infxns* **Acts:** Bacteriostatic; interferes w/ protein synth. *Spectrum:* Streptococci (eg, pneumococci), *Staphylococci*, & gram(+) & (–) anaerobes; no activity against gram(–) aerobes **Dose:** *Adults.* *PO:* 150–450 mg PO q6–8h *IV:* 300–600 mg IV q6h or 900 mg IV q8h *Vag cream:* 1 applicator hs × 7 d *Vag supp:* Insert 1 qhs × 3 d *Topical:* Apply 1% gel, lotion, or soln bid. **Peds** *Neonates.* (Avoid use; contains benzyl alcohol) 10–15 mg/kg/24 h ÷ q8–12h *Children > 1 mo.* 10–30 mg/kg/24 h ÷ q6–8h, to a max of 1.8 g/d PO and 4.8 g/d IV *Topical:* Apply 1% gel, lotion, or soln bid; ↓ in severe hepatic impair **W/P:** [B, +] Can cause fatal colitis **CI:** Hx pseudomembranous colitis **Disp:** Caps 75, 150, 300 mg; susp 75 mg/5 mL; Inj 300 mg/2 mL; Vag cream 2%; topical soln 1%; gel 1%; lotion 1%; Vag supp 100 mg **SE:** D may be *C. difficile* pseudomembranous colitis, rash, ↑ LFTs **Notes:** D/C drug w/ D, evaluate for *C. difficile*

Clindamycin/Benzoyl Peroxide (Benzaclin, Onexton, Generic) **Uses:** *Topical for acne vulgaris* **Acts:** Bacteriostatic antibiotic w/ keratolytic **Dose:** Apply bid (A.M. & P.M.) **W/P:** [C, ?] Pseudomembranous colitis reported **CI:** Component sens, Hx UC/abx-associated colitis **Disp:** *Clindamycin/benzoyl peroxide:* 1%/5% gel 25-g jar or 35/50-g pump, 1.2%/5% gel 45-g tube; *Onexton:* 1.2%/3.75% gel **SE:** Dry skin, pruritus, peeling, erythema, sunburn, allergic Rxns **Notes:** May bleach hair/fabrics; not approved in peds

Clindamycin/Tretinoin (Veltin Gel, Ziana) **Uses:** *Acne vulgaris* **Acts:** Lincosamide abx (↓ protein synthesis) w/ a retinoid. *Spectrum:* P. acnes **Dose:** *Adults & Peds > 12 y.* Apply pea-size amount to area qd **W/P:** [C, ?/–] Do not use w/ erythromycin products **CI:** Hx regional enteritis/UC/abx-associated colitis **Disp:** Topical gel (clindamycin 1.2%/tretinoin 0.025%) **SE:** Dryness, irritation, erythema, pruritus, exfoliation, dermatitis, sunburn **Notes:** Avoid eyes, lips, mucous membranes

Clobazam (Onfi) [C-IV] **Uses:** *Szs assoc w/ Lennox-Gastaut synd* **Acts:** Potentiates GABA neurotransmission; binds to benzodiazepine GABA$_A$ receptor **Dose:** *Adults & Peds ≥ 2 y. ≤ 30 kg.* 5 mg PO/d, titrate weekly 20 mg/d max *> 30 kg.* 5 mg bid 10 mg daily, titrate weekly 40 mg/d max; ÷ dose bid if > 5 mg/d; may crush & mix w/ applesauce; ↓ dose in geriatric pts, CYP2C19 poor metabolizers, & mild–mod hepatic impair; ↓ dose weekly by 5–10 mg/d w/ D/C **W/P:** [C, ±]

physical/psychological dependence & suicidal ideation/behavior; withdrawal Sxs w/ rapid dose ↓; alcohol ↑ clobazam levels by 50%; adjust w/ CYP2C19 inhib, ↓ dose of drugs metabolized by CYP2D6; may ↓ contraceptive effect; SJS and TEN **Disp:** Tabs 5, 10, 20 mg; susp 2.5 mg/mL **SE:** Somnolence, sedation, cough, V, constipation, drooling, UTI, aggression, dysarthria, fatigue, insomnia, ataxia, pyrexia, lethargy, ↑/↓ appetite

Clofarabine (Clolar) **Uses:** Rx relapsed/refractory ALL after at least 2 regimens in children 1–21 y **Acts:** Antimetabolite; ↓ ribonucleotide reductase w/ false nucleotide base-inhibiting DNA synth **Dose:** 52 mg/m² IV over 2 h daily × 5 d (repeat q2–6wk); per protocol; ↓ w/ renal impair **W/P:** [D, –] **Disp:** Inj 20 mg/20 mL **SE:** N/V/D, anemia, leukopenia, thrombocytopenia, neutropenia, Infxn, ↑ AST/ALT **Notes:** Monitor for tumor lysis synd & SIRS/capillary leak synd; hydrate well

Clomiphene (Generic) **Uses:** *Tx ovulatory dysfunction in women desiring PRG* **Acts:** Nonsteroidal ovulatory stimulant; estrogen antagonist **Dose:** 50 mg × 5 d; if no ovulation ↑ to 100 mg × 5 d @ 30 d later; ovulation usually 5–10 d post-course, time coitus w/ expected ovulation time; use ↓ dose/shorter course w/ ovarian hypersens (ie, PCOS) **W/P:** [X, /–] r/o PRG & ovarian hyperstimulation synd **CI:** Hypersens, uterine bleeding, PRG, ovarian cysts (not d/t PCOS), liver Dz, thyroid/adrenal dysfunction **Disp:** Tabs 50 mg **SE:** Ovarian enlargement, vasomotor flushes

Clomipramine (Anafranil) **BOX:** Closely monitor for suicidal ideation or unusual behavior changes **Uses:** *OCD*, depression, chronic pain, panic attacks **Acts:** TCA; ↑ synaptic serotonin & norepinephrine **Dose:** *Adults.* Initial 25 mg/d PO in ÷ doses; ↑ over few wk 250 mg/d max QHS **Peds > 10 y.** Initial 25 mg/d PO in ÷ doses; ↑ over few wk 200 mg/d or 3 mg/kg/d max given ÷hs **W/P:** [C, +/–] **CI:** w/ MAOI, linezolid, IV methylene blue (risk serotonin synd), TCA allergy, during AMI recovery **Disp:** Caps 25, 50, 75 mg **SE:** Anticholinergic (xerostomia, urinary retention, constipation), somnolence

Clonazepam (Klonopin, Generic) [C-IV] **Uses:** *Lennox-Gastaut synd, akinetic & myoclonic Szs, absence Szs, panic attacks*, RLS, neuralgia, parkinsonian dysarthria, bipolar disorder **Acts:** Benzodiazepine; anticonvulsant **Dose:** *Adults.* 1.5 mg/d PO in 3 ÷ doses; ↑ by 0.5–1 mg/d q3d PRN up to 20 mg/d **Peds.** 0.01–0.03 mg/kg/24 h PO ÷ tid; ↑ to 0.1–0.2 mg/kg/24 h ÷ tid; 0.2 mg/kg/d max; avoid abrupt D/C **W/P:** [D, M] Elderly pts, resp Dz, CNS depression, severe hepatic impair, NAG **CI:** Severe liver Dz, acute NAG **Disp:** Tabs 0.5, 1, 2 mg; oral disintegrating tabs 0.125, 0.25, 0.5, 1, 2 mg **SE:** CNS (drowsiness, dizziness, ataxia, memory impair) **Notes:** Can cause anterograde amnesia; a CYP3A4 substrate

Clonidine, Epidural (Duraclon) **BOX:** Dilute 500 mcg/mL before use; not rec for OB, postpartum, or periop pain management due to ↓ BP/HR **Uses:** *w/ Opiates for severe pain in CA pts uncontrolled by opiates alone* **Acts:** Centrally acting analgesic **Dose:** 30 mcg/h by epidural Inf **W/P:** [C, ?/M] May ↓ HR/resp **CI:** See Box; clonidine sens, Inj site Infxn, anticoagulants, bleeding diathesis, use above C4 dermatome **Disp:** 500 mcg/mL; dilute to 100 mcg/mL w/ NS (preservative free) **SE:** ↓

BP, dry mouth, N/V, somnolence, dizziness, confusion, sweating, hallucinations, tinnitus **Notes:** Avoid abrupt D/C; may cause nervousness, rebound ↑ BP

Clonidine, Oral (Catapres, Generic) Uses: *HTN*; opioid, EtOH, & tobacco withdrawal, ADHD **Acts:** Centrally acting α-adrenergic stimulant **Dose:** *Adults.* 0.1 mg PO bid, adjust daily by 0.1–0.2-mg increments (max 2.4 mg/d) *Peds.* 5–10 mcg/kg/d ÷ q8–12h (max 0.9 mg/d); ↓ in renal impair **W/P:** [C, +/–] Avoid w/ β-blocker, elderly, severe CV Dz, renal impair; use w/ agents that affect sinus node may cause severe ↓ HR **CI:** Component sens **Disp:** Tabs 0.1, 0.2, 0.3 mg **SE:** Drowsiness, orthostatic ↓ BP, xerostomia, constipation, ↓ HR, dizziness **Notes:** More effective for HTN if combined w/ diuretics; withdraw slowly, rebound HTN w/ abrupt D/C of doses > 0.2 mg bid; ADHD use in peds needs CV assessment before starting epidural clonidine (*Duraclon*) used for chronic CA pain

Clonidine, Oral, ER (Kapvay, Generic) Uses: *ADHD alone or as adjunct* **Acts:** Central α-adrenergic stimulant **Dose:** *Adults & Peds > 6 y.* Initial 0.1 mg qhs, then adjust weekly to bid; split dose based on table; do not crush/chew; do not substitute other products as mg dosing differs; > 0.4 mg/d not rec

Kapvay Total Daily Dose	Morning Dose	Bedtime Dose
0.1 mg	N/A	0.1 mg
0.2 mg	0.1 mg	0.1 mg
0.3 mg	0.1 mg	0.2 mg
0.4 mg	0.2 mg	0.2 mg

W/P: [C, +/–] May cause severe ↓ HR and ↓ BP; w/ BP meds **CI:** Component sens **Disp:** Tabs ER 0.1, 0.2 mg **SE:** Somnolence, fatigue, URI, irritability, sore throat, insomnia, nightmares, emotional disorder, constipation, congestion, ↑ temperature, dry mouth, ear pain **Notes:** On D/C, ↓ no more than 0.1 mg q3–7d

Clonidine, Transdermal (Catapres-TTS) Uses: *HTN* **Acts:** Centrally acting α-adrenergic stimulant **Dose:** 1 patch q7d to hairless area (upper arm/torso); titrate to effect; ↓ w/ severe renal impair **W/P:** [C, +/–] Avoid w/ β-blocker, withdraw slowly, in elderly, severe CV Dz, and w/ renal impair; use w/ agents that affect sinus node may cause severe ↓ HR **CI:** Component sens **Disp:** TTS-1, TTS-2, TTS-3 (delivers 0.1, 0.2, 0.3 mg, respectively, of clonidine/d for 1 wk) **SE:** Drowsiness, orthostatic ↓ BP, xerostomia, constipation, ↓ HR **Notes:** Do not D/C abruptly (rebound HTN); doses > 2 TTS-3 usually not associated w/ ↑ efficacy; steady state in 2–3 d

Clopidogrel (Plavix, Generic) Uses: *Reduce atherosclerotic events*, administer ASAP in ECC setting w/ high-risk ST depression or T-wave inversion

Acts: ↓ Plt aggregation **Dose:** 75 mg/d *ECC 2010. ACS:* 300–600 mg PO loading dose, then 75 mg/d PO; full effects take several days **W/P:** [B, ?] Active bleeding; risk of bleeding from trauma & other; TTP; liver Dz; other CYP2C19 (eg, fluconazole); OK w/ ranitidine, famotidine **CI:** Coagulation disorders, active intracranial bleeding; CABG planned w/in 5–7 d **Disp:** Tabs 75, 300 mg **SE:** ↑ bleeding time, GI intolerance, HA, dizziness, rash, thrombocytopenia, ↓ WBC **Notes:** Plt aggregation to baseline ~ 5 d after D/C, plt transfusion to reverse acutely; clinical response highly variable

Clorazepate (Tranxene T-TAB, Generic) [C-IV]
Uses: *Acute anxiety disorders, acute EtOH withdrawal Sxs, adjunctive therapy Rx partial Szs* **Acts:** Benzodiazepine; antianxiety agent **Dose:** *Adults.* 15–60 mg/d PO single or ÷ doses *Elderly & debilitated pts:* Initial 7.5–15 mg/d in ÷ doses *EtOH withdrawal:* day 1: Initial 30 mg, then 30–60 mg ÷ doses; day 2: 45–90 mg ÷ doses; day 3: 22.5–45 mg ÷ doses; day 4: 15–30 mg ÷ doses; after day 4: 15–30 mg ÷ doses, then 7.5–15 mg/d ÷ doses *Peds > 9 y.* 3.75–7.5 mg/dose build to 60 mg/d max ÷ bid-tid **W/P:** [D, ?/–] Elderly; Hx depression **CI:** NAG; Component hypersens **Disp:** Tabs 3.75, 7.5, 15 mg **SE:** CNS depressant effects (drowsiness, dizziness, ataxia, memory impair), ↓ BP **Notes:** Monitor pts w/ renal/hepatic impair (drug may accumulate); avoid abrupt D/C; may cause dependence

Clotrimazole (Lotrimin, Mycelex, Others) [OTC]
Uses: *Candidiasis & tinea Infxns* **Acts:** Antifungal; alters cell wall permeability. *Spectrum:* Oropharyngeal candidiasis, dermatophytoses, superficial mycoses, cutaneous candidiasis, & vulvovaginal candidiasis **Dose:** *PO: Prophylaxis:* 1 troche dissolved in mouth tid *Rx:* 1 troche dissolved in mouth 5×/d for 14 d *Vag 1% cream:* 1 applicator-full hs for 7 d *2% cream:* 1 applicator-full hs for 3 d *Tabs:* 100 mg vaginally hs for 7 d or 200 mg (2 tabs) vaginally hs for 3 d or 500-mg tab vaginally hs once *Topical:* Apply bid 10–14 d **W/P:** [B (C if PO), ?] Not for systemic fungal Infxn; safety in children < 3 y not established **CI:** Component allergy **Disp:** 1% cream; soln; troche 10 mg; Vag cream 1%, 2% **SE:** *Topical:* Local irritation *PO:* N/V, ↑ LFTs **Notes:** PO prophylaxis immunosuppressed pts

Clotrimazole/Betamethasone (Lotrisone)
Uses: *Fungal skin Infxns* **Acts:** Imidazole antifungal & anti-inflam. *Spectrum:* Tinea pedis, cruris, & corporis **Dose:** *Adults & Peds ≥ 17 y.* Apply & massage into area bid for 2–4 wk **W/P:** [C, ?] Varicella Infxn **CI:** Children < 12 y **Disp:** Cream 1/0.05% 15, 45 g; lotion 1/0.05% 30 mL **SE:** Local irritation, rash **Notes:** Not for diaper dermatitis or under occlusive dressings

Clozapine (Clozaril, FazaClo, Versacloz)
BOX: Myocarditis, agranulocytosis, Szs, & orthostatic ↓ BP associated w/ clozapine; ↑ mortality in elderly w/ dementia-related psychosis **Uses:** *Refractory severe schizophrenia*; childhood psychosis; OCD, bipolar disorder **Acts:** "Atypical" antipsychotic **Dose:** 12.5 mg daily or bid initial; ↑ to 300–450 mg/d over 2 wk; maintain lowest dose possible; do not D/C abruptly **W/P:** [B, +/–] Monitor for psychosis & cholinergic rebound **CI:** Uncontrolled epilepsy; comatose state; WBC < 3500 cells/mm³ and

ANC < 2000 cells/mm^3 before Rx or < 3000 cells/mm^3 during Rx; EOS > 3000/mm^2 **Disp:** ODTs 12.5, 25, 100, 150, 200 mg; tabs 25, 100 mg; susp 50 mg/mL **SE:** Sialorrhea, tachycardia, drowsiness, ↑ Wt, constipation, incontinence, rash, Szs, CNS stimulation, hyperglycemia **Notes:** Avoid activities where sudden loss of consciousness could cause harm; benign temperature ↑ may occur during the 1st 3 wk of Rx; weekly CBC mandatory 1st 6 mo, then q other wk

Cobicistat (Tybost) **Uses:** *HIV; ↑ exposure to atazanavir or darunavir* **Acts:** CYP3A4 inhib **Dose:** 150 mg PO ad w/ azatanavir or darunavir; w/ food **W/P:** [B, –]; false Cr ↑; many drug interactions; not interchangeable w/ ritonavir; not rec w/ darunavir 600 mg bid, fosamprenavir, saquinavir, or tipranavir **CI:** w/ Drugs w/ altered plasma conc can cause serious effects (w/atazanavir or darunavir and alfuzosin, dronanderone, ergot derivatives, indanivir, irinotecan, lovastatin, midazolam, nevirapine, pimozide, rifampin, sildenafil, simvastatin, St. John's wort, triazolam) **Disp:** Tabs 150 mg **SE:** ↑ bili, jaundice, icterus; rash

Cocaine [C-II] **Uses:** *Topical anesthetic for mucous membranes* **Acts:** Narcotic analgesic, local vasoconstrictor **Dose:** Lowest topical amount that provides relief; 3 mg/kg max **W/P:** [C, ?] **CI:** ocular anesthesia **Disp:** Topical soln & viscous preparations 4–10%; powder **SE:** CNS stimulation, nervousness, loss of taste/smell, chronic rhinitis, CV tox, abuse potential **Notes:** Use only on PO, laryngeal, & nasal mucosa; do not use on extensive areas of broken skin

Codeine [C-II] **Uses:** *Mild–mod pain; symptomatic relief of cough* **Acts:** Narcotic analgesic; ↓ cough reflex **Dose:** *Adults. Analgesic:* 15–60 mg PO q4h PRN; 360 mg max/24 h *Antitussive:* 10–20 mg PO q4h PRN; max 120 mg/d *Peds. Analgesic:* 0.5–1 mg/kg/dose PO q4–6h PRN *Antitussive:* 1–1.5 mg/kg/24 h PO ÷ q4h; max 30 mg/24 h; ↓ in renal/hepatic impair **W/P:** [C (D if prolonged use or high dose at term), +/–] CNS depression, Hx drug abuse, severe hepatic impair **CI:** Component sens **Disp:** Tabs 15, 30, 60 mg; soln 30 mg/5 mL; **SE:** Drowsiness, constipation, ↓ BP **Notes:** Usually combined w/ APAP for pain or w/ agents (eg, terpin hydrate) as an antitussive

Colchicine (Colcrys, Mitigare, Generic) **Uses:** *Acute gouty arthritis & prevention of recurrences; familial Mediterranean fever*; primary biliary cirrhosis* **Acts:** ↓ migration of leukocytes; ↓ leukocyte lactic acid production **Dose:** *Acute gout:* 1.2 mg load, 0.6 mg 1 h later, then prophylactic 0.6 mg/qd-bid *FMF: Adult* 1.2–2.4 mg/d *Peds > 4 y see label* **W/P:** [C, +/–] P-glycoprotein or CYP3A4 inhib in pts w/ renal or hepatic impair, ↓ renal or avoid in elderly or w/ indinavir **CI:** Serious renal, GI, hepatic, or cardiac disorders; blood dyscrasias **Disp:** Tabs 0.6 mg **SE:** N/V/D, Abd pain, BM suppression, hepatotox

Colesevelam (Welchol) **Uses:** *↓ LDL & total chol alone or in combo w/ an HMG-CoA reductase inhib, improve glycemic control in type 2 DM* **Acts:** Bile acid sequestrant **Dose:** 3 tabs PO bid or 6 tabs daily w/ meals **W/P:** [B, ?] Severe GI motility disorders; in pts w/ triglycerides > 300 mg/dL (may ↑ levels); use not established in peds **CI:** Bowel obst, serum triglycerides > 500; Hx hypertriglyceridemia-pancreatitis **Disp:** Tabs 625 mg; oral susp 3.75 g **SE:** Constipation, dyspepsia, myalgia, weakness **Notes:** May ↓ absorption of fat-soluble vits

Colestipol (Colestid) **Uses:** *Adjunct to ↓ serum chol in primary hypercholesterolemia, relieve pruritus associated w/ ↑ bile acids* **Acts:** Binds intestinal bile acids to form insoluble complex **Dose:** *Granules:* 5–30 g/d ÷ 2–4 doses; *tabs:* 2–16 g/d ÷ daily-bid **W/P:** [C, ?] Avoid w/ high triglycerides, GI dysfunction **CI:** Bowel obst **Disp:** Tabs 1 g; granules 5 g/pack or scoop **SE:** Constipation, Abd pain, bloating, HA, GI irritation & bleeding **Notes:** Do not use dry powder; mix w/ beverages, cereals, etc; may ↓ absorption of other meds and fat-soluble vits

Conivaptan HCl (Vaprisol) **Uses:** *Euvolemic & hypervolemic hyponatremia* **Acts:** Dual arginine vasopressin V$_{1A}$/V$_2$ receptor antag **Dose:** 20 mg IV × 1 dose over 30 min, then 20 mg cont IV Inf over 24 h; 20 mg/d cont IV Inf for 1–3 more d; may ↑ to 40 mg/d if Na$^+$ not responding; 4 d max use; use large vein, change site q24h **W/P:** [C, ?/–] Rapid ↑ Na$^+$ (> 12 mEq/L/24 h) may cause osmotic demyelination synd; impaired renal/hepatic Fxn; may ↑ digoxin levels; CYP3A4 inhib (Table 10, p 356) **CI:** Hypovolemic hyponatremia; w/ CYP3A4 inhib; anuria **Disp:** Inj 20 mg/100 mL **SE:** Inf site Rxns, HA, N/V/D, constipation, ↓ K$^+$, orthostatic ↓ BP, thirst, dry mouth, pyrexia, pollakiuria, polyuria, Infxn **Notes:** Monitor Na$^+$, vol and neurologic status; D/C w/ very rapid ↑ Na$^+$; mix only w/ 5% dextrose

Conjugated Estrogens/Bazedoxifene (Duavee) **BOX:** Do not use w/ additional estrogen; ↑ risk endometrial CA; do not use to prevent CV Dz or dementia; ↑ risk of stroke & DVT in postmenopausal (50–79 y); ↑ dementia risk in postmenopausal (≥ 65 y) **Uses:** *Tx mod/severe menopausal vasomotor Sx; Px postmenopausal osteoporosis* **Acts:** Conj estrogens w/ estrogen agonist/antag **Dose:** One tab PO daily **W/P:** [X, –] w/ CYP3A4 inhib may ↑ exposure; do not use w/ progestins, other estrogens; w/ Hx of CV Dz; ↑ risk gallbladder Dz; D/C w/ vision loss, severe ↑ TG; jaundice; monitor thyroid function if on thyroid Rx **CI:** Hepatic impair; deficiency of protein C or S, antithrombin, other thrombophilic Dz; AUB; Hx breast CA; estrogen-dependent neoplasia; Hx of TE; PRG, childbearing potential, nursing mothers; component hypersens **Disp:** Tabs (conjugated estrogens mg/bazedoxifene mg) 0.45/20 **SE:** N/D, dyspepsia, Abd pain, oropharyngeal/neck pain, dizziness, muscle spasms, hot flush **Notes:** Use for shortest duration for benefit; not rec ≥ 75 y

Copper IUD (ParaGard T 380A) **Uses:** *Contraception, long-term (up to 10 y)* **Acts:** ?, interfere w/ sperm survival/transport **Dose:** Insert any time during menstrual cycle; replace at 10 y max **W/P:** [C, ?] Remove w/ intrauterine PRG, increased risk of comps w/ PRG if device in place **CI:** Acute PID or in high-risk behavior, postpartum endometritis, cervicitis **Disp:** 313.4 mg IUD **SE:** PRG, ectopic PRG, pelvic Infxn w/ or w/o immunocompromised, embedment, perforation, expulsion, Wilson Dz, fainting w/ insert, Vag bleeding **Notes:** Counsel pt does not protect against STD/HIV; see PI for detailed instructions; 99% effective

Cortisone, Systemic, Topical See Steroids, pp 287 & 288, and Tables 2 & 3, pp 335 and 336

Crizotinib (Xalkori) Uses: *Locally advanced/metastatic NSCLC ALK-positive* Acts: TKI Dose: 250 mg PO bid; swallow whole; see label for tox adjustments W/P: [D, ?/–] w/ Hepatic impair & CrCl < 30 mL/min; may cause ↑ QT (monitor); ↓ dose w/ CYP3A substrates; avoid w/ strong CYP3A inducers/inhib & CYP3A substrates w/ narrow therapeutic index Disp: Caps 200, 250 mg SE: N/V/D, constipation, Abd pain, stomatitis, edema, vision disorder, hepatotox, pneumonitis, pneumonia, PE, neutropenia, thrombocytopenia, lymphopenia, HA, dizziness, fatigue, cough, dyspnea, URI, fever, arthralgia, ↓ appetite, rash, neuropathy Notes: ✓ CBC & LFTs monthly

Crofelemer (Fulyzaq) Uses: *Noninfectious diarrhea w/ HIV on anti-retrovirals* Acts: Inhibits cAMP-stimulated CF transmembrane conductance regulator Cl⁻ channel and Ca-activated Cl⁻ channels of intestinal epithelial cells, controls Cl⁻ and fluid secretion Dose: 125 mg bid W/P: [C, –] CI: Ø Disp: Tabs 125 mg DR SE: Flatulence, cough, bronchitis, URI, ↑ bili Notes: r/o infectious D before; do not crush/chew tabs; minimal absorption, drug interaction unlikely

Cromolyn Sodium (Intal, NasalCrom, Opticrom, Others) Uses: *Adjunct to the Rx of asthma; prevent exercise-induced asthma; allergic rhinitis; ophthal allergic manifestations*; food allergy, systemic mastocytosis, IBD Acts: Antiasthmatic; mast cell stabilizer Dose: *Adults & Peds > 12 y.* Inh: 20 mg (as powder in caps) inhaled qid *Nasal instillation:* Spray once in each nostril 3–6×/d *Ophthal:* 1–2 gtt in each eye 4–6 × d *Peds.* Inh: 2 puffs qid of metered-dose inhaler *PO:* W/P: [B, ?] w/ Renal/hepatic impair CI: Acute asthmatic attacks Disp: soln for nebulizer 20 mg/2 mL; nasal soln 5.2 mg/actuation; ophthal soln 4% SE: Unpleasant taste, hoarseness, coughing Notes: No benefit in acute Rx; 2–4 wk for maximal effect in perennial allergic disorders Oral form "Gastrocrom" used for mastocytosis

Cyanocobalamin [Vitamin B₁₂] (Nascobal) Uses: *Pernicious anemia & other vit B₁₂ deficiency states; ↑ requirements d/t PRG; thyrotoxicosis; liver or kidney Dz* Acts: Dietary vit B₁₂ supl Dose: *Adults.* 1000–2000 mcg PO qd × 1–2 wk, then 1000 mcg/d *Intranasal:* 500 mcg in 1 nostril once/wk 100 mcg IM or SQ daily for 6–7 d, then 100 mcg IM 2×/wk for 1 mo, then 100 mcg IM monthly *Peds.* Use 0.2 mcg/kg × 2 d test dose; if OK 30–50 mcg/d for 2 or more wk (total 1000 mcg), then maint: 100 mcg/mo W/P: [A (C if dose exceeds RDA), +] CI: Allergy to cobalt; hereditary optic nerve atrophy; Leber Dz Disp: Tabs 50, 100, 250, 500, 1000, 2500, 5000 mcg; Inj 1000 mcg/mL; intranasal (*Nascobal*) gel 500 mcg/0.1 mL SE: Itching, D, HA, anxiety Notes: PO absorption erratic; OK for use w/ hyperalimentation; added to many oral supls

Cyclobenzaprine (Flexeril) Uses: *Relief of muscle spasm* Acts: Centrally acting skeletal muscle relaxant; reduces tonic somatic motor activity Dose: 5–10 mg PO bid–qid (2–3 wk max) W/P: [B, ?] Shares the toxic potential of the

TCAs; urinary hesitancy, NAG **CI:** Do not use concomitantly or w/in 14 d of MAOIs; hyperthyroidism; heart failure; arrhythmias **Disp:** Tabs 5, 7.5, 10 mg **SE:** Sedation & anticholinergic effects **Notes:** May inhibit mental alertness or physical coordination

Cyclobenzaprine, ER (Amrix) **Uses:** *Muscle spasm* **Acts:** ? Centrally acting long-term muscle relaxant **Dose:** 15–30 mg PO daily 2–3 wk; 30 mg/d max **W/P:** [B, ?] w/ urinary retention, NAG, w/ EtOH/CNS depressant **CI:** MAOI w/in 14 d, elderly, arrhythmias, heart block, CHF, MI recovery phase, ↑ thyroid **Disp:** Caps ER 15, 30 mg **SE:** Dry mouth, drowsiness, dizziness, HA, N, blurred vision, dysgeusia **Notes:** Avoid abrupt D/C w/ long-term use

Cyclopentolate, Ophthalmic (Cyclogyl, Cylate) **Uses:** *Cycloplegia, mydriasis* **Acts:** Cycloplegic mydriatic, anticholinergic inhibits iris sphincter and ciliary body **Dose:** *Adults.* 1 gtt in eye 40–50 min preprocedure, may repeat × 1 in 5–10 min **Peds.** As adult, children 0.5%; infants use 0.5% **W/P:** [C (may cause late-term fetal anoxia/↓ HR), ?], w/ premature infants, HTN, Down synd, elderly, **CI:** NAG **Disp:** Ophthal soln 0.5, 1, 2% **SE:** Tearing, HA, irritation, eye pain, photophobia, arrhythmia, tremor, ↑ IOP, confusion **Notes:** Compress lacrimal sac for several min after dose; heavily pigmented irises may require ↑ strength; peak 25–75 min, cycloplegia 6–24 h, mydriasis up to 24 h; 2% soln may result in psychotic Rxns and behavioral disturbances in peds

Cyclopentolate/Phenylephrine (Cyclomydril) **Uses:** *Mydriasis greater than cyclopentolate alone* **Acts:** Cycloplegic mydriatic, α-adrenergic agonist w/ anticholinergic to inhibit iris sphincter **Dose:** 1 gtt in eye q 5–10 min (max 3 doses) 40–50 min preprocedure **W/P:** [C (may cause late-term fetal anoxia/↓ HR), ?] HTN, w/ elderly w/ CAD **CI:** NAG **Disp:** Ophthal soln cyclopentolate 0.2%/phenylephrine 1% (2, 5 mL) **SE:** Tearing, HA, irritation, eye pain, photophobia, arrhythmia, tremor **Notes:** Compress lacrimal sac for several min after dose; heavily pigmented irises may require ↑ strength; peak 25–75 min, cycloplegia 6–24 h, mydriasis up to 24 h

Cyclophosphamide (Cytoxan, Neosar) **Uses:** *Hodgkin Dz & NHLs; multiple myeloma; SCLC, breast & ovarian CAs; mycosis fungoides; neuroblastoma; retinoblastoma; acute leukemias; allogeneic & ABMT in high doses; severe rheumatologic disorders (SLE, JRA, Wegner granulomatosis)* **Acts:** Alkylating agent **Dose:** *Adults.* (per protocol) 500–1500 mg/m²; single dose at 2- to 4-wk intervals; 1.8 g/m²–160 mg/kg (or at 12 g/m² in 75-kg individual) in the BMT setting (per protocols) **Peds.** *SLE:* 500 mg–1g/m² q mo *JRA:* 10 mg/kg q 2 wk; ↓ w/ renal impair **W/P:** [D, –] w/ BM suppression, hepatic Insuff **CI:** Component sens **Disp:** Tabs 25, 50 mg; Inj 500 mg, 1, 2 g **SE:** ↓ BM; hemorrhagic cystitis, SIADH, alopecia, anorexia; N/V; hepatotx; rare interstitial pneumonitis; irreversible testicular atrophy possible; cardiotox rare; 2nd malignancies (bladder, ALL), risk 3.5% at 8 y, 10.7% at 12 y **Notes:** Hemorrhagic cystitis prophylaxis: cont bladder irrigation & MESNA uroprotection; encourage hydration, long-term bladder CA screening

Cyclosporine (Gengraf, Neoral, Sandimmune) BOX: ↑ Risk neoplasm, ↑ risk skin malignancies, ↑ risk HTN and nephrotox Uses: *Organ rejection in kidney, liver, heart, & BMT w/ steroids; RA; psoriasis* Acts: Immunosuppressant; reversible inh of immunocompetent lymphocytes Dose: *Adults & Peds.* PO: 15 mg/kg/12h pretransplant; after 2 wk, taper by 5 mg/wk to 3–5 mg/kg/d *IV:* If NPO, give 1/3 PO dose IV; ↓ in renal/hepatic impair W/P: [C, −] Dose-related risk of nephrotox/hepatotox/serious fatal Infxns; live, attenuated vaccines may be less effective; may induce fatal malignancy; many drug interactions; ↑ risk of Infxns after D/C CI: Renal impair; uncontrolled HTN; w/ lovastatin, simvastatin Disp: Caps 25, 100 mg; PO soln 100 mg/mL; Inj 50 mg/mL SE: May ↑ BUN & Cr & mimic transplant rejection; HTN; HA; hirsutism Notes: Administer in glass container; *Neoral & Sandimmune* not interchangeable; monitor BP, Cr, CBC, LFTs, interaction w/ St. John's wort; Levels: *Trough:* Just before next dose, *Therapeutic:* Variable 150–300 ng/mL RIA

Cyclosporine, Ophthalmic (Restasis) Uses: *↑ Tear production suppressed d/t ocular inflam* Acts: Immune modulator, anti-inflam Dose: 1 gtt bid each eye 12 h apart; OK w/ artificial tears, allow 15 min between W/P: [C, ?] CI: Ocular Infxn, component allergy Disp: Single-use vial 0.05% SE: Ocular burning/hyperemia Notes: Mix vial well

Cyproheptadine (Periactin) Uses: *Allergic Rxns; itching* Acts: Phenothiazine antihistamine; serotonin antag Dose: *Adults.* 4–20 mg PO ÷ q8h; max 0.5 mg/kg/d *Peds 2–6 y.* 2 mg bid-tid (max 12 mg/24 h) *7–14 y.* 4 mg bid-tid; ↓ in hepatic impair W/P: [B, −] Elderly, CV Dz, asthma, thyroid Dz, BPH CI: Neonates or < 2 y; NAG; BOO; acute asthma; GI obst; w/ MAOI Disp: Tabs 4 mg; syrup 2 mg/5 mL SE: Anticholinergic, drowsiness Notes: May stimulate appetite

Cytarabine [ARA-C] (Cytosar-U) BOX: Administration by experienced physician in properly equipped facility; potent myelosuppressive agent Uses: *Acute leukemias, CML, NHL; IT for leukemic meningitis or prophylaxis* Acts: Antimetabolite; interferes w/ DNA synth Dose: 100–150 mg/m²/d for 5–10 d (low dose); 3 g/m² q12h for 6–12 doses (high dose); 1 mg/kg 1–2/wk (SQ maint); 5–75 mg/m² up to 3/wk IT (per protocols); ↓ in renal/hepatic impair W/P: [D, ?] in elderly, w/ marked BM suppression, ↓ dosage by ↓ the number of days of administration CI: Component sens Disp: Inj 100, 500 mg, 1, 20, 100 mg/mL SE: ↓ BM, N/V/D, stomatitis, flu-like synd, rash on palms/soles, hepatic/cerebellar dysfunction w/ high doses, noncardiogenic pulm edema, neuropathy, fever Notes: Little use in solid tumors; high-dose tox limited by corticosteroid ophthal soln

Cytarabine Liposome (DepoCyt) BOX: Can cause chemical arachnoiditis (N/V, HA, fever) ↓ severity w/ dexamethasone. Administer by experienced physician in properly equipped facility Uses: *Lymphomatous meningitis* Acts: Antimetabolite; interferes w/ DNA synth Dose: 50 mg IT q14d for 5 doses, then 50 mg IT q28d × 4 doses; use dexamethasone prophylaxis W/P: [D, ?] May cause neurotox; blockage to CSF flow may ↑ the risk of neurotox; use in peds not established **CI:** Active meningeal Infxn **Disp:** IT Inj 50 mg/5 mL **SE:** Neck pain/rigidity, HA, confusion, somnolence, fever, back pain, N/V, edema, neutropenia, ↓ plt, anemia **Notes:** Cytarabine liposomes are similar in microscopic appearance to WBCs; caution in interpreting CSF studies

Cytomegalovirus Immune Globulin [CMV-IG IV] (CytoGam)   Uses: *Prophylaxis/attenuation CMV Dz w/ transplantation* **Acts:** IgG antibodies to CMV **Dose:** 150 mg/kg/dose w/in 72 h of transplant; wk 2, 4, 6, 8: 100–150 mg/kg/dose; wk 12, 16 posttransplant: 50–100 mg/kg/dose **W/P:** [C, ?] Anaphylactic Rxns; renal dysfunction **CI:** Allergy to immunoglobulins; IgA deficiency **Disp:** Inj 50 mg/mL **SE:** Flushing, N/V, muscle cramps, wheezing, HA, fever, non-cardiogenic pulm edema, renal Insuff, aseptic meningitis **Notes:** IV only in separate line; do not shake

Dabigatran (Pradaxa)   BOX: Pradaxa D/C w/o adequate anticoagulation ↑ stroke risk Uses: *↓ Risk stroke/systemic embolism w/ NVAF* **Acts:** Thrombin inhib **Dose:** CrCl > 30 mL/min: 150 mg PO bid; CrCl 15–30 mL/min: 75 mg PO bid; do not chew/break/open caps **W/P:** [C, ?/–] Avoid w/ P-glycoprotein inducers (i.e., rifampin) **CI:** Active bleeding, prosthetic valve **Disp:** Caps 75, 150 mg **SE:** Bleeding, gastritis, dyspepsia **Notes:** See label to convert between anticoagulants; caps sensitive to humidity (caps stable after opening bottle); routine coagulants not needed; ↑ PTT/INR/TT; w/ nl TT, no drug activity; ½ life 12–17 h

Dabrafenib (Tafinlar)   Uses: *Met melanoma (single agent) w/ BRAF V600E mutation; combo w/ trametinib w/ BRAF V600E or V600K mutation* **Acts:** TKI **Dose:** As single agent: 150 mg PO twice daily; Combo: 150 mg PO 2 ×/d + trametinib 2 mg PO 1 ×/d; 1 h ac or 2 h pc; see label dosage mods w/ tox **W/P:** [D, –] Embryo-fetal tox; may cause new malignancies, tumor promotion in BRAF wild-type melanoma, ↑ bleeding risk, cardiomyopathy, VTE, ocular tox, skin tox, ↑ glu, febrile Rxn; risk of hemolytic anemia w/ G6PD deficiency; avoid w/ strong inhib/inducing CYP3A4 & CYP2C8; use w/ substrates of CYP3A4, CYP2C8, CYP2C9, CYP2C19, or CYP2B6 may ↓ efficacy of these agents **CI:** Ø **Disp:** Caps 50, 75 mg **SE:** See W/P; single agent: hyperkeratosis, pyrexia, arthralgia, papilloma, alopecia, HA, palmar-plantar erythrodysesthesia synd; w/ trametinib: N/V/D, constipation, Abd pain, pyrexia, chills, fatigue, rash, edema, cough, HA, arthralgia, night sweats, ↓ appetite, myalgia **Notes:** Use non-hormonal contraception w/ Tx and for 2 wk after D/C of single therapy or 4 mo after D/C w/ trametinib; may ↓ spermatogenesis

Dacarbazine (DTIC-Dome)   BOX: Causes hematopoietic depression, hepatic necrosis, may be carcinogenic, teratogenic Uses: *Melanoma, Hodgkin Dz, sarcoma* **Acts:** Alkylating agent; antimetabolite as a purine precursor; ↓ protein synth, RNA, & especially DNA **Dose:** 250 mg/m²/d for 5 d or 375 mg/m² on d 1 & 15 (per protocols); ↓ in renal impair **W/P:** [C, –] In BM suppression; renal/hepatic impair **CI:** Component sens **Disp:** Inj 100, 200 mg **SE:** ↓ BM, N/V, hepatotox, flu-like synd, ↓ BP, photosens, alopecia, facial flushing, facial paresthesias, urticaria, phlebitis at Inj site **Notes:** Avoid extrav, ✓ CBC, plt

Daclizumab (Zenapax) BOX: Administer under skilled supervision in properly equipped facility Uses: *Prevent acute organ rejection* **Acts:** IL-2 receptor antag **Dose:** 1 mg/kg/dose IV; 1st dose pretransplant, then 1 mg/kg q14d × 4 doses **W/P:** [C, ?] **CI:** Component sens **Disp:** Inj 5 mg/mL **SE:** Hyperglycemia, edema, HTN, ↓ BP, constipation, HA, dizziness, anxiety, nephrotox, pulm edema, pain, anaphylaxis/hypersens **Notes:** Administer w/in 4 h of preparation

Dactinomycin (Cosmegen) BOX: Administer under skilled supervision in properly equipped facility; powder and soln tox, corrosive, mutagenic, carcinogenic, and teratogenic; avoid exposure and use precautions **Uses:** *Choriocarcinoma, Wilms tumor, Kaposi and Ewing sarcomas, rhabdomyosarcoma, uterine and testicular CA* **Acts:** DNA-intercalating agent **Dose:** *Adults.* 15 mcg/kg/d for 5 d q3–6 wk or 400–600 mcg/m² for 5d q3–6 wk *Peds.* Sarcoma (per protocols); ↓ in renal impair **W/P:** [D, ?] **CI:** Concurrent/recent chickenpox or herpes zoster; infants < 6 mo **Disp:** Inj 0.5 mg **SE:** Myelo-/immunosuppression, severe N/V/D, alopecia, acne, hyperpigmentation, radiation recall phenomenon, tissue damage w/ extrav, hepatotox **Notes:** Classified as abx but not used as antimicrobial

Dalbavancin (Dalvance) Uses: *Acute bacterial skin and skin structure Infxns* **Acts:** Glycopeptide antibacterial (blocks cell wall synth). *Spectrum:* Methicillin-susceptible/resistant strains, *S. aureus, Streptococcus* spp (*agalactiae, anginosus, pyogenes*), *Enterococcus* **Dose:** *Two-dose regimen:* 1000 mg IV, followed by 500 mg 1 wk later; ↓ in renal impair **W/P:** [C, ?/–] Anaphylaxis reported; avoid rapid Inf; ↑ ALT, *Clostridium difficile*-associated D reported **CI:** Component hypersens **Disp:** 500 mg powder to reconstitute **SE:** N/D, HA **Notes:** Not approved in peds

Dalfampridine (Ampyra) Uses: *Improve walking w/ MS* **Acts:** K⁺ channel blocker **Dose:** 10 mg PO q12h; max dose/d 20 mg **W/P:** [C, ?/–] Not w/ other 4-aminopyridines **CI:** Hx Sz; w/ CrCl ≤ 50 mL/min **Disp:** Tab ER 10 mg **SE:** HA, N, constipation, dyspepsia, dizziness, insomnia, UTI, nasopharyngitis, back pain, pharyngolaryngeal pain, asthenia, balance disorder, MS relapse, paresthesia, Sz **Notes:** Do not cut/chew/crush/dissolve tab

Dalteparin (Fragmin) BOX: ↑ Risk of spinal/epidural hematoma w/ LP **Uses:** *Unstable angina, non–Q-wave MI, prevent & Rx DVT following surgery (hip, Abd), pts w/ restricted mobility, extended therapy Rx for PE DVT in CA pts* **Acts:** LMW heparin **Dose:** *Angina/MI:* 120 units/kg (max 10,000 units) SQ q12h w/ ASA *DVT prophylaxis:* 2500–5000 units SQ 1–2 h preop, then daily for 5–10 d *Systemic anticoagulation:* 200 units/kg/d SQ or 100 units/kg bid SQ *CA:* 200 Int units/kg (max 18,000 Int units) SQ q24h × 30 d, mo 2–6 150 Int units/kg SQ q24h (max 18,000 Int units) **W/P:** [B, ?] In renal/hepatic impair, active hemorrhage, cerebrovascular Dz, cerebral aneurysm, severe HTN **CI:** HIT; pork product allergy; **Disp:** Inj multiple ranging from 2500 units (16 mg/0.2 mL) to 25,000 units/mL (3.8 mL) prefilled vials **SE:** Bleeding, pain at site, ↓ plt **Notes:** Predictable effects eliminate lab monitoring; not for IM/IV use

Dantrolene (Dantrium, Revonto, Ryanodex, Generic) BOX: Hepatotox reported; D/C after 45 d if no benefit observed **Uses:** *Rx spasticity d/t upper motor neuron disorders (eg, spinal cord injuries, stroke, CP, MS); malignant hyperthermia* **Acts:** Skeletal muscle relaxant **Dose:** *Adults.* Spasticity: 25 mg PO daily; ↑ 25 mg to effect to 100 mg PO q8h (400 mg/d max) *Peds.* 0.5 mg/kg/dose/d; ↑ by 0.5 mg/kg dose tid to 2 mg/kg/dose tid (max 400 mg/d) *Adults & Peds. Malignant hyperthermia: Rx:* Cont maint IV, start 2.5 mg/kg until Sxs subside or 10 mg/kg is reached *Postcrisis follow-up:* 4–8 mg/kg/d in 3–4 ÷ doses for 1–3 d to prevent recurrence **W/P:** [C, ?] Impaired cardiac/pulm/hepatic Fxn **CI:** Active hepatic Dz; where spasticity needed to maintain posture or balance **Disp:** Caps 25, 50, 100 mg; powder for Inj 250 mg/5 mL vial **SE:** Hepatotox, ↑ LFTs, drowsiness, dizziness, rash, muscle weakness, N/V/D, pleural effusion w/ pericarditis, blurred vision, hep, photosens **Notes:** Monitor LFTs; avoid sunlight/EtOH/CNS depressants

Dapagliflozin (Farxiga) **Uses:** *Type 2 DM* **Acts:** SGLT2 inhib **Dose:** 5–10 mg PO qam; do not use if GFR < 60 ml/min **W/P:** [C, −] ↓ BP d/t ↓ intravascular vol; ↑ Cr, ✓ renal fxn; ↓ BS risk w/ insulin/insulin secretagogue; genital mycotic Infxn; ↑ LDL; bladder CA **CI:** Hypersens Rxn; severe renal impair (< 30 ml/min), end-stage renal Dz, dialysis **Disp:** Tabs 5, 10 mg **SE:** UTI, female genital mycotic Infxn, nasopharyngitis, see W/P **Notes:** No clinical trials to date to show ↓ in macrovascular complications

Dapagliflozin/Metformin (Xigduo XR) BOX: Associated w/ lactic acidosis, risk ↑ w/ sepsis, dehydration, renal/hep impair, ↑ alcohol, acute CHF; lactic acidosis Sxs include myalgias, malaise, resp distress, Abd pain, somnolence; labs: ↓ pH, ↑ anion gap, ↑ lactate; D/C immediately & hospitalize if suspected. **Uses:** *Type 2 DM, adjunct to diet & exercise* **Acts:** (*Dapagliflozin*) SGLT2 inhib w/ (*metformin*) biguanide, ↓ hep glu & absorption of glu **Dose:** Based on pt regimen; ↑ dose slowly w/ typical (dapagliflozin mg/metformin mg) 5/5 to 10/2000 PO qd; do not use ≥ 80 y unless nl renal fxn **W/P:** [C, −] ↓ BP; metformin not rec w/ hepatic Dz; not for type 1 DM or DKA; temp D/C metformin w/ contrast media; avoid w/ ethanol; ✓ B₁₂ levels; do not use w/ bladder CA; dapagliflozin can ↑ SCr (>30) **CI:** Component hypersens, mod/severe renal impair, DKA, metabolic acidosis **Disp:** Combo tabs: (dapagliflozin mg/metformin mg) 5/500, 5/1000, 10/500, 10/1000 **SE:** HA, N, GU fungal Infxn, UTI, back pain, nasopharyngitis **Notes:** Take in A.M. w/ food to ↓ GI effects; do not crush/cut/chew tabs; ✓ blood glu, HbA₁c

Dapsone, Oral **Uses:** *Rx & prevent PCP; toxoplasmosis prophylaxis; leprosy* **Acts:** PABA antag, ↓ bacterial folic acid synth, bactericidal **Dose:** *Adults.* PCP prophylaxis 50–100 mg PO daily; Rx PCP 100 mg/d PO w/ TMP 15–20 mg/kg/d for 21 d *Peds. PCP prophylaxis alternated dose:* (> 1 mo) 4 mg/kg/dose once/wk (max 200 mg); Rx *PCP:* 2 mg/kg/24 h PO daily; max 100 mg/d **W/P:** [C, −] G6PD deficiency; severe anemia **CI:** Component sens **Disp:** Tabs 25, 100 mg **SE:** Hemolysis, methemoglobinemia, agranulocytosis, rash, cholestatic jaundice **Notes:** Absorption ↑ by an acidic environment; for leprosy, combine w/ rifampin & other agents

Dapsone, Topical (Aczone) Uses: *Topical for acne vulgaris* Acts: Unknown; bactericidal Dose: Apply pea-size amount and rub into areas bid; wash hands after W/P: [C, –] G6PD deficiency; severe anemia CI: Component sens Disp: 5% gel SE: Skin oiliness/peeling, dryness erythema Notes: Not for oral, ophthal, or intravag use; check G6PD levels before use; follow CBC if G6PD deficient

Daptomycin (Cubicin) Uses: *Complicated skin/skin structure Infxns d/t gram(+) organisms* S. aureus, bacteremia, MRSA endocarditis Acts: Cyclic lipopeptide; rapid membrane depolarization & bacterial death. Spectrum: S. aureus (including MRSA), S. pyogenes, S. agalactiae, S. dysgalactiae subsp Equisimilis, & E. faecalis (vancomycin-susceptible strains only) Dose: Skin: 4 mg/kg IV daily × 7–14 d (over 2 min) Bacteremia & Endocarditis: 6 mg/kg q24h; ↓ w/ CrCl < 30 mL/min or dialysis: q48h W/P: [B, ?] w/ HMG-CoA inhib Disp: Inj 500 mg/10 mL SE: Anemia, constipation, N/V/D, HA, rash, site Rxn, muscle pain/weakness, edema, cellulitis, hypo-/hyperglycemia, ↑ alk phos, cough, back pain, Abd pain, ↓ K+, anxiety, CP, sore throat, cardiac failure, confusion, Candida Infxns Notes: ✓ CPK baseline & weekly; consider D/C HMG-CoA reductase inhib to ↓ myopathy risk; not for Rx PNA

Darbepoetin Alfa (Aranesp) BOX: Associated w/ ↑ CV, thromboembolic events and/or mortality; D/C if Hgb > 12 g/dL; may increase tumor progression and death in CA pts Uses: *Anemia associated w/ CRF*, anemia in nonmyeloid malignancy w/ concurrent chemotherapy Acts: ↑ Erythropoiesis, recombinant erythropoietin variant Dose: 0.45 mcg/kg single IV or SQ qwk; titrate, do not exceed Hgb of 12 g/dL; use lowest doses possible, see PI to convert from Epogen W/P: [C, ?] May ↑ risk of CV &/or neurologic SE in renal failure; HTN; w/ Hx Szs CI: Uncontrolled HTN, component allergy Disp: 25, 40, 60, 100, 200, 300 mcg/mL, 150 mcg/0.75 mL in polysorbate or albumin excipient SE: May ↑ cardiac risk, CP, hypo-/hypertension, N/V/D, myalgia, arthralgia, dizziness, edema, fatigue, fever, ↑ risk Infxn Notes: Longer half-life than Epogen; ✓ weekly CBC until stable

Darifenacin (Enablex) Uses: *OAB* Acts: urinary antispasmodic Acts: Muscarinic receptor antag Dose: 7.5 mg/d PO; 15 mg/d max (7.5 mg/d w/ mod hepatic impair or w/ CYP3A4 inhib); w/ drugs metabolized by CYP2D (Table 10, p 356); swallow whole W/P: [C, ?/–] w/ Hepatic impair CI: Urinary/gastric retention, uncontrolled NAG, paralytic ileus Disp: Tabs ER 7.5, 15 mg SE: Xerostomia/eyes, constipation, dyspepsia, Abd pain, retention, abn vision, dizziness, asthenia

Darunavir (Prezista) Uses: *Rx HIV w/ resistance to multiple protease inhib* Acts: HIV-1 protease inhib Dose: Adults. Rx-naïve w/ no darunavir resistance substitutions: 800 mg w/ ritonavir 100 mg qd; Rx experienced w/ 1 darunavir resistance: 600 mg w/ ritonavir 100 mg BID w/ food Peds 6–18 y > 20 kg. Dose based on BW (see label); do not exceed the Rx experienced adult dose; do not use qd dosing in peds; w/ food W/P: [C, ?/–] Hx sulfa allergy, CYP3A4 substrate, changes levels of many meds (↑ amiodarone, ↑ dihydropyridine, ↑ HMG-CoA reductase inhib [statins], ↓ SSRIs, ↓ methadone); do not use w/ salmeterol, colchicine (w/ renal impair; do not use w/ severe hepatic impair); adjust dose w/ bosentan, tadalafil for PAH **CI**: w/ Astemizole, rifampin, St. John's Wort, terfenadine, ergotamines, lovastatin, simvastatin, methylergonovine, pimozide, midazolam, triazolam, alpha 1-adrenoreceptor antag (alfuzosin), PDE5 inhib (eg, sildenafil) **Disp**: Tabs 75, 150, 400, 600, 800 mg **SE**: ↑ glu, cholesterol, triglycerides, central redistribution of fat (metabolic synd), N, ↓ neutrophils, ↑ amylase

Darunavir/Cobicistat (Prezcobix) Uses: *HIV-1 Infxn in Tx-naïve & Tx-experienced pts w/ no darunavir resistance–associated substitutions* **Acts**: HIV-1 antiviral w/ CYP3A inhib **Dose**: *Adults*. 800/150 mg qd w/ food **W/P**: [C, ?/–] w/ Risk factors for liver Dz; severe skin Rxns, including SJS, reported **CI**: w/ Meds whose altered concentrations are associated w/ serious effects **Disp**: Tabs 800/150 mg **SE**: N/V/D, rash, HA, Abd pain **Notes**: HIV genotype testing rec for Tx-experienced pts

Dasatinib (Sprycel) Uses: CML, Ph + ALL **Acts**: Multi-TKI **Dose**: 100–140 mg PO qd; adjust w/ CYP3A4 inhib/inducers (Table 10, p 356) **W/P**: [D, ?/–] **CI**: Ø **Disp**: Tabs 20, 50, 70, 80, 100, 140 mg **SE**: ↓ BM, edema, fluid retention, pleural effusions, N/V/D, Abd pain, bleeding, fever, ↑ QT **Notes**: Replace K⁺, Mg²⁺ before Rx

Daunorubicin (Cerubidine) **BOX**: Cardiac Fxn should be monitored d/t potential risk for cardiac tox & CHF, renal/hepatic dysfunction Uses: *Acute leukemias* **Acts**: DNA-intercalating agent; ↓ topoisomerase II; generates oxygen-free radicals **Dose**: 45–60 mg/m²/d for 3 consecutive d; 25 mg/m²/wk (per protocols); ↓ w/ renal/hepatic impair **W/P**: [D, ?] **CI**: Component sens **Disp**: Inj 20, 50 mg **SE**: ↓ BM, mucositis, N/V, orange urine, alopecia, radiation recall phenomenon, hepatotox (↑ bili), tissue necrosis w/ extrav, cardiotox (1–2% CHF w/ 550 mg/m² cumulative dose) **Notes**: Prevent cardiotox w/ dexrazoxane (w/ > 300 mg/m² daunorubicin cum dose); IV use only; allopurinol prior to ↓ hyperuricemia

Decitabine (Dacogen) Uses: *MDS* **Acts**: Inhib DNA methyltransferase **Dose**: 15 mg/m² cont Inf over 3 h; repeat q8h × 3 d; repeat cycle q6wk, min 4 cycles; delay Tx and ↓ dose if inadequate hematologic recovery at 6 wk (see PI); delay Tx w/ Cr > 2 mg/dL or bili > 2× ULN **W/P**: [D, ?/–]; avoid PRG; males should not father a child during or 2 mo after; renal/hepatic impair **Disp**: Powder 50 mg/vial **SE**: ↓ WBC, ↓ HgB, ↓ plt, febrile neutropenia, edema, petechiae, N/V/D, constipation, stomatitis, dyspepsia, cough, fever, fatigue, ↑ LFTs/bili, hyperglycemia, Infxn, HA **Notes**: ✓ CBC & plt before cycle and PRN; premedicate w/ antiemetic

Deferasirox (Exjade) **BOX**: May cause renal and hepatic tox/failure, GI bleeding; follow labs Uses: *Chronic iron overload d/t transfusion in pts > 2 y* **Acts**: Oral iron chelator **Dose**: 20 mg/kg PO/d; adjust by 5–10 mg/kg q3–6mo based on monthly ferritin; 40 mg/kg/d max; on empty stomach 30 min ac; hold dose w/ ferritin < 500 mcg/L; dissolve in water/orange/apple juice (< 1 g/3.5 oz; > 1 g in 7 oz), drink immediately; resuspend residue and swallow; do not chew/swallow whole tabs or take w/ aluminum-containing antacids **W/P:** [C, ?/–] Elderly, renal impair, heme disorders; ↑ MDS in pt ≥ 60 y **Disp:** Tabs for oral susp 125, 250, 500 mg **SE:** N/V/D, Abd pain, skin rash, HA, fever, cough, ↑ Cr & LFTs, Infxn, hearing loss, dizziness, cataracts, retinal disorders, ↑ IOP **Notes:** ARF, cytopenias possible; ✓ Cr weekly 1st mo, then qmo, ✓ CBC, urine protein, LFTs; do not use w/ other iron-chelator therapies; dose to nearest whole tab; initial auditory/ophthal testing, then q12mo

Deferiprone (Ferriprox) **BOX:** May cause neutropenia & agranulocytosis w/ Infxn & death; monitor baseline ANC & weekly; D/C if Infxn develops; advise pts to report any Sx of Infxn **Uses:** *Transfusion iron overload in thalassemia synds* **Acts:** Iron chelator **Dose:** 25 mg/kg PO tid (75 mg/kg/d); max round dose to nearest 1/2 tab **W/P:** [D, –] D/C w/ ANC < 1.5×10^9/L **CI:** Hypersens **Disp:** Tabs (scored) 500 mg **SE:** N/V, Abd pain, chromaturia, arthralgia, ↑ ALT, neutropenia, agranulocytosis, ↑ QT, HA **Notes:** Separate by 4 h antacids & mineral supplements w/ polyvalent cations; ✓ plasma zinc

Degarelix (Firmagon) **Uses:** *Advanced PCa* **Acts:** Reversible LHRH antag, ↓ LH and testosterone w/o flare seen w/ LHRH agonists (transient ↑ in testosterone) **Dose:** Initial 240 mg SQ in two 120 mg doses (40 mg/mL); maint 80 mg SQ (20 mg/mL) q28d **W/P:** Anaphylaxis, may ↑ QT **CI:** Women; comp hypersens **Disp:** Inj vial 120 mg (initial); 80 mg (maint) **SE:** Inj site Rxns, hot flashes, ↑ Wt, ↑ serum GGT **Notes:** Requires 2 Inj initially; 44% testosterone castrate (< 50 ng/dL) at d 1, 96% d 3

Delavirdine (Rescriptor) **Uses:** *HIV Infxn* **Acts:** Nonnucleoside RT inhib **Dose:** 400 mg PO tid **W/P:** [C, ?] CDC rec: HIV-infected mothers not breast-feed (transmission risk); w/ renal/hepatic impair **CI:** w/ Drugs dependent on CYP3A (Table 10, p 356) **Disp:** Tabs 100, 200 mg **SE:** Fat redistribution, immune reconstitution synd, HA, fatigue, rash, ↑ transaminases, N/V/D **Notes:** Avoid antacids; ↓ cytochrome P450 enzymes; numerous drug interactions; monitor LFTs

Demeclocycline (Declomycin) **Uses:** *SIADH* **Acts:** Abx, antag ADH action on renal tubules **Dose:** 600–1200 mg/d PO on empty stomach; ↓ in renal failure; avoid antacids **W/P:** [D, ?/–] Avoid in hepatic/renal impair & children **CI:** Tetracycline allergy **Disp:** Tabs 150, 300 mg **SE:** D, Abd cramps, photosens, DI **Notes:** Avoid sunlight, numerous drug interactions

Denosumab (Prolia, Xgeva) **Uses:** *Tx osteoporosis in postmenopausal women, ↑ BMD in men on ADT (Prolia); prevent skeletal events w/ bone mets from solid tumors & hypercalcemia of malignancy refractory to bisphosphonates (Xgeva)* **Acts:** RANKL inhibitor (human IgG2 MoAb); inhib osteoclasts **Dose:** *Prolia:* 60 mg SQ q6mo; *Xgeva:* 120 mg SQ q4wk; in upper arm, thigh, Abd **W/P:** [D (*Xgeva*), X (*Prolia*), ?/–] **CI:** Hypocalcemia **Disp:** Inj *Prolia* 60 mg/mL; *Xgeva* 120 mg/1.7 mL **SE:** ↓ Ca^{2+}, hypophosphatemia, serious Infxns, dermatitis, rashes, eczema, ONJ, pancreatitis, pain (musculoskeletal, back), fatigue, asthenia, dyspnea, N, Abd pain, flatulence, hypercholesterolemia, anemia, cystitis **Notes:** Give w/ Ca 1000 mg & vit D 400 Int units/d

Desipramine (Norpramin) **BOX:** Closely monitor for worsening depression or emergence of suicidality **Uses:** *Endogenous depression*, chronic pain, peripheral neuropathy **Acts:** TCA; ↑ synaptic serotonin or norepinephrine in CNS **Dose:** *Adults.* 100–200 mg/d single or ÷ dose; usually single hs dose (max 300 mg/d); ↓ dose in elderly *Peds 6–12 y.* 1–3 mg/kg/d ÷ dose (max 5 mg/kg/d) **W/P:** [C, ?/–] w/ CV Dz, Sz disorder, hypothyroidism, elderly, liver impair **CI:** MAOIs w/in 14 d; during AMI recovery phase w/ linezolid or IV methylene blue (↑ risk serotonin synd) **Disp:** Tabs 10, 25, 50, 75, 100, 150 mg **SE:** Anticholinergic (blurred vision, urinary retention, xerostomia); orthostatic ↓ BP; ↑ QT, arrhythmias **Notes:** Numerous drug interactions; blue-green urine; avoid sunlight

Desirudin (Iprivask) **BOX:** Recent/planned epidural/spinal anesthesia, ↑ epidural/spinal hematoma risk w/ paralysis; consider risk vs benefit before neuraxial intervention **Uses:** *DVT Px in hip replacement* **Acts:** Thrombin inhibitor **Dose:** 15 mg SQ q12h, initial 5–15 min prior to surgery; CrCl 31–60 mL/min: 5 mg SQ q12h; CrCl < 31 mL/min: 1.7 mg SQ q12h; ✓ aPTT & SCr daily for dosage mod **W/P:** [C, ?/–] **CI:** Active bleeding, irreversible coagulants, hypersens to hirudins **Disp:** Inj 15 mg **SE:** Hemorrhage, N/V, Inj site mass, wound secretion, anemia, thrombophlebitis, ↓ BP, dizziness, anaphylactic Rxn, fever

Desloratadine (Clarinex, Generic) **Uses:** *Seasonal & perennial allergic rhinitis; chronic idiopathic urticaria* **Acts:** Active metabolite of Claritin, H₁-antihistamine, blocks inflam mediators **Dose:** *Adults & Peds > 12 y.* 5 mg PO daily; 5 mg PO q other day w/ hepatic/renal impair **W/P:** [C, ?/–] *RediTabs* contain phenylalanine **Disp:** Tabs 5 mg; *RediTabs* (rapid dissolving) 2.5, 5 mg; syrup 0.5 mg/mL **SE:** Allergy, anaphylaxis, somnolence, HA, dizziness, fatigue, pharyngitis, xerostomia, N, dyspepsia, myalgia

Desloratadine/Pseudoephedrine (Clarinex-D 12 Hour) **Uses:** *Seasonal allergic rhinitis/nasal congestion* **Acts:** Selective H1-receptor histamine antag w/ sympathomimetic amine/decongestant **Dose:** *Adults & Peds > 12 y.* 1 tab PO bid w/ or w/o food **W/P:** [C, ?/–] CV/CNS effects, w/ DM, hyperthyroidism, BPH, ↑ IOP, do not use w/in 14 days of MAOI, rare hypersens, avoid w/ renal/hepatic impair **Disp:** Tabs 5 mg; *RediTabs* (rapid dissolving) 2.5, 5 mg; syrup 0.5 mg/mL **SE:** See W/P; dry mouth, N, fatigue, anorexia, HA, somnolence, dizziness, insomnia, pharyngitis

Desmopressin (DDAVP, Stimate) **BOX:** Not for hemophilia B or w/ factor VIII antibody; not for hemophilia A w/ factor VIII levels < 5% **Uses:** *DI; bleeding d/t uremia, hemophilia A, & type I von Willebrand Dz (parenteral); nocturnal enuresis* **Acts:** Synthetic analog of vasopressin (human ADH); ↑ factor VIII **Dose:** *DI: Intranasal: Adults.* 0.1–0.4 mL (10–40 mcg/d in 1–3 ÷ doses) *Peds 3 mo–12 y.* 0.05–0.3 mL (5 mcg/d) in 1 or 2 doses *Parenteral: Adults.* 0.5–1 mL (2–4 mcg/d in 2 ÷ doses); converting from nasal to parenteral, use 1/10 nasal dose *PO: Adults.* 0.05 mg bid; ↑ to max of 1.2 mg *Hemophilia A & von Willebrand Dz (type I): Adults & Peds > 10 kg.* 0.3 mcg/kg in 50 mL NS, Inf over 15–30 min

Peds < 10 kg. As above w/ dilution to 10 mL w/ NS *Nocturnal enuresis: Peds > 6 y.* 20 mcg PO hs **W/P:** [B, M] Avoid overhydration **CI:** Hemophilia B; CrCl < 50 mL/min, severe classic von Willebrand Dz; pts w/ factor VIII antibodies; hyponatremia **Disp:** Tabs 0.1, 0.2 mg; Inj 4 mcg/mL; nasal spray 0.1 mg/mL (10 mcg/spray) 1.5 mg/mL (150 mcg/spray) **SE:** Facial flushing, HA, dizziness, vulval pain, nasal congestion, pain at Inj site, ↓ Na+, H$_2$O intoxication **Notes:** In very young & old pts, ↓ fluid intake to avoid H$_2$O intoxication & ↓ Na+; ↓ urine output, ↑ urine osmolality, ↓ plasma osmolality

Desvenlafaxine (Khedezla, Pristiq, Generic) **BOX:** Monitor for worsening or emergence of suicidality, particularly in peds, adolescent, and young adult pts; not approved in peds **Uses:** *MDD* **Acts:** Selective serotonin and norepinephrine reuptake inhib **Dose:** 50 mg PO daily; w/ renal impair 50 mg/d max; w/ hepatic impair 10 mg/d max; take tabs whole **W/P:** [C, −] serotonin synd w/ other agents (triptans, TCAs, fentanyl, lithium, tramadol, tryptophan, buspirone, St. John's Wort); monitor for ↑ BP; ↑ bleeding risk; use w/ NAG; may activate bipolar Dz; taper slowly; Sz; ↓ Na+ and interstitial lung Dz reported **CI:** Hypersens, MAOI w/in 14 d of stopping MAOI w/ methylene blue, w/ linezolid **Disp:** ER Tabs 50, 100 mg **SE:** N, dizziness, insomnia, hyperhidrosis, constipation, somnolence, decreased appetite, anxiety, male sexual Fxn disorders

Dexamethasone, Ophthalmic (AK-Dex Ophthalmic, Decadron Ophthalmic, Maxidex) **Uses:** *Inflam or allergic conjunctivitis* **Acts:** Anti-inflam corticosteroid **Dose:** Instill 1–2 gtt tid-qid **W/P:** [C, ?/−] **CI:** Active untreated bacterial, viral, & fungal eye Infxns **Disp:** Susp & soln 0.1% **SE:** Long-term use associated w/ cataracts

Dexamethasone, Ophthalmic Implant (Ozurdex) **Uses:** *Macular edema d/t retinal vein occlusions* **Acts:** Anti-inflam corticosteroid **Dose:** 1 intravitreal implant **W/P:** [C, ?/−] Endophthalmitis, eye inflam, ↑ IOP, retinal detachments; monitor after Inj **CI:** Ocular Infxns, glaucoma, torn lens capsule, hypersens **Disp:** Implant w/ 0.7 mg dexamethasone **SE:** Cataracts, ↑ IOP, conjunctival hemorrhage

Dexamethasone, Systemic, Topical (Decadron) See Steroids, Systemic, p 287, and Steroids, Topical, p 288 *Peds. ECC 2010. Croup:* 0.6 mg/kg IV/IM/PO once; max dose 16 mg; *Asthma:* 0.6 mg/kg IV/IM/PO q24h; max dose 16 mg

Dexlansoprazole (Dexilant) **Uses:** *Heal and maint of EE, GERD* PUD **Acts:** PPI, DR **Dose:** *EE:* 60 mg qd up to 8 wk; *Maint healed EE:* 30 mg qd up to 6 mo; *GERD:* 30 mg qd × 4 wk; ↓ w/ hepatic impair **W/P:** [B, +/−] Do not use w/ clopidogrel/atazanavir or drugs w/ pH-based absorption (eg, ampicillin, iron salts, ketoconazole); may alter warfarin and tacrolimus levels **CI:** Component hypersens **Disp:** Caps 30, 60 mg **SE:** N/V/D, flatulence, Abd pain, URI **Notes:** w/ or w/o food; take whole or sprinkle on tsp applesauce; clinical response does not r/o gastric malignancy; see also Lansoprazole; ? ↑ risk of fractures w/ all PPI; risk of hypomagnesemia w/ long-term use, monitor

Dexmedetomidine (Precedex) Uses: *Sedation in intubated & nonintubated pts* Acts: Sedative; selective α_2-agonist Dose: *ICU Sedation:* 1 mcg/kg IV over 10 min, then 0.2–0.7 mcg/kg/h; *Procedural sedation:* 0.5–1 mcg/kg IV over 10 min, then 0.2–1 mcg/kg/h; ↓ in elderly, liver Dz W/P: [C, ?/–] CI: Ø Disp: Inj 200 mcg/2 mL SE: Hypotension, bradycardia Notes: Tachyphylaxis & tolerance associated w/ exposure > 24 h

Dexmethylphenidate (Focalin, Focalin XR)[C-II] BOX: Caution w/ Hx drug dependence/alcoholism; chronic abuse may lead to tolerance, psychological dependence & abnormal behavior; monitor closely during withdrawal Uses: *ADHD* Acts: CNS stimulant, blocks reuptake of norepinephrine & DA Dose: *Adults. Focalin:* 2.5 mg PO twice daily, ↑ by 2.5–5 mg weekly; max 20 mg/d *Focalin XR:* 10 mg PO daily, ↑ 10 mg weekly; max 40 mg/d *Peds ≥ 6 y. Focalin:* 2.5 mg PO bid, ↑ 2.5–5 mg weekly; max 20 mg/d *Focalin XR:* 5 mg PO daily, ↑ 5 mg weekly; max 30 mg/d; if already on methylphenidate, start w/ half of current total daily dose W/P: [C, ?/–] Avoid w/ known cardiac abn; may ↓ metabolism of warfarin/anticonvulsants/antidepressants CI: Agitation, anxiety, tension, glaucoma, Hx motor tic, fam Hx/diagnosis Tourette's, w/in 14 d of MAOI; hypersens to methylphenidate Disp: Tabs 2.5, 5, 10 mg; caps ER 5, 10, 15, 20, 25, 30, 35, 40 mg SE: HA, anxiety, dyspepsia, ↓ appetite, Wt loss, dry mouth, visual disturbances, ↑ HR, HTN, MI, stroke, sudden death, Szs, growth suppression, aggression, mania, psychosis Notes: ✓CBC w/ prolonged use; swallow ER caps whole or sprinkle contents on applesauce (do not crush/chew)

Dexpanthenol (Ilopan-Choline Oral, Ilopan) Uses: *Minimize paralytic ileus, Rx postop distention* Acts: Cholinergic agent Dose: *Prevent postop ileus:* 250–500 mg IM stat, repeat in 2 h, then q6h PRN *Ileus:* 500 mg IM stat, repeat in 2 h, then q6h, PRN W/P: [C, ?] CI: Hemophilia, mechanical bowel obst Disp: Inj 250 mg/mL; cream 2% (Panthoderm Cream [OTC]) SE: GI cramps

Dexrazoxane (Totect, Zinecard) Uses: *Prevent anthracycline-induced (eg, doxorubicin) cardiomyopathy (Zinecard), extrav of anthracycline chemotherapy (Totect)* Acts: Chelates heavy metals; binds intracellular iron & prevents anthracycline-induced free radicals Dose: *Systemic for cardiomyopathy (Zinecard):* 10:1 ratio dexrazoxane: doxorubicin 30 min before each dose, 5:1 ratio w/ CrCl < 40 mL/min *Extrav (Totect):* IV Inf over 1–2 h daily × 3 d, w/in 6 h of extrav; *Day 1:* 1000 mg/m² (max 2000 mg); *Day 2:* 1000 mg/m² (max 2000 mg); *Day 3:* 500 mg/m² (max 1000 mg); w/ CrCl < 40 mL/min, ↓ dose by 50% W/P: [D, –] CI: Component sens Disp: Inj powder 250, 500 mg (10 mg/mL) SE: ↓ BM, fever, Infxn, stomatitis, alopecia, N/V/D; ↑ LFTs, Inj site pain

Dextran 40 (Gentran 40, Rheomacrodex) Uses: *Shock, prophylaxis of DVT & thromboembolism, adjunct in peripheral vascular surgery* Acts: Expands plasma vol; ↓ blood viscosity Dose: *Shock:* 10 mL/kg Inf rapidly; 20 mL/kg max 1st 24 h; beyond 24 h 10 mL/kg max; D/C after 5 d *Prophylaxis of DVT & thromboembolism:* 10 mL/kg IV day of surgery, then 500 mL/d IV for 2–3 d, then

500 mL IV q2–3d based on risk for up to 2 wk **W/P:** [C, ?] Inf Rxns; w/ corticosteroids **CI:** Major hemostatic defects; cardiac decompensation; renal Dz w/ severe oliguria/anuria **Disp:** 10% dextran 40 in 0.9% NaCl or 5% dextran **SE:** Allergy/ anaphylactoid Rxn (observe during 1st min of Inf), arthralgia, cutaneous Rxns, ↓ BP, fever **Notes:** Monitor Cr & lytes; keep well hydrated

Dextroamphetamine (Dexedrine, Dexedrine Spansules, ProCentra, Zenzedi) [C-II] **BOX:** Amphetamines have a high potential for abuse; long-term use may lead to dependence; serious CV events, including death, w/ preexisting cardiac cond **Uses:** *ADHD, narcolepsy* **Acts:** CNS stimulant; ↑ DA & norepinephrine release **Dose:** *Adults & Peds ≥ 6 y. ADHD:* 5 mg daily-bid, ↑ by 5 mg/d weekly PRN, max 60 mg/d ÷ bid-tid *Peds 3–5 y.* 2.5 mg PO daily, ↑ 2.5 mg/d weekly PRN to response *< 3 y.* Not recommended *Narcolepsy: Peds 6–12 y. 5 mg daily,* ↑ by 5 mg/d weekly PRN; max 60 mg/d ÷ bid-tid *≥ 12 y.* 10-60 mg/d ÷ bid-tid; ER caps once daily **W/P:** [C, +/–] Hx drug abuse; separate 14 d from MAOIs **CI:** Advanced arteriosclerosis, CVD, mod–severe HTN, hyperthyroidism, glaucoma **Disp:** Tabs 5, 10 mg; ER caps 5, 10, 15 mg; *ProCentra* soln 5 mg/mL; *Dexedrine Spansules* ER caps 5, 10, 15 mg; *Zenzedi* tabs 2.5, 5, 7.5, 10, 15, 20, 30 mg **SE:** HTN, ↓ appetite, insomnia **Notes:** May open ER capsules, do not crush beads

Dextromethorphan (Benylin DM, Delsym, Mediquell, PediaCare 1, Others) [OTC] **Uses:** *Control nonproductive cough* **Acts:** Suppresses medullary cough center **Dose:** *Adults.* 10–20 mg PO q4h or 30 mg q6h PRN; ER 60 mg PO bid (max 120 mg/d). *Peds 4–6 y.* 2.5–7.5 mg q4–8h (max 30 mg/24 h) *7–12 y.* 5–10 mg q4–8h (max 60 mg/24 h) **W/P:** [C, ?/–] Not for persistent or chronic cough **CI:** < 2 y; w/in 2 wk of or w/ MAOI **Disp:** Caps 15 mg; caps ER 30 mg; lozenges 2.5, 5, 7.5, 15 mg; syrup 15 mg/15 mL, 10 mg/5 mL; liq 10 mg/15 mL, 3.5, 7.5, 15 mg/5 mL; sustained-action liq 30 mg/5 mL **SE:** GI disturbances **Notes:** Found in combo OTC products w/ guaifenesin; deaths reported in pts < 2 y; no longer OTC for < 4 y; abuse potential; efficacy in children debated; do not use w/in 14 d of D/C MAOI

Dextrose 50%/25% **Uses:** *Hypoglycemia, insulin OD* **Acts:** Sugar source in the form of D-glu **Dose:** *Adults.* One 50-mL amp of 50% soln IV *Peds. ECC 2010. Hypoglycemia:* 0.5–1 g/kg (25% max IV/IO conc); 50% Dextrose (0.5 g/mL): 1–2 mL/kg; 25% Dextrose (0.25 g/mL): 2–5 mL/kg; 10% Dextrose (0.1 g/mL): 5–10 mL/kg; 5% Dextrose (0.95 g/mL): 10–20 mL/kg if vol tolerated **W/P:** [C, M] w/ Suspected intracranial bleeding can ↑ ICP **CI:** Ø if used w/ documented hypoglycemia **Disp:** Inj forms **SE:** Burning at IV site, local tissue necrosis w/ extrav; neurologic Sxs (Wernicke encephalopathy) if pt thiamine deficient **Notes:** If pt well enough to protect airway, use oral glu first; do not routinely use in altered mental status w/o low glu; can worsen outcome in stroke; lower-conc dextrose used in IV fluids

Diazepam (Diastat rectal gel, Valium) [C-IV] **Uses:** *Anxiety, EtOH withdrawal, muscle spasm, status epilepticus, panic disorders, amnesia, preop sedation* **Acts:** Benzodiazepine **Dose:** *Adults. Status epilepticus:* 5–10 mg IV q10–15 min to 30 mg max in 8-h period Adjunct to periodic incr Sz activity: *Adults & Peds > 12 yr*

0.2 mg/kg rectal gel *Anxiety, muscle spasm:* 2–10 mg PO bid-qid or IM/IV q3–4h PRN *Preop:* 5–10 mg PO or IM 20–30 min or IV just prior to procedure *EtOH withdrawal:* 10 mg tid-qid × 24 h, then 5 mg PO tid-qid PRN or 5–10 mg IV q10–15min for CIWA withdrawal score ≥ 8, 100 mg/h max; titrate to agitation; avoid excessive sedation; may lead to aspiration or resp arrest *Peds. Status epilepticus:* < *5 y.* 0.05–0.3 mg/kg/dose IV q15–30min up to a max of 5 mg > *5 y.* to max of 10 mg Adjunct to periodic incr Sz activity Peds 2-5 yrs: 0.5 mg/kg, 6-11 yrs 0.3 mg/kg *Sedation, muscle relaxation:* 0.04–0.3 mg/kg/dose q2–4h IM or IV to max of 0.6 mg/kg in 8 h, or 0.12–0.8 mg/kg/24 h PO ÷ tid-qid; ↓ w/ hepatic impair **W/P:** [D, ?/–] **CI:** Coma, CNS depression, resp depression, NAG, severe uncontrolled pain, PRG **Disp:** Tabs 2, 5, 10 mg; soln 5 mg/mL; Inj 5 mg/mL; Diastat rectal gel (AcuDial syringe system) 2.5, 5, 7.5, 10, 12.5, 15, 17.5, 20 mg **SE:** Sedation, amnesia, ↓ HR, ↓ BP, rash, ↓ resp rate **Notes:** 5 mg/min IV max in adults or 1–2 mg/min in peds (resp arrest possible); IM absorption erratic; avoid abrupt D/C

Diazoxide (Proglycem) Uses: *Hypoglycemia d/t hyperinsulinism* **Acts:** ↓ Pancreatic insulin release; antihypertensive **Dose:** *Hypoglycemia: Adults & Peds.* 3–8 mg/kg/24 h PO ÷ q8–12h *Neonates.* 8–15 mg/kg/24 h PO in 2–3 equal doses **W/P:** [C, ?] ↓ Effect w/ phenytoin; ↑ effect w/ diuretics, warfarin **CI:** Allergy to thiazides or other sulfonamide-containing products **Disp:** PO susp 50 mg/mL **SE:** Hyperglycemia, ↓ BP, dizziness, Na⁺ & H₂O retention, N/V, weakness **Notes:** Can give false(–) insulin response to glucagons

Dibucaine (Nupercainal, Others [OTC]) Uses: *Hemorrhoids, temporary relief of pain/ itching* **Acts:** Topical anesthetic **Dose:** *Adults & Peds > 12 y. Hemorrhoids:* Insert PR w/ applicator bid & after each BM *Adults & Peds > 2 y. Pain/itching:* Apply sparingly to skin bid-qid max **W/P:** [C, ?] topical use only **CI:** Component sens **Disp:** 1% oint w/ or w/o rectal applicator **SE:** Local irritation, rash

Diclofenac, Inj (Dyloject) BOX: May ↑ risk of CV events & GI bleeding; CI in postop CABG Uses: *Mild/mod pain; mod/severe pain alone or w/ opioid analgesics* **Acts:** NSAID **Dose:** 37.5 mg IV bolus over 15 s; repeat q6h PRN; max 150 mg* **W/P:** [C (avoid after 30 wk, D), M] ↑ Risk of MI/CVA; GI bleeding/perf/ulceration; renal Insuff, papillary necrosis; hepatic injury; ↑ BP, edema, fluid retention; anaphylactic w/ aspirin react; skin Rxns, including SJS, TEN **CI:** NSAID/aspirin ASA allergy; following CABG; periop mod/severe renal insuff w/ risk for vol depletion **Disp:** Inj single-use vial, 37.5 mg/mL **SE:** N/V, constipation, flatulence, HA, dizziness, insomnia, IV site pain **Notes:** Use for shortest duration possible; ✓ BP; D/C w/local skin Rxn; can cause premature closure of ductus arteriosus

Diclofenac, Ophthalmic (Voltaren Ophthalmic) Uses: *Inflam post-cataract or pain/photophobia post–corneal refractive surgery* **Acts:** NSAID **Dose:** *Postop cataract:* 1 gtt qid, start 24 h postop × 2 wk *Postop refractive:* 1–2 gtt w/in 1 h preop and w/in 15 min postop, then qid up to 3 d **W/P:** [C, ?] May ↑ bleeding risk in ocular tissues **CI:** NSAID/ASA allergy **Disp:** Ophthal soln 0.1% 2.5-mL bottle **SE:** Burning/stinging/itching, keratitis, ↑ IOP, lacrimation, abn vision, conjunctivitis, lid swelling, discharge, iritis

Diclofenac, Oral (Cataflam, Voltaren, Voltaren-XR, Zorvolex) BOX: May ↑ risk of CV events & GI bleeding; CI in postop CABG Uses: *Arthritis (RA/OA) & pain, oral and topical; actinic keratosis* Acts: NSAID Dose: *RA/OA:* 150–200 mg/d ÷ 2–4 doses DR; 100 mg/d XR *Zorvolex:* 18 or 35 mg PO tid w/ food or milk W/P: [C (avoid after 30 wk), ?/–] CHF, HTN, renal/hepatic dysfunction; Hx PUD, asthma; different forms not interchangeable; ↑ risk of MI/CVA CI: NSAID/aspirin ASA allergy; porphyria; following CABG Disp: Tabs 50 mg; tabs DR 25, 50, 75, 100 mg; XR tabs 100 mg; *Zorvolex* caps 18, 35 mg SE: Abd cramps, heartburn, GI ulceration, rash, interstitial nephritis Notes: Do not crush tabs; watch for GI bleeding; ✓CBC, LFTs

Diclofenac, Topical (Flector Patch, Pennsaid, Solaraze, Voltaren Gel) BOX: May ↑ risk of CV events & GI bleeding; CI in postop CABG Uses: *Arthritis of the knee (Pennsaid); arthritis of knee/hands (Voltaren Gel); pain due to strain, sprain, and contusions (Flector Patch); actinic keratosis (Solaraze)* Acts: NSAID Dose: *Flector Patch:* 1 patch to painful area bid *Pennsaid:* 10 drops spread around knee; repeat until 40 drops applied; usual dose 40 drops/knee qid; wash hands; wait until dry before dressing *Solaraze:* 0.5 g to each 5 × 5 cm lesion 60–90 d; apply bid *Voltaren Gel:* Upper extremity 2 g qid (max 8 g/d); lower extremity 4 g qid (max 16 g/d) W/P: [C < 30 wk gest; D > 30 wk; ?/–] Avoid nonintact skin; ↑ risk of MI/CVA; ↑ BP, renal/hepatic dysfunct, w/ Hx PUD, asthma; avoid w/ PO NSAID CI: NSAID/ASA allergy; following CABG; component allergy Disp: *Flector Patch:* 180 mg (10 × 14 cm); *Voltaren Gel* 1%; *Solaraze* 3%; *Pennsaid* 2% soln SE: Pruritus, dermatitis, burning, dry skin, N, HA Notes: Do not apply patch/gel to damaged skin or while bathing; ✓CBC, LFTs periodically; no box warning on *Solaraze*

Diclofenac/Misoprostol (Arthrotec 50, Arthrotec 75) BOX: May induce abortion, birth defects; do not take if PRG; may ↑ risk of CV events & GI bleeding; CI in postop CABG Uses: *OA and RA w/ ↑ risk of GI bleeding* Acts: NSAID w/ GI-protective PGE₁ Dose: *OA:* 50–75 mg PO bid-tid *RA:* 50 mg bid-qid or 75 mg bid; w/ food or milk W/P: [X, ?] CHF, HTN, renal/hepatic dysfunction, & Hx PUD, asthma; avoid w/ porphyria; ↑ risk of MI/CVA CI: PRG; GI bleeding; renal/hepatic failure; severe CHF; NSAID/aspirin ASA allergy; following CABG Disp: Tabs *Arthrotec 50:* 50 mg diclofenac w/ 0.2 mg misoprostol; *Arthrotec:* 75 mg diclofenac w/ 0.2 mg misoprostol SE: Abd cramps, heartburn, GI ulcers, rash, interstitial nephritis Notes: Do not crush tabs; watch for GI bleeding; ✓CBC, LFTs; PRG test females before use

Dicloxacillin (Generic) Uses: *Rx of pneumonia, skin, & soft-tissue Infxns, & osteomyelitis caused by penicillinase-producing staphylococci* Acts: Bactericidal; ↓ cell wall synth. Spectrum: *S. aureus & Streptococcus* Dose: *Adults.* 125–500 mg qid (2 g/d max) *Peds < 40 kg.* 12.5–100 mg/kg/d ÷ qid; take on empty stomach W/P: [B, ?] CI: Component or PCN sens Disp: Caps 125, 250, 500 mg SE: N/D, Abd pain Notes: Monitor PTT if pt on warfarin

Dicyclomine (Bentyl) Uses: *Functional IBS* **Acts:** Smooth-muscle relaxant **Dose:** 20 mg PO qid; ↑ to 160 mg/d max or 20 mg IM q6h, 80 mg/d ÷ qid, then ↑ to 160 mg/d, max 2 wk **W/P:** [B, –] **CI:** Infants < 6 mo, NAG, MyG, severe UC, BOO, GI obst, reflux esophagitis **Disp:** Caps 10 mg; tabs 20 mg; syrup 10 mg/5 mL; Inj 10 mg/mL **SE:** Anticholinergic SEs may limit dose **Notes:** Take 30–60 min ac; avoid EtOH, do not administer IV

Didanosine [ddI] (Videx) **BOX:** Allergy manifested as fever, rash, fatigue, GI/resp Sxs reported; stop drug immediately & do not rechallenge; lactic acidosis & hepatomegaly/steatosis reported Uses: *HIV Infxn in zidovudine-intolerant pts* **Acts:** NRTI **Dose:** *Adults.* **> 60 kg.** 400 mg/d PO or 200 mg PO bid < **60 kg.** 250 mg/d PO or 125 mg PO bid; adults should take 2 tabs/administration **Peds 2 wk–8 mo.** 100 mg/m² bid > **8 mo.** 120 mg/m² PO bid; on empty stomach; ↓ w/ renal impair **W/P:** [B, –] CDC rec: HIV-infected mothers not breast-feed **CI:** Component sens; w/ allopurinol or ribavirin **Disp:** Chew tabs 100, 150, 200 mg; DR caps 125, 200, 250, 400 mg; powder for soln 2, 4 g **SE:** Pancreatitis, peripheral neuropathy, D, HA **Notes:** Do not take w/ meals; thoroughly chew tabs; do not mix w/ fruit juice or acidic beverages; reconstitute powder w/ H₂O; many drug interactions

Diflunisal (Dolobid) **BOX:** May ↑ risk of CV events & GI bleeding; CI in postop CABG Uses: *Mild–mod pain; OA; RA* **Acts:** NSAID **Dose:** *Pain:* 500 mg PO bid *OA/RA:* 500–1000/mg/d PO bid (max 1.5 g/d); ↓ in renal impair, take w/ food/milk **W/P:** [C (D 3rd tri or near delivery), ?/–] CHF, HTN, renal/hepatic dysfunction, Hx PUD, ↑ risk of MI/CVA **CI:** Allergy to NSAIDs or ASA, active GI bleeding, post-CABG **Disp:** Tabs 500 mg **SE:** May ↑ bleeding time; HA, Abd cramps, heartburn, GI ulceration, rash, interstitial nephritis, fluid retention

Digoxin (Digitek, Lanoxin, Lanoxin Pediatric, Generic) Uses: *CHF, AF & atrial flutter, PAT* **Acts:** Positive inotrope; AV node refractory period **Dose:** *Adults.* PO digitalization: 0.5–0.75 mg PO, then 0.25 mg PO q6–8h to total 1–1.5 mg *IV or IM digitalization:* 0.25–0.5 mg IM or IV, then 0.25 mg q4–6h to total 0.125–0.5 mg PO, IM, or IV (average daily dose 0.125–0.25 mg) *Peds. Preterm infants.* Digitalization: 30 mcg/kg PO or 25 mcg/kg IV; give 1/2 of dose initial, then 1/4 of dose at 8–12 h intervals for 2 doses *Maint:* 5–7.5 mcg/kg/24 h PO or 4–6 mcg/kg/24 h IV ÷ q12h *Term infants.* Digitalization: 25–35 mcg/kg PO or 20–30 mcg/kg IV; give 1/2 the initial dose, then 1/3 of dose at 8–12 h *Maint:* 6–10 mcg/kg/24 h PO or 5–8 mcg/kg/24 h ÷ q12h *2–5 y.* Digitalization: 30–40 mcg/kg PO or 25–35 mcg/kg IV *Maint:* 7.5–10 mcg/kg/24 h PO or 6–9 mcg/kg IV ÷ q12h. *5–10 y.* Digitalization: 25–35 mcg/kg PO or 15–30 mcg/kg IV *Maint:* 5–10 mcg/kg/24 h PO or 4–8 mcg/kg q12 h *>10 y.* 10–15 mcg/kg PO or 8–12 mcg/kg IV *Maint:* 2.5-5 mcg/kg PO or 2–3 mcg/kg IV q 24 h; ↓ in renal impair **W/P:** [C, +/–] w/ K+, Mg2+, renal failure **CI:** AV block; IHSS; constrictive pericarditis **Disp:** Tabs 0.125, 0.25 mg; elixir 0.05 mg/mL; Inj 0.1, 0.25 mg/mL **SE:** Can cause heart block; ↓ K⁺ potentiates tox; N/V, HA, fatigue, visual disturbances (yellow-green halos around lights); cardiac arrhythmias **Notes:** Multiple drug interactions; IM Inj painful, has erratic absorption & should not be used. *Levels: Trough:* Just before next dose; *Therapeutic:* 0.8–2 ng/mL; *Toxic:* > 2 ng/mL; *Half-life:* 36 h

Digoxin Immune Fab (DigiFab) Uses: *Life-threatening digoxin intoxication* Acts: Antigen-binding fragments bind & inactivate digoxin Dose: *Adults & Peds.* Based on serum level & pt's Wt; see charts provided w/ drug W/P: [C, ?] CI: Sheep product allergy Disp: Inj 40 mg/vial SE: Worsening of cardiac output or CHF, ↓ K⁺, facial swelling, redness Notes: Each vial binds ~ 0.5 mg of digoxin; renal failure may require redosing in several days

Diltiazem (Cardizem, Cardizem CD, Cardizem LA, Cardizem SR, Cartia XT, Dilacor XR, Dilt-XR, Taztia XT, Tiazac) Uses: *Angina, prevention of reinfarction, HTN, AF or atrial flutter, PAT* Acts: CCB Dose: *Stable angina PO:* Initial, 30 mg PO qid; ↑ to 120–320 mg/d in 3–4 ÷ doses PRN; XR 120 mg/d (540 mg max) *LA:* 180–360 mg/d *HTN:* SR: 60–120 mg PO bid; ↑ to 360 mg/d max *CD or XR:* 120–360 mg/d (max 540 mg/d) or LA 180–360 mg/d *AF, atrial flutter, PSVT:* 0.25 mg/kg IV bolus over 2 min; may repeat in 15 min at 0.35 mg/kg; begin Inf 5–15 mg/h *ECC 2010. Acute rate control:* 0.25 mg/kg (15–20 mg) over 2 min, followed in 15 min by 0.35 mg/kg (20–25 mg) over 2 min; maint Inf 5–15 mg/h W/P: [C, +/−] ↑ Effect w/ amiodarone, cimetidine, fentanyl, Li, cyclosporine, digoxin, β-blockers, theophylline CI: SSS, AV block, ↓ BP, AMI, pulm congestion Disp: *Cardizem CD:* Caps 120, 180, 240, 300, 360 mg; *Cardizem LA:* Tabs 120, 180, 240, 300, 360, 420 mg; *Cardizem SR:* Caps 60, 90, 120 mg; *Cardizem:* Tabs 30, 60, 90, 120 mg; *Cartia XT:* Caps 120, 180, 240, 300 mg; *Dilacor XR:* Caps 120, 180, 240 mg; *Dilt-XR:* Caps 120, 180, 240 mg; *Tiazac:* Caps 120, 180, 240, 300, 360, 420 mg; Inj 5 mg/mL; *Taztia XT:* 120, 180, 240, 300, 360 mg SE: Gingival hyperplasia, ↓ HR, AV block, ECG abnormalities, peripheral edema, dizziness, HA Notes: *Cardizem CD, Dilacor XR, & Tiazac* **not** interchangeable

Dimenhydrinate (Dramamine, Others) Uses: *Prevention & Rx of N/V, dizziness, & vertigo of motion sickness* Acts: Antiemetic, histamine antag Dose: *Adults.* 50–100 mg PO q4–6h, max 400 mg/d; 50 mg IM/IV PRN *Peds 2–6 y.* 12.5–25 mg PO q6–8h max 75 mg/d *6–12 y.* 25–50 mg q6–8h, max 150 mg/d W/P: [B, ?] CI: Component sens; neonates (contains benzyl alcohol) Disp: Tabs 50 mg; chew tabs 50 mg; Inj 50 mg/mL SE: Anticholinergic SE Notes: Take 30 min before travel for motion sickness

Dimethyl Fumarate (Tecfidera) Uses: *Relapsing MS* Acts: Activates the Nrf2 pathway, exact mechanism unknown Dose: 120 mg PO bid × 7 d, then ↑ to 240 mg PO bid; swallow whole W/P: [C, ?/−] May cause lymphopenia, ✓ CBC at baseline, annually & PRN; withhold Tx w/ severe Infxn CI: Ø Disp: Caps DR 120, 240 mg SE: N/D, Abd pain, flushing, pruritus, rash, ↑ LFTs

Dimethyl Sulfoxide [DMSO] (Rimso-50) Uses: *Interstitial cystitis* Acts: Unknown Dose: Intravesical, 50 mL, retain for 15 min; repeat q2wk until relief W/P: [C, ?] CI: Component sens Disp: 50% soln SE: Cystitis, eosinophilia, GI & taste disturbance

Dinoprostone (Cervidil Insert, Prepidil Gel, Prostin E2)   BOX: Should only be used by trained personnel in an appropriate hospital setting Uses: *Induce labor; terminate PRG (12–20 wk); evacuate uterus in missed abortion or fetal death* Acts: Prostaglandin; changes consistency, dilatation, & effacement of the cervix; induces uterine contraction Dose: *Gel:* 0.5 mg; if no cervical/uterine response, repeat 0.5 mg q6h (max 24-h dose 1.5 mg) *Vag insert:* 1 insert (10 mg = 0.3 mg dinoprostone/h over 12 h); remove w/ onset of labor or 12 h after insertion *Vag supp:* 20 mg repeated q3–5h; adjust PRN supp: 1 high in vagina, repeat at 3–5-h intervals until abortion (240 mg max) W/P: [X, ?] CI: Ruptured membranes, allergy to prostaglandins, placenta previa or AUB, when oxytocic drugs CI or if prolonged uterine contractions are inappropriate (Hx C-section, cephalopelvic disproportion, etc) Disp: *Vag gel:* 0.5 mg in 3-g syringes (w/ 10- & 20-mm shielded catheter); *Vag supp:* 20 mg; *Vag insert, CR:* 10 mg SE: N/V/D, dizziness, flushing, HA, fever, abn uterine contractions

Dinutuximab (Unituxin)   BOX: Severe/fatal inf Rxns (26%); prehydrate and premedicate; monitor during and 4 h after Inf; stop Inf w/ severe Rxns; permanently D/C w/ anaphylaxis; neuropathic pain in most; give IV opioid before, during, & for 2 h after Inf; D/C w/ severe pain, neuropathy Uses: *High-risk neuroblastoma in peds w/ partial response to multiagent regimen* Acts: Binds to disialoganglioside GD2 Dose: *Peds.* 17.5 mg/m²/d IV × 4 d (max 5 cycles); use w/ sargramostim, aldesleukin, isotretinoin; part of a 28-d cycle multidrug regimen W/P: [N/A, N/A] Inf Rxns; pain, neuropathy, ↓ BP, electrolyte abn, capillary leak, Infxn, HUS, ↓ BM, ocular tox, many drug interactions: do not give w/ BCG, belimurab, clozapine, dipyrone, pimecrolimus, tacrolimus, tofacitinib, live vaccines CI: Hx dinutuximab anaphylaxis Disp: 17.5 mg/5 mL (3.5 mg/mL) single-use vial SE: Weakness, fatigue, insomnia, HA, skin rash, night sweats, N /V/D, ↑ ALT/AST, hepatotox, fever, cough, pneumonia, URI, peripheral edema; rare anaphylaxis, hypersens Rxns, intestinal perf, TEN Notes: Sound-alikes/look-alikes: obinutuzumab, rituximab; Inf only; not IV push or bolus

Diphenhydramine (Benadryl) [OTC]   Uses: *Rx & prevent allergic Rxns, motion sickness, potentiate narcotics, sedation, cough suppression, Rx of extrapyramidal Rxns* Acts: Antihistamine, antiemetic Dose: *Adults.* 25–50 mg PO q4–6h (max 300 mg/d); 10–50 mg IM/IV (max 400 mg/d) *Peds > 2 y.* 5 mg/kg/24 h PO or IM ÷ q6h (max 300 mg/d); ↑ dosing interval w/ mod–severe renal Insuff W/P: [B, −] Elderly, NAG, BPH, w/ MAOI CI: Acute asthma Disp: Tabs & caps 25, 50 mg; chew tabs 12.5 mg; elixir 12.5 mg/5 mL; syrup 12.5 mg/5 mL; liq 12.5 mg/5 mL; Inj 50 mg/mL, cream, gel, liq 2% SE: Anticholinergic (xerostomia, urinary retention, sedation)

Diphenoxylate/Atropine (Lomotil, Lonox) [C-V]   Uses: *D* Acts: Constipating meperidine congener, ↓ GI motility Dose: *Adults.* Initial, 5 mg PO tid-qid until controlled, then 2.5–5 mg PO bid; 20 mg/d max *Peds > 2 y.* 0.3–0.4 mg/kg/24 h (of diphenoxylate) bid-qid; 20 mg/d max W/P: [C, ?/−] Elderly, w/ renal impair

CI: Obstructive jaundice, D d/t bacterial Infxn; children < 2 y **Disp:** Tabs 2.5 mg diphenoxylate/0.025 mg atropine; liq 2.5 mg diphenoxylate/0.025 mg atropine/5 mL **SE:** Drowsiness, dizziness, xerostomia, blurred vision, urinary retention, constipation

Diphtheria/Tetanus Toxoids [DT] (Generic Only) (Ages < 7 y)
Uses: *Primary immunization, ages < 7 y (DTaP is recommended vaccine) *Acts:** Active immunization **Dose:** 0.5 mL IM × 1, 5-dose series for primary immunization if DTaP CI W/P: [C, N/A] **CI:** Component sens **Disp:** Single-dose syringes 0.5 mL **SE:** Inj site pain, redness, swelling; fever, fatigue, myalgias/arthralgias, N/V, Sz, other neurological SE rare; syncope, apnea in preterm infants **Notes:** If IM, use only preservative-free Inj; do not confuse DT (for children < 7 y) w/ Td (for adults); DTaP is recommended for primary immunization

Diphtheria/Tetanus Toxoids [Td] (Decavac, Tenivac) (Ages > 7 y)
Uses: *Primary immunization, booster (peds 7–9 y; peds 11–12 y if 5 y since last shot, then q10y); tetanus protection after wound *Acts:** Active immunization **Dose:** 0.5 mL IM × 1 W/P: [C, ?/–] **CI:** Component sens **Disp:** Single-dose syringes 0.5 mL **SE:** Inj site pain, redness, swelling; fever, fatigue, HA, malaise, neurologic disorders rare **Notes:** If IM, use preservative-free Inj; use DTaP (*Adacel*) rather than TT or Td all adults 19–64 y who have **not** previously received 1 dose of DTaP (protection adult pertussis) and Tdap for ages 10–18 y (*Boostrix*); do not confuse Td (for adults) w/ DT (for children < 7 y)

Diphtheria/Tetanus Toxoids/Acellular Pertussis, Adsorbed [Tdap] (Ages < 7 y) (Daptacel, Infanrix, Tripedia)
Uses: Primary vaccination; 5 Inj at 2, 4, 6, 15–18 mo and 4–6 y **Acts:** Active immunization **Dose:** 0.5 mL IM × 1 W/P: [C, N/A] **CI:** Component sens; if previous pertussis vaccine caused progressive neurologic disorder/encephalopathy w/in 7 d of shot **Disp:** Single-dose vials 0.5 mL **SE:** Inj site nodule/pain/swelling/redness; drowsiness, fatigue, fever, fussiness, irritability, lethargy, V, prolonged crying; rare ITP and neurologic disorders **Notes:** If IM, use only preservative-free Inj; DTaP recommended for primary immunization age < 7 y, if age 7–9 y use Td, ages > 10–11 y use Tdap; if encephalopathy or other neurologic disorder w/in 7 d of previous dose DO NOT USE DTaP: use DT or Td depending on age

Diphtheria/Tetanus Toxoids/Acellular Pertussis, Adsorbed [Tdap] (Ages > 10–11 y) (Boosters: Adacel, Boostrix)
Uses: *"Catch-up" vaccination if 1 or more of the 5 childhood doses of DTP or DTaP missed; all adults 19–64 y who have **not** received 1 dose previously (adult pertussis protection) or if around infants < 12 mo; booster q10y; tetanus protection after fresh wound **Acts:** Active immunization, ages > 10–11 y *Acts:** Active immunization **Dose:** 0.5 mL IM × 1 W/P: [C, ?/–] w/ Latex allergy **CI:** Component sens; if previous pertussis vaccine caused progressive neurologic disorder/encephalopathy w/in 7 d of shot **Disp:** Single-dose vials 0.5 mL **SE:** Inj site pain, redness, swelling; Abd pain, arthralgias/myalgias, fatigue, fever, HA, N/V/D, rash, tiredness **Notes:** If IM, use only preservative-free Inj; ACIP rec: Tdap for ages 10–18 y

(*Boostrix*) or 10–64 y (*Adacel*); Td should be used in children 7–9 y; CDC rec pts > age 65 who have close contact w/ infants get a dose of Tdap (protection against pertussis)

Diphtheria/Tetanus Toxoids/Acellular Pertussis, Adsorbed/IPV (Kinrix, Quadracel) Uses: *Immunization against diphtheria, tetanus, pertussis, & polio as 5th dose in DTaP series and 4th dose in IPV, ages 4–6 y* Acts: Active immunization Dose: *Peds 4–6 y.* 0.5 mL IM Inj × 1 into deltoid W/P: Anaphylactoid/hypersens Rxns; syncope; current mod–severe acute illness; w/ anticoagulant; Hx severe local reaction to tetanus toxoid, bleeding disorder, Guillain-Barré synd, Szs, neurologic Dz; predisposition to Szs; immunocompromised CI: Allergic Rxn after previous DTaP/IPV; encephalopathy w/ previous pertussis vaccine; progressive neurologic Dz Disp: Single Inj 0.5 mL SE: Limb swelling, malaise, drowsiness, HA, ↓ appetite, pain, Inj site erythema, myalgia, fever Notes: Refrigerate; discard if frozen; do not mix w/ other vaccine/Inj; tetanus/diphtheria antibodies ↓ w/ age; give initial series to elderly w/o primary immunization or at risk; monitor for syncope for 15 min

Diphtheria/Tetanus Toxoids/Acelluar Pertussis, Adsorbed/Hep B (Recombinant)/IPV, Combined (Pediarix) Uses: *Immunization against diphtheria, tetanus, pertussis, HBV, polio (types 1, 2, 3) as a 3-dose primary series in infants & children < 7 y, born to HBsAg(−) mothers* Acts: Active immunization Dose: *Infants.* Three 0.5-mL doses IM, at 6–8-wk intervals, start at 2 mo; children given 1 dose of hep B vaccine, same; previously vaccinated w/ 1 or more doses IPV, use to complete series W/P: [C, N/A] w/ Bleeding disorders CI: HBsAg(+) mother, adults, children > 7 y, immunosuppressed, component sens or allergy to yeast/neomycin/polymyxin B, encephalopathy, progressive neurologic disorders Disp: Single-dose syringes 0.5 mL SE: Drowsiness, restlessness, fever, fussiness, ↓ appetite, Inj site pain/swelling/nodule/redness Notes: If IM, use only preservative-free Inj

Diphtheria/Tetanus Toxoids/Acellular Pertussis, Adsorbed/IPV/ Haemophilus b Conjugate Vaccine, Combined (Pentacel) Uses: *Immunization against diphtheria, tetanus, pertussis, poliomyelitis and invasive Dz due to Haemophilus influenzae type b* Acts: Active immunization Dose: *Infants.* 0.5 mL IM at 2, 4, 6, and 15–18 mo W/P: [C, N/A] w/ Fever > 40.5°C (105°F), HHE or persistent, inconsolable crying > 3 h w/in 48 h after a previous pertussis-containing vaccine; Sz w/in 3 d after a previous pertussis-containing vaccine; Guillain-Barré synd w/in 6 wk of previous tetanus toxoid vaccine; w/ Hx Sz antipyretic may be administered w/ vaccine × 24 h; w/ bleeding disorders CI: Allergy to any components; encephalopathy w/in 7 d of previous pertussis vaccine; w/ progressive neurologic disorders Disp: Single-dose vials 0.5 mL SE: Fussiness/irritability and inconsolable crying; fever > 38.0°C; Inj site Rxn

Dipivefrin (Propine) Uses: *Open-angle glaucoma* Acts: α-Adrenergic agonist Dose: 1 gtt in eye q12h W/P: [B, ?/−] CI: NAG Disp: 0.1% soln SE: HA, local irritation, blurred vision, photophobia, HTN

Dipyridamole (Persantine) Uses: *Prevent postop thromboembolic disorders, often in combo w/ ASA or warfarin (eg, CABG, vascular graft); w/ warfarin after artificial heart valve; chronic angina; w/ ASA to prevent coronary artery thrombosis; dipyridamole IV used in place of exercise stress test for CAD* Acts: Anti-plt activity; coronary vasodilator Dose: *Adults & Peds > 12 y.* 75–100 mg PO qid; stress test 0.14 mg/kg/min (max 60 mg over 4 min) W/P: [B, ?/–] w/ Other drugs that affect coagulation CI: Component sens Disp: Tabs 25, 50, 75 mg; Inj 5 mg/mL SE: HA, ↓ BP, N, Abd distress, flushing, rash, dizziness, dyspnea Notes: IV use can worsen angina

Dipyridamole/Aspirin (Aggrenox) Uses: *↓ Reinfarction after MI; prevent occlusion after CABG; ↓ risk of stroke* Acts: ↓ Plt aggregation (both agents) Dose: 1 cap PO bid W/P: [D, ?/–] CI: Ulcers, bleeding diathesis Disp: Dipyridamole (XR) 200 mg/ASA 25 mg SE: ASA component: allergic Rxns, skin Rxns, ulcers/GI bleeding, bronchospasm; dipyridamole component: dizziness, HA, rash Notes: Swallow caps whole

Disopyramide (Norpace, Norpace CR, Generic) BOX: Excessive mortality or nonfatal cardiac arrest rate w/ use in asymptomatic non–life-threatening ventricular arrhythmias w/ MI 6 d–2 y prior; restrict use to life-threatening arrhythmias only Uses: *Suppression & Px of VT* Acts: Class IA antiarrhythmic; stabilizes membranes, ↓ action potential Dose: *Adults.* Immediate < 50 kg 200 mg, > 50 kg 300 mg, maint 400–800 mg/d ÷ q6h or q12h for CR, max 1600 mg/d *Peds < 1 y.* 10–30 mg/kg/24 h PO (÷ qid) *1–4 y.* 10–20 mg/kg/24 h PO (÷ qid) *4–12 y.* 10–15 mg/kg/24 h PO (÷ qid) *12–18 y.* 6–15 mg/kg/24 h PO (÷ qid); ↓ in renal/hepatic impair W/P: [C, –] Elderly, w/ abn ECG, lytes, liver/renal impair, NAG CI: AV block, cardiogenic shock, ↓ BP, CHF Disp: Caps 100, 150 mg; CR caps 100, 150 mg SE: Anticholinergic SEs; negative inotrope, may induce CHF Notes: Levels: *Trough:* just before next dose; *Therapeutic:* 2–5 mcg/mL; *Toxic* > 7 mcg/mL; *Half-life:* 4–10 h

Dobutamine (Dobutrex, Generic) Uses: *Short-term in cardiac decompensation secondary to ↓ contractility* Acts: Positive inotrope Dose: *Adults. ECC 2010.* 2.5–20 mcg/kg/min; titrate to HR not > 10% of baseline *Peds. ECC 2010. Shock w/ high SVR:* 2–20 mcg/kg/min; titrate W/P: [B, ?/–] w/ Arrhythmia, MI, severe CAD, ↓ vol CI: Sens to sulfites, IHSS Disp: Inj 250 mg/20 mL, 500 mg/40 mL SE: CP, HTN, dyspnea Notes: Monitor PWP & cardiac output if possible; ✓ ECG for ↑ HR, ectopic activity; follow BP

Docetaxel (Docefrez, Taxotere, Generic) BOX: Do not administer if neutrophil count < 1500 cells/mm³; severe Rxns possible in hepatic dysfunction; hypersens & severe fluid retention possible Uses: *Breast (anthracycline-resistant), ovarian, lung, & prostate CA* Acts: Antimitotic agent; promotes microtubular aggregation; semisynthetic taxoid Dose: 100 mg/m² over 1 h IV q3wk (per protocols); dexamethasone 8 mg bid prior & continue for 3–4 d; ↓ dose w/ ↑ bili levels W/P: [D, –] Infusion contains ethanol; can cause intoxication CI: Sens to meds w/ polysorbate 80, component sens **Disp:** Inj (mg/mL): 20/0.5, 80/2, 20/1, 80/4, 160/8, 140/7; *Docefrez:* vial 20, 80 mg **SE:** ↓ BM, neuropathy, N/V, alopecia, fluid retention synd; cumulative doses of 300–400 mg/m² w/o steroid prep & post-Tx & 600–800 mg/m² w/ steroid prep; allergy possible (rare w/ steroid prep) **Notes:** ✓ Bili/SGOT/SGPT prior to each cycle; frequent CBC during Tx

Docusate Calcium (Surfak)/Docusate Potassium (Dialose)/ Docusate Sodium (Colace, DOSS) **Uses:** *Constipation; adjunct to painful anorectal conditions (hemorrhoids)* **Acts:** Stool softener **Dose:** *Adults.* 50–500 mg PO ÷ daily-qid *Peds Infants–3 y.* 10–40 mg/24 h ÷ daily-qid *3–6 y.* 20–60 mg/24 h ÷ daily-qid *6–12 y.* 40–150 mg/24 h ÷ daily-qid **W/P:** [A, +] Use w/ mineral oil; intestinal obst, acute Abd pain, N/V **Disp:** *Ca:* Caps 50, 240 mg; *K:* Caps 100, 240 mg; *Na:* Caps 50, 100, 250 mg; syrup 60 mg/15 mL; liq 150 mg/15 mL; soln 50 mg/mL; enema 283 mg/mL **SE:** Rare Abd cramping, D **Notes:** Take w/ full glass of water; no laxative action; do not use > 1 wk

Dofetilide (Tikosyn) **BOX:** To minimize the risk of induced arrhythmia, hospitalize for minimum of 3 d to provide evaluation of CrCl, cont ECG monitoring, & cardiac resuscitation **Uses:** *Maintain nl sinus rhythm in AF/A flutter after conversion* **Acts:** Class III antiarrhythmic, prolongs action potential **Dose:** Based on CrCl & QTc; CrCl > 60 mL/min 500 mcg PO q12h, ✓ QTc 2–3 h after; if QTc > 15% over baseline or > 500 ms, ↓ to 250 mcg q12h, ✓ QTc after each dose; if CrCl < 60 mL/min, see PI; D/C if QTc > 500 ms after dosing adjustments **W/P:** [C, −] w/ AV block, renal Dz, electrolyte imbalance **CI:** Baseline QTc > 440 ms, CrCl < 20 mL/min; w/ verapamil, cimetidine, trimethoprim, ketoconazole, quinolones, HCTZ **Disp:** Caps 125, 250, 500 mcg **SE:** Ventricular arrhythmias, QT ↑, torsades de pointes, rash, HA, CP, dizziness **Notes:** Avoid w/ other drugs that ↑ QT interval; hold class I/III antiarrhythmics for 3 half-lives prior to dosing; amiodarone level should be < 0.3 mg/L before use, do not initiate if HR < 60 BPM; restricted to participating prescribers; correct K⁺ and Mg²⁺ before use

Dolasetron (Anzemet) **Uses:** *Prevent chemotherapy and postop-associated N/V* **Acts:** 5-HT₃ receptor antag **Dose:** *Adults. PO:* 100 mg PO as a single dose 1 h prior to chemotherapy *Postop:* 12.5 mg IV, or 100 mg PO 2 h preop *Peds 2–16 y.* 1.8 mg/kg PO (max 100 mg) as single dose *Postop:* 0.35 mg/kg IV or 1.2 mg/kg PO **W/P:** [B, ?] w/ Cardiac conduction problems **CI:** IV use w/ chemo component sens **Disp:** Tabs 50, 100 mg; Inj 20 mg/mL **SE:** ↑ QT interval, D, HTN, HA, Abd pain, urinary retention, transient ↑ LFTs **Notes:** IV form no longer approved for chemo-induced N/V due to heart rhythm abnormalities

Dolutegravir (Tivicay) **Uses:** *HIV-1 Infxn w/ other antiretrovirals* **Acts:** INSTI **Dose:** *Adults. Tx-naïve or Tx-experienced INSTI naïve:* 50 mg PO 1 ×/d; *Tx-naïve or Tx-experienced INSTI naïve w/ a potent UGT1A/CYP3A inducer (efavirenz, fosamprenavir/ritonavir, tipranavir/ritonavir, or rifampin):* 50 mg PO 2 ×/d; *INSTI-experienced with certain INSTI-associated resistance substitutions or suspected INSTI resist:* 50 mg PO 2 ×/d *Peds ≥ 12 y & ≥ 40 kg. Tx-naïve or*

Tx-experienced INSTI-naïve: 50 mg PO 1 ×/d; *w/ efavirenz, fosamprenavir/ritonavir, tipranavir/ritonavir, or rifampin:* 50 mg PO 2 ×/d **W/P:** [B, ?/–] CDC rec HIV-infected mothers not breast-feed; D/C w/ hypersens Rxn (rash, constitutional findings, organ dysfunction); ↑ LFTs w/ underlying hep B or C (monitor LFTs); w/ other antiretroviral therapy, may cause fat redistribution/accumulation and immune reconstitution synd **CI:** w/ Dofetilide **Disp:** Tabs 50 mg **SE:** HA, insomnia, N/V/D, Abd pain, ↑ serum lipase, hypersens Rxn, ↑ glu, ↑ bili, pruritus **Notes:** Take 2 h before or 6 h after antacids or laxatives, sucralfate, iron & calcium supl, buffered meds

Dolutegravir/Abacavir/Lamivudine (Triumeq) BOX: Hypersens Rxns more likely w/ HLAB*5701 allele and abacavir; lactic acidosis & hepato-megaly/steatosis w/ fatalities; exacerbations of hep B after D/C lamivudine compo-nent; ✓ LFTs **Uses:** *HIV Infxn* **Acts:** INSTI w/ 2 NRTI **Dose:** 1 tab qd w/ efavirenz, fosamprenavir/ritonavir, tipranavir/ritonavir, or rifampin; give additional 50 mg dolutegravir tab 12 h after Triumeq **W/P:** [C, –] Not rec w/ mild hepatic impair, CrCl < 50 mL/min; many drug interactions; pancreatitis w/ abacavir & lamivudine; hypersens Rxns possible (rash, hep tox); D/C w/ severe Rxns **CI:** HLA-B*5701 allele, component hypersens, mod/severe liver Dz, w/ dofetilide **Disp:** Combo tabs dolutegravir 50 mg/abacavir 600 mg/lamivudine 300 mg **SE:** HA, fatigue, insomnia, ↑ ALT/AST (✓ LFTs at baseline, monitor w/ liver Dz, HBV, HCV) **Notes:** w/ or w/o Food; screen for HLA-B*5701 before use

Donepezil (Aricept, Generic) **Uses:** *Mild/mod/severe Alzheimer dementia*; ADHD; behavioral synds in dementia; dementia w/ Parkinson Dz; Lewy-body dementia **Acts:** ACH inhib **Dose:** 5 mg qhs, ↑ to 10 mg PO qhs after 4–6 wk **W/P:** [C, ?] Risk for ↓ HR w/ preexisting conduction abnormalities, may exaggerate succi-nylcholine-type muscle relaxation w/ anesthesia, ↑ gastric acid secretion **CI:** Hyper-sens **Disp:** Tabs 5, 10, 23 mg; ODT tabs 5, 10 mg **SE:** N/V/D, insomnia, Infxn, muscle cramp, fatigue, anorexia **Notes:** N/V/D dose-related & resolves in 1–3 wk

Dopamine (Generic) BOX: Tissue vesicant, give phentolamine w/ extrav **Uses:** *Short-term use in cardiac decompensation secondary to ↓ contractility; ↑ organ perfusion (at low dose)* **Acts:** Positive inotropic agent w/ dose response: 1–5 mcg/kg/min renal effects; 5–15 mcg/kg/min β1 agonist (↑ CO); > 15 mcg/kg/min α1 agonist (peripheral vasoconstriction, pressor; **Dose:** *Adults.* 5 mcg/kg/min by cont Inf, ↑ by 5 mcg/kg/min to 50 mcg/kg/min max to effect *ECC 2010.* 2–20 mcg/kg/min **Peds.** *ECC 2010. Shock w/ adequate intravascular volume and stable rhythm:* 2–20 mcg/kg/min; titrate, if > 20 mcg/kg/min needed, consider alternative adrenergic **W/P:** [C, ?] ↓ Dose w/ MAOI **CI:** Pheochromocytoma, VF, sulfite sens **Disp:** Inj 40, 80, 160 mg/mL; premixed 0.8, 1.6, 3.2 mg/mL **SE:** Tachycardia, vasoconstriction, ↓ BP, HA, N/V, dyspnea **Notes:** > 10 mcg/kg/min ↓ renal perfu-sion; monitor urinary output & ECG for ↑ HR, BP, ectopy; monitor PCWP & car-diac output if possible; phentolamine used for extrav 10–15 mL NS w/ 5–10 mg of phentolamine

Doripenem (Doribax) Uses: *Complicated intra-Abd Infxn and UTI, including pyelo* Acts: Carbapenem, ↓ cell wall synth, a β-lactam. *Spectrum:* Excellent gram(+) (except MRSA and *Enterococcus* sp), excellent gram(−) coverage, including β-lactamase producers, good anaerobic Dose: 500 mg IV q8h, ↓ w/ renal impair W/P: [B, ?] Not indicated for ventilator-associated bacterial pneumonia CI: Carbapenem β-lactams hypersens Disp: 250, 500 mg vial SE: HA, N/D, rash, phlebitis Notes: May ↓ valproic acid levels; overuse may ↑ bacterial resistance; monitor for *C. difficile*-associated D

Dornase Alfa (DNase, Pulmozyme) Uses: *↓ Frequency of resp Infxns in CF* Acts: Enzyme cleaves extracellular DNA, ↓ mucous viscosity Dose: *Adults & Peds > 5 y.* Inh 2.5 mg/2.5 mg qd-bid dosing w/ FVC > 85% w/ recommended nebulizer W/P: [B, ?] CI: Chinese hamster product allergy Disp: Soln for Inh 1 mg/mL SE: Pharyngitis, voice alteration, rash

Dorzolamide (Trusopt) Uses: *Open-angle glaucoma, ocular hypertension* Acts: Carbonic anhydrase inhib Dose: 1 gtt in eye(s) tid W/P: [C, ?] w/ NAG, CrCl < 30 mL/min CI: Component sens Disp: 2% soln SE: Irritation, bitter taste, punctate keratitis, ocular allergic Rxn

Dorzolamide/Timolol (Cosopt) Uses: *Open-angle glaucoma, ocular hypertension* Acts: Carbonic anhydrase inhib w/ β-adrenergic blocker Dose: 1 gtt in eye(s) bid W/P: [C, ?/−] CrCl < 30 mL/min CI: Component sens, asthma, severe COPD, sinus bradycardia, AV block Disp: Soln dorzolamide 2% & timolol 0.5% SE: Irritation, bitter taste, superficial keratitis, ocular allergic Rxn

Doxazosin (Cardura, Cardura XL) Uses: *HTN & symptomatic BPH* Acts: α₁-Adrenergic blocker; relaxes bladder neck smooth muscle Dose: *HTN:* Initial 1 mg/d PO, may ↑ to 16 mg/d PO *BPH:* Initial 1 mg/d PO, may ↑ to 8 mg/d; XL 4–8 mg qam W/P: [C, ?] w/ Liver impair CI: Component sens; use w/ PDE5 inhib (eg, sildenafil) can cause ↓ BP Disp: Tabs 1, 2, 4, 8 mg; XL 4, 8 mg SE: Dizziness, HA, drowsiness, fatigue, malaise, sexual dysfunction, doses > 4 mg ↑ postural ↓ BP risk; intraoperative floppy iris synd Notes: 1st dose hs; syncope may occur w/in 90 min of initial dose

Doxepin, Caps, Soln (Generic) BOX: Closely monitor for worsening depression or emergence of suicidality Uses: *Depression, anxiety, chronic pain* Acts: TCA; ↑ synaptic CNS serotonin or norepinephrine Dose: 25–150 mg/d PO, usually hs but can ÷ doses; up to 300 mg/d for depression; ↓ in hepatic impair W/P: [C, ?/−] w/ EtOH abuse, elderly, w/ MAOI CI: NAG, urinary retention, MAOI use w/in 14 d, in recovery phase of MI Disp: Caps 10, 25, 50, 75, 100, 150 mg; soln 4-oz container calibrated 5, 10, 15, 20, 25 mg SE: Anticholinergic SEs, ↓ BP, tachycardia, drowsiness, dizziness Notes: Caps for depression, etc

Doxepin, Tabs (Silenor) Uses: *Insomnia* Acts: TCA Dose: Take w/in 30 min HS 6 mg qd; 3 mg in elderly; 6 mg/d max; not w/in 3 h of a meal W/P: [C, ?/−] w/ EtOH abuse/elderly/sleep apnea/CNS depressants; may cause abnormal thinking and hallucinations; may worsen depression CI: NAG, urinary retention,

MAOI w/in 14 d **Disp:** Tabs 3, 6 mg **SE:** Somnolence/sedation, N, URI **Notes:** Tabs for insomnia

Doxepin, Topical (Prudoxin, Zonalon) Uses: *Short-term Rx pruritus (atopic dermatitis or lichen simplex chronicus)* Acts: Antipruritic; H_1- & H_2-receptor antag Dose: Apply thin coating tid-qid, 8 d max W/P: [B, ?/–] CI: Component sens Disp: 5% cream SE: ↓ BP, tachycardia, drowsiness, photosens Notes: Limit application area to avoid systemic tox

Doxorubicin (Generic) Uses: *Acute leukemias; Hodgkin Dz & NHLs; soft tissue, osteo- & Ewing sarcoma; Wilms tumor; neuroblastoma; bladder, breast, ovarian, gastric, thyroid, & lung CAs* Acts: Intercalates DNA; ↓ DNA topoisomerase I & II Dose: 60–75 mg/m² q3wk; ↓ w/ hepatic impair; IV use only; ↓ cardiotox w/ weekly (20 mg/m²/wk) or cont Inf (60–90 mg/m² over 96 h); (per protocols) W/P: [D, ?/–] CI: Severe CHF, cardiomyopathy, preexisting ↓ BM, previous Rx w/ total cumulative doses of doxorubicin, idarubicin, daunorubicin Disp: Inj 10, 20, 50 mg; soln 2 mg/mL SE: ↓ BM, venous streaking & phlebitis, N/V/D, mucositis, radiation recall phenomenon, cardiomyopathy rare (dose-related) Notes: Limit of 550 mg/m² cumulative dose (400 mg/m² w/ prior mediastinal irradiation); dexrazoxane may limit cardiac tox; tissue damage w/ extrav; red/orange urine; tissue vesicant w/ extrav, Rx w/ dexrazoxane; liposomal formulations available (*Doxil, Lipodox, Lipodox 50*)

Doxycycline (Acticlate, Adoxa, Oracea, Periostat, Vibramycin, Vibra-Tabs) Uses: *Acne vulgaris, uncomplicated GC, chlamydia, PID, Lyme Dz, skin Infxns, anthrax, malaria prophylaxis* Acts: Tetracycline; bacteriostatic; ↓ protein synth. Spectrum: Limited gram(+) and (–), *Rickettsia* sp, *Chlamydia*, *M. pneumoniae*, *B. anthracis* Dose: Adults. 100 mg PO q12h on 1st d, then 100 mg PO daily-bid or 100 mg IV q12h; acne qd, chlamydia × 7 d, Lyme × 21 d, PID × 14 d *Peds > 8 y.* 5 mg/kg/24 h PO, 200 mg/d max ÷ daily-bid W/P: [D, –] Hepatic impair CI: Children < 8 y, severe hepatic dysfunction Disp: Tabs 20, 50, 75, 100, 150 mg; caps 50, 75, 100, 150 mg; *Oracea* 40 mg caps (30 mg timed release, 10 mg DR); syrup 50 mg/5 mL; susp 25 mg/5 mL; Inj 100/vial SE: D, GI disturbance, photosens Notes: ↓ Effect w/ antacids; tetracycline of choice w/ renal impair; for inh anthrax use w/ 1–2 additional abx; not for CNS anthrax

Doxylamine/Pyridoxine (Diclegis) Uses: *Morning sickness* Acts: Antihistamine & vit B_6 Dose: 2 tabs PO qhs; max 4 tabs/d (1 qam, 1 mid-afternoon, 2 qhs) W/P: [A, –] CNS depression; anticholinergic (caution w/ asthma, ↑ IOP, NAG, peptic ulcer, pyloroduodenal or bladder neck obst) CI: Component hypersens, w/ MAOIs Disp: Tabs DR (doxylamine/pyridoxine) 10/10 mg SE: Somnolence, dizziness, HA, urinary retention, blurred vision, palpitation, ↑ HR, dyspnea

Dronabinol (Marinol) [C-III] Uses: *N/V associated w/ CA chemotherapy; appetite stimulation* Acts: Antiemetic; ↓ V center in the medulla Dose: Adults & Peds. Antiemetic: 5–15 mg/m²/dose q4–6h PRN. Adults. Appetite stimulant: 2.5 mg PO before lunch & dinner; max 20 mg/d W/P: [C, –] Elderly, Hx psychological disorder, Sz disorder, substance abuse CI: Hx schizophrenia, sesame oil hypersens

Disp: Caps 2.5, 5, 10 mg **SE:** Drowsiness, dizziness, anxiety, mood change, hallucinations, depersonalization, orthostatic ↓ BP, tachycardia **Notes:** Principal psychoactive substance present in marijuana

Dronedarone (Multaq) **BOX:** CI w/ NYHA Class IV HF or NYHA Class II-III HF w/ decompensation; CI in AF if cannot be converted to NSR **Uses:** *AF/atrial flutter* **Acts:** Antiarrhythmic **Dose:** 400 mg PO bid w/ A.M. and P.M. meal **W/P:** [X, –] w/ Other drugs (see PI); increased risk of death and serious CV events **CI:** See Box; 2nd-/3rd-degree AV block or SSS (unless w/ pacemaker), HR < 50 BPM, w/ strong CYP3A inhib, w/ drugs/herbals that ↑ QT interval, QTc interval ≥ 500 ms, severe hepatic impair, PRG **Disp:** Tabs 400 mg **SE:** N/V/D, Abd pain, asthenia, heart failure, ↑ K^+, ↑ Mg^{2+}, ↑ QTc, ↓ HR, ↑ SCr, rash **Notes:** Avoid grapefruit juice

Droperidol (Inapsine) **BOX:** Cases of QT interval prolongation and torsades de pointes (some fatal) reported **Uses:** *N/V;* anesthetic premedication* **Acts:** Tranquilizer, sedation, antiemetic **Dose:** *Adults.* *N:* initial max 2.5 mg IV/IM, may repeat 1.25 mg based on response **Peds.** *Premed:* 0.01–0.015 mg/kg/dose (max 1.25 mg) *N:* 0.1 mg/kg/dose (max 2.5 mg) **W/P:** [C, ?] w/ Hepatic/renal impair **CI:** Component sens; ↑ QT **Disp:** Inj 2.5 mg/mL **SE:** Drowsiness, ↓ BP, occasional tachycardia & extrapyramidal Rxns, ↑ QT interval, arrhythmias **Notes:** Give IV push slowly over 2–5 min

Droxidopa (Northera) **BOX:** Monitor supine BP (↓ dose or D/C if raising head of bed does not ↓ supine BP) **Uses:** *Neurogenic orthostatic hypotension* **Acts:** Norepinephrine precursor w/ peripheral arterial/venous vasoconstriction **Dose:** 100 mg PO tid; max 600 mg PO tid; last dose 3 h prior to hs & elevate head of bed **W/P:** [C, –] Supine HTN may ↑ CV risk; w/ h/o CHF, arrhythmias, ischemic heart Dz; w/ DOPA decarboxylase inhib **CI:** Ø **Disp:** Caps 100, 200, 300 mg **SE:** HA, dizziness, N, HTN, fatigue, syncope, hyperpyrexia, confusion, UTI **Notes:** Contains FD&C Yellow No. 5 (tartrazine), may cause allergic-type Rxn

Dulaglutide (Trulicity) **BOX:** In animals, ↑ incidence of thyroid tumors **Uses:** *Adjunct to diet and exercise to ↑ glycemic control in type 2 DM* **Acts:** GLP-1 receptor agonist **Dose:** *Adults.* 0.5 mg SQ 1 × wk; not rec 1st line **W/P:** [C, –] Hypersens Rxns; pancreatitis; caution w/ renal impair; not for type 1 DM **CI:** Personal or family Hx thyroid carcinoma, MEN 2 synd **Disp:** Pen injector 0.5, 0.75, 1.5 mL/0.5 mL **SE:** N/V/D, Abd pain, ↓ appetite **Notes:** Not a replacement for insulin; self-administer w/ Inj Abd, thigh, upper arm; w/ missed dose, take if > 3 days until next dose; otherwise wait until next dose

Duloxetine (Cymbalta) **BOX:** Antidepressants may ↑ risk of suicidality; consider risks/benefits of use; closely monitor for clinical worsening, suicidality, or behavior changes **Uses:** *Depression, DM peripheral neuropathic pain, general GAD, fibromyalgia, chronic OA & back pain* **Acts:** SSNRI **Dose:** *Depression:* 40–60 mg/d PO ÷ bid *DM neuropathy:* 60 mg/d PO *GAD:* 60 mg/d, max 120 mg/d *Fibromyalgia, OA/back pain:* 30–60 mg/d, 60 mg/d max **W/P:** [C, ?/–]; Use in 3rd tri; avoid if CrCl < 30 mL/min, NAG, w/ fluvoxamine, inhib of CYP2D6

(Table 10, p 356), TCAs, phenothiazines, type class 1C antiarrhythmics (Table 9, p 355) **CI:** ↑ Risk serotonin synd w/ MAOI (linezolid or IV meth blue) use w/in 14 d, w/ thioridazine, NAG, hepatic Insuff **Disp:** Caps DR 20, 30, 60 mg **SE:** N, dry mouth, somnolence, fatigue, constipation, ↓ appetite, hyperhydrosis **Notes:** Swallow whole; monitor BP; avoid abrupt D/C

Dutasteride (Avodart) **Uses:** *Symptomatic BPH to improve Sxs, ↓ risk of retention and BPH surgery alone or in combo w/ tamsulosin* **Acts:** 5α-Reductase inhib; ↓ intracellular DHT **Dose:** *Monotherapy:* 0.5 mg PO/d *Combo:* 0.5 mg PO qd w/ tamsulosin 0.4 mg qd **W/P:** [X, –] Hepatic impair; PRG women should not handle pills; R/O CA before starting **CI:** Women, peds **Disp:** Caps 0.5 mg **SE:** ↑ Testosterone, ↑ TSH, impotence, ↓ libido, gynecomastia, ejaculatory disturbance, may ↑ risk of high-grade PCa **Notes:** No blood donation until 6 mo after D/C; ↓ PSA, ✓ new baseline PSA at 6 mo (corrected PSA × 2); any PSA rise on dutasteride suspicious for CA; now available in fixed-dose combo w/ tamsulosin (see *Jalyn*)

Dutasteride/Tamsulosin (Jalyn) **Uses:** *Symptomatic BPH to improve Sxs* **Acts:** 5α-Reductase inhib (↓ intracellular DHT) w/ α-blocker **Dose:** 1 cap daily after same meal **W/P:** [X, –] w/ CYP3A4 and CYP2D6 inhib may ↑ SEs; PRG women should not handle pills; R/O CA before starting; IFIS (tamsulosin) discuss w/ ophthalmologist before cataract surgery; rare priapism; w/ warfarin; may ↑ risk of high-grade PCa **Disp:** Caps women, peds, component sens **Disp:** Caps 0.5 mg dutasteride w/ 0.4 mg tamsulosin **SE:** Impotence, decreased libido, ejaculation disorders, breast disorders **Notes:** No blood donation until 6 mo after D/C; ↓ PSA, ✓ new baseline PSA at 6 mo (corrected PSA × 2); any PSA rise on dutasteride suspicious for CA (see also Dutasteride and Tamsulosin)

Ecallantide (Kalbitor) **BOX:** Anaphylaxis reported, administer in a setting able to manage anaphylaxis and HAE, monitor closely **Uses:** *Acute attacks of HAE* **Acts:** Plasma kallikrein inhib **Dose:** *Adults & Peds > 16 y.* 30 mg SQ in three 10-mg injections; if attack persists may repeat 30-mg dose w/in 24 h **W/P:** [C, ?/–] Hypersens Rxns **CI:** Hypersens to ecallantide **Disp:** Inj 10 mg/mL **SE:** HA, N/V/D, pyrexia, Inj site Rxn, nasopharyngitis, fatigue, Abd pain

Echothiophate Iodide, Ophthalmic (Phospholine iodide) **Uses:** *Glaucoma* **Acts:** Cholinesterase inhib **Dose:** 1 gtt in eye(s) bid w/ 1 dose hs **W/P:** [C, ?] **CI:** Active uveal inflam, inflam Dz of iris/ciliary body, glaucoma iridocyclitis **Disp:** Powder for reconstitution 6.25 mg/5 mL (0.125%) **SE:** Local irritation, myopia, blurred vision, ↓ BP, ↓ HR

Econazole (Ecoza, Spectazole, Generic) **Uses:** *Tinea, cutaneous Candida, & tinea versicolor Infxns* **Acts:** Topical antifungal **Dose:** Apply to areas bid for Candida (daily for tinea versicolor) for 2–4 wk **W/P:** [C, ?] **CI:** Component sens **Disp:** Topical cream 1%; (*Ecoza*) foam 1% **SE:** Local irritation, pruritus, erythema **Notes:** Early Sx/clinical improvement; complete course to avoid recurrence

Eculizumab (Soliris) **BOX:** ↑ Risk of meningococcal Infxns (give meningococcal vaccine 2 wk prior to 1st dose and revaccinate per guidelines) **Uses:** *Rx paroxysmal nocturnal hemoglobinuria* **Acts:** Complement inhib **Dose:** 600 mg IV q7d × 4 wk, then 900 mg IV 5th dose 7 d later, then 900 mg IV q14d **W/P:** [C, ?] **CI:** Active *N. meningitidis* Infxn; if not vaccinated against *N. meningitidis* **Disp:** 300-mg vial **SE:** Meningococcal Infxn, HA, nasopharyngitis, N, back pain, Infxns, fatigue, severe hemolysis on D/C **Notes:** IV over 35 min (2-h max Inf time); monitor for 1 h for S/Sx of Inf Rxn

Edrophonium (Enlon) **Uses:** *Diagnosis of MyG; acute MyG crisis; curare antag, reverse of nondepolarizing neuromuscular blockers* **Acts:** Anticholinesterase inhib **Dose:** *Adults.* Test for MyG: 2 mg IV in 1 min; if tolerated, give 8 mg IV; (+) test is brief ↑ in strength *Peds.* See label **W/P:** [C, ?] **CI:** GI or GU obst; allergy to sulfite **Disp:** Inj 10 mg/mL **SE:** N/V/D, excessive salivation, stomach cramps, ↑ aminotransferases **Notes:** Can cause severe cholinergic effects; keep atropine available, 0.4–0.5 mg IV to Rx muscarinic SE (fasciculations, muscle weakness); Enlon-Plus contains atropine for reversal only

Edoxaban (Savaysa) **BOX:** ↑ Risk of ischemic events w/ premature D/C in the absence of anticoagulation; do not use in NVAF pts w/ CrCl > 95 mL/min (↑ ischemic stroke risk); epidural or spinal hematomas w/ neuraxial anesthesia or spinal puncture **Uses:** *DVT and PE after 5–10 d of initial parenteral anticoagulant; ↓ CVA/systemic embolism in NVAF* **Acts:** Factor Xa inhib, ↓ prothrombinase activity & thrombin-induced plt aggregation **Dose:** Tabs 60 mg PO qd after 5–10 d of initial therapy w/ a parenteral anticoagulant *Wt ≤ 60kg.* Tabs 30 mg PO qd; w/ P-gp inhib: 30 mg PO qd; *NVAF:* 60 mg PO qd **W/P:** ↑ bleeding risk (eg, w/ ASA, other antiplatelet/antithrombotic agents, chronic NSAID use); not rec w/ mod/severe liver impair, w/ CrCl < 15 mL/min, w/ mechanical heart valves or mod/severe mitral stenosis; ↓ dose w/ CrCl 15–50 mL/min or Wt ≤ 60 kg; D/C > 24 h prior to surgery **CI:** Active bleeding **Disp:** Tabs 15, 30, 60 mg **SE:** Hemorrhage, dermal hemorrhage, skin rash, bleeding (GI, Vag, hematuria, urethral, oral, nasal, pharyngeal, puncture site), ↓ Hgb, ↑ LFTs **Notes:** Substrate of P-gp; coagulation tests not required but may ↑ PT/aPTT

Efavirenz (Sustiva) **Uses:** *HIV Infxns* **Acts:** Antiretroviral; nonnucleoside RT inhib **Dose:** *Adults.* 600 mg/d PO qhs *Peds ≥ 3 y 10–< 15 kg.* 200 mg PO qd *15–< 20 kg.* 250 mg PO qd *20–< 25 kg.* 300 mg PO qd *25–< 32.5 kg.* 350 mg PO qd *32.5–< 40 kg.* 400 mg PO qd *≥ 40 kg.* 600 mg PO qd; on empty stomach **W/P:** [D, –] CDC rec: HIV-infected mothers not breast-feed **CI:** w/ Astemizole, bepridil, cisapride, midazolam, pimozide, triazolam, ergot derivatives, voriconazole **Disp:** Caps 50, 200; tabs 600 mg **SE:** Somnolence, vivid dreams, depression, CNS Sxs, dizziness, rash, N/V/D **Notes:** ✓ LFTs (especially w/ underlying liver Dz), cholesterol; not for monotherapy

Efavirenz/Emtricitabine/Tenofovir (Atripla) **BOX:** Lactic acidosis and severe hepatomegaly w/ steatosis, including fatal cases, reported w/ nucleoside analogs alone or combo w/ other antiretrovirals **Uses:** *HIV Infxns* **Acts:** Triple fixed-dose combo nonnucleoside RT inhib/nucleoside analog **Dose:** 1 tab qd on empty stomach; hs dose may ↓ CNS SE **W/P:** [D, –] CDC rec: HIV-infected mothers not breast-feed, w/ obesity **CI:** < 12 y or < 40 kg, w/ astemizole, midazolam, triazolam, or ergot derivatives (CYP3A4 competition by efavirenz could cause serious/life-threatening SE) **Disp:** Tabs efavirenz 600 mg/emtricitabine 200 mg/tenofovir 300 mg **SE:** Somnolence, vivid dreams, HA, dizziness, rash, N/V/D, ↓ BMD **Notes:** Monitor LFTs, cholesterol; see individual agents for additional info, not for HIV/hep B coinfection

Efinaconazole (Jublia) Uses: *Onychomycosis* **Acts:** Azole antifungal. *Spectum: Trichophyton rubrum, Trichophyton mentagrophytes* **Dose:** Apply to entire surface and under tip of affected toenail(s) qd × 48 wk **W/P:** [C, ?/–] Local irritation **CI:** Ø **Disp:** Topical soln 10% **SE:** Pain, dermatitis, vesicles at application site; ingrown toenails

Eletriptan (Relpax) Uses: *Acute Rx of migraine* **Acts:** Selective serotonin receptor (5-HT$_{1B/1D}$) agonist **Dose:** 20–40 mg PO, may repeat in 2 h; 80 mg/24 h max **W/P:** [C, +/–] **CI:** Hx ischemic heart Dz, coronary artery spasm, stroke or TIA, peripheral vascular Dz, IBD, uncontrolled HTN, hemiplegic or basilar migraine, severe hepatic impair, w/in 24 h of another 5-HT$_1$ agonist or ergot, w/in 72 h of CYP3A4 inhib **Disp:** Tabs 20, 40 mg **SE:** Dizziness, somnolence, N, asthenia, xerostomia, paresthesias; pain, pressure, or tightness in chest, jaw, or neck; serious cardiac events

Eltrombopag (Promacta) **BOX:** May cause hepatotox; ✓ baseline ALT/AST/bili q2wk w/ dosage adjustment, then monthly; D/C if ALT is > 3× ULN w/ ↑ bili, or Sx of liver injury Uses: *Tx ↓ plt in idiopathic thrombocytopenia refractory to steroids, immune globulins, splenectomy* **Acts:** Thrombopoietin receptor agonist **Dose:** 50 mg PO daily, adjust to keep plt ≥ 50,000 cells/mm³; 75 mg/d max; start 25 mg/d if East-Asian or w/ hepatic impair; on an empty stomach; not w/in 4 h of product w/ polyvalent cations **W/P:** [C, ?/–] ↑ Risk for BM reticulin fiber deposition, heme malignancies, rebound ↓ plt on D/C, thromboembolism **CI:** Ø **Disp:** Tabs 12.5, 25, 50, 75 mg **SE:** Rash, bruising, menorrhagia, N/V, dyspepsia, ↓ plt, ↑ ALT/AST, limb pain, myalgia, paresthesia, cataract, conjunctival hemorrhage **Notes:** D/C if no ↑ plt count after 4 wk; restricted distribution *Promacta Cares (1-877-9-PROMACTA)*

Elvitegravir (Vitekta) Uses: *HIV Infxn; used w/ HIV protease inhib w/ ritonavir & another antiretroviral drug for HIV-1 Tx-experienced adults* *Acts:* Viral INSTI **Dose:** 85 or 150 mg PO qd w/ food (based on specific antiretroviral used w/ ritonavir); see PI) **W/P:** [B, –] Breast-feeding by HIV-infected women not rec; not rec w/ severe hepatic Dz; do not use w/ rifabutin, rifampin, rifapentine, St. John's Wort **CI:** Ø **Disp:** Tabs 85, 150 mg **SE:** N/D, HA, immune reconstitution synd, suicidal ideation **Notes:** ✓ CBC w/ differential, reticulocyte/CD4 counts, HIV RNA plasma levels, LFTs; ✓ HBV status before

Emedastine (Emadine) Uses: *Allergic conjunctivitis* **Acts:** Antihistamine; selective H$_1$-antag **Dose:** 1 gtt in eye(s) up to qid **W/P:** [B, ?] **CI:** Allergy to ingredients (preservatives benzalkonium, tromethamine) **Disp:** 0.05% soln **SE:** HA, blurred vision, burning/stinging, corneal infiltrates/staining, dry eyes, foreign body sensation, hyperemia, keratitis, tearing, pruritus, rhinitis, sinusitis, asthenia, bad taste, dermatitis, discomfort **Notes:** Do not use contact lenses if eyes are red

Empagliflozin (Jardiance) **Uses:** * Adjunct to diet/exercise w/ type 2 DM* **Acts:** SGLT2 inhib **Dose:** 10 mg PO qam, to 25 mg QD PRN; do not use w/ eGFR < 45 **W/P:** [C, –] X/eGFR < 45; monitor/correct vol, especially in elderly; follow Cr, ↓ insulin or insulin secretagogue to limit hypoglycemia risk **CI:** Hypersens, severe renal impair, dialysis, ESRD **Disp:** Tabs 10, 25 mg **SE:** UTI, female genital mycotic Infxn

Empagliflozin/Linagliptin (Glyxambi) **Uses:** *Adjunct to diet/exercise w/ type 2 DM* **Acts:** SGLT2 inhib (empagliflozin) w/ DPP-4 inhib (linagliptin) **Dose:** 10 mg/5 mg PO qam; max 25 mg/5 mg daily; do not use if eGFR is < 45 mL/min/1.73 m² **W/P:** [C, –] Pancreatitis; hypersens; ↑ LDL; ✓ renal Fxn; ↓ BP (monitor vol status) **CI:** Severe renal impair, ESRD, dialysis; component hypersens **Disp:** Tabs (empagliflozin mg/linagliptin mg) 10/5, 25/5 **SE:** UTI, URI, nasopharyngitis, ↓ BP, genital mycotic Infxn, hypersens

Emtricitabine (Emtriva) **BOX:** Lactic acidosis & severe hepatomegaly w/ steatosis reported; not for HBV Infxn **Uses:** HIV-1 Infxn **Acts:** NRTI **Dose:** 200-mg caps or 240-mg soln PO daily; ↓ w/ renal impair **W/P:** [B, –] Risk of liver Dz **CI:** Component sens **Disp:** Soln 10 mg/mL; caps 200 mg **SE:** HA, N/D, rash, rare hyperpigmentation of feet & hands, posttreatment exacerbation of hep B, do not use w/ HIV & HBV coinfection **Notes:** 1st once-daily NRTI; caps/soln not equivalent; not OK as monotherapy; screen for hep B, do not use w/ HIV & HBV coinfection

Enalapril (Enalaprilat, Epaned Kit, Vasotec) **BOX:** ACE inhib used during PRG can cause fetal injury & death **Uses:** *HTN, CHF, LVD, DN* **Acts:** ACE inhib **Dose:** *Adults.* 2.5–40 mg/d PO; 1.25 mg IV q6h **Peds.** 0.05–0.08 mg/kg/d PO q12–24h; ↓ w/ renal impair **W/P:** [C (1st tri; D 2nd & 3rd tri), +/–] D/C immediately w/ PRG, w/NSAIDs, K⁺ supls **CI:** Bilateral RAS, angioedema **Disp:** Tabs 2.5, 5, 10, 20 mg; *Enalaprilat:* IV 1.25 mg/mL; *Epaned Kit:* powder for oral (1 mg/mL) **SE:** ↓ BP w/ initial dose (especially w/ diuretics), ↑ K⁺, ↑ Cr, cough, angioedema **Notes:** Monitor Cr; D/C diuretic for 2–3 d prior to start

Enfuvirtide (Fuzeon) **BOX:** Rarely causes allergy; never rechallenge **Uses:** *w/ Antiretroviral agents for HIV-1 in Tx-experienced pts w/ viral replication despite ongoing Rx* **Acts:** Viral fusion inhib **Dose:** *Adults.* 90 mg (1 mL) SQ bid in upper arm, anterior thigh, or Abd; rotate site **Peds.** See PI **W/P:** [B, –] **CI:** Previous allergy to drug **Disp:** 90 mg/mL recons; pt kit w/ supplies × 1 mo **SE:** Inj site Rxns; pneumonia, D, N, fatigue, insomnia, peripheral neuropathy **Notes:** Available via restricted distribution system; use immediately on recons or refrigerate (24 h max)

Enoxaparin (Lovenox) **BOX:** Recent or anticipated epidural/spinal anesthesia, ↑ risk of spinal/epidural hematoma w/ subsequent paralysis **Uses:** *Prevention & Rx of DVT; Rx PE; unstable angina & non–Q-wave MI* **Acts:** LMW heparin; inhibit thrombin by complexing w/ antithrombin III **Dose:** *Adults. Prevention:*

30 mg SQ bid or 40 mg SQ q24h *DVT/PE Rx:* 1 mg/kg SQ q12h or 1.5 mg/kg SQ q24h *Angina:* 1 mg/kg SQ q12h *Ancillary to AMI fibrinolysis:* 30 mg IV bolus, then 1 mg/kg SQ bid; CrCl < 30 mL/min, ↓ to 1 mg/kg SQ qd *Peds. Prevention:* 0.5 mg/kg SQ q12h *DVT/PE Rx:* 1 mg/kg SQ q12h; ↓ dose w/ CrCl < 30 mL/min **W/P:** [B, ?] Not for prophylaxis in prosthetic heart valves **CI:** Active bleeding, HIT Ab, heparin, pork sens **Disp:** Inj (30-, 40-, 60-, 80-, 100-, 120-, 150-mg syringes); 300-mg/mL multi-dose vial **SE:** Bleeding, hemorrhage, bruising, thrombocytopenia, fever, pain/hematoma at site, ↑ AST/ALT **Notes:** No effect on bleeding time, plt Fxn, PT, or aPTT; monitor plt for HIT, clinical bleeding; may monitor antifactor Xa; not for IM

Entacapone (Comtan) **Uses:** *Parkinson Dz* **Acts:** Selective & reversible catechol-O-methyltransferase inhib **Dose:** 200 mg w/ each levodopa/carbidopa dose; max 1600 mg/d; ↓ levodopa/carbidopa dose 25% w/ levodopa dose > 800 mg **W/P:** [C, ?] Hepatic impair **CI:** Use w/ MAOI **Disp:** Tabs 200 mg **SE:** Dyskinesia, hyperkinesia, N/D, dizziness, hallucinations, orthostatic ↓ BP, brown-orange urine **Notes:** ✓ LFTs; do not D/C abruptly

Enzalutamide (Xtandi) **Uses:** *Metastatic CRPC pre- or post-docetaxel* **Acts:** Androgen receptor inhib **Dose:** *(men only):* 160 mg daily, do not chew/open caps **W/P:** [X, –] Sz risk **CI:** PRG **Disp:** Caps 40 mg **SE:** HA, dizziness, insomnia, fatigue, anxiety, MS pain, muscle weakness, paresthesia, back pain, spinal cord compression, cauda equina synd, arthralgias, edema, URI, lower resp Infxn, hematuria, ↑ BP, falls **Notes:** Avoid w/ strong CYP2C8 inhib, strong/mod CYP3A4 or CYP2C8 induc, avoid CPY3A4, CYP2C9, CYP2C19 substrates w/ narrow therapeutic index; if on warfarin ✓ INR

Ephedrine (Generic) **Uses:** *Acute bronchospasm, bronchial asthma, nasal congestion*, ↓ BP, narcolepsy, enuresis, & MyG **Acts:** Sympathomimetic; stimulates α- & β-receptors; bronchodilator **Dose:** *Adults. Congestion:* 12.5–25 mg PO q4h PRN w/ expectorant; ↓ *BP:* 25–50 mg IV q5–10min; 150 mg/d max *Peds.* 0.1–0.2 mg/kg/dose IV q4–6h PRN **W/P:** [C, ?/–] **CI:** Arrhythmias, NAG **Disp:** Caps 25 mg; Inj 50 mg/mL **SE:** CNS stimulation (nervousness, anxiety, trembling), tachycardia, arrhythmia, HTN, xerostomia, dysuria **Notes:** Protect from light; monitor BP, HR, urinary output; can cause false(+) amphetamine EMIT; take last dose 4–6 h before hs; abuse potential, OTC sales mostly banned/ restricted

Epinastine (Elestat) **Uses:** *Itching w/ allergic conjunctivitis* **Acts:** Antihistamine *Dose:* 1 gtt bid **W/P:** [C, ?/–] **Disp:** Soln 0.05% **SE:** Burning, folliculosis, hyperemia, pruritus, URI, HA, rhinitis, sinusitis, cough, pharyngitis **Notes:** Remove contacts before, reinsert in 10 min

Epinephrine (Adrenalin, Auvi-Q, EpiPen, EpiPen Jr, Others) **Uses:** *Cardiac arrest, anaphylactic Rxn, bronchospasm, open-angle glaucoma* **Acts:** non-selective α- and β-adrenergic agonist **Dose:** *Adults & Peds. Anaphylaxis:* Auto-injectors for self-administration; Inj into anterior lateral thigh > *30 kg (66 kg).* *Auvi-Q:* 0.3 mg; *EpiPen:* 0.3 mg *15–30 kg. Auvi-Q:* 0.15 mg; *EpiPen Jr:* 0.15 mg

Adults. ECC 2010. 1 mg (10 mL of 1:10,000 soln) IV/IO push; repeat q3–5min (0.2 mg/kg max) if 1-mg dose fails; *Inf:* 0.1–0.5 mcg/kg/min, titrate; ET 2–2.5 mg in 5–10 mL NS *Profound bradycardia/hypotension:* 2–10 mcg/min (1 mg in 250 mL D5W) *Allergic Rxn:* 0.3–0.5 mg (0.3–0.5 mL of 1:1000 soln) SQ *Anaphylaxis:* 0.3–0.5 mg (0.3–0.5 mL of 1:10,000 soln) IV *Asthma:* 0.1–0.5 mL SQ of 1:1000 soln; repeat q20min to 4 h; or 1 Inh (metered-dose), repeat in 1–2 min; or susp 0.1–0.3 mL SQ for extended effect **Peds. ECC 2010.** *Pulseless arrest:* (0.1 mL/kg 1:10,000) IV/ IO q3–5min; max dose 1 mg; OK via ET tube (0.1 mL/kg 1:1,000) until IV/IO access *Symptomatic bradycardia:* 0.01 mg/kg (0.1 mL/kg 1:10,000) cont Inf: typical 0.1–1 mcg/kg/min, titrate *Anaphylaxis/status asthmaticus:* 0.01 mg/kg (0.01 ml/kg 1:1000) SQ/IM, repeat PRN; max single dose 0.3 mg **W/P:** [C, ?] ↓ Bronchodilation w/ β-blockers **CI:** Cardiac arrhythmias, NAG **Disp:** Inj 1:1000, 1:2000, 1:10,000; nasal inhal 0.1%; oral Inh 2.25% soln; *EpiPen/EpiPen Jr* 1 dose = 0.30 mg; *EpiPen Jr* 1 dose = 0.15 mg; *Auvi-Q* auto-injector 0.3 mg/0.3 mL, 0.15 mg/0.15 mL **SE:** CV (tachycardia, HTN, vasoconstriction), CNS stimulation (nervousness, anxiety, trembling), ↓ renal blood flow **Notes:** Can give via ET tube if no central line (use 2–2.5 × IV dose); *EpiPen & Auvi-Q* (voice prompt device) for pt self-Inj

Epirubicin (Ellence) **BOX:** Do not give IM or SQ; extrav causes tissue necrosis; potential cardiotox; severe myelosuppression; ↓ dose w/ hepatic impair **Uses:** *Adjuvant Rx for (+) axillary nodes after resection of primary breast CA secondary AML* **Acts:** Anthracycline cytotoxic agent **Dose:** Per protocols; ↓ dose w/ hepatic impair **W/P:** [D, –] **CI:** Baseline neutrophil count < 1500 cells/mm³, severe cardiac Insuff, recent MI, severe arrhythmias, severe hepatic dysfunction, previous anthracyclines Rx to max cumulative dose **Disp:** Inj 50 mg/25 mL, 200 mg/100 mL **SE:** Mucositis, N/V/D, alopecia, ↓ BM, cardiotox, secondary AML, tissue necrosis w/ extrav (see Adriamycin for Rx), lethargy **Notes:** ✓ CBC, bili, AST, Cr, cardiac Fxn before/during each cycle

Eplerenone (Inspra) **Uses:** *HTN, ↑ survival after MI w/ LVEF < 40% and CHF* **Acts:** Selective aldosterone antag **Dose:** 50 mg PO daily-bid, doses > 100 mg/d no benefit w/ ↑ K⁺; ↓ to 25 mg PO daily if giving w/ CYP3A4 inhib **W/P:** [B, ?/–] w/ CYP3A4 inhib (Table 10, p 356); monitor K⁺ w/ ACE inhib, ARBs, NSAIDs, K⁺-sparing diuretics; grapefruit juice, St. John's Wort **CI:** K⁺ > 5.5 mEq/L; NIDDM w/ microalbuminuria; SCr > 2 mg/dL (males), > 1.8 mg/dL (females); CrCl < 30 mL/min; w/ K⁺ supls/K⁺-sparing diuretics, ketoconazole **Disp:** Tabs 25, 50 mg **SE:** ↑ cholesterol/triglycerides, ↑ K⁺, HA, dizziness, gynecomastia, D, orthostatic ↓ BP **Notes:** May take 4 wk for full effect

Epoetin Alfa [Erythropoietin, EPO] (Epogen, Procrit) **BOX:** ↑ Mortality, serious CV/thromboembolic events, and tumor progression. Renal failure pts experienced ↑ greater risks (death/CV events) on ESAs to target Hgb levels 11 g/dL; maintain Hgb 10–12 g/dL; in CA pts, ESAs ↓ survival/time to progression in some CA when dosed Hgb ≥ 12 g/dL; use lowest dose needed; use only for myelosuppressive chemotherapy; D/C following chemotherapy; preop ESA ↑

DVT; consider DVT prophylaxis **Uses:** *CRF-associated anemia, zidovudine Rx in HIV-infected pts, CA chemotherapy; ↓ transfusions associated w/ surgery* **Acts:** Induces erythropoiesis **Dose:** *Adults & Peds.* 50–150 units/kg IV/SQ 3×/wk; adjust dose q4–6wk PRN *Surgery:* 300 units/kg/d × 10 d before to 4 d after; ↓ dose if Hct ~36% or Hgb, ↑ > ≅ 12 g/dL or Hgb ↑ > 1 g/dL in 2-wk period; hold dose if Hgb > 12 g/dL **W/P:** [C, ?/–] **CI:** Uncontrolled HTN **Disp:** Inj 2000, 3000, 4000, 10,000, 20,000, 40,000 units/mL **SE:** HTN, HA, fatigue, fever, tachycardia, N/V **Notes:** Refrigerate; monitor baseline & posttreatment Hct/Hgb, BP, ferritin

Epoprostenol (Flolan, Veletri, Generic) **Uses:** *Pulm HTN* **Acts:** Dilates pulm/systemic arterial vascular beds; ↓ plt aggregation **Dose:** Initial 2 ng/kg/min; ↑ by 2 ng/kg/min q15min until dose-limiting SE (CP, dizziness, N/V, HA, ↓ BP, flushing); IV cont Inf 4 ng/kg/min < max tolerated rate; adjust based on response; see PI **W/P:** [B, ?] ↑ tox w/ diuretics, vasodilators, acetate in dialysis fluids, anticoagulants **CI:** Chronic use in CHF 2nd degree, if pt develops pulm edema w/ dose initiation, severe LVSD **Disp:** Inj 0.5, 1.5 mg **SE:** Flushing, tachycardia, CHF, fever, chills, nervousness, HA, N/V/D, jaw pain, flu-like Sxs **Notes:** Abrupt D/C can cause rebound pulm HTN; monitor bleeding w/ other antiplatelet/anticoagulants; watch ↓ BP w/ other vasodilators/diuretics

Eprosartan (Teveten) **BOX:** Fetal toxicity **Uses:** *HTN*, DN, CHF **Acts:** ARB **Dose:** 400–800 mg/d single dose or bid **W/P:** [C (1st tri); D (2nd & 3rd tri), D/C immediately w/PRG] w/ Li, ↑ K⁺ w/ K⁺-sparing diuretics/supls/high-dose trimethoprim **CI:** Bilateral RAS, 1st-degree aldosteronism **Disp:** Tabs 400, 600 mg **SE:** Fatigue, depression, URI, UTI, Abd pain, rhinitis/pharyngitis/cough, hypertriglyceridemia

Eptifibatide (Integrilin) **Uses:** *ACS, PCI* **Acts:** Glycoprotein IIb/IIIa inhib **Dose:** 180 mcg/kg IV bolus, then 2 mcg/kg/min cont Inf; ↓ in renal impair (CrCl < 50 mL/min: 180 mcg/kg, then 1 mcg/kg/min) **Dose:** *ECC 2010. ACS:* 180 mcg/kg/min IV bolus over 1–2 min, then 2 mcg/kg/min, then repeat bolus in 10 min; continue Inf 18–24 h post-PCI **W/P:** [B, ?] Monitor bleeding w/ other anticoagulants **CI:** Other glycoprotein IIb/IIIa inhib, Hx abn bleeding, hemorrhagic stroke (w/in 30 d), severe HTN, major surgery (w/in 6 wk), plt count < 100,000 cells/mm³, renal dialysis **Disp:** Inj 0.75, 2 mg/mL **SE:** Bleeding, ↓ BP, Inj site Rxn, thrombocytopenia **Notes:** Monitor bleeding, coagulants, plts, SCr, activated coagulation time (ACT) w/ prothrombin consumption index (keep ACT 200–300 s)

Eribulin (Halaven) **Uses:** *Met breast CA after 2 chemo regimens (including anthracycline & taxane)* **Acts:** Microtubule inhib **Dose:** 1.4 mg/m² IV (over 2–5 min) d 1 & 8 of 21-d cycle; ↓ dose w/ hepatic & mod renal impair; delay/↓ for tox (see label) **W/P:** [D, –] **CI:** Ø Inj 0.5 mg/mL **SE:** ↓ WBC/Hct/plt, fatigue/asthenia, neuropathy, N/V/D, constipation, pyrexia, alopecia, ↑ QT, arthralgia/myalgia, back/pain, cough, dyspnea, UTI **Notes:** ✓ CBC & for neuropathy before dose

Erlotinib (Tarceva) **Uses:** *NSCLC after failing 1 chemotherapy; maint NSCLC who have not progressed after 4 cycles cisplatin-based therapy, CA pancreas* **Acts:**

HER1/EGFR TKI **Dose:** *CA pancreas:* 100 mg; *Others:* 150 mg/d PO 1 h ac or 2 h pc; ↓ (in 50-mg decrements) w/ severe Rxn or w/ CYP3A4 inhib (Table 10, p 356); per protocols **W/P:** [D, ?/–] Avoid pregnancy; w/ CYP3A4 inhib (Table 10, p 356) **Disp:** Tabs 25, 100, 150 mg **SE:** Rash, N/V/D, anorexia, Abd pain, fatigue, cough, dyspnea, edema, stomatitis, conjunctivitis, pruritus, skin/nail changes, Infxn, ↑ LFTs, interstitial lung Dz **Notes:** May ↑ INR w/ warfarin, monitor INR

Ertapenem (Invanz) **Uses:** *Complicated intra-Abd, acute pelvic, & skin Infxns, pyelonephritis, CAP* **Acts:** α-carbapenem; β-lactam antibiotic, ↓ cell wall synth. *Spectrum:* Good gram(+/–) & anaerobic coverage, not *Pseudomonas*, PCN-resistant pneumococci, MRSA, *Enterococcus*, β-lactamase (+) *H. influenzae*, *Mycoplasma*, *Chlamydia* **Dose:** *Adults.* 1 g IM/IV daily; 500 mg/d in CrCl < 30 mL/min *Peds 3 mo–12 y.* 15 mg/kg bid IM/IV, max 1 g/d **W/P:** [B, ?/–] Sz Hx, CNS disorders, β-lactam & multiple allergies; probenecid ↓ renal clearance **CI:** component hypersens or amide anesthetics **Disp:** Inj 1 g/vial **SE:** HA, N/V/D, Inj site Rxn, thrombocytosis, ↑ LFTs **Notes:** Can give IM × 7 d, IV × 14 d; 137 mg Na⁺ (6 mEq)/g ertapenem

Erythromycin, Oral (E-Mycin, E.E.S., Ery-Tab, EryPed, Generic) **Uses:** *Bacterial Infxns; bowel prep*; ↑ GI motility (*prokinetic*); *acne vulgaris* **Acts:** Bacteriostatic; interferes w/ protein synth. *Spectrum:* Group A streptococci (*S. pyogenes*), *S. pneumoniae, N. gonorrhoeae* (if PCN-allergic), *Legionella, M. pneumoniae* **Dose:** *Adults.* Base 250–500 mg PO q6–12h or ethylsuccinate 400–800 mg q6–12h; 500 mg–1 g IV q6h *Prokinetic:* 250 mg PO tid 30 min ac *Peds.* 30–50 mg/kg/d PO ÷ q6–12h or 15–50 mg/kg/d IV ÷ q6h, max 4 g/d **W/P:** [B, +/?] Pseudomembranous colitis risk, ↑ tox of carbamazepine, cyclosporine, digoxin, methylprednisolone, theophylline, felodipine, warfarin, simvastatin/lovastatin; ↓ sildenafil dose w/ use **CI:** Hepatic impair, preexisting liver Dz (estolate), use w/ pimozide ergotamine dihydroergotamine **Disp:** *Lactobionate (Ilotycin): Powder for Inj* 500 mg, 1 g. *Base:* Tabs 250, 333, 500 mg; caps 250 mg. *Stearate (Erythrocin):* Tabs 250, 500 mg. *Ethylsuccinate (EES, EryPed):* Chew tabs 200 mg; tabs 400 mg; susp 200, 400 mg/5 mL **SE:** HA, Abd pain, N/V/D, ↑ QT, torsades de pointes, ventricular arrhythmias/tachycardias (rarely); cholestatic jaundice (estolate) **Notes:** 400 mg ethylsuccinate = 250 mg base/estolate; w/ food minimizes GI upset; lactobionate contains benzyl alcohol (caution in neonates)

Erythromycin, Ophthalmic (Ilotycin, Romycin) **Uses:** *Conjunctival/corneal Infxns* **Acts:** Macrolide antibiotic **Dose:** 1/2 in 2–6×/d **W/P:** [B, +/?] **CI:** Erythromycin hypersens **Disp:** 0.5% oint **SE:** Local irritation

Erythromycin, Topical (Akne-Mycin, Ery, Erythra-Derm, Generic) **Uses:** *Acne vulgaris* **Acts:** Macrolide antibiotic **Dose:** Wash & dry area, apply 2% product over area bid **W/P:** [B, +] Pseudomembranous colitis possible **CI:** Component sens **Disp:** Soln 2%; gel 2%; pads & swabs 2% **SE:** Local irritation

Erythromycin/Benzoyl Peroxide (Benzamycin) Uses: *Topical for acne vulgaris* **Acts:** Macrolide antibiotic w/ keratolytic **Dose:** Apply bid (A.M. & P.M.) **W/P:** [C, ?] **CI:** Component sens **Disp:** Gel erythromycin 30 mg/benzoyl peroxide 50 mg/g **SE:** Local irritation, dryness

Escitalopram (Lexapro, Generic) **BOX:** Closely monitor for worsening depression or emergence of suicidality, particularly in ped pts Uses: *Depression, anxiety* **Acts:** SSRI **Dose:** 10–20 mg PO daily; 10 mg/d in elderly & hepatic impair **W/P:** [C, +/–] Serotonin synd (Table 11, p 358); use of escitalopram w/ NSAID, ASA, or other drugs affecting coagulation associated w/ ↑ bleeding risk **CI:** w/in 14 d of MAOI **Disp:** Tabs 5, 10, 20 mg; soln 1 mg/mL **SE:** N/V/D, sweating, insomnia, dizziness, xerostomia, sexual dysfunction **Note:** Full effects may take 3 wk

Eslicarbazepine (Aptiom) Uses: *Partial-onset Sz* **Acts:** Inhib voltage-gated Na⁺ channels **Dose:** 400 mg PO daily × 1 wk, then 800 mg PO daily; max 1200 mg/d; CrCl < 50 mL/min: 200 mg PO daily × 2 wk, then 400 mg PO daily, max 600 mg/d **W/P:** [C, –] Suicidal behavior/ideation; TEN; SJS; DRESS; ↓ Na⁺; anaphylactic Rxn/angioedema; hepatotox **CI:** Hypersens to eslicarbazepine, oxcarbazepine **Disp:** Tabs 200, 400, 600, 800 mg **SE:** See W/P, N/V, dizziness, somnolence, HA, diplopia, fatigue, vertigo, ataxia, blurred vision, tremor, abn TFTs **Notes:** w/ PRG enroll in the North American Antiepileptic Drug Pregnancy Registry (1-888-233-2334 or http://www.aedpregnancyregistry.org/); w/ D/C withdrawal gradually

Esmolol (Brevibloc, Generic) Uses: *SVT & noncompensatory sinus tachycardia, AF/A flutter* **Acts:** β₁-Adrenergic blocker; class II antiarrhythmic **Dose:** *Adults & Peds. ECC 2010.* 0.5 mg/kg (500 mcg/kg) over 1 min, then 0.05 mg/kg/min (50 mcg/kg/min) Inf; if inadequate response after 5 min, repeat 0.5 mg/kg bolus, then titrate Inf up to 0.2 mg/kg/min (200 mcg/kg/min); max 0.3 mg/kg/min (300 mcg/kg/min) **W/P:** [C (1st tri; D 2nd or 3rd tri), ?] **CI:** Sinus bradycardia, heart block, uncompensated CHF, cardiogenic shock, ↓ BP **Disp:** Inj 10, 250 mg/mL; premix Inf 10 mg/mL **SE:** ↓ BP; ↓ HR, diaphoresis, dizziness, pain on Inj **Notes:** Hemodynamic effects back to baseline w/in 30 min after D/C Inf

Esomeprazole Magnesium, Sodium, Strontium (Nexium, Nexium IV, Nexium 24HR [OTC], Generic) Uses: *Rx GERD; ↓ risk NSAID gastric ulcer; H. pylori Infxn in combo w/ abx ("triple therapy") to ↓ risk duodenal ulcer recurrence; hypersecretory cond (Zollinger-Ellison synd)* **Acts:** PPI, ↓ gastric acid **Dose:** *Adults. GERD:* 20–40 mg/d PO × 4–8 wk; 20–40 mg IV 10–30 min Inf or > 3 min IV push, 10 d max; *NSAID ulcer:* 20–40 mg qd up to 6 mo; *H. pylori Infxn:* 40 mg/d PO, plus clarithromycin 500 mg PO bid & amoxicillin 1000 mg/bid for 10 d; *hypersecretory:* 40 mg PO bid *Peds 1 mo–1 y.* 2.5/5/10 mg based on Wt 1 ×/d × 6 wk for erosive esophagitis *1–11 y.* 10–20 mg qd up to 8 wk *12–17 y.* 20–40 mg qd up to 8 wk **W/P:** [C, ?/–] w/ Severe liver Dz 20 mg max;

caution w/ meds that pH affects absorption, including digoxin; caution w/ cilostazol, tacrolimus, MTX **CI:** PPI sens; do not use w/ clopidogrel, atazanavir, nelfinavir; ? ↑ risk of fractures w/ all PPI **Disp:** All oral products *DR: Nexium 24HR (OTC):* caps 20; *Nexium:* caps 20, 40 mg; *Strontium form:* 24.65 mg = 20 mg of esomeprazole; 49.3 mg = 40 mg of esomeprazole; *oral susp* 10 mg/packet; IV 20, 40 mg **SE:** *Adults.* HA, N/D, flatulence, Abd pain, constipation, dry mouth *Peds 1–17 y.* HA, Abd pain, N/D, somnolence *<1y.* Abd pain, regurgitation, tachypnea, ↑ ALT **Notes:** Do not chew; may open caps & sprinkle on applesauce; risk of hypomagnesemia w/ long-term use, monitor; sodium form for IV; all others PO

Estazolam (ProSom, Generic) [C-IV] Uses: *Short-term management of insomnia* **Acts:** Benzodiazepine **Dose:** 1–2 mg PO qhs PRN; ↓ in hepatic impair/elderly/debilitated **W/P:** [X, −] ↑ Effects w/ CNS depressants; cross-sens w/ other benzodiazepines **CI:** PRG, component hypersens, w/ itraconazole or ketoconazole **Disp:** Tabs 1, 2 mg **SE:** Somnolence, weakness, palpitations, anaphylaxis, angioedema, amnesia **Notes:** May cause psychological/physical dependence; avoid abrupt D/C after prolonged use

Esterified Estrogens (Menest) **BOX:** ↑ Risk endometrial CA; do not use in the prevention of CV Dz or dementia; ↑ risk of MI, stroke, breast CA, PE, DVT, in postmenopausal **Uses:** *Vasomotor Sxs or vulvar/Vag atrophy w/ menopause; female hypogonadism, PCa* **Acts:** Estrogen supl **Dose:** *Menopausal vasomotor Sx:* 1.25 mg/d, cyclically 3 wk on, 1 wk off; add progestin 10–14 d w/ 28-d cycle w/ uterus intact; *Hypogonadism:* 2.5–7.5 mg/d in ÷ doses PO × 20 d, off × 10 d; add progestin 10–14 d w/ 28-d cycle w/ uterus intact **W/P:** [X, −] **CI:** Undiagnosed genital bleeding, breast CA, estrogen-dependent tumors, thromboembolic disorders, thrombophlebitis, recent MI, PRG, severe hepatic Dz **Disp:** Tabs 0.3, 0.625, 1.25, 2.5 mg **SE:** N, HA, bloating, breast enlargement/tenderness, edema, venous thromboembolism, hypertriglyceridemia, gallbladder Dz **Notes:** Use lowest dose for shortest time (see WHI data [www.whi.org])

Estradiol, Gel (Divigel) **BOX:** ↑ Risk endometrial CA; do not use to prevent CV Dz or dementia; ↑ risk MI, stroke, breast CA, PE, and DVT in postmenopausal (50–79 y); ↑ dementia risk in postmenopausal (≥ 65 y) **Uses:** *Vasomotor Sx in menopause* **Acts:** Estrogen **Dose:** 0.25 g qd on right or left upper thigh (alternate) **W/P:** [X, +/−] May ↑ w/ thyroid Dz **CI:** Undiagnosed genital bleeding, breast CA, estrogen-dependent tumors, thromboembolic disorders, thrombophlebitis, recent MI, PRG, severe hepatic Dz **Disp:** 0.1% gel 0.25/0.5/1 g single-dose foil packets w/ 0.25-, 0.5-, 1-mg estradiol, respectively **SE:** N, HA, bloating, breast enlargement/tenderness, edema, venous thromboembolism, ↑ BP, hypertriglyceridemia, gallbladder Dz **Notes:** If person other than pt applies, glove should be used, keep dry immediately after, rotate site; contains alcohol, caution around flames until dry, not for Vag use

Estradiol, Metered Gel (Elestrin, Estrogel) BOX: ↑ Risk endometrial CA; do not use to prevent CV Dz or dementia; ↑ risk MI, stroke, breast CA, PE, and DVT in postmenopausal (50–79 y); ↑ dementia risk in postmenopausal (≥ 65 y) Uses: *Postmenopausal vasomotor Sxs* Acts: Estrogen Dose: Apply 0.87–1.7 g to upper arm skin qd; add progestin × 10–14 d/28-d cycle w/ intact uterus; use lowest effective estrogen dose W/P: [X, ?] CI: AUB, breast CA, estrogen-dependent tumors, hereditary angioedema, thromboembolic disorders, recent MI, PRG, severe hepatic Dz Disp: Gel 0.06%; metered dose/activation SE: Thromboembolic events, MI, stroke, ↑ BP, breast/ovarian/endometrial CA, site Rxns, Vag spotting, breast changes, Abd bloating, cramps, HA, fluid retention Notes: Wait > 25 min before sunscreen; avoid concomitant use for > 7 d; BP, breast exams

Estradiol, Oral (Delestrogen, Estrace, Femtrace, Others) BOX: ↑ Risk endometrial CA; do not use to prevent CV Dz or dementia; ↑ risk MI, stroke, breast CA, PE, and DVT in postmenopausal (50–79 y); ↑ dementia risk in postmenopausal (≥ 65 y) Uses: *Atrophic vaginitis, menopausal vasomotor Sxs, prevent osteoporosis, ↑ low estrogen levels, palliation breast and PCa* Acts: Estrogen Dose: *PO:* 1–2 mg/d, adjust PRN to control Sxs; *Vag cream:* 2–4 g/d × 2 wk, then 1 g 1–3×/wk; *Vasomotor Sx/Vag atrophy:* 10–20 mg IM q4wk, D/C or taper at 3- to 6-mo intervals; *Hypoestrogenism:* 10–20 mg IM q4wk; *PCa:* 30 mg IM q12wk W/P: [X, –] CI: Genital bleeding of unknown cause, breast CA, porphyria, estrogen-dependent tumors, thromboembolic disorders, thrombophlebitis; recent MI; hepatic impair Disp: Tabs 0.5, 1, 2 mg; depot Inj (*Delestrogen*) 10, 20, 40 mg/mL SE: N, HA, bloating, breast enlargement/tenderness, edema, ↑ triglycerides, venous thromboembolism, gallbladder Dz Notes: When estrogen used in postmenopausal w/ uterus, use w/ progestin

Estradiol, Spray (Evamist) BOX: ↑ Risk endometrial CA; do not use to prevent CV Dz or dementia; ↑ risk MI, stroke, breast CA, PE, and DVT in postmenopausal (50–79 y); ↑ dementia risk in postmenopausal (≥ 65 y) Uses: *Vasomotor Sx in menopause* Acts: Estrogen supl Dose: 1 spray on inner surface of forearm W/P: [X, +/–] May ↑ PT/PTT/plt aggregation w/ thyroid Dz CI: Undiagnosed genital bleeding, breast CA, estrogen-dependent tumors, thromboembolic disorders, thrombophlebitis, recent MI, PRG, severe hepatic Dz Disp: 1.53 mg/spray (56-spray container) SE: N, HA, bloating, breast enlargement/tenderness, edema, venous thromboembolism, ↑ BP, hypertriglyceridemia, gallbladder Dz Notes: Contains alcohol, caution around flames until dry; not for Vag use

Estradiol, Transdermal (Alora, Climara, Estraderm, Minivelle, Vivelle Dot) BOX: ↑ Risk endometrial CA; do not use to prevent CV Dz or dementia; ↑ risk MI, stroke, breast CA, PE, and DVT in postmenopausal (50–79 y); ↑ dementia risk in postmenopausal (≥ 65 y) Uses: *Severe menopausal vasomotor Sxs; female hypogonadism; Minivelle also approved for postmenopausal osteoporosis* Acts: Estrogen supl Dose: Start 0.025–0.05 mg/d patch 1–2×/wk based on product (*Climara* 1×/wk; *Alora* 2×/wk) adjust PRN to control Sxs; w/ intact uterus cycle 3 wk on, 1 wk off or use cyclic progestin 10–14 d **W/P:** [X, –] See Estradiol, Oral **CI:** PRG, AUB, porphyria, breast CA, estrogen-dependent tumors, Hx thrombophlebitis, thrombosis **Disp:** Transdermal patches (mg/24 h) 0.025, 0.0375, 0.05, 0.06, 0.075, 0.1 **SE:** N, bloating, breast enlargement/tenderness, edema, HA, hypertriglyceridemia, gallbladder Dz **Notes:** Do not apply to breasts, place on trunk, rotate sites; see Estradiol, Oral notes

Estradiol, Vaginal (Estring, Femring, Vagifem) **BOX:** ↑ Risk endometrial CA; do not use to prevent CV Dz or dementia; ↑ risk MI, stroke, breast CA, PE, and DVT in postmenopausal (50–79 y); ↑ dementia risk in postmenopausal (≥ 65 y) **Uses:** *Postmenopausal Vag atrophy (Estring)* *vasomotor Sxs and vulvar/Vag atrophy associated w/ menopause (Femring)* *atrophic vaginitis (Vagifem)* **Acts:** Estrogen supl **Dose:** *Estring:* Insert ring into upper third of Vag vault; remove and replace after 90 d; reassess 3–6 mo; *Femring:* Use lowest effective dose, insert vaginally, replace q3mo; *Vagifem:* 1 tab vaginally qd × 2 wk, then maint 1 tab 2×/wk, D/C or taper at 3–6 mo **W/P:** [X, –] May ↑ PT/PTT/plt aggregation w/ thyroid Dz, toxic shock reported **CI:** Undiagnosed genital bleeding, breast CA, estrogen-dependent tumors, thromboembolic disorders, thrombophlebitis, recent MI, PRG, severe hepatic Dz **Disp:** *Estring ring:* 2 mg/24 h; *Femring ring:* 0.05 and 0.1 mg/24 h; *Vagifem tab (Vag):* 10 mcg **SE:** HA, leukorrhea, back pain, candidiasis, vaginitis, Vag discomfort/hemorrhage, arthralgia, insomnia, Abd pain; see Estradiol, Oral notes

Estradiol/Levonorgestrel, Transdermal (Climara Pro) **BOX:** ↑ Risk endometrial CA; do not use to prevent CV Dz or dementia; ↑ risk MI, stroke, breast CA, PE, and DVT in postmenopausal (50–79 y); ↑ dementia risk in postmenopausal (≥ 65 y) **Uses:** *Menopausal vasomotor Sx; prevent postmenopausal osteoporosis* **Acts:** Estrogen & progesterone **Dose:** 1 patch 1×/wk **W/P:** [X, –] w/ ↓ Thyroid **CI:** AUB, estrogen-sensitive tumors, Hx thromboembolism, liver impair, PRG, hysterectomy **Disp:** Estradiol 0.045 mg/levonorgestrel 0.015 mg day patch **SE:** Site Rxn, Vag bleed/spotting, breast changes, Abd bloating/cramps, HA, retention fluid, edema, ↑ BP **Notes:** Apply lower Abd; for osteoporosis give Ca²⁺/vit D supl; follow breast exams

Estradiol/Norethindrone (Activella, Lopreeza, Mimvey, Mimvey Lo, Generic) **BOX:** ↑ Risk endometrial CA; do not use to prevent CV Dz or dementia; ↑ risk MI, stroke, breast CA, PE, and DVT in postmenopausal (50–79 y); ↑ dementia risk in postmenopausal (≥ 65 y) **Uses:** *Menopause vasomotor Sxs; prevent osteoporosis* **Acts:** Estrogen/progestin; plant derived **Dose:** 1 tab/d, start w/ lowest dose combo **W/P:** [X, –] w/ ↓ Ca²⁺/thyroid **CI:** PRG; Hx breast CA; estrogen-dependent tumor; abn genital bleeding; Hx DVT, PE, or related disorders; recent (w/in past year) arterial thromboembolic Dz (CVA, MI) **Disp:** *Femhrt:* Tabs 2.5/0.5, 5 mcg/1 mg; *Activella:* Tabs 1/0.5, 0.5 mg/0.1 mg **SE:** Thrombosis, dizziness, HA, libido changes, insomnia, emotional instability, breast pain **Notes:** Use in women w/ intact uterus; caution in heavy smokers; combo also used as OCP

Estramustine Phosphate (Emcyt) Uses: *Advanced PCa* Acts: Estradiol w/ nitrogen mustard; exact mechanism unknown Dose: 14 mg/kg/d in 3–4 ÷ doses; on empty stomach, no dairy products W/P: [NA, not used in females] CI: Active thrombophlebitis or thromboembolic disorders Disp: Caps 140 mg SE: N/V, exacerbation of preexisting CHF, edema, hepatic disturbances, thrombophlebitis, MI, PE, gynecomastia in 20–100% Notes: Low-dose breast irradiation before may ↓ gynecomastia

Estrogen, Conjugated (Premarin) BOX: ↑ Risk endometrial CA; do not use to prevent CV Dz or dementia; ↑ risk MI, stroke, breast CA, PE, and DVT in postmenopausal (50–79 y); ↑ dementia risk in postmenopausal (≥ 65 y) Uses: *Mod–severe menopausal vasomotor Sxs; atrophic vaginitis, dyspareunia*; palliative advanced PCa; Px & Tx of estrogen-deficiency osteoporosis Acts: Estrogen replacement Dose: 0.3–1.25 mg/d PO; intravaginal cream 0.5–2g × 21 d, then off × 7 d or 0.5 mg twice weekly W/P: [X, –] CI: Severe hepatic impair, genital bleeding of unknown cause, breast CA, estrogen-dependent tumors, thromboembolic disorders, thrombosis, thrombophlebitis, recent MI Disp: Tabs 0.3, 0.45, 0.625, 0.9, 1.25 mg; Vag cream 0.625 mg/g SE: ↑ Risk of endometrial CA, gallbladder Dz, thromboembolism, HA, & possibly breast CA Notes: Generic products not equivalent

Estrogen, Conjugated/Medroxyprogesterone (Premphase, Prempro) BOX: ↑ Risk endometrial CA; do not use to prevent CV Dz or dementia; ↑ risk MI, stroke, breast CA, PE, and DVT in postmenopausal (50–79 y); ↑ dementia risk in postmenopausal (≥ 65 y) Uses: *Mod–severe menopausal vasomotor Sxs; atrophic vaginitis; prevent postmenopausal osteoporosis* Acts: Hormonal replacement Dose: Prempro 1 tab PO daily; Premphase 1 tab PO daily W/P: [X, –] CI: Severe hepatic impair, genital bleeding of unknown cause, breast CA, estrogen-dependent tumors, thromboembolic disorders, thrombosis, thrombophlebitis Disp: (As estrogen/medroxyprogesterone) Prempro: Tabs 0.3/1.5, 0.45/1.5, 0.625/2.5, 0.625/5 mg; Premphase: Tabs 0.625/0 (d 1–14) & 0.625/5 mg (d 15–28) SE: Gallbladder Dz, thromboembolism, HA, breast tenderness Notes: See WHI (www.whi.org); use lowest dose/shortest time possible

Estrogen, Conjugated Synthetic (Enjuvia) BOX: ↑ Risk endometrial CA; do not use to prevent CV Dz or dementia; ↑ risk MI, stroke, breast CA, PE, and DVT in postmenopausal (50–79 y); ↑ dementia risk in postmenopausal (≥ 65 y) Uses: *Vasomotor menopausal Sxs, vulvovaginal atrophy* Acts: Multiple estrogen replacement Dose: For all w/ intact uterus progestin × 10–14 d/28-d cycle; Vasomotor: 0.3–1.25 mg PO daily (Enjuvia); Vag atrophy: 0.3 mg/d; W/P: [X, –] CI: See Estrogen, Conjugated Disp: Enjuvia Tabs ER 0.3, 0.45, 0.625, 0.9, 1.25 mg SE: ↑ Risk endometrial/breast CA, gallbladder Dz, thromboembolism

Eszopiclone (Lunesta, Generic) [C-IV] Uses: *Insomnia* Acts: Nonbenzodiazepine hypnotic Dose: Start 1 mg, may ↑ to 2–3 mg hs if needed Elderly: 1–2 mg/d hs; w/ hepatic impair use w/ CYP3A4 inhib (Table 10, p 356): 1 mg/d hs only if necessary W/P: [C, ?/–] Disp: Tabs 1, 2, 3 mg SE: HA, xerostomia, dizziness, somnolence, hallucinations, rash, Infxn, unpleasant taste, anaphylaxis, angioedema **Notes:** High-fat meals ↓ absorption; dose > 2 mg may cause next day impairment

Etanercept (Enbrel) **BOX:** Serious Infxns (bacterial sepsis, TB, reported); D/C w/ severe Infxn; evaluate for TB risk; test for TB before use; lymphoma/other CA possible in children/adolescents possible **Uses:** *↓ Sxs of RA in pts who fail other DMARD*, Crohn Dz, plaque psoriasis **Acts:** TNF-receptor blocker **Dose:** *Adults*. RA: 50 mg SQ weekly or 25 mg SQ 2×/wk (separated by at least 72–96 h) *Peds 4–17 y*. 0.8 mg/kg/wk (max 50 mg/wk) or 0.4 mg/kg (max 25 mg/dose) 2×/wk 72–96 h apart **W/P:** [B, ?] w/ Predisposition to Infxn (ie, DM); may ↑ risk of malignancy in peds and young adults **CI:** Active Infxn **Disp:** Inj 25 mg/vial, 50 mg/mL syringe **SE:** HA, rhinitis, Inj site Rxn, URI, new-onset psoriasis **Notes:** Rotate Inj sites

Ethambutol (Myambutol, Generic) **Uses:** *Pulm TB* & other mycobacterial Infxns, MAC **Acts:** ↓ RNA synth **Dose:** *Adults & Peds > 12 y*. 15–25 mg/kg/d PO single dose; ↓ in renal impair, take w/ food, avoid antacids **W/P:** [C, +/?] **CI:** Unconscious pts, optic neuritis **Disp:** Tabs 100, 400 mg **SE:** HA, hyperuricemia, acute gout, Abd pain, ↑ LFTs, optic neuritis, GI upset

Ethinyl Estradiol/Norelgestromin Patch (Ortho Evra, Xulane) **BOX:** Cigarette smoking ↑ risk of serious CV events; ↑ risk w/ age & no. of cigarettes smoked; hormonal contraceptives should not be used by women who are > 35 y and smoke; different from OCP pharmacokinetics **Uses:** *Contraceptive patch* **Acts:** Estrogen & progestin **Dose:** Apply patch to Abd, buttocks, upper torso (not breasts), or upper outer arm at the beginning of the menstrual cycle; new patch is applied weekly for 3 wk; wk 4 is patch-free **W/P:** [X, +/–] **CI:** PRG, Hx or current DVT/PE, stroke, MI, CV Dz, CAD; SBP ≥ 160 systolic mm Hg or DBP ≥ 100 diastolic mm Hg severe HTN; severe HA w/ focal neurologic Sx; breast/endometrial CA; estrogen-dependent neoplasms; hepatic dysfunction; jaundice; major surgery w/ prolonged immobilization; heavy smoking if > 35 y **Disp:** *Ortho Evra:* 20 cm² patch (6-mg norelgestromin [active metabolite norgestimate] & 0.75 mg of ethinyl estradiol); *Xulane:* 4.86 mg norelgestromin/0.53 mg ethinyl estradiol **SE:** Breast discomfort, HA, site Rxns, N, menstrual cramps; thrombosis risks similar to OCP **Notes:** Less effective in women > 90 kg; instruct pt does not protect against STD/HIV; discourage smoking

Ethosuximide (Zarontin, Generic) **Uses:** *Absence (petit mal) Szs* **Acts:** Anticonvulsant; ↑ Sz threshold **Dose:** *Adults & Peds > 6 y*. Initial, 500 mg PO ÷ bid; ↑ by 250 mg/d q4–7d PRN (max 1500 mg/d); usual maint 20–30 mg/kg *Peds 3–6 y*. 250 mg/d; ↑ by 250 mg/d q4–7d PRN; maint 20–30 mg/kg/d ÷ bid; max 1500 mg/d **W/P:** [C, +/?] In renal/hepatic impair; antiepileptics may ↑ risk of suicidal behavior or ideation **CI:** Component sens **Disp:** Caps 250 mg; syrup 250 mg/5 mL **SE:** Blood dyscrasias, GI upset, drowsiness, dizziness, irritability **Notes:** Levels: *Trough:* just before next dose; *Therapeutic: Peak:* 40–100 mcg/mL; *Toxic Trough:* > 100 mcg/mL; *Half-life:* 25–60 h

Etidronate Disodium (Didronel, Generic) Uses: *↑ Ca^{2+} of malignancy, Paget Dz, & heterotopic ossification* Acts: ↓ Nl & abn bone resorption **Dose:** *Paget Dz:* 5–10 mg/kg PO ÷ doses (for 3–6 mo); ↑ Ca^{2+}: 20 mg/kg IV × 30–90 d **W/P:** [B if PO (C if parenteral), ?] Bisphosphonates may cause severe musculoskeletal pain **CI:** Overt osteomalacia, SCr > 5 mg/dL **Disp:** Tabs 200, 400 mg **SE:** GI intolerance (↓ by ÷ daily doses); hyperphosphatemia, hypomagnesemia, bone pain, abn taste, fever, convulsions, nephrotox **Notes:** Take PO on empty stomach 2 h before or 2 h pc

Etodolac BOX: May ↑ risk of CV events & GI bleeding; may worsen ↑ BP Uses: *OA & pain*, RA Acts: NSAID **Dose:** 200–400 mg PO bid-qid (max 1000 mg/d) **W/P:** [C (D 3rd tri), ?] ↑ Bleeding risk w/ ASA, warfarin; ↑ nephrotox w/ cyclosporine; Hx CHF, HTN, renal/hepatic impair, PUD; ↑ risk of MI/CVA **CI:** Active GI ulcer **Disp:** Tabs 400, 500 mg; ER tabs 400, 500, 600 mg; caps 200, 300 mg **SE:** N/V/D, gastritis, abd cramps, dizziness, HA, depression, edema, renal impair **Notes:** Do not crush tabs

Etomidate (Amidate, Generic) Uses: *Induce general or short-procedure anesthesia* Acts: Short-acting hypnotic **Dose:** *Adults & Peds > 10 y.* Induce anesthesia 0.2–0.6 mg/kg IV over 30–60 s *Peds < 10 y.* Not recommended Peds. *ECC 2010.* Rapid sedation: 0.2–0.4 mg/kg IV/IO over 30–60 s; max dose 20 mg **W/P:** [C, ?] **CI:** Hypersens **Disp:** Inj 2 mg/mL **SE:** Inj site pain, myoclonus

Etonogestrel, Implant (Implanon) Uses: *Contraception* Acts: Transforms endometrium from proliferative to secretory **Dose:** 1 implant subdermally q3y **W/P:** [X, +] Exclude PRG before implant **CI:** PRG, hormonally responsive tumors, breast CA, AUB, hepatic tumor, active liver Dz, Hx thromboembolic Dz **Disp:** 68-mg implant 4 cm long **SE:** Spotting, irregular periods, amenorrhea, dysmenorrhea, HA, tender breasts, N, Wt gain, acne, ectopic PRG, PE, ovarian cysts, stroke, ↑ BP **Notes:** 99% effective; remove implant and replace; restricted distribution; physician must register and train; does not protect against STDs; site nondominant arm 8–10 cm above medial epicondyle of humerus; implant must be palpable after placement

Etonogestrel/Ethinyl Estradiol, Vaginal Insert (NuvaRing) BOX: Cigarette smoking ↑ risk of serious CV events; ↑ Risk w/ age & no. cigarettes smoked; hormonal contraceptives should not be used by women who are > 35 y and smoke; different from OCP pharmacokinetics Uses: *Contraceptive* Acts: Estrogen & progestin combo **Dose:** Rule out PRG first; insert ring vaginally for 3 wk, remove for 1 wk; insert new ring 7 d after last removed (even if bleeding) at same time of day ring removed. 1st day of menses is day 1, insert before day 5 even if bleeding; use other contraception for first 7 d of starting Rx; see PI if converting from other contraceptive; after delivery or 2nd tri Ab, insert 4 wk postpartum (if not breast-feeding) **W/P:** [X, ?/–] HTN, gallbladder Dz, ↑ lipids, migraines, sudden HA **CI:** PRG, heavy smokers > 35 y, DVT, PE, cerebro-/CV Dz, estrogen-dependent neoplasm, undiagnosed abn genital bleeding, hepatic tumors, cholestatic jaundice **Disp:** Intravag ring: ethinyl estradiol 0.015 mg/d & etonogestrel 0.12 mg/d **Notes:** If ring removed, rinse w/ cool/lukewarm H_2O (not hot) & reinsert ASAP; if not reinserted w/in 3 h, effectiveness ↓; do not use w/ diaphragm

Etoposide [VP-16] (Etopophos, Toposar, Vepesid, Generic) Uses: *Testicular CA, NSCLC, Hodgkin Dz, NHLs, peds ALL, allogeneic/autologous BMT in high doses* Acts: Topoisomerase II inhib Dose: 50 mg/m²/d IV for 3–5 d; 50 mg/m²/d IV for 21 d (PO availability = 50% of IV); 2–6 g/m² per course or 25–70 mg/kg in BMT (per protocols); ↓ in renal/hepatic impair W/P: [D, –] CI: IT administration Disp: Caps 50 mg; Inj 20 mg/mL SE: N/V (emesis in 10–30%), ↓ BM, alopecia, ↓ BP w/ rapid IV, anorexia, anemia, leukopenia, ↑ risk secondary leukemias

Etravirine (Intelence) Uses: *HIV Infxn* Acts: Non-NRTI Dose: Adults. 200 mg PO bid after a meal Peds. 16–20 kg: 100 mg, 20–25 kg: 125 mg, 25–30 kg: 150 mg, > 30 kg: 200 mg; all PO bid after a meal W/P: [B, ±] Many interactions: substrate/inducer (CYP3A4), substrate/inhib (CYP2C9, CYP2C19); do not use w/ tipranavir/ritonavir, fosamprenavir/ritonavir, atazanavir/ritonavir, protease inhib w/o ritonavir, and non-NRTIs CI: Ø Disp: Tabs 25, 100, 200 mg SE: N/V/D, rash, severe/potentially life-threatening skin Rxns, fat redistribution

Everolimus (Afinitor, Afinitor Disperz) Uses: *Advanced RCC w/ sunitinib or sorafenib failure, subependymal giant cell astrocytoma and PNET in nonsurgical candidates w/ tuberous sclerosis*, renal angiomyolipoma w/ tuberous sclerosis Acts: mTOR inhib Dose: 10 mg PO daily, ↓ to 5 mg w/ SE or hepatic impair; avoid w/ high-fat meal W/P: [D, ?] Avoid w/ or if received live vaccines; w/ CYP3A4 inhib CI: Compound/ rapamycin derivative hypersens Disp: Tabs 2.5, 5, 7.5, 10 mg; Disperz for suspen 2, 3, 5 mg SE: Noninfectious pneumonitis, ↑ Infxn risk, oral ulcers, asthenia, cough, fatigue, diarrhea, ↑ glu/SCr/lipids; ↓ hemoglobin/WBC/plt Notes: Follow CBC, LFT, glu, lipids; see also Everolimus (Zortress)

Everolimus (Zortress) Uses: *Px renal and liver transplant rejection; combo w/ basiliximab w/ ↓ dose of steroids and cyclosporine* Acts: mTOR inhib Dose: 0.75 mg PO bid, adjust to trough levels 3–8 ng/mL W/P: [C, ?] CI: Compound/ rapamycin-derivative hypersens Disp: Tabs 0.25, 0.5,0.75 mg SE: Peripheral edema, constipation, ↑ BP, N, ↓ Hct, UTI, ↑ lipids Notes: Follow CBC, LFT, glu, lipids; see also Everolimus (Afinitor); trough level 3–8 ng/mL w/ cyclosporine

Exemestane (Aromasin, Generic) Uses: *Advanced breast CA in postmenopausal women w/ progression after tamoxifen* Acts: Irreversible, steroidal aromatase inhib; ↓ estrogens Dose: 25 mg PO daily after a meal W/P: [X, ?/–] CI: PRG, component sens Disp: Tabs 25 mg SE: Hot flashes, N, fatigue, ↑ alkaline phosphate

Exenatide (Byetta) Uses: *Type 2 DM combined w/ metformin &/or sulfonylurea Acts: GLP-1 receptor agonist; incretin mimetic: ↑ insulin release, ↓ glucagon secretion, ↓ gastric emptying, promotes satiety Dose: 5 mcg SQ bid w/in 60 min before A.M. & P.M. meals; ↑ to 10 mcg SQ bid after 1 mo PRN; do not give pc W/P: [C, ?/–] May ↓ absorption of other drugs (take abx/contraceptives 1 h before) CI: CrCl < 30 mL/min Disp: Soln 5, 10 mcg/dose in prefilled pen SE: Hypoglycemia, N/V/D, dizziness, HA, dyspepsia, ↓ appetite, jittery; acute pancreatitis

Notes: Consider ↓ sulfonylurea to ↓ risk of hypoglycemia; discard pen 30 d after 1st use; monitor Cr

Exenatide, ER (Bydureon, Bydureon Pen) **BOX:** Causes thyroid C-cell tumors in rats, ? human relevance; CI in pts w/ Hx or family Hx MTC or MEN2; counsel pts on thyroid tumor risk & Sx **Uses:** *Type 2 DM* **Acts:** GLP-1 receptor agonist **Dose:** 2 mg SQ 1 × wk; w/ or w/o meals **W/P:** [C, ?/–] w/ Mod renal impair; w/ severe GI Dz; may cause acute pancreatitis and absorption of PO meds, may ↑ INR w/ warfarin **CI:** MTC, MEN2, hypersens; CrCl < 30 mL/min **Disp:** Inj 2 mg/ vial *Bydureon Pen* 2 mg w/ 23 g, 5/16 needle **SE:** N/V/D, constipation, dyspepsia, ↓ appetite, hypoglycemia, HA, Inj site Rxn, pancreatitis, renal impair, hypersens

Ezetimibe (Zetia) **Uses:** *Hypercholesterolemia alone or w/ an HMG-CoA reductase inhib* **Acts:** ↓ Cholesterol & phytosterols absorption **Dose:** *Adults & Peds > 10 y.* 10 mg/d PO **W/P:** [C, ?/–] Bile acid sequestrants ↓ bioavailability **CI:** Hepatic impair **Disp:** Tabs 10 mg **SE:** HA, D, Abd pain, ↑ transaminases w/ HMG-CoA reductase inhib, erythema multiforme **Notes:** See Ezetimibe/Simvastatin

Ezetimibe/Atorvastatin (Liptruzet) **Uses:** *Tx primary & mixed hyperlipidemia* **Acts:** Cholesterol absorption inhib & HMG-CoA reductase inhib **Dose:** 10/10–10/80 mg/d PO; w/ clarithromycin, itraconazole, saquinavir/ritonavir, darunavir/ritonavir, fosamprenavir, fosamprenavir/ritonavir: 10/20 mg/d max; w/ nelfinavir, boceprevir: 10/40 mg/d max; use caution/lowest effective dose w/ tipranavir/ritonavir; start 10/40 mg/day for > 55% ↓ in LDL-C **W/P:** [X, –] w/ CYP3A4 inhib, fenofibrates, niacin > 1 g/d **CI:** Liver Dz, ↑ LFTs; PRG/lactation; w/cyclosporine, tipranavir/ritonavir, telaprevir, gemfibrozil; component hypersens **Disp:** Tabs (mg ezetimibe/mg simvastatin) 10/10, 10/20, 10/40, 10/80 **SE:** ↑ LFTs, musculoskeletal pain, myopathy, Abd pain, dizziness, N/D, HA, insomnia, hot flash, ↑ K⁺ **Notes:** Instruct pt to report unusual muscle pain/weakness

Ezetimibe/Simvastatin (Vytorin) **Uses:** *Hypercholesterolemia* **Acts:** ↓ Absorption of cholesterol & phytosterols w/ HMG-CoA-reductase inhib **Dose:** 10/10–10/80 mg/d PO; w/ diltiazem/amiodarone or verapamil: 10/10 mg/d max; w/ amlodipine/ranolazine 10/20 max; ↓ w/ severe renal Insuff; give 2 h before or 4 h after bile acid sequestrants **W/P:** [X, –]; w/ CYP3A4 inhib (Table 10, p 356), gemfibrozil, niacin > 1 g/d, danazol, amiodarone, verapamil; avoid high dose w/ diltiazem; w/ Chinese pt on lipid-modifying meds **CI:** PRG/lactation; w/ cyclosporine & danazol; liver Dz, ↑ LFTs **Disp:** Tabs (mg ezetimibe/mg simvastatin) 10/10, 10/20, 10/40, 10/80 **SE:** HA, GI upset, myalgia, myopathy (muscle pain, weakness, or tenderness w/ creatine kinase 10 × ULN), rhabdomyolysis, hep, Infxn **Notes:** Monitor LFTs, lipids; ezetimibe/simvastatin combo lowered LDL more than simvastatin alone in ENHANCE study, but was no difference in carotid-intima media thickness; pts to report muscle pain

Ezogabine (Potiga) **BOX:** Retinal abnormalities possible; abn visual acuity/ loss possible; D/C if inadequate clinical benefit; baseline q6mo visual monitoring by an ophthalmic professional (acuity & dilated fundus photography); w/ retinal pigment abnormalities/vision changes D/C drug **Uses:** *Partial-onset Szs* **Acts:** ↑ Transmembrane K^+ currents & augment GABA mediated currents **Dose:** 100 mg PO tid; ↑ dose by 50 mg tid qwk, max dose 400 mg tid (1200 mg/d); ↓ dosage in elderly, renal/hepatic impair (see PI); swallow whole **W/P:** [C, ?/–] May need to ↑ dose when used w/ phenytoin & carbamazepine; monitor digoxin levels **Disp:** Tabs 50, 200, 300, 400 mg **SE:** Dizziness, somnolence, fatigue, abnormal coordination, gait disturbance, confusion, psychotic Sxs, hallucinations, attention disturbance, memory impair, vertigo, tremor, blurred vision, aphasia, dysarthria, urinary retention, ↑ QT interval, suicidal ideation/behavior, withdrawal Szs **Notes:** Withdraw over minimum of 3 wk

Famciclovir (Famvir, Generic) **Uses:** *Acute herpes zoster (shingles) & genital herpes* **Acts:** ↓ Viral DNA synth **Dose:** *Zoster:* 500 mg PO q8h × 7 d *Simplex:* 125–250 mg PO bid; ↓ w/ renal impair **W/P:** [B, –] **CI:** Component sens **Disp:** Tabs 125, 250, 500 mg **SE:** Fatigue, dizziness, HA, pruritus, N/D **Notes:** Best w/in 72 h of initial lesion

Famotidine (Pepcid, Pepcid AC, Generic) [OTC] **Uses:** *Short-term Tx of duodenal ulcer & benign gastric ulcer; maint for duodenal ulcer, hypersecretory conditions, GERD, & heartburn* **Acts:** H₂-antagonist; ↓ gastric acid **Dose:** *Adults.* *Ulcer:* 20 mg IV q12h or 20–40 mg PO qhs × 4–8 wk *Hypersecretion:* 20–160 mg PO q6h *GERD:* 20 mg PO bid × 6 wk; maint: 20 mg PO bid *Heartburn:* 10 mg PO PRN q12h *Peds.* 0.5–1 mg/kg/d; ↓ in severe renal Insuff **W/P:** [B, M] **CI:** Component sens **Disp:** Tabs 10, 20, 40 mg; chew tabs 10 mg; susp 40 mg/5 mL; gelatin caps 10 mg; Inj 10 mg/mL **SE:** Dizziness, HA, constipation, N/V/D, ↓ plt, hep **Notes:** Chew tabs contain phenylalanine

Febuxostat (Uloric) **Uses:** *Hyperuricemia and gout* **Acts:** Xanthine oxidase inhib (enzyme that converts hypoxanthine to xanthine to uric acid) **Dose:** 40 mg PO qd; ↑ 80 mg if uric acid not < 6 mg/dL after 2 wk **W/P:** [C, ?/–] **CI:** Use w/ azathioprine, mercaptopurine, theophylline **Supplied:** Tabs 40, 80 mg **SE:** ↑ LFTs, rash, myalgia **Notes:** OK to continue w/ gouty flare or use w/ NSAIDs

Felodipine (Plendil, Generic) **Uses:** *HTN & CHF* **Acts:** CCB **Dose:** 2.5–10 mg PO daily; swallow whole; ↓ in hepatic impair **W/P:** [C, ?/–] ↑ Effect w/ azole antifungals, erythromycin, grapefruit juice **CI:** Component sens **Disp:** ER tabs 2.5, 5, 10 mg **SE:** Peripheral edema, flushing, tachycardia, HA, gingival hyperplasia **Notes:** Follow BP in elderly & w/ hepatic impair

Fenofibrate (Antara, Lipofen, Lofibra, TriCor, Triglide, Generic) **Uses:** *Hypertriglyceridemia, hypercholesteremia* **Acts:** ↓ Triglyceride synth **Dose:** 43–160 mg/d; ↓ w/ renal impair; take w/ meals **W/P:** [C, –] **CI:** Hepatic/severe renal Insuff, primary biliary cirrhosis, unexplained ↑ LFTs, gallbladder Dz **Disp:** Caps 35, 40, 43, 48, 50, 54, 67, 105, 107, 130, 134, 145, 160, 200 mg **SE:** GI disturbances, cholecystitis, arthralgia, myalgia, dizziness, ↑ LFTs **Notes:** Monitor LFTs

Fenofibric Acid (Fibricor, Trilipix, Generic) Uses: *Adjunct to diet for ↑ triglycerides; to ↓ LDL-C, cholesterol, triglycerides, and apo B; to ↑ HDL-C in hypercholesterolemia/mixed dyslipidemia; adjunct to diet w/ a statin to ↓ triglycerides and ↑ HDL-C w/ CHD or w/ CHD risk* Acts: PPAR-α agonist, causes ↑ VLDL catabolism, fatty acid oxidation, and clearing of triglyceride-rich particles w/ ↓ VLDL, triglycerides; ↑ HDL in some Dose: *Mixed dyslipidemia w/ a statin:* 135 mg PO qd *Hypertriglyceridemia:* 45–135 mg qd; maint based on response *Primary hypercholesterolemia/mixed dyslipidemia:* 135 mg PO qd; 135 mg/d max; 35 mg w/ renal impair W/P: [C, –] Multiple interactions, ↑ embolic phenomenon CI: Severe renal impair, pt on dialysis, active liver/gall bladder Dz, nursing Disp: DR caps 45, 135 mg; tabs 35, 105 mg SE: HA, back pain, nasopharyngitis, URI, N/D, myalgia, gall stones, ↓ CBC (usually stabilizes), rare myositis/rhabdomyolysis Notes: ✓CBC, lipid panel, LFTs; D/C if LFT > 3× ULN

Fenoldopam (Corlopam, Generic) Uses: *Hypertensive emergency* Acts: Rapid vasodilator Dose: Initial 0.03–0.1 mcg/kg/min IV Inf, titrate q15min by 0.05–0.1 mcg/kg/min to max 1.6 mcg/kg/min W/P: [B, ?] ↓ BP w/ β-blockers CI: Ø Disp: Inj 10 mg/mL SE: ↓ BP, edema, facial flushing, N/V/D, atrial flutter/fibrillation, ↑ IOP Notes: Avoid concurrent β-blockers

Fenoprofen (Nalfon, Generic) BOX: May ↑ risk of CV events and GI bleeding Uses: *Arthritis & pain* Acts: NSAID Dose: 200–600 mg q4–8h, to 3200 mg/d max; w/ food W/P: [C (D 3rd tri), +/–] CHF, HTN, renal/hepatic impair, Hx PUD, ↑ risk of MI/CVA CI: NSAID sens Disp: Caps 400, 600 mg SE: GI disturbance, dizziness, HA, rash, edema, renal impair, hep Notes: Swallow whole

Fentanyl (Sublimaze, Generic) [C-II] Uses: *Short-acting analgesic* in anesthesia & PCA Acts: Narcotic analgesic Dose: *Adults.* 1–2 mcg/kg *or* 25–100 mcg/dose IV/IM titrated *Anesthesia:* 5–15 mcg/kg Peds: 200 mcg over 15 min, titrate to effect Peds: 1–2 mcg/kg IV/IM q1–4h, titrate; ↓ in renal impair W/P: [C, +/–] CI: Paralytic ileus ↑ ICP, resp depression, severe renal/hepatic impair Disp: Inj 0.05 mg/mL SE: Sedation, ↓ BP, ↓ HR, constipation, N, resp depression, miosis Notes: 0.1 mg fentanyl = 10 mg morphine IM

Fentanyl, Transdermal (Duragesic, Generic) [C-II] BOX: Potential for abuse and fatal OD Uses: *Persistent mod–severe chronic pain in pts already tolerant to opioids* Acts: Narcotic Dose: Apply patch to upper torso q72h; dose based on narcotic requirements in previous 24 h; start 25 mcg/h patch q72h; ↓ in renal impair W/P: [C, +/–] w/ CYP3A4 inhib (Table 10, p 356) may ↑ fentanyl effect, w/ Hx substance abuse CI: Not opioid tolerant, short-term pain management, postop outpatient pain in outpatient surgery, mild pain, PRN use, ↑ ICP, resp depression, severe renal/hepatic impair, peds < 2 y Disp: Patches 12.5, 25, 50, 75, 100 mcg/h SE: Resp depression (fatal), sedation, ↓ BP, ↓ HR, constipation, N, miosis Notes: 0.1 mg fentanyl = 10 mg morphine IM; do not cut patch; peak level in PRG 24–72 h

Fentanyl, Transmucosal (Abstral, Actiq, Fentora, Lazanda, Onsolis, Generic) [C-II] BOX: Potential for abuse and fatal OD; use only in pts w/ chronic pain who are opioid tolerant; CI in acute/postop pain; do not substitute for other fentanyl products; fentanyl can be fatal to children, keep away; use w/ strong CYP3A4 inhib may ↑ fentanyl levels; Many have restricted distribution **Uses:** *Breakthrough CA pain w/ tolerance to opioids* **Acts:** Narcotic analgesic, transmucosal absorption **Dose:** Titrate to effect

- *Abstral:* Start 100 mcg SL, 2 doses max per pain breakthrough episode; wait 2 h for next breakthrough dose; limit to < 4 breakthrough doses w/ successful baseline dosing
- *Actiq:* Start 200 mcg PO × 1, may repeat × 1 after 30 min
- *Fentora:* Start 100 mcg buccal tab × 1, may repeat in 30 min, 4 tabs/dose max
- *Lazanda:* Through TIRF REMS Access Program; initial 1 × 100 mcg spray; if no relief, titrate for breakthrough pain as follows: 2 × 100 mcg spray (1 in each nostril); 1 × 400 mcg; 2 × 400 mcg (1 in each nostril); wait 2 h before another dose; max 4 doses/24h
- *Onsolis:* Start 200 mcg film, ↑ 200 mcg increments to max four 200-mcg films or single 1200-mcg film

W/P: [C, +/−] resp/CNS depression possible; CNS depressants/CYP3A4 inhib may ↑ effect; may impair tasks (driving, machinery); w/ severe renal/hepatic impair **CI:** Opioid intolerant pt, acute/postop pain **Disp:**

- *Abstral:* SL tabs 100, 200, 300, 400, 600, 800 mcg
- *Actiq:* Lozenges on stick 200, 400, 600, 800, 1200, 1600 mcg
- *Fentora:* Buccal tabs 100, 200, 400, 600, 800 mcg
- *Lazanda:* Nasal spray metered dose audible and visual counter, 8 doses/ bottle, 100/400 mcg/spray
- *Onsolis:* Buccal soluble film 200, 400, 600, 800, 1200 mcg

SE: Sedation, ↓ BP, ↓ HR, constipation, N/V, ↓ resp, dyspnea, HA, miosis, anxiety, confusion, depression, rash dizziness **Notes:** 0.1 mg fentanyl = 10 mg IM morphine

Ferric Carboxymaltose (Injectafer) Uses: *Iron-deficiency anemia* **Acts:** Fe Supl **Dose:** ≥ 50 kg: 2 doses 750 mg IV separated by 7 d; < 50 kg: 2 doses of 15 mg/kg IV separated by 7 d **W/P:** [C, M] Hypersens Rxn (monitor during & 30 min after Inf) **CI:** Component hypersens **Disp:** Inj 750 mg iron/15 mL single-use vial **SE:** N, HTN, flushing, hypophosphatemia, dizziness, HTN

Ferric Citrate (Auryxia) Uses: *↓ PO_4^{-3} in ESRD* **Acts:** GI PO_4^{-3} binder **Dose:** 2 tabs PO TID w/ meals; adjust 1–2 tabs to PO_4^{-3} target level (Nl: 2.4–4.1 mg/dL) **W/P:** [B, +/−] ✓ Ferritin & transferrin **CI:** Iron overload synd **Disp:** Tabs 210 mg ferric iron **SE:** N/V/D, constipation, discolored stools **Notes:** May need to adjust timing of other meds (eg, doxycycline, take 1 h before)

Ferrous Gluconate (Ferate, Fergon [OTC], Others) BOX: Accidental OD of iron-containing products is a leading cause of fatal poisoning in children < 6 y; keep out of reach of children **Uses:** *Iron-deficiency anemia* & Fe supl **Acts:**

Dietary supl **Dose:** *Adults.* 60 mg qd-qid *Peds.* 4–6 mg/kg/d ÷ doses; on empty stomach (OK w/ meals if GI upset occurs); avoid antacids **W/P:** [A, ?] **CI:** Hemochromatosis, hemolytic anemia **Disp:** Tabs *Ferate* 240 mg (27 mg Fe); *Fergon* 240 (27 mg Fe), 324 mg (38 mg Fe) **SE:** GI upset, constipation, dark stools, discoloration of urine, may stain teeth **Notes:** 12% Elemental Fe; false(+) stool guaiac; keep away from children; severe tox in OD

Ferrous Gluconate Complex (Ferrlecit) **Uses:** *Iron-deficiency anemia or supl to erythropoietin Rx therapy* **Acts:** Fe supl **Dose:** *Test dose:* 2 mL (25 mg Fe) IV over 1 h, if OK, 125 mg (10 mL) IV over 1 h *Usual cumulative dose:* 1 g Fe over 8 sessions (until favorable Hct) **W/P:** [B, ?] **CI:** Non–Fe-deficiency anemia; CHF; Fe overload **Disp:** Inj 12.5 mg/mL **SE:** ↓ BP, serious allergic Rxns, GI disturbance, Inj site Rxn **Notes:** Dose expressed as mg Fe; may infuse during dialysis

Ferrous Sulfate [OTC] **Uses:** *Iron-deficiency anemia & Fe supl* **Acts:** Dietary supl **Dose:** *Adults.* 300 mg qd-qid. *Peds.* 1–6 mg/kg/d ÷ qd–tid; on empty stomach (OK w/ meals if GI upset occurs); avoid antacids **W/P:** [A, ?] ↑ Absorption w/ vit C; ↓ absorption w/ tetracycline, fluoroquinolones, antacids, H₂ blockers, PPI **CI:** Hemochromatosis, hemolytic anemia **Disp:** Tabs 140 (45 mg Fe), 142 (45 mg Fe), 324 (65 mg Fe), 325 mg (65 mg Fe); SR caps & tabs 160 (50 mg Fe); gtt 75 mg/0.6 mL (15 mg Fe/0.6 mL); elixir 220 mg/5 mL (44 mg Fe/5 mL); syrup 300 mg/5 mL (50 mg Fe/5 mL) **SE:** GI upset, constipation, dark stools, discolored urine

Ferumoxytol (Feraheme) **BOX:** Risk for fatal hypersens Rxn **Uses:** *Iron-deficiency anemia in chronic kidney Dz* **Acts:** Fe replacement **Dose:** 510 mg IV × 1, then 510 mg IV × 1 3–8 d later; give over at least 15 min **W/P:** [C, ?/–] Monitor for hypersens & ↓ BP for 30 min after dose, may alter MRI studies **CI:** Iron overload; hypersens to ferumoxytol **Disp:** IV soln 30 mg/mL (510 mg elemental Fe/17 mL) **SE:** N/D, constipation, dizziness, hypotension, peripheral edema, hypersens Rxn **Notes:** ✓ hematologic response 1 month after 2nd dose

Fesoterodine (Toviaz) **Uses:** * OAB w/ urge urinary incontinence, urgency, frequency* **Acts:** Competitive muscarinic receptor antag, ↓ bladder muscle contractions **Dose:** 4 mg PO qd, ↑ to 8 mg PO daily PRN **W/P:** [C, ?/–] Avoid > 4 mg w/ severe renal Insuff or w/ CYP3A4 inhib (eg, ketoconazole, clarithromycin); w/ BOO, ↓ GI motility/constipation, NAG, MyG **CI:** Urinary/gastric retention or uncontrolled NAG, hypersens to class **Disp:** Tabs 4, 8 mg **SE:** Dry mouth, constipation, ↓ sweating can cause heat prostration

Fexofenadine (Allegra, Allegra-D, Generic) **Uses:** *Allergic rhinitis; chronic idiopathic urticaria* **Acts:** Selective antihistamine, H₁-receptor antag; Allegra-D contains pseudoephedrine **Dose:** *Adults & Peds > 12 y.* 60 mg PO bid or 180 mg/d; 12-h ER form bid, 24-h ER form qd *Peds 2–11 y.* 30 mg PO bid; ↓ in renal impair **W/P:** [C, +/?] w/ Nevirapine **CI:** Component sens **Disp:** Tabs 30, 60, 180 mg; susp 6 mg/mL; *Allegra-D* 12-h ER tab (60 mg fexofenadine/120 mg pseudoephedrine), *Allegra-D* 24-h *ER* (180 mg fexofenadine/240 mg pseudoephedrine) **SE:** Drowsiness (rare), HA, ischemic colitis

Fidaxomicin (Dificid) Uses: **C. difficile-associated D** Acts: Macrolide abx Dose: 200 mg PO bid × 10 d W/P: [B, +/–] Not for systemic Infxn or < 18 y; to ↓ resistance, use only when diagnosis suspected/proven Disp: Tabs 200 mg SE: N/V, Abd pain, GI bleed, anemia, neutropenia

Filgrastim [G-CSF] (Granix, Neupogen, Zarxio) Uses: *↓ Incidence of Infxn in febrile neutropenic pts; Rx chronic neutropenia (ie, BMT, lethal radiation dose)** Acts: Recombinant G-CSF Dose: *Adults & Peds.* 5 mcg/kg/d SQ or IV (over 30 min) single daily dose; D/C when ANC > 10,000 cells/mm³; *Zarxio* also 10 mcg/kg/day IV w/ BMT, leukopheresis W/P: [C, ?] w/ Component hypersens CI: Allergy to *E. coli*-derived proteins or G-CSF Disp: *Granix:* pre-filled syringe 300 mcg/0.5 mL, 480 mcg/0.8 mL; *Neupogen:* Inj vial and pre-filled syringe 300 mcg/mL, 480 mg/1.6 mL SE: Fever, alopecia, N/V/D, splenomegaly, bone pain, HA, rash Notes: ✓ CBC & plt; monitor for cardiac events; no benefit w/ ANC > 10,000 cells/mm³; *Granix* OK for pt self-Inj

Finafloxacin Otic (Xtoro Otic) Uses: **Acute otitis externa** Acts: Quinolone abx; ↓ DNA gyrase. *Spectrum:* P. aeruginosa, S. aureus Dose: *Adults & Peds >1 y.* 4 gtt bid in ear(s) × 7 d W/P: [C, –/±] Quinolone allergy CI: Ø Disp: Otic susp 0.3% 8 mL bottle SE: Ear pruritus, N Notes: Shake well; warm bottle in hands 1–2 min before use; w/ otowick, use 8 ggt w/ insertion, then 4 gtt bid × 7 d

Finasteride (Propecia, Proscar [Generic]) Uses: **BPH & androgenetic alopecia** Acts: ↓ 5-alpha-reductase Dose: *BPH:* 5 mg/d PO *Alopecia:* 1 mg/d PO; food ↓ absorption W/P: [X, –] Hepatic impair CI: Pregnant women should avoid handling pills, teratogen to male fetus Disp: Tabs 1 mg (*Propecia*), 5 mg (*Proscar*) SE: ↓ Libido, vol ejaculate, ED, gynecomastia; may slightly ↑ risk of high-grade PCa Notes: Both ↓ PSA by ~50%; reestablish PSA baseline 6 mo (double PSA for "true" reading); 3–6 mo for effect on urinary Sxs; continue to maintain new hair, not for use in women

Fingolimod (Gilenya) Uses: **Relapsing MS** Acts: Sphingosine 1-phosphate receptor modulator; ↓ lymphocyte migration into CNS Dose: 0.5 mg PO qd; monitor for 6 h after 1st dose for bradycardia W/P: [C, –] Monitor w/ severe hepatic impair and if on Class 1a or III antiarrhythmics/beta-blockers/ CCBs (rhythm disturbances); avoid live vaccines during & 2 mo after D/C; ketoconazole ↑ level PML possible Disp: Caps 0.5 mg SE: HA, D, back pain, dizziness, bradycardia, AV block, HTN, Infxns, macular edema, ↑ LFTs, cough, dyspnea Notes: Obtain baseline ECG, CBC, LFTs & eye exam; women of childbearing potential should use contraception during & 2 mo after D/C

Flavoxate (Generic) Uses: **Relief of Sx of dysuria, urgency, nocturia, suprapubic pain, urinary frequency, incontinence** Acts: Antispasmodic Dose: 100–200 mg PO tid-qid W/P: [B, ?] CI: GI obst, GI hemorrhage, ileus, achalasia, BPH Disp: Tabs 100 mg SE: Drowsiness, blurred vision, xerostomia

Flecainide (Tambocor, Generic) BOX: ↑ Mortality in pts w/ ventricular arrhythmias and recent MI; pulm effects reported; ventricular proarrhythmic effects in AF/A flutter, not OK for chronic AF **Uses:** Px AF/A flutter & PSVT, *prevent/suppress life-threatening ventricular arrhythmias* **Acts:** Class 1C antiarrhythmic **Dose:** *Adults.* Start 50 mg PO q12h; ↑ by 50 mg q12h q4d, to max 400 mg/d max **Peds.** 3–6 mg/kg/d in 3 ÷ doses; ↓ w/ renal impair **W/P:** [C, +] Monitor w/ hepatic impair, ↑ conc w/ amiodarone, digoxin, quinidine, ritonavir/amprenavir, β-blockers, verapamil; may worsen arrhythmias **CI:** 2nd-/3rd-degree AV block, right BBB w/ bifascicular or trifascicular block, cardiogenic shock, CAD, ritonavir/amprenavir, alkalinizing agents **Disp:** Tabs 50, 100, 150 mg **SE:** Dizziness, visual disturbances, dyspnea, palpitations, edema, CP, tachycardia, CHF, HA, fatigue, rash, N **Notes:** Initiate Rx in hospital; dose q8h if pt is intolerant/uncontrolled at q12h; *Levels: Trough:* Just before next dose; *Therapeutic:* 0.2–1 mcg/mL; *Toxic:* > 1 mcg/mL; *half-life:* 7–22 h

Flibanserin (ADDYI) **BOX:** Hypotension and syncope in certain settings (w/ EtOH and strong CYP3A4 inhib; limited distribution **Uses:** *Premenopausal women w/acquired, generalized hypoactive sexual desire disorder (HSDD) not due to a medical/psych condition* **Acts:** Unknown, interacts w/ serotonin receptors **Dose:** 100 mg PO QHS **W/P:** [?, –] ↓ BP/syncope w/ EtOH, CNS depression **CI:** W/ EtOH, CYP3A4 inhibitors, hepatic impair **Disp:** tabs 100 mg **SE:** Dizziness, somnolence, N, fatigue, insomnia, dry mouth **Notes:** Available only through REMS Program; does not enhance sexual performance.

Floxuridine (Generic) **BOX:** Administration by experienced physician only; pts should be hospitalized for 1st course d/t risk for severe Rxn **Uses:** *GI adenoma, liver, renal CAs*; colon & pancreatic CAs **Acts:** Converted to 5-FU; thymidylate synthase; inhib ↓ DNA synthase (S-phase specific) **Dose:** 0.1–0.6 mg/kg/d for 1–6 wk (per protocols) usually intraarterial for liver mets **W/P:** [D, –] Interaction w/ vaccines **CI:** BM suppression, poor nutritional status, serious Infxn, PRG, component sens **Disp:** Inj 500 mg **SE:** ↓ BM, anorexia, Abd cramps, N/V/D, mucositis, alopecia, skin rash, & hyperpigmentation; rare neurotox (blurred vision, depression, nystagmus, vertigo, & lethargy); intraarterial catheter-related problems (ischemia, thrombosis, bleeding, & Infxn) **Notes:** Need effective birth control; palliative Rx for inoperable/incurable pts

Fluconazole (Diflucan, Generic) **Uses:** *Candidiasis (esophageal, oropharyngeal, urinary tract, Vag, prophylaxis); cryptococcal meningitis; prophylaxis w/ BMT* **Acts:** Antifungal; ↓ cytochrome P-450 sterol demethylation. *Spectrum:* All Candida sp except *C. krusei, C. glabrata* **Dose:** *Adults.* 100–400 mg/d PO or IV *Vaginitis:* 150 mg PO daily *Crypto:* Doses up to 800 mg/d reported; 400 mg d 1, then 200 mg ×10–12 wk after CSF (–) *Peds.* 3–6 mg/kg/d PO or IV; 12 mg/kg/d/systemic Infxn; ↓ in renal impair **W/P:** [C, Vag candidiasis (D high or prolonged dose), –] Do not use w/ clopidogrel (↓ effect) **CI:** Ø **Disp:** Tabs 50, 100, 150, 200 mg; susp 10, 40 mg/mL; Inj 2 mg/mL **SE:** HA, rash, GI upset, ↓ K⁺, ↑ LFTs **Notes:** PO (preferred) = IV levels; congenital anomalies w/ high dose 1st tri

Fludarabine (Generic) **BOX:** Administer only under supervision of qualified physician experienced in chemotherapy; can ↓ BM and cause severe CNS effects (blindness, coma, and death); severe/fatal autoimmune hemolytic anemia reported, monitor for hemolysis; use w/ pentostatin not OK (fatal pulm tox) **Uses:** *Autoimmune hemolytic anemia, CLL, cold agglutinin hemolysis*, low-grade lymphoma, mycosis fungoides **Acts:** ↓ Ribonucleotide reductase; blocks DNA polymerase-induced DNA repair **Dose:** 20–30 mg/m²/d for 5 d, as a 30-min Inf (per protocols); ↓ w/ renal impair **W/P:** [D, –] Give cytarabine before fludarabine (↓ its metabolism) **CI:** w/ Pentostatin, severe Infxns, CrCl < 30 mL/min, hemolytic anemia **Disp:** Inj 50 mg **SE:** ↓ BM, N/V/D, ↑ LFTs, edema, CHF, fever, chills, fatigue, dyspnea, nonproductive cough, pneumonitis, severe CNS tox rare in leukemia, autoimmune hemolytic anemia

Fludrocortisone Acetate (Florinef, Generic) **Uses:** *Adrenocortical Insuff, Addison Dz, salt-wasting synd* **Acts:** Mineralocorticoid **Dose:** *Adults.* 0.1–0.2 mg/d PO *Peds.* 0.05–0.1 mg/d PO **W/P:** [C, ?] **CI:** Systemic fungal Infxns; known allergy **Disp:** Tabs 0.1 mg **SE:** HTN, edema, CHF, HA, dizziness, convulsions, acne, rash, bruising, hyperglycemia, hypothalamic-pituitary-adrenal suppression, cataracts **Notes:** For adrenal Insuff, use w/ glucocorticoid; dose changes based on plasma renin activity

Flumazenil (Romazicon, Generic) **Uses:** *Reverse sedative effects of benzodiazepines & general anesthesia* **Acts:** Benzodiazepine receptor antag **Dose:** *Adults.* 0.2 mg IV over 15 s; repeat PRN, to 1 mg max (5 mg max in benzodiazepine OD) *Peds.* 0.01 mg/kg (0.2 mg/dose max) IV over 15 s; repeat 0.005 mg/kg at 1-min intervals to max 1 mg total; ↓ in hepatic impair **W/P:** [C, ?] **CI:** TCA OD; if pts given benzodiazepines to control life-threatening conditions (ICP/status epilepticus) **Disp:** Inj 0.1 mg/mL **SE:** N/V, palpitations, HA, anxiety, nervousness, hot flashes, tremor, blurred vision, dyspnea, hyperventilation, withdrawal synd **Notes:** Does not reverse narcotic Sx or amnesia, use associated w/ Szs

Fluorouracil, Inj [5-FU] (Adrucil, Generic) **BOX:** Administration by experienced chemotherapy physician only; pts should be hospitalized for 1st course d/t risk for severe Rxn **Uses:** *Colorectal, gastric, pancreatic, breast, basal cell*, head, neck, bladder CAs **Acts:** thymidylate synthetase inhib (↓ DNA synth, S-phase specific) **Dose:** 200–1200 mg/m²/d × 1–5 d IV push to 24-h cont Inf; protracted venous Inf of 200–300 mg/m²/d (per protocol); 800 mg/d max **W/P:** [D, ?] ↑ Tox w/ allopurinol; do not give live vaccine before 5-FU **CI:** Poor nutritional status, depressed BM Fxn, serious Infxn, bili > 5 mg/dL **Disp:** Inj 50 mg/mL **SE:** Stomatitis, esophago-pharyngitis, N/V/D, anorexia, ↓ BM, rash/dry skin/photosens, tingling in hands/feet w/ pain (palmar-plantar erythrodysesthesia), phlebitis/discoloration at Inj sites **Notes:** ↑ Thiamine intake; contraception OK

Fluorouracil, Topical [5-FU] (Carac, Efudex, Fluoroplex, Generic) **Uses:** *Basal cell carcinoma (when standard therapy impractical); actinic/solar keratosis* **Acts:** Inhibits thymidylate synthetase (↓ DNA synth, S-phase specific) **Dose:** 5% cream bid × 2–6 wk **W/P:** [X, ?/–] Irritant chemotherapy **CI:** Component sens **Disp:** Cream 0.5, 1, 5%; soln 2, 5% **SE:** Rash, dry skin, photosens **Notes:** Healing may not be evident for 1–2 mo; wash hands thoroughly; avoid occlusive dressings; do not overuse

Fluoxetine (Prozac, Prozac Weekly, Sarafem, Generic) BOX: Closely monitor for worsening depression or emergence of suicidality, particularly in ped pt **Uses:** *Depression, OCD, panic disorder, bulimia (*Prozac*)* *PMDD (*Sarafem*)* **Acts:** SSRI **Dose:** 20 mg PO (max 80 mg/d ÷ dose); weekly 90 mg/wk after 1–2 wk of standard dose *Bulimia:* 60 mg q A.M. *Panic disorder:* 20 mg/d *OCD:* 20–80 mg/d *PMDD:* 20 mg/d or 20 mg intermittently, start 14 d prior to menses, repeat w/ each cycle; ↓ in hepatic failure **W/P:** [C, ?/–] Serotonin synd w/ MAOI, SSRI, serotonin agonists, linezolid; QT prolongation w/ phenothiazines; do not use w/ clopidogrel (↓ effect) **CI:** w/ MAOI/thioridazine (wait 5 wk after D/C before MAOI) **Disp:** *Prozac:* Caps 10, 20, 40 mg; scored tabs 10, 20 mg; SR weekly caps 90 mg; soln 20 mg/5 mL. *Sarafem:* Tabs 10, 20 mg **SE:** N, nervousness, Wt loss, HA, insomnia

Flurazepam (Dalmane, Generic) [C-IV] Uses: *Insomnia* **Acts:** Benzodiazepine **Dose:** *Adults & Peds > 15 y.* 15–30 mg PO qhs PRN; ↓ in elderly **W/P:** [X, ?/–] Elderly, low albumin, hepatic impair **CI:** NAG; PRG **Disp:** Caps 15, 30 mg **SE:** "Hangover" d/t accumulation of metabolites, apnea, anaphylaxis, angioedema, amnesia **Notes:** May cause dependency

Flurbiprofen (Ansaid, Ocufen, Generic) BOX: May ↑ risk of CV events and GI bleeding **Uses:** *Arthritis, ocular surgery* **Acts:** NSAID **Dose:** *Ansaid* 100–300 mg/d ÷ bid-qid, max 300 mg/d w/ food; *Ocufen:* Ocular 1 gtt q30 min × 4, beginning 2 h preop **W/P:** [C (D in 3rd tri), ?/–]; ↑ risk of MI/CVA **CI:** PRG (3rd tri); ASA allergy **Disp:** Tabs 50, 100 mg; *Ocufen:* 0.03% ophthal soln **SE:** Dizziness, GI upset, peptic ulcer Dz, ocular irritation

Flutamide (Generic) BOX: Liver failure & death reported; measure LFTs before, monthly, & periodically after; D/C immediately if ALT 2 × ULN or jaundice develops **Uses:** Advanced *PCa* (w/ LHRH agonists, eg, leuprolide or goserelin); w/ radiation & GnRH for localized CAP **Acts:** Nonsteroidal antiandrogen **Dose:** 250 mg PO tid (750 mg total) **W/P:** [D, ?] **CI:** Severe hepatic impair **Disp:** Caps 125 mg **SE:** Hot flashes, loss of libido, impotence, N/V/D, gynecomastia, hepatic failure **Notes:** ✓ LFTs, avoid EtOH

Fluticasone Furoate, Inh (Arnuity Ellipta) Uses: *Prophylactic maint Tx asthma > 12 y* **Acts:** Steroid, anti-inflam **Dose:** 100 Inh qd; ↑ 200 mcg w/ poor response after 2 wk **W/P:** [C, M] *Candida* Infxn (throat, mouth); worsening asthma, paradoxical bronchospasm; immune/adrenal suppression, hypercorticism; ↓ BMD; glaucoma, cataracts **CI:** Status asthmaticus/acute asthma; component hypersens **Disp:** Inh powder 100, 200 mcg/Inh **SE:** HA, nasopharyngitis, URI, bronchitis **Notes:** Caution w/ strong P450 3A4 inhib

Fluticasone Furoate, Nasal (Veramyst) Uses: *Seasonal allergic rhinitis* **Acts:** Topical steroid **Dose:** *Adults & Peds > 12 y.* 2 sprays/nostril/d, then 1 spray/d maint *Peds 2–11 y.* 1–2 sprays/nostril/d **W/P:** [C, M] Avoid w/ ritonavir, other steroids, recent nasal surgery/trauma **CI:** Ø **Disp:** Nasal spray 27.5 mcg/actuation **SE:** HA, epistaxis, nasopharyngitis, pyrexia, pharyngolaryngeal pain, cough, nasal ulcers, back pain, anaphylaxis

Fluticasone Propionate, Inh (Flovent Diskus, Flovent HFA) Uses: *Chronic asthma* **Acts:** Topical steroid **Dose:** *Adults & Peds > 12 y.* 2–4 puffs bid *Peds 4–11 y.* 88 mcg bid **W/P:** [C, M] **CI:** Status asthmaticus **Disp:** *Diskus:* dry powder 50, 100, 250 mcg/action; *HFA:* MDI 44/110/220 mcg/Inh **SE:** HA, dysphonia, oral candidiasis **Notes:** Risk of thrush, rinse mouth after; counsel on use of devices

Fluticasone Propionate, Nasal (Flonase, Generic [OTC]) Uses: *Seasonal allergic rhinitis* **Acts:** Topical steroid **Dose:** *Adults & Peds > 12 y.* 2 sprays/nostril/d *Peds 4–11 y.* 1–2 sprays/nostril/d **W/P:** [C, M] **CI:** Primary Rx of status asthmaticus **Disp:** Nasal spray 50 mcg/actuation **SE:** HA, dysphonia, oral candidiasis

Fluticasone Furoate/Vilanterol Trifenatate (Breo Ellipta) BOX: LABAs may ↑ risk of asthma-related death; not indicated for Tx of asthma Uses: *COPD* **Acts:** Inh steroid & LABA **Dose:** 1 Inh qd **W/P:** [C, ?/–] Not for acute Sx; ↑ risk pneumonia & other Infxns; adrenal suppression/hypercorticism w/ high doses; w/ CV Dz, Sz disorders, thyrotoxicosis, DM, ketoacidosis; w/ strong CYP3A4 inhib, MAOIs, TCAs, beta-blockers, diuretics, other LABAs **CI:** Hypersens to milk protein/components **Disp:** Inh powder (*fluticasone/vilanterol*) 100 mcg/25 mcg blister **SE:** Nasopharyngitis, URI, HA, oral candidiasis, ↑ glu, ↓ K+, glaucoma, cataracts, ↓ BMD, paradoxical bronchospasm **Notes:** After Inh rinse mouth w/o swallowing to ↓ risk of candidiasis

Fluticasone Propionate/Salmeterol Xinafoate (Advair Diskus, Advair HFA) BOX: ↑ Risk of worsening wheezing or asthma-related death w/ long-acting β₂-adrenergic agonists; use only if asthma not controlled on agent such as inhaled steroid Uses: *Maint Rx for asthma & COPD* **Acts:** Corticosteroid w/ LA bronchodilator β₂ agonist **Dose:** *Adults & Peds > 12 y.* 1 Inh bid q12h; titrate to lowest effective dose (4 Inh or 920/84 mcg/d max) **W/P:** [C, M] **CI:** Acute asthma attack; conversion from PO steroids; w/ phenothiazines **Disp:** *Diskus:* metered-dose Inh powder (mcg fluticasone/mcg salmeterol) 100/50, 250/50, 500/50; *HFA:* aerosol 45/21, 115/21, 230/21 mg **SE:** URI, pharyngitis, HA **Notes:** Combo of Flovent & Serevent; do not wash mouthpiece, do not exhale into device; Advair HFA for pts not controlled on other meds (eg, low-medium dose Inh steroids) or whose Dz severity warrants 2 maint therapies

Fluvastatin (Lescol, Generic) Uses: *Atherosclerosis, primary hypercholesterolemia, heterozygous familial hypercholesterolemia, hypertriglyceridemia* **Acts:** HMG-CoA reductase inhib **Dose:** 20–40 mg bid PO or ER 80 mg/d; ↓ w/ hepatic impair **W/P:** [X, –] **CI:** Active liver Dz, ↑ LFTs, PRG, breast-feeding **Disp:** Caps 20, 40 mg; ER 80 mg **SE:** HA, dyspepsia, N/D, Abd pain, myalgia **Notes:** Dose no longer limited to hs; ✓ LFTs; OK w/ grapefruit

Fluvoxamine (Luvox CR, Generic) **BOX:** Closely monitor for worsening depression or emergence of suicidality, particularly in ped pts **Uses:** *OCD, SAD* **Acts:** SSRI **Dose:** Initial 50-mg single qhs dose, ↑ to 300 mg/d in ÷ doses; *CR:* 100–300 mg PO qhs, may ↑ by 50 mg/d qwk, max 300 mg/d; ↓ in elderly/hepatic impair, titrate slowly; ÷ doses > 100 mg **W/P:** [C, ?/–] Multiple interactions (see PI: MAOIs, phenothiazines, SSRIs, serotonin agonists, others); do not use w/ clopidogrel **CI:** MAOI w/in 14 d, w/ alosetron, tizanidine, thioridazine, pimozide, ramelteon **Disp:** Tabs 25, 50, 100 mg; caps ER 100, 150 mg **SE:** HA, N/D, somnolence, insomnia, ↓ Na⁺, **Notes:** Gradual taper to D/C

Folic Acid, Inj, Oral (Generic) **Uses:** *Megaloblastic anemia; folate deficiency* **Acts:** Dietary supl **Dose:** *Adults.* *Supl:* 0.4 mg/d PO *PRG:* 0.8 mg/d PO *Folate deficiency:* 1 mg PO daily–tid *Peds.* *Supl:* 0.04–0.4 mg/24 h PO, IM, IV, or SQ *Folate deficiency:* 0.5–1 mg/24 h PO, IM, IV, or SQ **W/P:** [A, +] **CI:** Not appropriate for pernicious, aplastic, normocytic anemias **Disp:** Tabs 0.4, 0.8, 1 mg; Inj 5 mg/mL **SE:** Well tolerated **Notes:** OK for all women of childbearing age; ↓ fetal neural tube defects by 50%; no effect on normocytic anemias

Fondaparinux (Arixtra) **BOX:** When epidural/spinal anesthesia or spinal puncture is used, pts anticoagulated or scheduled to be anticoagulated w/ LMW heparins, heparinoids, or fondaparinux are at risk for epidural or spinal hematoma, which can result in long-term or permanent paralysis **Uses:** *DVT prophylaxis w/ hip fracture, hip or knee replacement, Abd surgery; Rx DVT or PE in combo w/ warfarin* **Acts:** Synth inhib of activated factor Xₐ **Dose:** *Prophylaxis* 2.5 mg SQ daily, up to 5–9 d; start > 6 h postop; *Tx:* 7.5 mg SQ daily (< 50 kg: 5 mg SQ daily; > 100 kg: 10mg SQ daily); ↓ w/ renal impair **W/P:** [B, ?] ↑ Bleeding risk w/ anticoagulants, anti-plts, NSAIDs **CI:** Wt < 50 kg, CrCl < 30 mL/min, active bleeding, SBE ↓ plt w/ anti-plt Ab **Disp:** Prefilled syringes w/ 27-gauge needle: 2.5/0.5, 5/0.4, 7.5 /0.6, 10/0.8 mg/mL **SE:** Thrombocytopenia, anemia, fever, N **Notes:** D/C if plts < 100,000 cells/mcL; only give SQ; may monitor antifactor Xa levels

Formoterol Fumarate (Foradil, Perforomist) **BOX:** May ↑ risk of asthma-related death **Uses:** *Long-term Rx of bronchoconstriction in COPD, EIB (only Foradil)* **Acts:** LA β₂-agonist **Dose:** *Adults.* *Perforomist:* 20-mcg Inh q12h; *Foradil:* 12-mcg Inh q12h, 24 mcg/d max; *EIB:* 12 mcg 15 min before exercise *Peds > 5y.* (Foradil) See Adults **W/P:** [C, M] Not for acute Sx, w/ CV Dz, w/ adrenergic meds, xanthine derivatives meds that ↑ QT; β-blockers may ↓ effect, D/C w/ ECG change **CI:** Status asthmaticus or other acute COPD episode, w/o use of long-term asthma med, such as Inh steroid **Disp:** *Foradil* caps 12 mcg for Aerolizer inhaler (12 & 60 doses); *Perforomist:* 20 mcg/2 mL for inhaler **SE:** N/D, nasopharyngitis, dry mouth, angina, HTN, ↓ BP, tachycardia, arrhythmias, nervousness, HA, tremor, muscle cramps, palpitations, dizziness **Notes:** Excess use may ↑ CV risks; not for oral use

Fosamprenavir (Lexiva) **Uses:** *HIV Infxn* **Acts:** Protease inhib **Dose:** *Adults.* Tx-naïve: 1400 mg PO bid w/o ritonavir or 1400 mg PO qd w/ ritonavir 200 mg qd or 1400 mg qd w/ ritonavir 100 mg qd or 700 mg bid w/ ritonavir 100 mg bid

Experienced: 700 mg bid w/ ritonavir 100 mg bid *Peds 4 wk–18 y. < 11 kg:* 45 mg/kg w/ ritonavir 7 mg/kg; *11–15 kg:* 30 mg/kg w/ ritonavir 3 mg/kg; *15–20 kg:* 23 mg/kg w/ ritonavir 3 mg/kg; *≥ 20 kg:* 18 mg/kg w/ ritonavir 3 mg/kg (do not exceed adult dose) **W/P:** [C, ?/–] Do not use w/ salmeterol, colchicine, w/ renal/hepatic failure, adjust dose w/ bosentan, tadalafil for PAH **CI:** w/ CYP3A4 drugs (Table 10, p 356) such as w/ rifampin, lovastatin, simvastatin, delavirdine, ergot alkaloids, midazolam, triazolam, or pimozide; sulfa allergy; w/ alpha 1-adrenoceptor antagonist (alfuzosin); w/ PDE5 inhibitor sildenafil **Disp:** Tabs 700 mg; susp 50 mg/mL **SE:** N/V/D, HA, fatigue, rash **Notes:** Numerous drug interactions because of hepatic metabolism; replaced amprenavir

Fosaprepitant (Emend for Injection) **Uses:** *Px chemotherapy-associated N/V* **Acts:** Substance P/neurokinin 1 receptor antag **Dose:** *Chemotherapy:* 150 mg IV 30 min before chemotherapy on d 1 (followed by aprepitant [*Emend, Oral*] 80 mg PO d 2 and 3) in combo w/ other antiemetics **W/P:** [B, ?/–] Potential for drug interactions, substrate and mod CYP3A4 inhib (dose-dependent); ↓ effect of OCP and warfarin **CI:** w/ Pimozide, terfenadine, astemizole, or cisapride; polysorbate 80 allergy **Disp:** Inj 150 mg **SE:** N/D, weakness, hiccups, dizziness, HA, dehydration, hot flushing, dyspepsia, Abd pain, neutropenia, ↑ LFTs, Inj site discomfort **Notes:** See also Aprepitant, Oral (Emend)

Foscarnet (Foscavir, Generic) **BOX:** Renal impair major tox; Sz related to electrolyte imbalance; use only w/ immunocompromised host and acyclovir-resistant HSV Infxn **Uses:** *CMV retinitis*; acyclovir-resistant *herpes Infxns* **Acts:** ↓ Viral DNA polymerase & RT **Dose:** *CMV retinitis: Induction:* 90 mg/kg IV q12h or 60 mg/kg q8h × 14–21 d *Maint:* 90–120 mg/kg/d IV (Mon–Fri) *Acyclovir-resistant HSV: Induction:* 40 mg/kg IV q8–12h × 14–21 d; use central line; ↓ w/ renal impair **W/P:** [C, –] ↑ Sz potential w/ fluoroquinolones; avoid nephrotoxic Rx (cyclosporine, aminoglycosides, amphotericin B, protease inhib) **CI:** CrCl < 0.4 mL/min/kg **Disp:** Inj 24 mg/mL **SE:** Nephrotox, electrolyte abnormalities **Notes:** Sodium loading (500 mL 0.9% NaCl) before & after helps minimize nephrotox; monitor ionized Ca^{2+}

Fosfomycin (Monurol) **Uses:** *Uncomplicated UTI* **Acts:** ↓ Cell wall synth. *Spectrum:* gram(+) *Enterococcus,* staphylococci, pneumococci; gram(–) (*E. coli, Salmonella, Shigella, H. influenzae, Neisseria,* indole(–) *Proteus, Providencia*); *B. fragilis* & anaerobic gram(–) cocci are resistant **Dose:** 3 g PO in 90–120 mL of H_2O single dose; ↓ in renal impair **W/P:** [B, ?] ↓ Absorption w/ antacids/Ca salts **CI:** Component sens **Disp:** Granule packets 3 g **SE:** HA, GI upset **Notes:** May take 2–3 d for Sxs to improve

Fosinopril (Monopril, Generic) **Uses:** *HTN, CHF*, DN **Acts:** ACE inhib **Dose:** 10 mg/d PO initial; max 40 mg/d PO; ↓ in elderly; ↓ in renal impair **W/P:** [D, +] ↑ K^+ w/ K^+ supls, ARBs, K^+-sparing diuretics; ↑ renal after-effects w/ NSAIDs, diuretics, hypovolemia **CI:** Hereditary/idiopathic angioedema or angioedema w/ ACE inhib, bilateral RAS **Disp:** Tabs 10, 20, 40 mg **SE:** Cough, dizziness, angioedema, ↑ K^+

Fosphenytoin (Cerebyx, Generic) **BOX:** Rapid Inf associated w/ CV risk Uses: *Status epilepticus* **Acts:** ↓ Sz spread in motor cortex **Dose:** As PE **Load:** 15–20 mg PE/kg **Maint:** 4–6 mg PE/kg/d; ↓ dosage, monitor levels in hepatic impair **W/P:** [D, +] May ↑ phenobarbital **CI:** Sinus bradycardia, SA block, 2nd-/3rd-degree AV block, Adams-Stokes synd, rash during Rx **Disp:** Inj 2 mL/100 mg PE, 10 mL/500 mg PE **SE:** ↓ BP, dizziness, ataxia, pruritus, nystagmus **Notes:** 15 min to convert fosphenytoin to phenytoin; administer < 150 mg PE/min to prevent ↓ BP; administer w/ BP monitoring; PE = phenytoin equivalent

Frovatriptan (Frova) Uses: *Rx acute migraine* **Acts:** Vascular serotonin receptor agonist **Dose:** 2.5 mg PO, repeat in 2 h PRN; max 7.5 mg/d **W/P:** [C, ?/–] **CI:** Angina, ischemic heart Dz, coronary artery vasospasm, hemiplegic or basilar migraine, uncontrolled HTN, ergot use, MAOI use w/in 14 d **Disp:** Tabs 2.5 mg **SE:** N/V, dizziness, hot flashes, paresthesias, dyspepsia, dry mouth, hot/cold sensation, CP, skeletal pain, flushing, weakness, numbness, coronary vasospasm, HTN

Fulvestrant (Faslodex) Uses: *HR(+) met breast CA in postmenopausal women w/ progression following antiestrogen Rx therapy* **Acts:** Estrogen receptor antag **Dose:** 500 mg d 1, 15, & 29; maint 500 mg IM mo Inj in buttocks **W/P:** [X, ?/–] ↑ Effects w/ CYP3A4 inhib (Table 10, p 356); w/ hepatic impair **CI:** PRG **Disp:** Prefilled syringes 500 mg/mL (single 5 mL, dual 2.5 mL) **SE:** N/V/D, constipation, Abd pain, HA, back pain, hot flushes, pharyngitis, Inj site Rxns **Notes:** Only use IM

Furosemide (Lasix, Generic) Uses: *CHF, HTN, edema*, ascites **Acts:** Loop diuretic; ↓ Na & Cl reabsorption in ascending loop of Henle & distal tubule **Dose:** **Adults.** 20–80 mg PO or IV bid **Peds.** 1 mg/kg/dose IV q6–12h; 2 mg/kg/dose PO q12–24h (max 6 mg/kg/dose); ↑ doses w/ renal impair **W/P:** [C, +] ↓ K⁺, ↑ risk digoxin tox & ototox w/ aminoglycosides, cisplatin **CI:** Sulfonylurea allergy; anuria; hepatic coma; electrolyte depletion **Disp:** Tabs 20, 40, 80 mg; soln 10 mg/mL, 40 mg/5 mL; Inj 10 mg/mL **SE:** ↓ BP, hyperglycemia, ↓ K⁺ **Notes:** ✓ Lytes, renal Fxn; high doses IV may cause ototox

Gabapentin (Gralise, Neurontin, Generic) Uses: *Adjunct in partial Szs; PHN*; chronic pain synds **Acts:** Anticonvulsant; GABA analog **Dose:** **Adults & Peds > 12 y.** Anticonvulsant: 300 mg PO tid, ↑ max 3600 mg/d PHN: 300 mg d 1, 300 mg bid d 2, 300 mg tid d 3, titrate (1800–3600 mg/d); Gralise: qd w/ P.M. meal: 300 mg d 1, 600 mg d 2, 900 mg d 3–6, 1200 mg d 7–10, 1500 mg d 11–14, 1800 mg d 15, then 1800 mg **Peds 3–12 y.** 10–15 mg/kg/d ÷ tid, ↑ over 3 d 3–4 y. 40 mg/kg/d tid ≥5 y. 25–35 mg/kg/d ÷ tid, 50 mg/kg/d-max; ↓ w/ renal impair **W/P:** [C, ?] Use in peds 3–12 y w/ epilepsy may ↑ CNS-related adverse events **CI:** Component sens **Disp:** Caps 100, 300, 400 mg; soln 250 mg/5 mL; scored tabs 600, 800 mg; Gralise 30-d starter pack **SE:** Somnolence, dizziness, ataxia, fatigue

Notes: Not necessary to monitor levels; taper ↑ or ↓ over 1 wk; Different forms not equivalent

Gabapentin Enacarbil (Horizant)   **Uses:** *RLS* **Acts:** GABA analog; ? mechanism **Dose:** CrCl > 60 mL/min: 600 mg PO qd; 30–59 mL/min: 300 mg qd (max 600 mg/d); 15–29 mL/min: 300 mg qd; < 15 mL/min: 300 mg q other day; not recommended w/ hemodialysis; take w/ food at 5 P.M.; swallow whole; max 1200 mg/d **W/P:** [C, ?/–] **Disp:** Tabs ER 300, 600 mg **SE:** Somnolence, sedation, fatigue, dizziness, HA, blurred vision, feeling drunk, disorientation, ↓ libido, depression, suicidal thoughts/behaviors, multiorgan hypersens

Galantamine (Razadyne, Razadyne ER, Generic)   **Uses:** *Mild–mod Alzheimer Dz* **Acts:** ? Acetylcholinesterase inhib **Dose:** *Razadyne* 4 mg PO bid, ↑ to 8 mg bid after 4 wk; may ↑ to 16 mg bid in 4 wk; target 16–24 mg/d ÷ bid *Razadyne ER* Start 8 mg/d, ↑ to 16 mg/d after 4 wk, then to 24 mg/d after 4 more wk; give q A.M. w/ food **W/P:** [B, ?] w/ Heart block, ↑ effect w/ succinylcholine, bethanechol, amiodarone, diltiazem, verapamil, NSAIDs, digoxin; ↓ effect w/ anticholinergics; ↑ risk of death w/ mild impair **CI:** Severe renal/hepatic impair **Disp:** *Razadyne* Tabs 4, 8, 12 mg; soln 4 mg/mL; *Razadyne ER* Caps 8, 16, 24 mg **SE:** GI disturbances, ↓ Wt, sleep disturbances, dizziness, HA **Notes:** Caution w/ urinary outflow obst, Parkinson Dz, severe asthma/COPD, severe heart Dz or ↓ BP

Gallium Nitrate (Ganite)   **BOX:** ↑ Risk of severe renal Insuff w/ concurrent use of nephrotox drugs (eg, aminoglycosides, amphotericin B); D/C if use of potentially nephrotox drug is indicated; hydrate several d after administration; D/C w/ SCr > 2.5 mg/dL **Uses:** *↑ Ca²⁺ of malignancy* **Acts:** ↓ Bone resorption of Ca²⁺ **Dose:** *↓ Ca²⁺*: 100–200 mg/m²/d × 5 d *CA:* 350 mg/m² cont Inf × 5 d to 700 mg/m² rapid IV Inf q2wk in antineoplastic settings (per protocols), Inf over 24 h **W/P:** [C, ?] Do not give w/ live or rotavirus vaccine **CI:** SCr > 2.5 mg/dL **Disp:** Inj 25 mg/mL **SE:** Renal Insuff, ↓ Ca²⁺, hypophosphatemia, ↓ bicarb, < 1% acute optic neuritis **Notes:** Bladder CA, use in combo w/ vinblastine & ifosfamide

Ganciclovir (Cytovene, Vitrasert, Generic)   **BOX:** Tox: granulocytopenia, anemia, & thrombocytopenia; animal studies: teratogenic, aspermatogenesis; use only in immunocompromised pts w/ CMV retinitis & in transplant pts at risk for CMV **Uses:** *Rx & prevent CMV retinitis, prevent CMV Dz* in transplant recipients **Acts:** ↓ viral DNA synth **Dose:** *Adults & Peds. IV:* 5 mg/kg IV q12h for 14–21 d, then maint 5 mg/kg IV × 7 d/wk or 6 mg/kg IV × 5 d/wk *Ocular implant:* 1 implant q5–8mo **W/P:** [C, –] ↑ Effect w/ immunosuppressives, imipenem/cilastatin, zidovudine, didanosine, other nephrotox Rx **CI:** ANC < 500 cells/mm³, plt < 25,000 cells/mm³, intravitreal implant **Disp:** Inj 500 mg, ocular implant 4.5 mg **SE:** Granulocytopenia & thrombocytopenia, fever, rash, GI upset **Notes:** Not a cure for CMV; handle Inj w/ cytotoxic cautions; no systemic benefit w/ implant

Ganciclovir, Ophthalmic Gel (Zirgan)   **Uses:** *Acute herpetic keratitis (dendritic ulcers)* **Acts:** ↓ Viral DNA synth **Dose:** *Adult & Peds ≥2 y.* 1 gtt into affected eye/s 5 × d (q3h while awake) until ulcer heals, then 1 gtt tid × 7 d **W/P:** [C, ?/–] Remove contacts during therapy **CI:** Ø **Disp:** Gel, 5-g tube **SE:** Blurred vision, eye irritation, punctate keratitis, conjunctival hyperemia **Notes:** Correct ↓ Ca^{2+} before use; ✓ Ca^{2+}

Gefitinib (Iressa) Uses: *NSCLC after chemo failure or up-front w/ EGFR exon 19 deletions or exon 21 (L858R) mutations (companion test) **Acts:** EGFR TKI **Dose:** 250 mg w/o regard to food **W/P:** [D/–] Hepatotox **CI:** Component hypersens **Disp:** Tabs 250 mg **SE:** Interstitial lung disease, N/V/D, rash, acne, dry skin, pruritus ↓ Wt/appetite, asthenia

Gemcitabine (Gemzar, Generic) Uses: *Pancreatic CA (single agent), breast CA w/ paclitaxel, NSCLC w/ cisplatin, ovarian CA w/ carboplatin*, gastric CA **Acts:** Antimetabolite; nucleoside metabolic inhib; ↓ ribonucleotide reductase; produces false nucleotide base-inhibiting DNA synth **Dose:** 1000–1250 mg/m² over 30 min–1 h IV Inf/wk × 3–4 wk or 6–8 wk; modify dose based on hematologic Fxn (per protocol) **W/P:** [D, ?/–] **CI:** PRG **Disp:** Inj 200 mg, 1, 2 g **SE:** ↓ BM, N/V/D, drug fever, skin rash **Notes:** Reconstituted soln 38 mg/mL; monitor hepatic/renal Fxn

Gemfibrozil (Lopid, Generic) Uses: *Hypertriglyceridemia, CHD* **Acts:** Fibric acid **Dose:** 1200 mg/d PO ÷ bid 30 min ac A.M. & P.M. **W/P:** [C, ?] ↑ Warfarin effect, sulfonylureas; ↑ risk of myopathy w/ HMG-CoA reductase inhib; ↑ effects w/ cyclosporine **CI:** Renal/hepatic impair (SCr > 2.0 mg/dL), gallbladder Dz, primary biliary cirrhosis, use w/ repaglinide (↓ glucose) **Disp:** Tabs 600 mg **SE:** Cholelithiasis, GI upset **Notes:** Avoid w/HMG-CoA reductase inhib; ✓ LFTs & serum lipids

Gemifloxacin (Factive) BOX: Fluoroquinolones ↑ risk of tendonitis/tendon rupture; ↑ risk w/ age > 60 y, w/ steroids, transplant pts Uses: *CAP, acute exacerbation of chronic bronchitis* **Acts:** ↓ DNA gyrase & topoisomerase IV. **Spectrum:** *S. pneumoniae* (including multidrug-resistant strains), *H. influenzae, H. parainfluenzae, M. catarrhalis, M. pneumoniae, C. pneumoniae, K. pneumoniae* **Dose:** 320 mg PO qd × 5–7 d; CrCl < 40 mL/min: 160 mg PO/d **W/P:** [C, ?/–]; Peds < 18 y; Hx of ↑ QTc interval, electrolyte disorders, w/ class IA/III antiarrhythmics, erythromycin, TCAs, antipsychotics, ↑ INR and bleeding risk w/ warfarin **CI:** Fluoroquinolone allergy **Disp:** Tab 320 mg **SE:** Rash, N/V/D, *C. difficile* enterocolitis, ↑ risk of Achilles tendon rupture, tendonitis, Abd pain, dizziness, xerostomia, arthralgia, allergy/anaphylactic Rxns, peripheral neuropathy, **Notes:** Take 3 h before or 2 h after Al/Mg antacids, Fe^{2+}, Zn^{2+} or other metal cations; ↑ rash risk w/ ↑ duration of Rx

Gentamicin, Injectable (Generic) BOX: Monitor for tox, especially w/ known/suspected ↓ renal function; potentially nephrotox; neurotox manifested by ototox (usually irreversible), also numbness, skin tingling, muscle twitching, & convulsions; monitor renal & 8th cranial nerve function; consider serial audiograms; monitor levels, avoid prolonged levels > 12 mcg/mL; w/ overdosage/tox, consider hemodialysis; in the newborn infant, exchange transfusions may also be considered; avoid w/ other systemic or topical neurotox/nephrotox drugs; avoid use w/ potent diuretics; teratogenic **Uses:** *Septicemia, serious bacterial Infxn of CNS, urinary tract, resp tract, GI tract, including peritonitis, skin, bone, soft tissue, including burns; severe Infxn *P. aeruginosa* w/ carbenicillin; group D streptococci endocarditis w/ PCN-type drug; serious staphylococcal Infxns, but not the antibiotic of 1st choice; mixed Infxn w/ staphylococci and gram(−)* **Acts:** Aminoglycoside, bactericidal; ↓ protein synth. *Spectrum:* gram(−) (not *Neisseria, Legionella, Acinetobacter*); weaker gram(+) but synergy w/ PCNs **Dose:** *Adults. Standard:* 1–2 mg/kg IV q8–12h or daily dosing 4–7 mg/kg q24h IV; *Gram(+) Synergy:* 1 mg/kg q8h **Peds. Infants < 7 d < 1200 g.** 2.5 mg/kg/dose q18–24h *Infants > 1200 g.* 2.5 mg/kg/dose q12–18h *Infants > 7 d.* 2.5 mg/kg IV q8–12h *Children.* 2.5 mg/kg/d IV q8h; ↓ w/ renal Insuff; if obese, dose based on IBW **W/P:** [C, +/−] Avoid other nephrotoxics **CI:** Aminoglycoside sens **Disp:** Premixed Inf 40, 60, 70, 80, 90, 100, 120 mg; ADD-Vantage Inj vials 10 mg/mL; Inj 40 mg/mL; IT preservative-free 2 mg/mL **SE:** Nephro-/oto-/neurotox **Notes:** Follow CrCl, SCr, & serum conc for dose adjustments; use IBW to dose (use adjusted if obese > 30% IBW); OK to use intraperitoneal for peritoneal dialysis-related Infxns *Levels: Peak:* 30 min after Inf; *Trough:* < 0.5 h before next dose; *Therapeutic: Peak:* 5–8 mcg/mL, *Trough:* < 2 mcg/mL, if > 2 mcg/mL associated w/ renal tox

Gentamicin, Ophthalmic (Garamycin, Genoptic, Gentak, Generic)

Uses: *Conjunctival Infxns* **Acts:** Bactericidal; ↓ protein synth **Dose:** *Oint:* Apply 1/2 in bid-tid *Soln:* 1–2 gtt q2–4h, up to 2 gtt/h for severe Infxn **W/P:** [C, ?] **CI:** Aminoglycoside sens **Disp:** Soln & oint 0.1% and 0.3% **SE:** Local irritation **Notes:** Do not use other eye drops w/in 5–10 min; do not touch dropper to eye

Gentamicin, Topical (Generic)

Uses: *Skin Infxns* caused by susceptible organisms **Acts:** Bactericidal; ↓ protein synth **Dose:** *Adults & Peds > 1 y.* Apply tid-qid **W/P:** [C, ?] **CI:** Aminoglycoside sens **Disp:** Cream & oint 0.1% **SE:** Irritation

Gentamicin/Prednisolone, Ophthalmic (Pred-G Ophthalmic)

Uses: *Steroid-responsive ocular & conjunctival Infxns* sensitive to gentamicin **Acts:** Bactericidal; ↓ protein synth w/ anti-inflam. *Spectrum: Staphylococcus, E. coli, H. influenzae, Klebsiella, Neisseria, Pseudomonas, Proteus, & Serratia* sp **Dose:** *Oint:* 1/2 in in conjunctival sac qd-tid. *Susp:* 1 gtt bid-qid, up to 1 gtt/h for severe Infxns **W/P:** [C, ?] **Disp:** Oint, ophthal: Prednisolone acetate 0.6% & gentamicin sulfate 0.3% (3.5 g); *Susp, ophthal:* Prednisolone acetate 1% & gentamicin sulfate 0.3% (2, 5, 10 mL) **SE:** Local irritation

Glimepiride (Amaryl, Generic)

Uses: *Type 2 DM* **Acts:** Sulfonylurea; ↑ pancreatic insulin release; ↑ peripheral insulin sens; ↓ hepatic glu output/production **Dose:** 1–4 mg/d, max 8 mg **W/P:** [C, −] **CI:** DKA **Disp:** Tabs 1, 2, 4 mg **SE:** HA, N, hypoglycemia **Notes:** Give w/ 1st meal of day

Glimepiride/Pioglitazone (Duetact) BOX: Thiazolidinediones, including pioglitazone, cause or exacerbate CHF; not recommended in pts w/ symptomatic heart failure; CI w/ NYHA Class III or IV heart failure Uses: *Adjunct to exercise in type 2 DM not controlled by single agent* Acts: Sulfonylurea (↓ glucose) w/ agent that ↑ insulin sens & ↓ gluconeogenesis Dose: Initial 30 mg/2 mg PO q A.M.; 45 mg pioglitazone/8 mg glimepiride/d max; w/ food W/P: [C, ?/–] w/ Liver impair, elderly, w/ Hx bladder CA CI: Component sensitivity, DKA Disp: Tabs 30/2, 30 mg/4 mg SE: Hct, ↑ ALT, ↓ glucose, URI, ↑ Wt, edema, HA, N/D, may ↑ CV mortality Notes: Monitor CBC, ALT, Cr, Wt

Glipizide (Glucotrol, Glucotrol XL, Generic) Uses: *Type 2 DM* Acts: Sulfonylurea; ↑ pancreatic insulin release; ↑ peripheral insulin sens; ↓ hepatic glu output/production; ↓ intestinal glu absorption Dose: 5 mg initial, ↑ by 2.5–5 mg/d, max 40 mg/d; XL max 20 mg; 30 min ac; hold if NPO W/P: [C, ?/–] Severe liver Dz CI: DKA, type 1 DM, sulfonamide sens Disp: Tabs 5, 10 mg; XL tabs 2.5, 5, 10 mg SE: HA, anorexia, N/V/D, constipation, fullness, rash, urticaria, photosens, hypoglycemia Notes: Counsel about DM management; wait several days before adjusting dose; monitor glu

Glucagon, Recombinant (GlucaGen) Uses: *Severe hypoglycemic Rxns in DM, radiologic GI tract diagnostic aid*; β-blocker/CCB OD Acts: Accelerates liver gluconeogenesis Dose: Adults. 0.5–1 mg SQ, IM, or IV; repeat in 20 min PRN. ECC 2010. β-Blocker or CCB overdose: 3–10 mg slow IV over 3–5 min; follow w/ Inf of 3–5 mg/h Hypoglycemia: 1 mg IV, IM, or SQ Peds. Neonates. 30 mcg/kg/dose SQ, IM, or IV q4h PRN. Children. 0.025–0.1 mg/kg/dose SQ, IM, or IV; repeat in 20 min PRN W/P: [B, M] CI: Pheochromocytoma Disp: Inj 1 mg SE: N/V, ↓ BP Notes: Administration of dextrose IV necessary; ineffective in starvation, adrenal Insuff, or chronic hypoglycemia

Glucarpidase (Voraxaze) Uses: *Tx toxic plasma MTX conc (> 1 micromole/L) in pts w/ ↓ clearance* Acts: Carboxypeptidase enzyme converts MTX to inactive metabolites Dose: 50 units/kg IV over 5 min × 1 W/P: [C, ?/–] Serious allergic/anaphylactic Rxns; do not administer leucovorin w/in 2 h before/after dose Disp: Inj (powder) 1000 units/vial SE: N/V/D, HA, ↓/↑ BP, flushing, paraesthesias, hypersens, blurred vision, rash, tremor, throat irritation Notes: Measure MTX conc by chromatographic method w/in 48 h of admin; continue leucovorin until methotrexate conc below leucovorin Tx threshold × 3 d; hydrate & alkalinize urine

Glyburide (DiaBeta, Glynase, Generic) Uses: *Type 2 DM* Acts: Sulfonylurea; ↑ pancreatic insulin release; ↑ peripheral insulin sens; ↓ hepatic glu output/production; ↓ intestinal glu absorption Dose: 1.25–10 mg qd-bid, max 20 mg/d Micronized: 0.75–6 mg qd-bid, max 12 mg/d W/P: [C, ?] Renal impair, sulfonamide allergy, ? ↑ CV risk CI: DKA, type 1 DM Disp: Tabs 1.25, 2.5, 5 mg; micronized tabs (Glynase) 1.5, 3, 6 mg SE: HA, hypoglycemia, cholestatic jaundice, and hepatitis may cause liver failure Notes: Not OK for CrCl < 50 mL/min;

hold dose if NPO; hypoglycemia may be difficult to recognize; many medications can enhance hypoglycemic effects

Glyburide/Metformin (Glucovance, Generic) BOX: Lactic acidosis w/ metformin accumulation; if suspected, D/C & hospitalize Uses: *Type 2 DM* Acts: Sulfonylurea: ↑ Pancreatic insulin release. Metformin: ↑ Peripheral insulin sens; ↓ hepatic glu output/production; ↓ intestinal glu absorption Dose: 1st line (naïve pts), 1.25/250 mg PO qd-bid; 2nd line, 2.5/500 or 5/500 mg bid (max 20/2000 mg); take w/ meals, slowly ↑ dose; hold before & 48 h after ionic contrast media W/P: [C, –] CI: SCr > 1.4 mg/dL in females or > 1.5 mg/dL in males; hypoxemic conditions (sepsis, recent MI); alcoholism; metabolic acidosis; liver Dz; Disp: Tabs (glyburide/metformin) 1.25/250, 2.5/500, 5/500 mg SE: HA, hypoglycemia, lactic acidosis, anorexia, N/V, rash Notes: Avoid EtOH; hold dose if NPO; monitor folate levels (megaloblastic anemia)

Glycerin Suppository Uses: *Constipation* Acts: Hyperosmolar laxative Dose: *Adults.* 1 Adult supp PR PRN *Peds.* 1 Infant supp PR qd-bid PRN W/P: [C, ?] Disp: Supp (adult, infant); liq 4 mL/applicator full SE: D, cramping, rectal irritation, tenesmus

Golimumab (Simponi, Simponi Aria) BOX: Serious Infxns (bacterial, fungal, TB, opportunistic) possible; D/C w/ severe Infxn/sepsis, test & monitor for TB before & during Rx; lymphoma/other CA possible in children/adolescents Uses: *Mod–severe RA w/ methotrexate (Simponi, Simponi Aria), PA w/ or w/o methotrexate, AS, mod–severe UC (steroid dependent, failing other agents) (Simponi)* Acts: TNF blocker Dose: *Arthritis/spondylitis:* 50 mg SQ monthly *Colitis:* 200 mg SQ wk 0, 100 mg wk 2, then maint 100 mg q4wk; test for HBV/TB before start W/P: [B, ?/–] Do use w/ active Infxn; w/ malignancies, CHF, demyelinating Dz; do use w/ abatacept, anakinra, live vaccines CI: Ø Disp: Prefilled syringe 50 mg/4mL (Simponi Aria); SmartJect auto-injector and prefilled syringes 50 mg/ 0.5 mL, 100 mg/1 mL (Simponi) SE: URI, nasopharyngitis, Inj site Rxn, ↑ LFTs, Infxn, HBV reactivation, new-onset psoriasis Notes: Self-Inj by pt w/ instruction

Goserelin (Zoladex) Uses: *Advanced PCa & w/ radiation and flutamide for localized high-risk Dz endometriosis, breast CA* Acts: LHRH agonist, transient ↑ then ↓ in LH, w/ ↓ testosterone Dose: 3.6 mg SQ (implant) q28d or 10.8 mg SQ q3mo; usually upper Abd wall W/P: [X, –] may ↑ QTc CI: PRG, breast-feeding, 10.8-mg implant not for ♀ Disp: SQ implant 3.6 (1 mo), 10.8 mg (3 mo) SE: Hot flashes, ↓ libido, gynecomastia, & transient exacerbation of CA-related bone pain ("flare Rxn" 7–10 d after 1st dose) Notes: Inject SQ into fat in Abd wall; do not aspirate; ♀ must use contraception; may cause inj site and vascular injury

Granisetron, Oral, Transdermal (Sancuso, Generic) Uses: *Rx and Px of N/V (chemo/radiation/postoperation)* Acts: Serotonin (5-HT₃) receptor antag Dose: *Adults & Peds. Chemotherapy:* 10 mcg/kg/dose IV 30 min prior to chemotherapy *Adults. Chemotherapy:* 2 mg PO qd 1 h before chemotherapy, then 12 h later or 1 patch up to 7 d *Postop N/V:* 1 mg IV over 30 s before end of case

W/P: [B, +/–] St. John's wort ↓ levels **CI:** Liver Dz, children < 2 y **Disp:** Tabs 1 mg; soln 2 mg/10 mL; IV 0.1 mg/mL; patch 3.1 mg/24 h (*Sancuso*) **SE:** HA, asthenia, somnolence, D, constipation, Abd pain, dizziness, insomnia, ↑ LFTs

Guaifenesin (Robitussin, Others, Generic [OTC]) Uses: *Relief of dry, nonproductive cough* **Acts:** Expectorant **Dose:** *Adults.* 200–400 mg (10–20 mL) PO q4h; SR 600–1200 mg PO bid (max 2.4 g/d) *Peds 6 mo–2 y.* 25–50 mg q4h (max 300 mg/d) *2–5 y.* 50–100 mg (2.5–5 mL) PO q4h (max 600 mg/d) *6–11 y.* 100–200 mg (5–10 mL) PO q4h (max 1.2 g/d) **W/P:** [C, ?] **Disp:** 100, 200, 600 mg; 1, 2 g; SR tabs 600, 1200 mg; caps 200 mg; SR caps 300 mg; liq 100/200 mg/5 mL **SE:** GI upset **Notes** Give w/ large amount of water; some dosage forms contain EtOH

Guaifenesin/Codeine (Robafen AC, Others, Generic) [C-V] Uses: *Relief of dry cough* **Acts:** Antitussive w/ expectorant **Dose:** *Adults.* 5–10 mL or 1 tab PO q6–8h (max 60 mL/24 h) *Peds > 6 y.* 1–1.5 mg/kg codeine/d ÷ dose q4–6h (max 30 mg/24 h) *6–12 y.* 5 mL q4h (max 30 mL/24 h) **W/P:** [C, +] **Disp:** Brontex tab 10 mg codeine/300 mg guaifenesin; liq 2.5 mg codeine/75 mg guaifenesin/5 mL; others 10 mg codeine/100 mg guaifenesin/5 mL **SE:** Somnolence, constipation **Notes:** Not recommended for children < 6 y

Guaifenesin/Dextromethorphan (Various OTC Brands) Uses: *Cough* d/t upper resp tract irritation **Acts:** Antitussive w/ expectorant **Dose:** *Adults & Peds > 12 y.* 10 mL PO q6–8h (max 40 mL/24 h) *Peds 2–6 y.* Dextromethorphan 1–2 mg/kg/24 h ÷ 3–4 × d (max 10 mL/d) *6–12 y.* 5 mL q6–8h (max 20 mL/d) **W/P:** [C, +] **Acts:** Administration w/ MAOI **Disp:** Many OTC formulations **SE:** Somnolence **Notes:** Give w/ plenty of fluids; some forms contain EtOH

Guanfacine (Intuniv, Tenex, Generic) Uses: *ADHD (peds > 6 y)*; *HTN (adults)* **Acts:** Central α_{2a}-adrenergic agonist **Dose:** *Adults.* 1–3 mg/d IR PO h (*Tenex*), ↑ by 1 mg q3–4wk PRN 3 mg/d max *Peds.* 1–4 mg/d XR PO (*Intuniv*), ↑ by 1 mg q1wk PRN; 4 mg/d max **W/P:** [B, +/–] **Disp:** Tabs IR 1, 2 mg; tabs XR 1, 2, 3, 4 mg **SE:** Somnolence, dizziness, HA, fatigue, constipation, Abd pain, xerostomia, hypotension, bradycardia, syncope **Notes:** Rebound ↑ BP, anxiety, nervousness w/ abrupt D/C; metabolized by CYP3A4

Haemophilus B Conjugate Vaccine (ActHIB, Hiberix, HibTITER, PedvaxHIB, Others) Uses: *Immunize children against H. influenzae type B Dzs* **Acts:** Active immunization **Dose:** *Peds.* 0.5 mL (25 mg) IM (deltoid or vastus lateralis muscle) 2 doses 2 and 4 mo; booster 12–15 mo or 2, 4, and 6 mo booster at 12–15 mo depending on formulation **W/P:** [C, +] **CI:** Component sens, febrile illness, immunosuppression, thimerosal allergy **Disp:** Inj 7.5, 10, 15, 25 mcg/0.5 mL **SE:** Fever, restlessness, fussiness, anorexia, pain/redness Inj site; observe for anaphylaxis; edema, ↑ risk of *Haemophilus* B Infxn the wk after vaccination **Notes:** *Prohibit* and *TriHIBit* cannot be used in children < 12 mo; *Hiberix* approved ages 15 mo–4 y, single dose; booster beyond 5 y not required; report SAE to VAERS: 1-800-822-7967; dosing varies, check w/ each product

Haloperidol (Haldol, Generic)   BOX: ↑ Mortality in elderly w/ dementia-related psychosis; risk for torsade de pointes and QT prolongation, death w/ IV administration at higher doses **Uses:** *Psychotic disorders, agitation, Tourette disorders, hyperactivity in children* **Acts:** Butyrophenone; antipsychotic, neuroleptic **Dose:** *Adults. Mod Sxs:* 0.5–2 mg PO bid-tid *Severe Sxs/agitation:* 3–5 mg PO bid-tid or 1–5 mg IM q4h PRN (max 100 mg/d) *ICU psychosis:* 2–10 mg IV q30min to effect, then 25% max dose q6h *Peds 3–6 y.* 0.01–0.03 mg/kg/24 h PO qd. *6–12 y.* Initial, 0.5–1.5 mg/24 h PO; ↑ by 0.5 mg/24 h to maint of 2–4 mg/24 h (0.05–0.1 mg/kg/24 h) or 1–3 mg/dose IM q4–8h to 0.1 mg/kg/24 h max; *Tourette Dz* may require up to 15 mg/24 h PO; ↓ in elderly **W/P:** [C, ?] ↑ Effects w/ SSRIs, CNS depressants, TCA, indomethacin, metoclopramide; avoid levodopa (↓ antiparkinsonian effects) **CI:** NAG, severe CNS depression, coma, Parkinson Dz, ↓ BM suppression, severe cardiac/hepatic Dz **Disp:** Tabs 0.5, 1, 2, 5, 10, 20 mg; conc liq 2 mg/mL; Inj 5 mg/mL; decanoate Inj 50, 100 mg/mL **SE:** EPS, tardive dyskinesia, neuroleptic malignant synd, ↓ BP, anxiety, dystonias, risk for torsades de pointes and QT prolongation; leukopenia, neutropenia and agranulocytosis **Notes:** Do not give decanoate IV; dilute PO conc liq w/ H₂O/juice; monitor for EPS; ECG monitoring w/ off-label IV use; follow CBC if WBC counts decreased

Heparin (Generic)   Uses: *Rx & Px of DVT & PE*, unstable angina, AF w/ emboli, & acute arterial occlusion **Acts:** w/ antithrombin III to inactivate thrombin & ↓ thromboplastin formation **Dose:** *Adults. Prophylaxis:* 3000–5000 units SQ q8–12h *DVT/PE Rx:* Load 50–80 units/kg IV (max 10,000 units), then 10–20 units/kg IV qh (adjust based on PTT) *ECC 2010. STEMI:* Bolus 60 units/kg (max 4000 units); then 12 units/kg/h (max 1000 units/h), round to nearest 50 units; keep aPTT 1.5–2 × control 48 h or until angiography *Peds Infants.* Load 50 units/kg IV bolus, then 20 units/kg/h IV by cont Inf *Children.* Load 50 units/kg IV, then 15–25 units/kg cont Inf or 100 units/kg/dose q4h IV intermittent bolus (adjust based on PTT) **W/P:** [C, +] ↑ Risk of hemorrhage w/ anticoagulants, ASA, anti-plt, cephalosporins w/ MTT side chain **CI:** Uncontrolled bleeding, severe thrombocytopenia, suspected ICH **Disp:** Unfractionated Inj 10, 100, 1000, 2000, 2500, 5000, 7500, 10,000, 20,000, 40,000 units/mL **SE:** Bruising, bleeding, thrombocytopenia **Notes:** Follow PTT, thrombin time, or activated clotting time; little PT effect; therapeutic PTT 1.5–2 control for most conditions; monitor for HIT w/ plt counts; new "USP" formulation heparin is approximately 10% less effective than older formulations

Hepatitis A Vaccine (Havrix, Vaqta)   Uses: *Px hep A* in high-risk individuals (eg, travelers, certain professions, day-care workers if 1 or more children or workers are infected, high-risk behaviors, children at ↑ risk); in chronic liver Dz **Acts:** Active immunity **Dose:** *Adults. Havrix:* 1.0-mL IM w/ 1.0-mL booster 6–12 mo later *Vaqta:* 1.0 mL IM w/ 1.0 mL IM booster 6–18 mo later *Peds > 12 mo. Havrix:* 0.5-mL IM, w/ 0.5-mL booster 6–18 mo later; *Vaqta:* 0.5 mL IM w/ booster 0.5 mL 6–18 mo later **W/P:** [C, +] **CI:** Component sens; syringes contain latex **Disp:** *Havrix:* Inj 720 EL.U./0.5 mL, 1440 EL.U./1 mL; *Vaqta* 50 units/mL **SE:** Fever, fatigue, HA, Inj site pain **Notes:** Give primary at least 2 wk before anticipated exposure; do not give *Havrix* in gluteal region; report SAE to VAERS: 1-800-822-7967

Hepatitis A (Inactivated)/Hepatitis B (Recombinant) Vaccine (Twinrix) **Uses:** *Active immunization against hep A/B in pts > 18 y* **Acts:** Active immunity **Dose:** 1 mL IM at 0, 1, & 6 mo; accelerated regimen 1 mL IM d 0, 7 and 21–30, then booster at 12 mo; Use deltoid, not gluteal region **W/P:** [C, +/–] fainting possible **CI:** Component sens **Disp:** Single-dose vials, syringes w/latex **SE:** Fever, fatigue, HA, pain/redness at site **Notes:** Booster OK 6–12 mo after vaccination; report SAE to VAERS: 1-800-822-7967

Hepatitis B Immune Globulin (H-BIG, HepaGam B, HyperHep B, Nabi-HB) **Uses:** *Exposure to HBsAg(+) material (eg, blood, accidental needle-stick, mucous membrane contact, PO or sexual contact), prevent hep B in HBsAg(+) liver Tx pt* **Acts:** Passive immunization **Dose:** *Adults & Peds.* 0.06 mL/kg IM 5 mL max; w/in 24 h of exposure; w/in 14 d of sexual contact; repeat 1 mo if nonresponder or refused initial Tx; liver Tx per protocols **W/P:** [C, ?] All: Allergies to γ-globulin, anti-immunoglobulin Ab, or thimerosal; IgA deficiency **Disp:** Inj **SE:** Inj site pain, dizziness, HA, myalgias, arthralgias, anaphylaxis **Notes:** IM anterolateral thigh or deltoid only; w/ continued exposure, give hep B vaccine; not for active hep B; ineffective for chronic hep B

Hepatitis B Vaccine (Engerix-B, Recombivax HB) **Uses:** *Px hep B*: men who have sex w/ men, people who inject street drugs; chronic renal/liver Dz, healthcare workers exposed to blood, body fluids; sexually active not in monogamous relationship, people seeking evaluation for or w/ STDs, household contacts and partners of hep B–infected persons, travelers to countries w/ ↑ hep B prevalence, clients/staff working w/ people w/ developmental disabilities **Acts:** Active immunization; recombinant DNA **Dose:** *Adults.* 3 IM doses 1 mL each; first 2 doses 1 mo apart; the third 6 mo after the first *Peds.* 0.5 mL IM adult schedule **W/P:** [C, +] ↓ Effect w/ immunosuppressives **CI:** Yeast allergy, component sens **Disp:** *Engerix-B:* Inj 20 mcg/mL; peds Inj 10 mcg/0.5 mL *Recombivax HB:* Inj 10 & 40 mcg/mL; peds Inj 5 mcg/0.5 mL **SE:** Fever, HA, Inj site pain **Notes:** Deltoid IM Inj adults/older peds; younger peds, use anterolateral thigh

Hetastarch (Hespan) **Uses:** *Plasma vol expansion*, adjunct for leukapheresis **Acts:** Synthetic colloid; acts similar to albumin **Dose:** *Vol expansion:* 500–1000 mL (1500 mL/d max) IV (20 mL/kg/h max rate) *Leukapheresis:* 250–700 mL; ↓ in renal failure **W/P:** [C, +] **CI:** Severe bleeding disorders, CHF, oliguric/anuric renal failure **Disp:** Inj 6 g/100 mL **SE:** Bleeding (↑ PT, PTT, bleeding time) **Notes:** Not blood or plasma substitute

Histrelin Acetate (Supprelin LA, Vantas) **Uses:** *Advanced PCa, precocious puberty* **Acts:** GNRH agonist; paradoxically ↑ release of GnRH w/ ↓ LH from anterior pituitary; in men ↓ testosterone **Dose:** *Supprelin LA:* 1 implant q12mo;

Vantas: PCa 50 mg SQ implant q12mo inner aspect of the upper arm **W/P:** [X, –] Transient "flare Rxn" at 7–14 d after 1st dose [LH/testosterone surge before suppression]); w/ impending cord compression or urinary tract obstruction; ↑ risk DM, CV Dz, MI **CI:** GNRH sens; PRG **Disp:** 50 mg 12-mo SQ implant **SE:** Hot flashes, fatigue, implant site Rxn, testis atrophy, gynecomastia **Notes:** Nonsteroidal antiandrogen (eg, bicalutamide) may block flare in men w/PCa

Human Papillomavirus Recombinant Vaccine (Cervarix [Types 16, 18], Gardasil [Types 6, 11, 16, 18], Gardasil 9) Uses: *Cervarix*: Girls 9–26 y prevent Dz due to HPV types 16 and 18: cervical CA, cervical CA in situ; *Gardasil*: Girls 9–26 y to prevent cervical, vulvar, vaginal CA; males/females 9–26 y to prevent anal CA, precancerous, or dysplastic lesions, genital warts due to HPV types 6, 11, 16, & 18; *Gardasil 9:* Girls 9–26 y to prevent cervical/vulvar/vaginal/anal CA due to HPV types 6, 11, 16, 18, 31, 33, 45, 52, 58; precancerous or dysplastic lesions due to HPV types 6, 11, 16, 18, 31, 33, 45, 52, 58; & genital warts due to HPV types 6, 11; boys 9–15 y to prevent anal CA due to HPV types 16, 18, 31, 33, 45, 52, 58; precancerous or dysplastic lesions due to HPV types 6, 11, 16, 18, 31, 33, 45, 52, 58; & genital warts due to HPV types 6, 11* **Acts:** Recombinant vaccine, passive immunity **Dose:** 0.5 mL IM (upper thigh or deltoid), then 1 and 6 mo (*Cervarix*) or 2 and 6 mo (*Gardasil*) **W/P:** [B, ?/–] **CI:** Component hypersens **Disp:** Single-dose vial & prefilled syringe 0.5 mL **SE:** Erythema, Inj site pain, fever, syncope, venous thromboembolism **Notes:** Syncope reported; observe 15 min after Inj; report AEs to VAERS: 1-800-822-7967; continue cervical CA screening; Hx of genital warts, abn Pap smear, or + HPV DNA test is not CI to vaccination

Hydralazine (Apresoline, Others, Generic) Uses: *Mod–severe HTN*; CHF (w/ *Isordil* in black patients) **Acts:** Peripheral vasodilator **Dose:** *Adults.* Initial 10 mg PO tid-qid, ↑ to 25 mg tid-qid, 300 mg/d max *Peds.* 0.75–3 mg/kg/24 h PO ÷ q6–12h; ↓ in renal impair; ✓ CBC & ANA before **W/P:** [C, +] ↓ Hepatic Fxn & CAD; ↑ tox w/ MAOI, indomethacin, β-blockers **CI:** Dissecting aortic aneurysm, mitral valve/rheumatic heart Dz **Disp:** Tabs 10, 25, 50, 100 mg; Inj 20 mg/mL **SE:** SLE-like synd w/ chronic high doses; SVT following IM route; peripheral neuropathy **Notes:** Compensatory sinus tachycardia eliminated w/ β-blocker; *Bidil* combo Isordil/hydralazine

Hydrochlorothiazide (HydroDIURIL, Esidrix, Others, Generic) Uses: *Edema, HTN*, prevent stones in hypercalciuria **Acts:** Thiazide diuretic; ↓ distal tubule Na^+ reabsorption **Dose:** *Adults.* 25–100 mg/d PO single or ÷ doses; 200 mg/d max *Peds < 6 mo.* 2–3 mg/kg/d in 2 ÷ doses *> 6 mo.* 2 mg/kg/d in 2 ÷ doses **W/P:** [D, +] **CI:** Anuria, sulfonamide allergy, renal Insuff **Disp:** Tabs 25, 50, mg; caps 12.5 mg; PO soln 50 mg/5 mL **SE:** ↓ K^+, hyperglycemia, hyperuricemia, ↓ Na^+; sun sens **Notes:** Follow K^+, may need supplementation

Hydrochlorothiazide/Amiloride (Moduretic, Generic) Uses: *HTN* **Acts:** Combined thiazide & K^+-sparing diuretic **Dose:** 1–2 tabs/d PO **W/P:** [D, ?]

CI: Renal failure, sulfonamide allergy **Disp:** Tabs (amiloride/HCTZ) 5 mg/50 mg **SE:** ↓ BP, photosens, ↑ K⁺/↓ K⁺, hyperglycemia, ↓ Na⁺, hyperlipidemia, hyperuricemia

Hydrochlorothiazide/Spironolactone (Aldactazide, Generic) Uses: *Edema, HTN* **Acts:** Thiazide & K⁺-sparing diuretic **Dose:** 25–200 mg each component/d, ÷ doses **W/P:** [D, +] **CI:** Sulfonamide allergy **Disp:** Tabs (HCTZ/spironolactone) 25/25, 50/50 mg **SE:** Photosens, ↓ BP, ↑ or ↓ K⁺, ↓ Na⁺, hyperglycemia, hyperlipidemia, hyperuricemia

Hydrochlorothiazide/Triamterene (Dyazide, Maxzide, Generic) Uses: *Edema & HTN* **Acts:** Combo thiazide & K⁺-sparing diuretic **Dose:** *Dyazide:* 1–2 caps PO qd. *Maxzide:* 1 tab/d PO **W/P:** [D, +/–] **CI:** Sulfonamide allergy **Disp:** (Triamterene/HCTZ) 37.5/25, 50/25, 75/50 mg **SE:** Photosens, ↓ BP, ↑ or ↓ K⁺, ↓ Na⁺, hyperglycemia, hyperlipidemia, hyperuricemia **Notes:** HCTZ component in *Maxzide* more bioavailable than in *Dyazide*

Hydrocodone, Extended Release (Hysingla ER, Zohydro) [C-II] BOX: Addiction risk, risk of resp depression; accidental consumption, especially peds, can be fatal; use during PRG can cause neonatal opioid withdrawal; contains acetaminophen, associated with liver failure, transplant, and death Uses: *Severe pain requiring around-the-clock long-term opiod treatment where alternatives are inadequate* **Acts:** Opioid agonist **Dose:** Opioid naïve/opioid intolerant 10 mg PO q12h; ↑ 10 mg q12h PRN every 3–7 d; do not crush/chew **W/P:** [C/M] Caution w/ other CNS depressants, MAOI, TCA, elderly, debilitated, w/ hepatitic impair; may ↑ ICP (✓ pupils); impairs mental/physical abilities; drugs that ↓ CYP3A4 may ↓ clearance; may prolong GI obstruction **CI:** Component hypersens; resp depression severe asthma/hypercarbia, ileus **Disp:** ER caps 10, 15, 20, 30, 40, 50 mg **SE:** Constipation, N/V, somnolence, fatigue, HA, dizziness, dry mouth, pruritus, Abd pain, edema, URI, spasms, UTI, back pain, tremor

Hydrocodone/Acetaminophen (Hycet, Lorcet, Vicodin, Others) [C-II] BOX: Acetaminophen hepatotox (acute liver failure, liver transplant, death) reported; often d/t acetaminophen > 4000 mg/d or more than one acetaminophen product Uses: *Mod–severe pain* **Acts:** Narcotic analgesic w/ nonnarcotic analgesic **Dose:** *Adults.* 1–2 caps or tabs PO q4–6h PRN; soln 15 mL q4–6h *Peds.* Soln (*Hycet*) 0.27 mL/kg q4–6h **W/P:** [C, M] **CI:** CNS depression, severe resp depression **Disp:** Many formulations; specify hydrocodone/APAP dose; caps/tabs 5/300, 5/325, 7.5/300, 7.5/325, 10/300, 10/325 mg; soln Hycet (fruit punch) 7.5 mg hydrocodone/325 mg acetaminophen/15 mL **SE:** GI upset, sedation, fatigue **Notes:** No longer disp w/ APAP > 325 mg/pill

Hydrocodone/Chlorpheniramine (Vituz), Hydrocodone/ Chlorpheniramine/Pseudoephedrine (Generic) [C-II] Uses: *Cough & nasal congestion* **Acts:** Narcotic antitussive w/ histamine-1 receptor antag (*Vituz*); antitussive, antihistamine, & nasal decongestant **Dose:** 5 mL q4–6h PRN (max 20 mL/24 h) **W/P:** [C, M] Resp depression, dependence, ↑ ICP; w/ anticholinergics, caution w/

DM, thyroid Dz, Addison Dz, BPH, asthma, acute Abd, severe renal/hepatic impair **CI:** Hypersens, w/in14 d of MAOI, NAG, urinary retention, severe ↑ BP or CAD **Disp** *Vituz:* Soln hydrocodone 5 mg/5 mL; soln hydrocodone 5 mg/chlorpheniramine 4 mg/pseudoephedrine 60 mg/5 mL **SE:** ↑ BP, GI upset, sedation, fatigue

Hydrocodone/Guaifenesin (Obredon) [C-II] Uses: *Cough & loosen mucus w/ URI* **Acts:** Narcotic cough suppressant w/ expectorant **Dose:** 10 mL q4–6h PRN; max 6 doses (60 mL) in 24 h **W/P:** [C, M] Resp depression, dependence, ↑ ICP; w/ anticholinergics, caution w/ DM, thyroid Dz, Addison Dz, BPH, asthma, acute Abd, severe renal/hepatic impair **CI:** Hypersens, w/in 14 d of MAOI **Disp:** Soln hydrocodone 2.5 mg/guaifenesin 200 mg/5 mL **SE:** HA, dizziness, sedation, N/D, ↓ BP, hot flush **Note:** Dependence risk, not for peds

Hydrocodone/Homatropine (Hycodan, Hydromet, Tussigon, Others, Generic) [C-II] Uses: *Relief of cough* **Acts:** Combo antitussive **Dose:** (Based on hydrocodone) *Adults.* 5–10 mg q4–6h PRN *Peds.* 0.6 mg/kg/d ÷ tid-qid PRN **W/P:** [C, M] **CI:** NAG, ↑ ICP, depressed ventilation **Disp:** Syrup 5 mg hydrocodone/5 mL; tabs 5 mg hydrocodone **SE:** Sedation, fatigue, GI upset **Notes:** Do not give < q4h; see individual drugs

Hydrocodone/Ibuprofen (Vicoprofen, Generic) [C-II] Uses: *Mod–severe pain (< 10 d)* **Acts:** Narcotic w/ NSAID **Dose:** 1–2 tabs q4–6h PRN **W/P:** [C, M] Renal Insuff; ↓ effect w/ ACE inhib & diuretics; ↑ effect w/ CNS depressants, EtOH, MAOI, ASA, TCA, anticoagulants **CI:** Component sens **Disp:** Tabs (mg hydrocodone/mg ibuprofen) 2.5/200, 5/200, 7.5/200, 10/200 **SE:** Sedation, fatigue, GI upset

Hydrocodone/Pseudoephedrine (Detussin, Histussin-D, Others, Generic) [C-II] Uses: *Cough & nasal congestion* **Acts:** Narcotic cough suppressant w/ decongestant **Dose:** 5 mL qid PRN **W/P:** [C, M] **CI:** MAOIs **Disp:** 5 mL soln (mg hydrocodone/mg pseudoephedrine) 3/15, 5/60; tabs 5/60 mg **SE:** ↑ BP, GI upset, sedation, fatigue

Hydrocortisone, Rectal (Anusol-HC Suppository, Cortifoam Rectal, Proctocort, Others, Generic) Uses: *Painful anorectal conditions*, radiation proctitis, UC **Acts:** Anti-inflam steroid **Dose:** *UC:* 10–100 mg PR qd-bid for 2–3 wk **W/P:** [B, ?/–] **CI:** Component sens **Disp:** *Hydrocortisone acetate:* Rectal aerosol 90 mg/applicator; 25, 30 mg; *Hydrocortisone base:* Rectal 0.5%, 1%, 2.5%; rectal susp 100 mg/60 mL **SE:** Minimal systemic effect

Hydrocortisone, Systemic, Topical (Cortef, Solu-Cortef, Generic) See Steroids, Systemic, p 287, & Topical, p 288 *Peds. ECC 2010.* Adrenal insufficiency: 2 mg/kg IV/IO bolus; max dose 100 mg **W/P:** [B, –] **CI:** Viral, fungal, or tubercular skin lesions; serious Infxns (except septic shock or TB meningitis) **SE:** *Systemic:* ↑ Appetite, insomnia, hyperglycemia, bruising **Notes:** May cause hypothalamic-pituitary-adrenal axis suppression

Hydromorphone (Dilaudid, Generic) [C–II] BOX: A potent Schedule II opioid agonist; highest potential for abuse and risk of resp depression;

HP formula is highly concentrated; do not confuse w/ standard formulations, OD and death could result; alcohol, other opioids, CNS depressants ↑ resp depressant effects neonatal withdrawal if used during PRG **Uses:** *Mod–severe pain* **Acts:** Narcotic analgesic **Dose:** 1–4 mg PO, IM, IV, or PR q4–6h PRN; 3 mg PR q6–8h PRN; ↓ w/ hepatic failure **W/P:** [B (D if prolonged use or high doses near term), ?] ↑ Resp depression and CNS effects, CNS depressants, phenothiazines, TCA **CI:** CNS lesion w/ ↑ ICP, COPD, cor pulmonale, emphysema, kyphoscoliosis, status asthmaticus; HP-Inj form in OB analgesia **Disp:** Scored tabs 2, 4, 8 mg scored; liq 5 mg/5 mL or 1 mg/mL; Inj 1, 2, 4 mg/ml; supp 3 mg **SE:** Sedation, dizziness, GI upset **Notes:** Morphine 10 mg IM = hydromorphone 1.5 mg IM

Hydromorphone, Extended Release (Exalgo) [C–II] BOX: Use in opioid tolerant only; high potential for abuse, criminal diversion and resp depression; not for postop pain or PRN use; OD and death especially in children; do not break/crush/chew tabs, may result in OD **Uses:** *Mod–severe chronic pain requiring around-the-clock opioid analgesic* **Acts:** Narcotic analgesic **Dose:** 8–64 mg PO/d titrate to effect; ↓ w/ hepatic/renal impair and elderly **W/P:** [C, –] Abuse potential; ↑ resp depression and CNS effects, w/ CNS depressants, pts susceptible to intracranial effects of CO_2 retention **CI:** Opioid-intolerant pts, ↓ pulmonary function, ileus, GI tract narrowing/obst, component hypersens; w/in 14 d of MAOI; anticholinergics may ↑ **SE Disp:** Tabs 8, 12, 16, 32 mg **SE:** constipation, N/V, somnolence, HA, dizziness **Notes:** See label for opioid conversion

Hydroxocobalamin (Cyanokit) Uses: *Cyanide poisoning* **Acts:** Binds cyanide to form nontoxic cyanocobalamin excreted in urine **Dose:** 5 g IV over 15 min, repeat PRN 5 g IV over 15 min–2 h, total dose 10 g **W/P:** [C, ?] **CI:** Ø known **Disp:** Kit: 2- to 2.5-g vials w/ Inf set **SE:** ↑ BP (can be severe) anaphylaxis, chest tightness, edema, urticaria, rash, chromaturia, N, HA, Inj site Rxns

Hydroxychloroquine (Plaquenil, Generic) BOX: Physicians should completely familiarize themselves w/ the complete contents of the FDA PI before prescribing **Uses:** *Malaria: Plasmodium vivax, malariae, ovale, and faliciparum* (**NOT** all strains of *falciparum*); malaria prophylaxis; discoid lupus, SLE, RA* **Acts:** Unknown/antimalarial **Dose:** *Acute Malaria: Adults.* 800 mg, then 400 mg at 6, 24, & 48 h *Peds.* 13 mg/kg, then 6.5 mg/kg at 6, 24, & 48 h; *Suppression Malaria: Adults.* 400 mg qd same d of wk, 2 wk before arrival through 8 wk leaving endemic area *Peds.* 5 mg base/kg, same dosing schedule; *Lupus*, 400 mg qd-bid, reevaluate at 4–12 wk, then 200–400 mg qd; *RA: Adults.* 400–600 mg qd, reevaluate at 4–12 wk, reduce by 50%; take w/ milk or food **W/P:** [D, ?/–] **CI:** Hx eye changes from any 4-aminoquinoline, hypersens **Disp:** Tabs 200 mg **SE:** HA, dizziness, N/V/D, Abd pain, anorexia, irritability, mood changes, psychosis, Szs, myopathy, blurred vision, corneal changes, visual field defects, retinopathy, aplastic anemia, leukopenia, derm Rxns, including SJS **Notes:** Do not use long-term in children; cardiomyopathy rare

Hydroxyurea (Droxia, Hydrea, Generic) Uses: *CML, head & neck, ovarian & colon CA, melanoma, ALL, sickle cell anemia, polycythemia vera, HIV* Acts: ↓ Ribonucleotide reductase Dose: (per protocol) 50–75 mg/kg for WBC > 100,000 cells/mL; 20–30 mg/kg in refractory CML; *HIV:* 1000–1500 mg/d in single or ÷ doses; ↓ in renal Insuff W/P: [D, –] ↑ Effects w/ zidovudine, zalcitabine, didanosine, stavudine, fluorouracil PRG Disp: Caps 200, 300, 400, 500 mg SE: ↓ BM suppression, BM suppression, WBC < 2500 cells/mL or plt < 100,000 cells/mm³, PRG Disp: Caps 200, 300, 400, 500 mg SE: ↓ BM (mostly leukopenia), N/V, rashes, facial erythema, radiation recall Rxns, renal impair Notes: Empty caps into H_2O

Hydroxyzine (Atarax, Vistaril, Generic) Uses: *Anxiety, sedation, itching* Acts: Antihistamine, antianxiety Dose: *Adults. Anxiety/sedation:* 50–100 mg PO or IM qid or PRN (max 600 mg/d); *Itching:* 25–50 mg PO or IM tid-qid. *Peds.* 0.5–1.0 mg/kg/24 h PO or IM q6h; ↓ w/ hepatic impair W/P: [C, +/–] ↑ Effects w/ CNS depressants, anticholinergics, EtOH CI: Component sens Disp: Tabs 10, 25, 50 mg; caps 25, 50 mg; syrup 10 mg/5 mL; susp 25 mg/5 mL; Inj 25, 50 mg/mL SE: Drowsiness, anticholinergic effects Notes: Used to potentiate narcotic effects; not for IV/SQ (thrombosis & digital gangrene possible)

Hyoscyamine (Anaspaz, Cystospaz, Levsin, Others, Generic) Uses: *Spasm w/ GI & bladder disorders* Acts: Anticholinergic Dose: 0.125–0.25 mg (1–2 tabs) SL/PO tid-qid, ac & hs; 1 SR caps q12h W/P: [C, +] ↑ Effects w/ amantadine, antihistamines, antimuscarinics, haloperidol, phenothiazines, TCA, MAOI CI: BOO, GI obst, NAG, MyG, paralytic ileus, UC, MI Disp: *(Cystospaz-M, Levsinex)* time-release caps 0.375 mg; elixir (EtOH); soln 0.125 mg/5 mL; Inj 0.5 mg/mL; tabs 0.125 mg; tabs *(Cystospaz)* 0.15 mg; XR tabs *(Levbid)* 0.375 mg; SL tabs *(Levsin SL)* 0.125 mg SE: Dry skin, xerostomia, constipation, anticholinergic SE, heat prostration w/ hot weather Notes: Administer tabs ac

Hyoscyamine/Atropine/Scopolamine/Phenobarbital (Donnatal, Others, Generic) Uses: *IB, spastic colitis, peptic ulcer, spastic bladder* Acts: Anticholinergic, antispasmodic Dose: 0.125–0.25 mg (1–2 tabs) tid-qid, 1 cap q12h (SR), 5–10 mL elixir tid-qid or q8h W/P: [D, M] CI: NAG Disp: Many combos/manufacturers. Caps *(Donnatal, others):* Hyoscyamine 0.1037 mg/atropine 0.0194 mg/scopolamine 0.0065 mg/phenobarbital 16.2 mg; Tabs *(Donnatal, others):* Hyoscyamine 0.1037 mg/atropine 0.0194 mg/scopolamine 0.0065 mg/phenobarbital 16.2 mg; *LA (Donnatal):* Hyoscyamine 0.311 mg/atropine 0.0582 mg/scopolamine 0.0195 mg/phenobarbital 48.6 mg; Elixirs *(Donnatal, others):* Hyoscyamine 0.1037 mg/atropine 0.0194 mg/scopolamine 0.0065 mg/phenobarbital 16.2 mg/5 mL SE: Sedation, xerostomia, constipation

Ibandronate (Boniva, Generic) Uses: *Rx & Px osteoporosis in postmenopausal women* Acts: Bisphosphonate, ↓ osteoclast-mediated bone resorption Dose: 2.5 mg PO qd or 150 mg 1 × mo on same day (do not lie down for 60 min after); 3 mg IV over 15–30 s q3mo **W/P:** [C, ?/–] Avoid w/ CrCl < 30 mL/min **CI:** Uncorrected ↓ Ca²⁺; inability to stand/sit upright for 60 min (PO) **Disp:** Tabs 2.5, 150 mg; Inj IV 3 mg/3 mL **SE:** ONJ (avoid extensive dental procedures) N/D, HA, dizziness, asthenia, HTN, Infxn, dysphagia, esophagitis, esophageal/gastric ulcer, musculoskeletal pain **Notes:** Take 1st thing in A.M. w/ water (6–8 oz) > 60 min before 1st food/beverage & any meds w/ multivalent cations; give adequate Ca²⁺ & vit D supls; possible association between bisphosphonates & severe muscle/bone/joint pain; may ↑ atypical subtrochanteric femur fractures

Ibrutinib (Imbruvica) Uses: *MCL & CLL after one prior therapy, Waldenstrom macroglobulinemia* Acts: TKI Dose: *MCL:* 560 mg PO qd; *CLL & Waldenstrom:* 420 mg PO qd; swallow whole; see PI; dose mod w/ tox **W/P:** [D, –] Embryo-fetal tox; may cause new primary malignancies, ↑ bleeding risk, Infxns, ↓ BM, renal tox; avoid w/ hepatic impair or w/ mod/strong CYP3A inhib & strong CYP3A inducers, ↓ dose w/ CYP3A inhib **CI:** Ø **Disp:** Caps 140 mg **SE:** N/V/D, constipation, Abd pain, ↓ plts/WBC, bruising, anemia, fatigue, MS pain, arthralgia, edema, URI, sinusitis, dyspnea, rash, ↓ appetite, pyrexia, stomatitis, dizziness

Ibuprofen, Oral (Advil, Motrin, Motrin IB, Rufen, Others, Generic) [OTC] **BOX:** May ↑ risk of MI/CVA & GI bleeding Uses: *Arthritis, pain, fever* Acts: NSAID Dose: *Adults.* 200–800 mg PO bid-qid (max 1.2 g/d pain/fever; max 3.2 g/d RA). *Peds.* 30–40 mg/kg/d in 3–4 ÷ doses (max 40 mg/kg/d); w/ food **W/P:** [C (D ≥ 30 wk gestation), +] May interfere w/ ASAs anti-plt effect if given < 8 h before ASA **CI:** 3rd-tri PRG, severe hepatic impair, allergy, use w/ other NSAIDs, upper GI bleeding, ulcers **Disp:** Tabs 100, 200, 400, 600, 800 mg; chew tabs 50, 100 mg; caps 200 mg; susp 50 mg/1.25 mL, 100 mg/2.5 mL, 100 mg/5 mL, 40 mg/mL (*Motrin IB & Advil OTC* 200 mg are the OTC forms) **SE:** Dizziness, peptic ulcer, plt inhibition, worsening of renal Insuff

Ibuprofen, Parenteral (Caldolor) **BOX:** May ↑ risk of MI/CVA & GI bleeding Uses: *Mild–mod pain, as adjunct to opioids, ↓ fever* Acts: NSAID Dose: *Pain:* 400–800 mg IV over 30 min q6h PRN; *Fever:* 400 mg IV over 30 min, then 400 mg q4–6h or 100–200 mg q4–6h PRN **W/P:** [C < 30 wk, D after 30 wk, ?/–] May ↓ ACE effects; avoid w/ ASA, and < 17 y **CI:** Hypersens NSAIDs; asthma, urticaria, or allergic Rxns w/ NSAIDs, periop CABG **Disp:** 10 mg/mL **SE:** N/V, HA, flatulence, hemorrhage, dizziness **Notes:** Make sure pt well hydrated; use lowest dose/shortest duration possible

Ibutilide (Convert, Generic) **BOX:** Potentially fatal arrhythmias; not best option w/ chronic AF Uses: *Rapid conversion of AF/A flutter* Acts: Class III antiarrhythmic Dose: > *60 kg:* 1 mg IV over 10 min; may repeat × 1; < 60 kg use 0.01 mg/kg *ECC 2010. SVT (AF/A flutter):* > *60 kg:* 1 mg (10 mL) over 10 min; a 2nd dose may be used; < 60 kg: 0.01 mg/kg over 10 min; consider DC cardioversion

W/P: [C, −] **CI:** w/ Class I/III antiarrhythmics (Table 9, p 355); QTc > 440 ms **Disp:** Inj 0.1 mg/mL **SE:** Arrhythmias, HA **Notes:** Give w/ ECG monitoring; ✓ K⁺, Mg²⁺; wait 10 min between doses

Icatibant (Firazyr) Uses: *Hereditary angioedema* Acts: Bradykinin B₂ receptor antag Dose: 30 mg SQ in Abd; repeat q6h × 3 doses/max/24 h W/P: [C, ?/−] Seek medical attn after Tx of laryngeal attack Disp: Inj 10 mg/mL (30 mg/ syringe) SE: Inj site Rxns, pyrexia, ↑ LFTs, dizziness, rash

Icosapent Ethyl (Vascepa) Uses: *Hypertriglyceridemia w/ triglycerides > 500 mg/dL* Acts: ↓ Hepatic VLDL-triglyceride synth/secretion & ↑ triglyceride clearance Dose: 2 caps bid w/ food W/P: [C, M] If hepatic Dx ✓ ALT/AST; caution w/ fish/shellfish allergy; may ↑ bleeding time CI: Component hypersens Disp: Caps 1 g SE: Arthralgias Notes: (Ethyl ester of eicosapentaenoic); ↓ risk of pancreatitis or CV morbidity/mortality not proven

Idarubicin (Idamycin, Generic) BOX: Administer only under supervision of a physician experienced in leukemia and in an institution w/ resources to maintain a pt compromised by drug tox; severe myelosuppression, vesicant; can cause cardiac tox; ↓ dose w/ renal/hepatic impair Uses: *Acute leukemias* (AML, ALL), *CML in blast crisis, breast CA* Acts: DNA-intercalating agent, ↓ DNA topoisomerase I & II Dose: (Per protocol) 10–12 mg/m²/d for 3–4 d; ↓ in renal/ hepatic impair W/P: [D, −] CI: Bilirubin > 5 mg/dL, PRG Disp: Inj 1 mg/mL (5-, 10-, 20-mg vials) SE: ↓ BM, cardiotox, N/V, mucositis, alopecia, & IV site Rxns, rarely ↓ renal/hepatic Fxn Notes: Avoid extrav, potent vesicant; IV only

Idelalisib (Zydelig) BOX: May cause fatal hepatotox; ✓ LFT before/during Rx; fatal/serious D/colitis/pneumonitis; intestinal perforation reported; monitor for all Uses: *CLL (relapsed), follicular B-cell NHL (relapsed), small lymphocytic lymphoma (relapsed)* Acts: Phosphatidylinositol 3-kinase inhib Dose: (Approved indications): 150 mg bid (use w/ rituximab for CLL) until Dz progression or tox; adjusted dose 100 mg PO bid W/P: [D, −] ✓ CBC q2wk for 1st 3 mo or wkly if ↓ WBC; D w/ poor response to antidiarrheals; D/C drug w/ serious hypersens Rxn; monitor for derm tox; a substrate of CYP3A4; avoid w/ other CYP3A4 substrate drugs; pts ≥ 65 yr ↑ risk of SEs CI: Component hypersens Disp: Tab: 100, 150 mg SE: Fatigue, insomnia, HA, rash, night sweats, N/V/D, Abd pain, ↓ appetite, ↓ WBC/HgB/plts, ↑ ALT/AST, hepatotox, weakness, cough, pneumonia, dyspnea, URI, fever, edema Notes: w/ or w/o food, swallow whole; sound-alike/look-alike: ibrutinib, idarubicin, imatinib & *Zydelig w/ Xtandi, Zytiga*

Ifosfamide (Ifex, Generic) BOX: Administer only under supervision by a physician experienced in chemotherapy; hemorrhagic cystitis; myelosupp; confusion, coma, nephrotox possible Uses: *Testis*, lung, breast, pancreatic, & gastric CA, Hodgkin lymphoma/NHL, soft-tissue sarcoma Acts: Alkylating agent Dose: (Per protocol) 1.2 g/m²/d for 5-d bolus or cont Inf; 2.4 g/m²/d for 3 d; w/ mesna uroprotection; ↓ in renal/hepatic impair W/P: [D, M] ↑ Effect w/ phenobarbital, carbamazepine, phenytoin; St. John's wort may ↓ levels CI: w/ BM Fxn, PRG

Disp: Inj 1, 3 g **SE:** Hemorrhagic cystitis, nephrotox, N/V, mild–mod leukopenia, lethargy & confusion, alopecia, ↑ LFT **Notes:** Administer w/ mesna to prevent hemorrhagic cystitis; WBC nadir 10–14 d; recovery 21–28 d

Iloperidone (Fanapt) **BOX:** Risk for torsades de pointes and ↑ QT; elderly pts at ↑ risk of death, CVA **Uses:** *Acute schizophrenia* **Acts:** Atypical antipsychotic **Dose:** *Initial:* 1 mg PO bid, then ↑ qd to goal 6–12 mg bid, max titration 4 mg/d **W/P:** [?/–] ↓ dose w/ strong CYP2D6, 3A4 inhib **CI:** Component hypersens **Disp:** Tabs 1, 2, 4, 6, 8, 10, 12 mg **SE:** Orthostatic ↓ BP, dizziness, dry mouth, ↑ Wt **Notes:** Titrate to ↓ BP risk; monitor QT interval

Iloprost (Ventavis) **Uses:** *NYHA class III/IV pulm arterial HTN* **Acts:** Prostaglandin analog **Dose:** Initial 2.5 mcg Inh; if tolerated, ↑ to 5 mcg Inh 6–9×/d at least 2 h apart while awake **W/P:** [C, ?/–] Anti-plt effects, ↑ bleeding risk w/ anticoagulants; additive hypotensive effects **CI:** SBP < 85 mm Hg **Disp:** Inh soln 10, 20 mcg/mL **SE:** Syncope, ↓ BP, vasodilation, cough, HA, trismus, D, dysgeusia, rash, oral irritation **Notes:** Requires *Pro-Dose AAD* or *I-neb ADD* system nebulizer; counsel on syncope risk; do not mix w/ other drugs; monitor vitals during initial Rx

Imatinib (Gleevec) **Uses:** *Rx CML Ph(+), CML blast crisis, ALL Ph(+), myelodysplastic/myeloproliferative Dz, aggressive systemic mastocytosis, chronic eosinophilic leukemia, GIST, dermatofibrosarcoma protuberans* **Acts:** ↓ BCL-ABL; TKI **Dose:** **Adults.** *Typical dose:* 400–600 mg PO qd; w/ meal **Peds.** *CML Ph(+) newly diagnosed:* 340 mg/m²/d, 600 mg/d max; *recurrent:* 260 mg/m²/d PO ÷ qd-bid, 340 mg/m²/d max **W/P:** [D, ?/–] w/ CYP3A4 meds (Table 10, p 356), warfarin **CI:** Component sens **Disp:** Tabs 100, 400 mg **SE:** GI upset, fluid retention, muscle cramps, musculoskeletal pain, arthralgia, rash, HA, neutropenia, thrombocytopenia **Notes:** Follow CBCs & LFTs baseline & monthly; w/ large glass of H₂O & food to ↓ GI irritation

Imipenem/Cilastatin (Primaxin, Generic) **Uses:** *Serious Infxns* d/t susceptible bacteria **Acts:** Bactericidal; ↓ cell wall synth. **Spectrum:** Gram(+) (*S. aureus*, group A & B streptococci), gram(–) (not *Legionella*), anaerobes **Dose:** **Adults.** 250–1000 mg (impenem) IV q6–8h, 500–750 mg IM **Peds.** 60–100 mg/kg/24 h IV ÷ q6h; ↓ if CrCl < 70 mL/min **W/P:** [C, +/–] Probenecid ↑ tox **CI:** Peds pts w/ CNS Infxn (↑ Sz risk) & < 30 kg or renal impair **Disp:** Inj (imipenem/cilastatin) 250/250, 500/500 mg **SE:** Szs if drug accumulates, GI upset, thrombocytopenia

Imipramine (Tofranil, Generic) **BOX:** Close observation for suicidal thinking or unusual changes in behavior **Uses:** *Depression, enuresis*, panic attack, chronic pain **Acts:** TCA; ↑ CNS synaptic serotonin or norepinephrine **Dose:** **Adults.** *Hospitalized:* Initial 100 mg/24 h PO in ÷ doses, ↑ over several wk, 300 mg/d max *Outpatient:* Maint 50–150 mg PO hs, 300 mg/24 h max **Peds.** *Antidepressant:* 1.5–5 mg/kg/24 h ÷ qd-qid *Enuresis:* > *6 y:* 10–25 mg PO qhs; ↑ by 10–25 mg at 1- to 2-wk intervals (max 50 mg for 6–12 y, 75 mg for > 12 y); Rx for 2–3 mo, then taper **W/P:** [D, ?/–] **CI:** Use w/ MAOIs, NAG, recovery from AMI, PRG, CHF, angina, CV Dz, arrhythmias **Disp:**

Tabs 10, 25, 50 mg; caps 75, 100, 125, 150 mg **SE:** CV Sxs, dizziness, xerostomia, discolored urine **Notes:** Less sedation than amitriptyline

Imiquimod Cream (Aldara, Zyclara) Uses: *Anogenital warts, HPV, condylomata acuminata (Aldara, Zyclara); actinic keratosis (Zyclara); basal cell carcinoma (Aldara)* **Acts:** Unknown; ? cytokine induction **Dose: Adults & Peds > 12 yr. Warts:** Apply qd up to 8 wk (Zyclara); Apply 3×/wk, leave on 6–10 h & wash off w/ soap & water, continue 16 wk max (Aldara); Actinic keratosis: Apply qd two 2 × wk cycles, separated by 2 wk; Basal cell: Apply 5 d/wk × 6 wk, dose based on lesion size cycles, separated (see PI) **W/P:** [B, ?] Topical only, not intra-vag or intra-anal **CI:** Component sens **Disp:** 2.5% packet, 3.75% packet or pump (Zyclara); single-dose packet 5% (250-mg cream Aldara) **SE:** Local skin Rxns, flu-like synd **Notes:** Not a cure; may weaken condoms/Vag diaphragms, wash hands before & after use

Immune Globulin G, Human, IV [IVIG] (Bivigam, Others) BOX: Thrombosis may occur; may cause renal dysfunction/failure; use minimum dose and Inf rate Uses: *Primary humoral immunodeficiency* **Acts:** IgG supl **Dose: Adults & Peds.** 300–800 mg/kg q3–4wk; Inf 0.5 mg/kg/min × 10 min, then ↑ 0.8 mg/kg/min q20min up to 6 mg/kg/min.; ↓ in renal Insuff **W/P:** [C, ?] ✓ Renal Fxn, aseptic meningitis, hemolytic anemia, pulmonary adverse reactions; from human blood, risk of Infxn (virus/CJD) **CI:** Component hypersens; IgA deficiency w/ Abs to IgA **Disp:** Soln for Inj 10% IgG (100 mg/mL) **SE:** HA, fatigue, Inj site Rxn, N/D, sinusitis, ↑ BP, dizziness, lethargy **Notes:** Monitor vitals during Inf; do not give if vol depleted

Immune Globulin G, Human, SQ (Hizentra,Vivaglobin, Others) Uses: *Primary immunodeficiency* **Acts:** IgG supl **Dose: Adults & Peds > 2 y.** See PI for dose calculation for SQ Inf only **W/P:** [C, ?] Not for IV, aseptic meningitis **CI:** Hx anaphylaxis to immune globulin; some IgA deficiency **Disp:** Soln for SQ Inj, Hizentra: 200 mg/mL (20%), Vivaglobin: 160 mg/mL (16%) **SE:** Inj site Rxn, HA, GI complaint, fever, N/D, rash, sore throat **Notes:** May instruct in home administration; keep refrigerated; discard unused drug; use up to 4 Inj sites, max flow rate not > 50 mL/h for all sites combined

Inamrinone [Amrinone] (Inocor) Uses: *Acute CHF, ischemic cardiomy-opathy* **Acts:** Inotrope w/ vasodilator **Dose: Adults.** IV bolus 0.75 mg/kg over 2–3 min; maint 5–10 mcg/kg/min, 10 mg/kg/d max; ↓ if CrCl < 30 mL/min **Peds. ECC 2010.** CHF in postop CV surg pts, shock w/ ↑ SVR: 0.75–1 mg/kg IV/IO load over 5 min; repeat × 2 PRN; max 3 mg/kg; cont Inf 5–10 mcg/kg/min **W/P:** [C, ?] **CI:** Bisulfite allergy **Disp:** Inj 5 mg/mL **SE:** Monitor fluid, lyte, & renal changes **Notes:** Incompatible w/ dextrose solns, ✓ LFTs, observe for arrhythmias

Indacaterol (Arcapta Neohaler) BOX: LABAs increase risk of asthma-related deaths; considered a class effect of all LABAs Uses: *Daily maint of COPD (chronic bronchitis/emphysema)* **Acts:** LABA **Dose:** 75-mcg cap Inh qd w/ Neohaler inhaler only **W/P:** [C, ?/–] Not for acute deterioration of COPD or asthma; paradoxical bronchospasm possible; excessive use or use w/ other LABA can cause cardiac effects and can be fatal; caution w/ Sz disorders, thyrotoxicosis or sympathomimetic sensitivity; w/ meds that can ↓ K+ or ↑ QTc; β-blockers may ↓ effect **CI:** All LABAs CI in asthma w/o use of long-term asthma control med; not indicated for asthma **Disp:** Inhal hard cap 75 mcg (30 blister pack w/ 1 Neohaler) **SE:** Cough, oropharyngeal pain, nasopharyngitis, HA, N **Notes:** Inform patient not to swallow caps

Indapamide (Lozol, Generic) **Uses:** *HTN, edema, CHF* **Acts:** Thiazide diuretic; ↑ Na, Cl, & H_2O excretion in distal tubule **Dose:** 1.25–5 mg/d PO **W/P:** [D, ?] ↑ Effect w/ loop diuretics, ACE inhib, cyclosporine, digoxin, Li **CI:** Anuria, thiazide/sulfonamide allergy, renal Insuff, PRG **Disp:** Tabs 1.25, 2.5 mg **SE:** ↓ BP, dizziness, photosens **Notes:** No additional effects w/ doses > 5 mg; take early to avoid nocturia; use sunscreen; OK w/ food/milk

Indinavir (Crixivan) **Uses:** *HIV Infxn* **Acts:** Protease inhib; ↓ maturation of noninfectious virions to mature infectious virus **Dose:** Typical 800 mg PO q8h in combo w/ other antiretrovirals (dose varies); on empty stomach; ↓ w/ hepatic impair **W/P:** [C, ?] Numerous interactions, especially CYP3A4 inhib (see Table 10, p 356) **CI:** w/ Triazolam, midazolam, pimozide, ergot alkaloids, simvastatin, lovastatin, sildenafil, St. John's wort, amiodarone, salmeterol, PDE5 inhib, alpha 1-adrenoreceptor antag (alfuzosin); colchicine **Disp:** Caps 200, 400 mg **SE:** Nephrolithiasis, dyslipidemia, lipodystrophy, N/V, ↑ bili **Notes:** Drink six 8-oz glasses of water/d

Indomethacin (Indocin, Tivorbex, Generic) **BOX:** May ↑ risk of MI/CVA events & GI bleeding; not for post-CABG pain **Uses:** *Arthritis (gouty, osteo, rheumatoid); ankylosing spondylitis; close-ductus arteriosus; Tivorbex: acute pain* **Acts:** ↓ Prostaglandins **Dose:** *Adults.* 25–50 mg PO bid-tid, max 200 mg/d *Infants.* 0.2–0.25 mg/kg/dose IV; may repeat in 12–24 h, max 3 doses; w/ food **W/P:** [C, +] **CI:** Periop pain w/ CABG, ASA/NSAID sens, peptic ulcer/active GI bleeding, precipitation of asthma/urticaria/rhinitis by NSAIDs/ASA, premature neonates w/ NEC, ↓ renal Fxn, active bleeding, thrombocytopenia, 3rd tri PRG **Disp:** Inj 1 mg/vial; caps 25, 50 mg; ER caps 75 mg; susp 25 mg/5 mL; supp 50 mg; *Tivorbex:* 20, 40 mg caps **SE:** GI bleeding or upset, dizziness, edema **Notes:** Monitor renal Fxn

Infliximab (Remicade) **BOX:** TB, invasive fungal Infxns, & other opportunistic Infxns reported, some fatal; perform TB skin testing prior to use; possible association w/ lymphoma, other malignancies **Uses:** *Mod–severe Crohn Dz; fistulizing Crohn Dz; UC; RA (w/ MTX) psoriasis, ankylosing spondylitis* **Acts:** IgG1K neutralizes TNF-α **Dose:** *Adults. Crohn Dz:* Induction: 5 mg/kg IV Inf, w/ doses 2 & 6 wk after. *Maint:* 5 mg/kg IV Inf q8wk *RA:* 3 mg/kg IV Inf at 0, 2, 6 wk, then q8wk *Peds > 6 y.* 5 mg/kg IV q8wk **W/P:** [B, ?/–] Active Infxn, hepatic impair, Hx or risk of TB, hep B **CI:** Murine allergy, mod–severe CHF, w/ live vaccines (eg, smallpox) **Disp:** 100-mg Inj **SE:** Allergic Rxns; HA, fatigue, GI upset, Inf Rxns; hepatotox; reactivation hep B, pneumonia, BM suppression, systemic vasculitis, pericardial effusion, new psoriasis **Notes:** Monitor LFTs, PPD at baseline, monitor hep B carrier, skin exam for malignancy w/ psoriasis; can premedicate w/ antihistamines, APAP, and/or steroids to ↓ Inf Rxns

Influenza Vaccine, Inactivated, Quadrivalent (IIV₄) (Fluarix Quadrivalent, Fluzone Quadrivalent, FluLaval Quadrivalent) See Table 13, p 362 **Uses:** *Prevent influenza* in all ≥ 6 mo **Acts:** Active immunization **Dose: Adults 18-64 y** *Fluzone,* 0.1 mL, intradermal annually **Adults and Peds > 3 y.** *Fluarix, FluLaval* 0.5 mL/dose IM annually **Peds 6–35 mo.** *(Fluzone)* 0.25 mL IM annually; 0.25 mL IM × 2 doses 4 wk apart for 1st vaccination; give 2 doses in 2nd vaccination year if only 1 dose given in 1st year. *3–8 y.* 0.5 mL IM annually; 0.5 mL IM × 2 doses 4 wk apart for 1st vaccination; **W/P:** [C, +] Hx Guillain-Barré synd w/in 6 wk of previous flu vaccine; syncope may occur w/ admin; immunocompromised w/ ↓ immune response **CI:** Previous life-threatening Rxn to any influenzae vaccine or reaction to any component of the vaccine (All); hx allergy to egg protein, *(Fluarix, FluLaval, Fluzone);* thimerosal allergy (multi-dose *FluLaval and Fluzone);* **Disp:** Based on manufacturer, 0.25-, 0.5-mL prefilled syringe, single-dose vial **SE:** Inj site soreness, fever, chills, HA, insomnia, myalgia, malaise, rash, urticaria, anaphylactoid Rxns, Guillain-Barré synd **Notes:** US Oct-Nov best, protection 1–2 wk after, lasts up to 6 mo; given yearly, vaccines based on predictions of flu season (Nov-April in US, w/ sporadic cases all year); refer to ACIP annual recs *(www.cdc.gov/vaccines/hcp/acip-recs/vacc-specific/flu.html)*

Influenza Vaccine, Inactivated, Trivalent (IIV₃) (Afluria, Flucelvax, Fluvirin, Fluzone, Fluzone High Dose) See Table 13, p 362 **Uses:** *Prevent influenza* in all ≥ 6 mo **Acts:** Active immunization **Dose: Adult/Peds > 9 y.** *Afluria* 0.5 mL/dose IM annually; *18-64 y* IM (can use *Afluria* jet injector) annually; *> 18 y Flucelvax* 0.5 mL IM annually; *> 65 y Fluzone High-Dose* 0.5 mL IM annually; **Peds > 4 yrs** *Fluvirin* 0.5 mL IM annually; **Peds 6–35 mo** *Fluzone* 0.25 mL IM annually; 0.25 mL IM × 2 doses 4 wk apart for 1st vaccination; give 2 doses in 2nd vaccination year if only 1 dose given in 1st year. **Peds 3–8 y.** *Fluzone* 0.5 mL IM annually; 0.5 mL IM × 2 doses 4 wk apart for 1st vaccination **W/P:** [B, +] Hx Guillain-Barré synd w/in 6 wk of previous influenza vaccine; syncope may occur w/ admin; immunocompromised w/ ↓ immune response **CI:** Previous life-threatening Rxn to any influenzae vaccine or reaction to any component of the vaccine (All); hx allergy to egg protein *(Afluria);* latex *(Flucelvax* [syringe cap may contain latex]); egg protein, latex, *(Fluvirin, Fluzone);* thimerosal allergy *(Fluvirin, & multi-dose Alfuria and Fluzone);* single-/multi-dose vials latex free; acute resp or febrile illness **Disp:** Based on manufacturer, 0.25, 0.5-mL prefilled syringe, single-/multi-dose vial; **SE:** Inj site soreness, fever, chills, HA, insomnia, myalgia, malaise, rash, urticaria, anaphylactoid Rxns, Guillain-Barré synd **Notes:** *Afluria* not for Peds 6mo – 8 y due to ↑ risk of febrile Rxn; however, if no other age appropriate vaccine available and concern over SE of influenza OK to used after risk/benefit discussion w/parents; US Oct-Nov best, protection 1–2 wk after, lasts up to

6 mo; given yearly, vaccines based on predictions of flu season (Nov–April in US, w/ sporadic cases all year); refer to ACIP annual recs *(www.cdc.gov/vaccines/hcp/ acip-recs/vacc-specific/flu.html)*

Influenza Vaccine, Live Attenuated, Quadrivalent (LAIV₄) (FluMist)
See Table 13, p 362 Uses: *Prevent influenza* Acts: Live attenuated vaccine **Dose:** *Adults and Peds 2–49 y.* 0.1 mL each nostril annually *Peds 2–8 y.* 0.1 mL each nostril annually; initial 0.1 mL each nostril × 2 doses 4 wk apart in 1st vaccination year W/P: [B, ?/–] Do not use if influenza antiviral meds w/in previous 48 hrs; Hx Guillain-Barré synd w/in 6 wk of previous influenza vaccine; ↑ risk of wheezing w/ asthma; use w/ influenza A/B antiviral drugs may ↓ efficacy CI: Hx allergy to egg protein, gentamicin, gelatin, or arginine; peds 2–17 y on ASA; PRG, known/suspected immune deficiency, asthma/reactive airway Dz, acute febrile illness, or reaction to previous dose of any influenzae vaccine Disp: Single-dose, nasal sprayer 0.2 mL; shipped frozen, store 35–46°F SE: Runny nose, nasal congestion, HA, cough, fever, sore throat Notes: Do not give w/ other vaccines; avoid contact w/ immunocompromised individuals for 7 d; should not take if influenzae antiviral meds w/in 48 hours; refer to ACIP annual recs *(www.cdc.gov/vaccines/ hcp/acip-recs/vacc-specific/flu.html)*

Influenza Vaccine, Recombinant, Trivalent (RIV₃) (FluBlok) See Table 13, p 362 Uses: *Px influenza* Acts: Active immunization Dose: *Adults > 18 y.* 0.5 mL/dose IM annually W/P: [B, ?/–] Hx Guillain-Barré synd w/in 6 wk of previous flu vaccine; immunocompromised w/ ↓ immune response CI: Hx component allergy (contains no egg protein, antibiotics, preservatives, latex) Disp: 0.5-mL single-dose vial SE: Inj site soreness, HA, fatigue, myalgia Notes: Adolescents/ adults >18 yrs w/egg allergy can receive the recombinant; US Oct–Nov best, protection 1–2 wk after, lasts up to 6 mo; given yearly, vaccines based on predictions of flu season (Nov–April in US, w/sporadic cases all year); refer to ACIP annual recs *(www.cdc.gov/vaccines/hcp/acip-recs/vacc-specific/flu.html)*

Ingenol Mebutate (Picato) Uses: *Actinic keratosis* Acts: Necrosis by neutrophil activation Dose: 25 cm² area (1 tube), evenly spread; 0.015% to face qd × 3 d; 0.05% to trunk/neck qd × 2 d W/P: [C, ?/–] CI: Ø Disp: Gel; 0.015%, 0.25 g/tube × 3 tubes; 0.05% 0.25 g/tube × 2 tubes SE: Local skin Rxns Notes: From plant sap Euphorbia peplus; allow to dry × 15 min; do not wash/ touch for 6 h; avoid eye contact

Insulin, Human Inhalation Powder (Afrezza) BOX: Acute bronchospasm possible; CI w/COPD; R/O lung disease Uses: *DM (types 1 & 2); w/type 1 use w/ long-acting insulin; not for DKA; not rec in smokers* Acts: rapid-acting insulin Dose: Individualize; 1 inhal/cartridge at start of meal; ↑ PRN W/P: [C, ?] H&P and spirometry (FEV1) before to R/O lung disease; w/ anti-adrenergic meds (beta-blockers, etc) may mask low blood sugar; w/ drugs that alter glu metabolism; do not use w/lung Ca; anaphylaxis possible; monitor for DKA; monitor for changes in insulin dose; fluid retention w/ thiazolidinediones (eg, pioglitazone, rosiglitazone);

↓ K+ **CI:** Component sens, w/ hypoglycemia, w/COPD **Disp:** Single-use cartridges 4, 8 units **SE:** ↓ glu, cough, throat pain/irritation **Notes:** Reassess PFT 6 mo after start

Insulin, Injectable (See Table 4, p 338)
Uses: *Type 1 or type 2 DM refractory to diet or PO hypoglycemic agents; acute life-threatening ↑ K+* **Acts:** Insulin supl **Dose:** Based on serum glu; usually SQ (upper arms, Abd wall [most rapid absorption site], upper legs, buttocks); can give IV (only regular)/IM; type 1 typical start dose 0.5–1 units/kg/d; type 2 0.2–0.4 units/kg/d; renal failure ↓ insulin needs **W/P:** [B, +] **CI:** Hypoglycemia **Disp:** See Table 4, p 338. Some are dispensed w/ preloaded insulin cartridge pens w/ 29-, 30-, or 31-gauge needles and dosing adjustments **SE:** Hypoglycemia; highly purified insulins ↑ free insulin; monitor for several weeks when changing doses/agents **Notes:** Specific agent/regimen based on pt and physician choices that maintain glycemic control Typical type 1 regimens use a basal daily insulin w/ premeal Inj of rapidly acting insulins. Insulin pumps may achieve basal insulin levels. ↑ malignancy risk w/ glargine controversial

Interferon Alpha-2b (Intron-A)
BOX: Can cause or aggravate fatal or life-threatening neuropsychiatric autoimmune, ischemic, and infectious disorders; monitor closely **Uses:** *HCL, Kaposi sarcoma, melanoma, CML, chronic hep B & C, follicular NHL, condylomata acuminata* **Acts:** Antiproliferative; modulates host immune response; ↓ viral replication in infected cells **Dose:** Per protocols. *Adults.* Per protocols. *HCL:* 2 mill units/m² IM/SQ 3×/wk for 2–6 mo. *Chronic hep B:* 5 mill units/d or 10 mill units 3×/wk IM/SQ × 16 wk *Follicular NHL:* 5 mill units SQ 3×/wk × 18 mo *Melanoma:* 20 mill units/m² IV × 5 d/wk × 4 wk, then 10 mill units/m² SQ 3×/wk × 48 wk *Kaposi sarcoma:* 30 mill units/m² IM/SQ 3×/wk until Dz progression or maximal response achieved *Chronic hep C (Intron-A):* 3 mill units IM/SQ 3×/wk × 16 wk (continue 18–24 mo if response) *Condyloma:* 1 mill units/lesion (max 5 lesions) 3×/wk (on alternate days) for 3 wk *Peds. Chronic hep B:* 3 mill units/m² SQ 3×/wk × 1 wk, then 6 mill units/m²-max 10 mill units/dose 3×/wk × 16–24 wk **CI:** Benzyl alcohol sens, decompensated liver Dz, autoimmune hep immunosuppressed, PRG, male w/ pregnant partner CrCl < 50 mL/min in combo w/ ribavirin **Disp:** Inj forms: powder 10/18/50 mill Int units; soln 6/10 mill Int units/mL (see also Peginterferon) **SE:** Flu-like Sxs, fatigue, anorexia, neurotox at high doses; up to 40% neutralizing Ab w/ Rx

Interferon Alphacon-1 (Infergen)
BOX: Can cause or aggravate fatal or life-threatening neuropsychiatric, autoimmune, ischemic, & infectious disorders; combo therapy w/ ribavirin; monitor closely **Uses:** *Chronic hep C* **Acts:** Biologic response modifier **Dose:** *Monotherapy:* 9 mcg 3×/wk × 24 wk (initial Rx) or 15 mcg 3×/wk up to 48 wk (retreatment) *Combo:* 15 mcg/d w/ ribavirin 1000 or 1200 mg (Wt < 75 kg and ≥ 75 kg) qd up to 48 wk (retreatment); ↓ dose w/ SAE **W/P:** [C, M] **CI:** E. coli product allergy, decompensated liver Dz, autoimmune hep **Disp:** Inj 30 mcg/mL **SE:** Flu-like synd, depression, blood

dyscrasias, colitis, pancreatitis, hepatic decompensation, ↑ SCr, eye disorders, ↓ thyroid **Notes:** Allow > 48 h between Inj; monitor CBC, plt, SCr, TFT

Interferon Beta-1a (Avonex, Rebif) **Uses:** *MS, relapsing* **Acts:** Biologic response modifier **Dose:** *(Avonex)* 30 mcg SQ 1x/wk; *(Rebif)* Give SQ for target dose 44 mcg 3×/wk: start 8.8 mcg 3×/wk × 2 wk, then 22 mcg 3×/wk × 2 wk, then 44 mcg 3×/wk × 2 wk; target dose 22 mcg: start 4.4 mcg 3×/wk × 2 wk, then 11 mcg 3×/wk × 2 wk, then 22 mcg SQ 3×/wk **W/P:** [C, ?/–] w/ Hepatic impair, depression, Sz disorder, thyroid Dz **CI:** Human albumin allergy **Disp:** 0.5-mL prefilled syringes w/ 29-gauge needle; *Titrate Pak:* 8.8 and 22 mcg; 22 or 44 mcg *Avonex pen:* 30 mcg/0.5 mL Inj **SE:** Inj site Rxn, HA, flu-like Sx, malaise, fatigue, rigors, myalgia, depression w/ suicidal ideation, hepatotox, ↓ BM **Notes:** Dose > 48 h apart; ✓ CBC 1, 3, 6 mo; ✓ TFTs q6mo w/ Hx thyroid Dz

Interferon Beta-1b (Betaseron, Extavia) **Uses:** *MS, relapsing/remitting/secondary progressive* **Acts:** Biologic response modifier **Dose:** 0.0625 mg (2 mill units) (0.25 mL) q other day SQ, ↑ by 0.0625 mg q2wk to target dose 0.25 mg (1 mL) q other day **W/P:** [C, –] **CI:** Human albumin allergy **Disp:** Powder for Inj 0.3 mg (9.6 mill units interferon) **SE:** Flu-like synd, depression, suicide, blood dyscrasias, ↑ AST/ALT/GGT, Inj site necrosis, anaphylaxis **Notes:** Teach pt self-Inj, rotate sites; ✓ LFTs, CBC 1, 3, 6 mo; TFT q6mo; consider stopping w/ depression

Interferon Gamma-1b (Actimmune) **Uses:** *↑↓ Incidence of serious Infxns in CGD, severe malignant osteopetrosis* **Acts:** Biologic response modifier **Dose:** 50 mcg/m^2 SQ (1.5 mill units/m^2) BSA > 0.5 m^2; if BSA < 0.5 m^2, give 1.5 mcg/kg/dose; given 3×/wk **W/P:** [C, –] **CI:** Allergy to *E. coli*-derived products **Disp:** Inj 100 mcg (2 mill units) **SE:** Flu-like synd, depression, blood dyscrasias, dizziness, altered mental status, gait disturbance, hepatic tox **Notes:** May ↑ deaths in interstitial pulm fibrosis

Ipilimumab (Yervoy) **BOX:** Severe fatal immune Rxns possible; D/C and Tx w/ high-dose steroids w/ severe Rxn; assess for enterocolitis, dermatitis, neuropathy, endocrinopathy before each dose **Uses:** *Unresectable/metastatic melanoma* **Acts:** Human CTLA-4-blocking Ab; ↑ T-cell proliferation/activation **Dose:** 3 mg/kg IV q3wk × 4 doses; Inf over 90 min **W/P:** [C, –] Can cause immune-mediated adverse Rxns; endocrinopathies may require Rx; hep dermatologic tox, heuramuscular tox, opthalmic tox **CI:** Ø **Disp:** IV 50 mg/10 mL, 200 mg/40 mL **SE:** Fatigue, D, pruritus, rash, colitis **Notes:** ✓ LFTs, TFT, chemistries baseline/pre-Inf

Ipratropium (Atrovent HFA, Atrovent Nasal, Generic) **Uses:** *Bronchospasm w/ COPD, rhinitis, rhinorrhea* **Acts:** Synthetic anticholinergic similar to atropine; antagonizes acetylcholine receptors, inhibits mucous gland secretions **Dose:** *Adults & Peds > 12 y.* 2–4 puffs qid, max 12 Inh/d; *Nasal:* 2 sprays/nostril bid-tid; *Nebulization:* 500 mcg 3–4×/d; *ECC 2010. Asthma:* 250–500 mcg by nebulizer/MDI q20min × 3 **W/P:** [B, ?/M] w/ Inh insulin **CI:** Allergy to soya lecithin-related foods **Disp:** *HFA:* MDI 17 mcg/dose; Inh soln 0.02%; nasal spray 0.03, 0.06% **SE:** Nervousness, dizziness, HA, cough, bitter taste, nasal dryness, URI, epistaxis **Notes:** Not for acute bronchospasm unless used w/ inhaled β-agonist; see also abuterol/ipratropium

Irbesartan (Avapro, Generic) BOX: D/C immediately if PRG detected **Uses:** *HTN, DN*, CHF **Acts:** Angiotensin II receptor antag **Dose:** 150 mg/d PO, may ↑ to 300 mg/d **W/P:** [C (1st tri); D 2nd/3rd tri), ?/–] **CI:** PRG, component sens **Disp:** Tabs 75, 150, 300 mg **SE:** Fatigue, ↓ BP, ↑ K

Irinotecan (Camptosar, Generic) BOX: D & myelosuppression; administer by experienced physician **Uses:** *Colorectal* & lung CA **Acts:** Topoisomerase I inhib; ↓ DNA synth **Dose:** Per protocol; 125–350 mg/m² qwk–q3wk (↓ hepatic dysfunction, as tolerated per tox) **W/P:** [D, –] **CI:** Allergy to component **Disp:** Inj 20 mg/mL **SE:** ↓ BM, N/V/D, Abd cramping, alopecia; D is dose limiting; Rx acute D w/ atropine; Rx subacute D w/ loperamide **Notes:** D correlated to levels of metabolite SN-38

Iron Dextran (Dexferrum, INFeD) BOX: Anaphylactic Rxn w/ death reported; proper personnel and equipment should be available; use test dose only if PO iron not possible **Uses:** *Iron-deficiency anemia where PO administration not possible* **Dose:** See also label for tables/formula to calculate dose. Estimate Fe deficiency; total dose (mL) = [0.0442 × (desired Hgb – observed Hgb) × lean body Wt] + (0.26 × lean body Wt); Fe replacement, blood loss: total dose (mg) = blood loss (mL) × Hct (as decimal fraction) max 100 mg/d **IV use:** *Test Dose:* 0.5 mL IV over 30 s, if OK, 2 mL or less daily IV over 1 mL/min to calculated total dose **IM use:** *Test Dose:* 0.5 mL deep IM in buttock. Administer calculated total dose not to exceed daily doses as follows: Infants < 5 kg: 0.5 mL; children < 10 kg: 1 mL all others: 2.0 mL (100 mg of iron) **W/P:** [C, M] w/Hx allergy/asthma; keep Epi available (1:1000) for acute Rxn **CI:** Component hypersens, non–Fe-deficiency anemia **Disp:** Inj 50 mg Fe/mL in 2 mL vials (*INFeD*) and 1 & 2 mL vials (*Dexferrum*) **Notes:** Not rec in infants < 4 mo; ✓ Hgb/Hct; also Fe, TIBC and % saturation transferrin may be used to monitor; reticulocyte count best early indicator of response (several days); IM use "Z-track" technique

Iron Sucrose (Venofer) Uses: *Iron-deficiency anemia in CKD, w/ or w/o dialysis, w/ wo erythropoietin* **Acts:** Fe supl **Dose:** 100 mg on dialysis; 200 mg slow IV over 25 min × 5 doses over 14 d; total cumulative dose 1000 mg **W/P:** [B, M] Hypersens, ↓ BP, Fe overload, may interfere w/ MRI **CI:** Non–Fe-deficiency anemia; Fe overload; component sens **Disp:** Inj 20 mg Fe/mL, 2.5, 5, 10 mL vials **SE:** Muscle cramps, N/V, strange taste in the mouth, diarrhea, constipation, HA, cough, back/jt pain, dizziness, swelling of the arms/legs **Notes:** Safety in peds not established

Isavuconazonium Sulfate (Cresemba) Uses: *Invasive aspergillosis & mucormycosis* **Acts:** Azole antifungal **Dose:** 372 PO or IV q8h × 6 doses, then 372 mg PO or IV qd, begin 12–24 h after last loading dose; IV dose over ≥ 1 h w/ in-line filter **W/P:** [C, –] Serious hepatic Rxn; Inf-related Rxn; embryo-fetal toxicity; multiple drug interactions **CI:** Hypersens Rxn; use w/ strong CYP3A4 inhib or inducer; familial short QT synd **Disp:** Caps 186 mg; single-dose vial 372 mg **SE:** N/V/D, HA, constipation, dyspnea, cough, edema, back pain, ↑ LFTs, ↓ K⁺ **Notes:** w/ or w/o food; D/C w/ Inf-related Rxn; monitoring and dose adjustments may be necessary

Isoniazid (INH) **BOX:** Severe & sometimes fatal hep may occur usually w/in 1st 3 mo of Tx, although may develop after mo of Tx **Uses:** *Rx & prophylaxis of TB* **Acts:** Bactericidal; interferes w/ mycolic acid synth, disrupts cell wall **Dose:** *Adults.* *Active TB:* 5 mg/kg/24 h PO or IM (usually 300 mg/d) or *DOT:* 15 mg/kg (max 900 mg) 3×/wk *Prophylaxis:* 300 mg/d PO for 6–12 mo or 900 mg 2×/wk **Peds.** *Active TB:* 10–15 mg/kg/d daily PO or IM 300 mg/d max *Prophylaxis:* 10 mg/kg/24 h PO; ↓ in hepatic/renal dysfunction **W/P:** [C, +] Liver Dz, dialysis; avoid EtOH **CI:** Acute liver Dz, Hx INH hep **Disp:** Tabs 100, 300 mg; syrup 50 mg/5 mL; Inj 100 mg/ mL **SE:** Hep, peripheral neuropathy, GI upset, anorexia, dizziness, skin Rxn **Notes:** Use w/ 2–3 other drugs for active TB, based on INH resistance patterns when TB acquired & sensitivity results; prophylaxis usually w/ INH alone. IM rarely used. ↓ Peripheral neuropathy w/ pyridoxine 50–100 mg/d. See CDC guidelines (http:// www.cdc.gov/tb/) for current TB recommendations

Isoproterenol (Isuprel) **Uses:** *Shock, cardiac arrest, AV nodal block* **Acts:** β₁- & β₂-receptor stimulants **Dose:** *Adults.* 2–10 mcg/min IV Inf; titrate; 2–10 mcg/min titrate **Peds.** 0.05–2 mcg/kg/min IV Inf; titrate **W/P:** [C, ?] **CI:** Angina, tachyarrhythmias (digitalis-induced or others) **Disp:** 0.02 mg/mL, 0.2 mg/mL **SE:** Insomnia, arrhythmias, HA, trembling, dizziness **Notes:** Pulse > 130 BPM may induce arrhythmias

Isosorbide Dinitrate (Dilatrate-SR, Isordil, Sorbitrate, Generic) **Uses:** *Rx & Px angina*, CHF (w/ hydralazine) **Acts:** Relaxes vascular smooth muscle **Dose:** *Acute angina:* 5–10 mg PO (chew tabs) q2–3h or 2.5–10 mg SL PRN q5–10 min; do not give > 3 doses in a 15- to 30-min period *Angina prophylaxis:* 5–20 mg PO bid-tid; maint 10–40 mg PO bid-tid; do not give nitrates on a chronic q6h or qid basis > 7–10 d; tolerance may develop; provide 10- to 12-h drug-free intervals; *dose in CHF:* initial 20 mg tid-qid, target 120–160 mg/d **W/P:** [C, ?] **CI:** Severe anemia, NAG, postural ↓ BP, cerebral hemorrhage, head trauma (can ↑ ICP), w/ sildenafil, tadalafil, vardenafil **Disp:** Tabs 5, 10, 20, 30; SR tabs 40 mg; SL tabs 2.5, 5 mg; SR caps 40 mg **SE:** HA, ↓ BP, flushing, tachycardia, dizziness **Notes:** Higher PO dose needed for same results as SL forms

Isosorbide Mononitrate (Imdur, Ismo, Monoket, Generic) **Uses:** *Rx & Px angina pectoris* **Acts:** Relaxes vascular smooth muscle **Dose:** 5–20 mg PO bid, w/ doses 7 h apart or XR (Imdur) 30–60 mg/d PO, max 240 mg **W/P:** [B, ?] Severe hypotension w/ paradoxical bradycardia, hypertrophic cardiomyopathy; head trauma/cerebral hemorrhage (can ↑ ICP) **CI:** W/ Sildenafil, tadalafil, vardenafil **Disp:** Tabs 10, 20 mg; XR 30, 60, 120 mg **SE:** HA, dizziness, ↓ BP

Isotretinoin (Amnesteem, Claravis, Myorisan, Sotret, Zentane, Generic) **BOX:** Do not use in pts who are/may become PRG; ↑ risk severe birth defects; available only through iPLEDGE restricted distribution program; pts, prescribers, pharmacies, and distributors must enroll **Uses:** *Severe nodular acne resistant to other Tx* **Acts:** Inhib sebaceous gland Fxn & keratinization **Dose: *Adults and Peds ≥ 12 y.*** 0.5–1 mg/kg/d 2 ÷ doses × 15–20 wk, do NOT take only qd; PRG test prior to Rx each mo, end of Tx, and 1 mo after D/C **W/P:** [X, –] Micro-dosed progesterone BCPs NOT an acceptable method of birth control; depression, suicidal thoughts and behaviors, psychosis/aggressive/violent behavior; pseudotumor cerbri; TEN, SJS; ↓ hearing, corneal opacities; ↓ night vision; IBD, pancreatitis, hepatic tox, ✓ lipids/LFTs regularly; back/jt pain, osteopenia, premature epiphyseal closure; ✓ chol, ↑ triglycerides, ↓ HDL; ↑ CK; ↑ glu **CI:** PRG, hypersens **Disp:** Caps 10, 20, 30, 40 mg **SE:** Dry/chapped lips, cheilitis, dry skin, dermatitis, dry eye, ↓ vision, HA, epistaxis, nasopharyngitis, URI, back pain **Notes:** ✓ Lipids/LFTs before; vit A may ↑ adverse events; avoid tetracyclines and any meds that may interfere w/ BCP effectiveness

Isradipine (DynaCirc, Generic) **Uses:** *HTN* **Acts:** CCB **Dose:** 2.5–5 mg PO bid; IR 2.5–10 mg bid; CR 5–20 qd **W/P:** [C, ?/–] **CI:** Severe heart block, sinus bradycardia, CHF, dosing w/in several hours of IV β-blockers **CI:** Hypotension < 90 mm Hg systolic **Disp:** Caps 2.5, 5 mg; tabs CR 5, 10 mg **SE:** HA, edema, flushing, fatigue, dizziness, palpitations

Itraconazole (Onmel, Sporanox, Generic) **BOX:** CI w/ cisapride, pimozide, quinidine, dofetilide, or levacetylmethadol. Serious CV events (eg, ↑ QT, torsades de pointes, VT, cardiac arrest, and/or sudden death) reported w/ these meds and other CYP3A4 inhib; do not use for onychomycosis w/ ventricular dysfunction; negative inotropic effects have been observed following IV administration; D/C/reasses use if S/Sxs of HF occur during Tx **Uses:** *Fungal Infxns (aspergillosis, blastomycosis, histoplasmosis, candidiasis, onychomycosis)* **Acts:** Azole antifungal, ↓ ergosterol synth **Dose:** Dose based on indication. 200 mg PO qd-tid (caps w/ meals or cola/grapefruit juice); PO soln on empty stomach; avoid antacids **W/P:** [C, –] Numerous interactions **CI:** see PI; PRG or considering PRG; ventricular dysfunction CHF **Disp:** Caps 100, 200 mg; soln 10 mg/mL **SE:** N/V, rash, hepatox, ↓ K+, CHF, ↑ BP, neuropathy **Notes:** Soln & caps not interchangeable; useful in pts who cannot take amphotericin B; follow LFTs

Ivacaftor (Kalydeco) **Uses:** *CF w/ G551D and others in label mutation transmembrane conductance regulator (CFTR) gene* **Acts:** ↑ Chloride transport **Dose: *Adults & Peds > 6 y.*** 150 mg bid; w/ fatty meal; ↓ hepatic impair w/ CYP3A inhib **W/P:** [B, ?/–] w/ CYP3A inhib (ketoconazole, itraconazole, clarithromycin); may ↑ digoxin, cyclosporin, tacrolimus, benzodiazepine levels; w/ hepatic impair Child-Pugh Class C; severe renal impair **Ø Disp:** Tabs 150 mg; granules 50, 75 mg **SE:** HA, URI, oropharyngeal pain, Abd pain, N/D, cataracts **Notes:** ✓ LFTs q3mo × 4, then yearly; D/C if AST/ALT 5 × ULN; use FDA-cleared CF mutation test

Ivermectin, Oral (Stromectol) **Uses:** *Strongyloidiasis (intestinal), onchocerciasis* **Acts:** Binds glutamate-gated chloride channels in nerve and muscle cells, paralysis and death of nematodes **Dose: *Adults & Peds.*** Based on Wt and condition. *Intestinal strongyloidiasis:* 1 tab 15–24 kg, 2 tabs 25–35 kg, 3 tabs 36–50 kg, 4 tabs 51–65 kg, 5 tabs 66–79 kg; ≥ 80 kg 200 mcg/kg *Onchocerciasis:* Repeat dose × 1 in 2 wk, 1 tab 15–25 kg, 2 tabs 26–44 kg, 3 tabs 45–64 kg, 4 tabs 65–84 kg; ≥ 85 kg 150 mcg/kg; on empty stomach **W/P:** [C, ?/–] Potential severe allergic/inflam Rxn Tx of onchocerciasis **CI:** Hypersens **Disp:** Tabs 3 mg **SE:** N/V/D, dizziness, pruritus ↑ AST/ALT; ↓ WBC, RBC **Notes:** From fermented *Streptomyces avermitilis*; does not kill adult onchocerca, requires redosing

Ivermectin, Topical (Sklice, Soolnatra) **Uses:** *Head lice (*Sklice*), rosacea (*Soolnatra*)* **Acts:** Paralysis/death of lice; roseacea ? **Dose: *Adults & Peds > 6 mo.*** *Sklice:* Coat hair & scalp **Adults.** *Soolnatra:* Apply pea-sized amount to affected areas of face qd **W/P:** [C, ?/–] **CI:** Ø **Disp:** *Sklice:* Lotion 0.5%, 4-oz tube; *Soolnatra:* 1% cream 30/45/60 mg tube **SE:** Conjunctivitis, red eye, dry skin (*Sklice*); skin burning/irritation (*Soolnatra*) **Notes:** *Sklice:* coat dry hair & scalp thoroughly; avoid eye contact; use w/ lice management plan

Ixabepilone (Ixempra) **BOX:** CI in combo w/ capecitabine w/ AST/ALT > 2.5 × ULN or bili > 1× ULN d/t ↑ tox and neutropenia-related death **Uses:** *Met/locally advanced breast CA after failure of an anthracycline, a taxane, and capecitabine* **Acts:** Microtubule inhib **Dose:** 40 mg/m² IV over 3 h q3wk, 88 mg max **W/P:** [D, ?/–] **CI:** Hypersens to Cremophor EL; baseline ANC < 1500 cells/mm³ or plt < 100,000 cells/mm³; AST/ or ALT > 2.5 × ULN, bili > 1 × ULN capecitabine **Disp:** Inj 15, 45 mg (use supplied diluent in kit) **SE:** Neutropenia, leukopenia, anemia, thrombocytopenia, peripheral sensory neuropathy, fatigue/asthenia, myalgia/arthralgia, alopecia, N/V/D, stomatitis/mucositis **Notes:** Substrate CYP3A4, adjust dose w/ strong CYP3A4 inhib/ inducers

Japanese Encephalitis Vaccine, Inactivated, Adsorbed (Ixiaro, Je-Vax) **Uses:** *Px Japanese encephalitis* **Acts:** Inactivated vaccine **Dose: Adults.** 0.5 mL IM, repeat 28 d later given at least 1 wk prior to exposure **Peds *1–3 y.*** Use Je-Vax: Three 0.5-mL SQ doses d 0, 7, 30 *> 3 y.* Three 1-mL SQ doses d 0, 7, 30 **W/P:** [B (Ixiaro)/ ?] Severe urticaria or angioedema may occur up to 10 d after vaccination **SE:** HA, fatigue, Inj site pain, flu-like synd, hypersens Rxns **Notes:** Abbrev administration schedules of 3 doses on day 0, 7, and 14; booster dose recommended after 2 y; avoid EtOH 48 h after dose; use is not recommended for all traveling to Asia

Ketamine (Ketalar, Generic) [C-III] **Uses:** *Induction/maintenance of anesthesia* (in combo w/ sedatives), sedation, analgesia **Acts:** Dissociative anesthesia; IV onset 30 s, duration 5–10 min **Dose: Adults.** 1–4.5 mg/kg IV, typical 2 mg/kg; 3–8 mg/kg IM **Peds.** 0.5–2 mg/kg IV; 0.5–1 mg/kg for minor procedures (also IM/PO regimens) **W/P:** w/ CAD, ↑ BP, tachycardia, EtOH use/abuse [C, ?/–] **CI:** When ↑ BP hazardous **Disp:** Soln 10, 50, 100 mg/mL **SE:** Arrhythmia, ↑ / ↓ HR, ↑ / ↓ BP, N/V, resp depression, emergence Rxn, ↑ CSF pressure; CYP2B6 inhibs w/ ↓ metabolism **Notes:** Used in RSI protocols; street drug of abuse

Ketoconazole, Oral (Nizoral, Generic)   **BOX:** (Oral use) Risk of fatal hepatotox; Concomitant terfenadine, astemizole, and cisapride are CI d/t serious CV adverse events **Uses:** *Systemic fungal Infxns (*Candida*, blastomycosis, histoplasmosis, etc); refractory topical dermatophyte Infxn*; PCa when rapid ↓ testosterone needed or hormone refractory **Acts:** Azole, ↓ fungal cell wall synth; high dose blocks P450, to ↓ testosterone production **Dose:** 200 mg PO daily; ↑ to 400 mg PO daily for serious Infxn *PCa:* 400 mg PO tid; best on empty stomach **W/P:** [C, −/−] w/ Any agent that ↑ gastric pH (↓ absorption); may enhance anticoagulants; w/ EtOH (disulfiram-like Rxn); numerous interactions, including statins, niacin; do not use w/ clopidogrel (↓ effect) **CI:** CNS fungal Infxns, w/ astemizole, triazolam **Disp:** Tabs 200 mg **SE:** N, rashes, hair loss, HA, ↑ Wt gain, dizziness, disorientation, fatigue, impotence, hepatox, adrenal suppression, acquired cutaneous adherence ("sticky skin synd") **Notes:** Monitor LFTs; can rapidly ↓ testosterone levels

Ketoconazole, Topical (Extina, Nizoral A-D Shampoo, Xolegel) [Shampoo OTC]   **Uses:** *Topical for seborrheic dermatitis, shampoo for dandruff* local fungal Infxns d/t dermatophytes & yeast **Acts:** Azole, ↓ fungal cell wall synth **Dose:** *Topical:* Apply qd-bid **W/P:** [C, +/−] **Disp:** Topical cream 2%; (*Xolegel*) gel 2%, (*Extina*) foam 2%, shampoo 2% **SE:** Irritation, pruritus, stinging **Notes:** Do not dispense foam into hands

Ketoprofen (Generic)   **BOX:** May ↑ risk of MI/CVA & GI bleeding; CI for periop pain in CABG surgery **Uses:** *Arthritis (RA/OA), pain* **Acts:** NSAID; ↓ prostaglandins **Dose:** 25–75 mg PO tid-qid, 300 mg/d/max; SR 200 mg/d; w/ food; ↓ w/ hepatic/renal impair, elderly **W/P:** [C (D 3rd tri), −] w/ ACE, diuretics; ↑ warfarin, Li, MTX, avoid EtOH **CI:** NSAID/ASA sens **Disp:** Caps 50, 75 mg; caps SR 200 mg **SE:** GI upset, peptic ulcers, dizziness, edema, rash, ↑ BP, ↑ LFTs, renal dysfunction

Ketorolac (Toradol, Generic)   **BOX:** For short-term (≤ 5 d) Rx of mod–severe acute pain; CI w/ PUD, GI bleeding, post-CABG, anticipated major surgery, severe renal Insuff, bleeding diathesis, L&D, nursing, and w/ ASA/NSAIDs; NSAIDs may cause ↑ risk of MI/CVA; PO CI in peds < 16 y; dose adjustments for < 50 kg **Uses:** *Pain* **Acts:** NSAID; ↓ prostaglandins **Dose:** *Adults.* 15–30 mg IV/IM q6h; 10 mg PO qid only as continuation of IM/IV; max IV/IM 120 mg/d, max PO 40 mg/d *Peds 2–16 y.* 1 mg/kg IM × 1 dose; 30 mg max; IV 0.5 mg/kg, 15 mg max; do not use for > 5 d; ↓ if > 65 y, elderly, w/ renal impair, < 50 kg **W/P:** [C (D 3rd tri), −] w/ ACE inhib, diuretics, BP meds, warfarin **CI:** see PI **Disp:** Tabs 10 mg; Inj 15 mg/mL, 30 mg/mL **SE:** Bleeding, peptic ulcer Dz, ↑ Cr & LFTs, ↑ BP, edema, dizziness, allergy

Ketorolac, Nasal (Sprix)   **BOX:** For short-term (≤ 5 d) use; CI w/ PUD, GI bleeding, suspected bleeding risk, post-CABG, advanced renal Dz or risk of renal failure w/ vol depletion; risk CV thrombotic events (MI, stroke); not indicated for use in children **Uses:** *Short-term (≤ 5 d) Rx pain requiring opioid-level analgesia*

Acts: NSAID; ↓ prostaglandins **Dose:** < 65 y. 31.5 mg (one 15.75-mg spray each nostril) q6–8h; max 126 mg/d *≥ 65 y, w/ renal impair or < 50 kg.* 15.75 mg (one 15.75-mg spray in only 1 nostril) q6–8h; max 63 mg/d **W/P:** [C (D 3rd tri), –] Do not use w/ other NSAIDs; can cause severe skin Rxns; do not use w/ critical bleeding risk; w/ CHF **CI:** see PI; prophylactic to major surgery/L&D, w/ Hx allergy to other NSAIDs recent or Hx of GI bleed or perforation **Disp:** Nasal spray 15.75 mg ketorolac/100 mcL spray (8 sprays/bottle) **SE:** Nasal discomfort/rhinitis, ↑ lacrimation, throat irritation, oliguria, rash, ↓ HR, ↓ urine output, ↑ ALT/AST, ↑ BP Notes: Discard open bottle after 24 h

Ketorolac, Ophthalmic (Acular, Acular LS, Acular PF, Acuvail) **Uses:** *Ocular itching w/ seasonal allergies; inflam w/ cataract extraction*; pain/ photophobia w/ incisional refractive surgery *(Acular PF)*; pain w/ corneal refractive surgery *(Acular LS)* **Acts:** NSAID **Dose:** 1 gtt qid **W/P:** [C, +] Possible cross-sens to NSAIDs, ASA **CI:** Hypersens **Disp:** *Acular LS:* 0.4% 5 mL; *Acular:* 0.5% 3, 5, 10 mL; *Acular PF:* Soln 0.5% Acuvail soln 0.45% **SE:** Local irritation, ↑ bleeding ocular tissues, hyphemas, slow healing, keratitis **Notes:** Do not use w/ contacts

Ketotifen (Alaway, Claritin Eye, Zaditor, Zyrtec Itchy Eye) [OTC] **Uses:** *Allergic conjunctivitis* **Acts:** Antihistamine H_1-receptor antag, mast cell stabilizer **Dose:** *Adults & Peds > 3 y.* 1 gtt in eye(s) q8–12h **W/P:** [C, ?/–] **Disp:** Soln 0.025%/5 & 10 mL **SE:** Local irritation, HA, rhinitis, keratitis, mydriasis **Notes:** Wait 10 min before inserting contacts

Kunecatechins [Sinecatechins] (Veregen) **Uses:** *External genital/ perianal warts* **Acts:** Unknown; green tea extract **Dose:** Apply 0.5-cm ribbon to each wart tid until all warts clear; not > 16 wk **W/P:** [C, ?] **Disp:** Oint 15% **SE:** Erythema, pruritus, burning, pain, erosion/ulceration, edema, induration, rash, phimosis **Notes:** Wash hands before/after use; not necessary to wipe off prior to next use; avoid on open wounds, may weaken condoms & Vag diaphragms, use in combo is not recommended

Labetalol (Trandate, Generic) **Uses:** *HTN* & hypertensive emergencies (IV) **Acts:** α- & β-Adrenergic blockers **Dose:** *Adults.* HTN: Initial 100 mg PO bid, then 200–400 mg PO bid *Hypertensive emergency:* 20–80 mg IV bolus, then 2 mg/ min IV Inf, titrate up to 300 mg *ECC 2010.* 10 mg IV over 1–2 min; repeat or double dose q10min (150 mg max); or initial bolus, then 2–8 mg/min **Peds.** PO: 1–3 mg/kg/d in ÷ doses, 1200 mg/d max *Hypertensive emergency:* 0.4–1.5 mg/kg/h IV cont Inf **W/P:** [C (D in 2nd or 3rd tri), +] **CI:** Asthma/COPD, cardiogenic shock, uncompensated CHF, heart block, sinus bradycardia **Disp:** Tabs 100, 200, 300 mg; Inj 5 mg/mL **SE:** Dizziness, N, ↓ BP, fatigue, CV effects

Lacosamide (Vimpat) **Uses:** *Adjunct in partial-onset Szs* **Acts:** Anticonvulsant **Dose:** *Initial:* 50 mg IV or PO bid, ↑ weekly; *Maint:* 200–400 mg/d; 300 mg/d max if CrCl < 30 mL/min or mild–mod hepatic Dz **W/P:** [C, ?] DRESS ↑ PR [C–V] Antiepileptics associated w/ ↑ risk of suicide ideation **CI:** Ø **Disp:** IV

200 mg/20 mL; tabs 50, 100, 150, 200 mg; oral soln 10 mg/mL **SE:** Dizziness, N/V, ataxia **Notes:** ✓ ECG before dosing

Lactic Acid/Ammonium Hydroxide [Ammonium Lactate] (Lac-Hydrin)
[OTC] Uses: *Severe xerosis & ichthyosis* **Acts:** Emollient moisturizer, humectant **Dose:** Apply bid **W/P:** [B, ?] **Disp:** Cream, lotion, lactic acid 12% w/ ammonium hydroxide **SE:** Local irritation, photosens **Notes:** Shake well before use

Lactobacillus (Lactinex Granules) [OTC] Uses: *Control of D*, especially after abx Rx **Acts:** Replaces nl intestinal flora, lactase production; *Lactobacillus acidophilus* and *Lactobacillus helveticus* **Dose:** *Adults & Peds > 3 y.* 1 packet, 1–2 caps, or 4 tabs qd-qid **W/P:** [A, +] Some products may contain whey **CI:** Milk/lactose allergy **Disp:** Tabs, caps, granules in packets (all OTC) **SE:** Flatulence **Notes:** May take granules on food

Lactulose (Constulose, Enulose, Generlac, Others) Uses: *Hepatic encephalopathy; constipation* **Acts:** Acidifies the colon, allows ammonia to diffuse into colon; osmotic effect to ↑ peristalsis **Dose:** *Adults. Acute hepatic encephalopathy:* 30–45 mL PO q1h until soft stools, then tid-qid, adjust 2–3 stool/d *Constipation:* 15–30 mL/d, ↑ to 60 mL/d 1–2 ÷ doses, adjust to 2–3 stools *Rectally:* 200 g in 700 mL of H₂O PR, retain 30–60 min q4–6h *Peds Infants.* 2.5–10 mL/24 h ÷ tid-qid *Other Peds.* 40–90 mL/24 h ÷ tid-qid *Constipation:* 1–3 mL/kg/d ÷ doses (max 60 mL/d) PO after breakfast **W/P:** [B, ?] **CI:** Galactosemia **Disp:** Syrup 10 g/15 mL, soln 10 g/15 mL, 10, 20 g/packet **SE:** Severe D, N/V, cramping, flatulence; life-threatening lyte disturbances

Lamivudine (Epivir, Epivir-HBV, 3TC [Many Combo Regimens])
BOX: Lactic acidosis & severe hepatomegal w/ steatosis reported w/ nucleoside analogs; do not use Epivir-HBV for Tx of HIV; monitor pts closely following D/C of therapy for hep B; HIV-1 resistance possible in pts w/ unrecognized/untreated HIV-1 **Uses:** *HIV Infxn, chronic hep B* **Acts:** NRTI, ↓ HIV RT & hep B viral polymerase, causes viral DNA chain termination **Dose:** *HIV: Adults & Peds > 16 y.* 150 mg PO bid or 300 mg PO daily *Peds able to swallow pills. 14–21 kg:* 75 mg bid; *22–29 kg:* 75 mg q A.M., 150 mg q P.M. *> 30 kg:* 150 mg bid *Neonates < 30 d:* 2 mg/kg bid; infants 1–3 mo: 4 mg/kg/dose; *3 mo–16 y.* 4 mg/kg/dose bid (max 150 mg bid) *Epivir-HBV: Adults.* 100 mg/d PO. *Peds 2–17 y.* 3 mg/kg/d PO, 100 mg max; ↓ w/ CrCl < 50 mL/min **W/P:** [C, ?] w/ Interferon-α and ribavirin may cause liver failure; do not use w/ zalcitabine or w/ ganciclovir/valganciclovir **Disp:** Tabs 100 mg (Epivir-HBV) 150 mg, 300 mg); soln 5 mg/mL (Epivir-HBV), 10 mg/mL **SE:** Malaise, fatigue, N/V/D, HA, pancreatitis, lactic acidosis, peripheral neuropathy, fat redistribution, rhabdomyolysis hyperglycemia, nasal Sxs **Notes:** Differences in formulations; do not use Epivir-HBV for hep in pt w/ unrecognized HIV d/t rapid emergence of HIV resistance

Lamotrigine (Lamictal) BOX: Life-threatening rashes, including SJS and toxic epidermal necrolysis, and/or rash-related death reported; D/C at 1st sign of rash **Uses:** *Epilepsy adjunct ≥ 2 y or monoRx ≥ 16 y; bipolar disorder ≥ 18 y*

Acts: Phenyltriazine antiepileptic, ↓ glutamate, stabilize neuronal membrane **Dose:** *Adults. Szs:* Initial 50 mg/d PO, then 50 mg PO bid × 1–2 wk, maint 300–500 mg/d in 2 ÷ doses *Bipolar:* Initial 25 mg/d PO × 1–2 wk, 50 mg PO daily for 2 wk, 100 mg PO daily for 1 wk, maint 200 mg/d *Peds.* 0.6 mg/kg in 2 ÷ doses for wk 1 & 2, then 1.2 mg/kg for wk 3 & 4, q1–2wk to maint 5–15 mg/kg/d (max 400 mg/d) in 1–2 ÷ doses; ↓ hepatic Dz or w/ enzyme inducers or valproic acid **W/P:** [C, –] ↑ suicide risk; ↓ for those w/ epilepsy vs psych use; interact w/ other antiepileptics, estrogen, rifampin **Disp:** (color-coded for use w/ interacting meds); starter titrate kits; tabs 25, 100, 150, 200 mg; chew tabs 2, 5, 25 mg; ODT 25, 50, 100, 200 mg **SE:** Photosens, HA, GI upset, dizziness, diplopia, blurred vision, blood dyscrasias, ataxia, rash (more life-threatening in peds vs adults), aseptic meningitis **Notes:** Value of therapeutic monitoring uncertain, taper w/ D/C

Lamotrigine, Extended Release (Lamictal XR) BOX: Life-threatening rashes, including SJS and toxic epidermal necrolysis, and/or rash-related death reported; D/C at 1st sign of rash **Uses:** *Adjunct primary generalized tonic-clonic Sz, conversion to monotherapy in pt > 13 y w/ partial Szs* **Acts:** Phenyltriazine antiepileptic, ↓ glutamate, stabilize neuronal membrane **Dose:** Adjunct target 200–600 mg/d; monotherapy conversion target dose 250–300 mg/d *Adults & Peds > 13 y. w/ Valproate:* 25 mg q other day wk 1–2, 25 mg qd wk 3–4, 50 mg qd wk 5, 100 mg qd wk 6, 150 mg qd wk 7, then maint 200–250 mg qd *w/o Carbamazepine, phenytoin, phenobarbital, primidone, or valproate:* 25 mg qd wk 1–2, 50 mg qd wk 3–4, 100 mg qd wk 5, 150 mg qd wk 6, 200 mg qd wk 7, then maint 300–400 mg qd *Convert IR to ER tabs:* Initial dose = total daily dose of IR. *Convert adjunctive to monotherapy:* Maint: 250–300 mg qd, see PI *w/OCP:* see PI **W/P:** [C, –] Interacts w/ other antiepileptics, estrogen (OCP), rifampin; valproic acid ↑ levels at least 2×; ↑ suicidal ideation; withdrawal Szs **CI:** Component hypersens (see PI) **Disp:** Tabs 25, 50, 100, 150, 200, 250, 300 mg **SE:** Dizziness, tremor/intention tremor, V, diplopia, rash (more life-threatening in peds than adults), aseptic meningitis, blood dyscrasias **Notes:** Taper over 2 wk w/ D/C

Lansoprazole (Prevacid, Prevacid 24HR [OTC]) **Uses:** *Duodenal ulcers, Px & Rx NSAID gastric ulcers, active gastric ulcers, H. pylori Infxn, erosive esophagitis, & hypersecretory conditions, GERD* **Acts:** PPI **Dose:** 15–30 mg/d PO *NSAID ulcer prevention:* 15 mg/d PO = 12 wk *NSAID ulcers:* 30 mg/d PO × 8 wk *Hypersecretory condition:* 60 mg/d before food; doses of 90 mg had been used; ↓ w/ severe hepatic impair **W/P:** [B, ?/–] w/ Clopidogrel **Disp:** *Prevacid:* DR caps 15, 30 mg; *Prevacid 24HR* [OTC] 15 mg; *Prevacid SoluTab* (ODT) 15, 30 mg (contains phenylalanine) **SE:** N/V, Abd pain, HA, fatigue **Notes:** Do not crush/chew; granules can be given w/ applesauce or apple juice (NG tube) only; ? ↑ risk of fractures w/ all PPI; caution w/ ODT in feeding tubes; risk of hypomagnesemia w/ long-term use; monitor

Lanthanum Carbonate (Fosrenol) **Uses:** *Hyperphosphatemia in end-stage renal Dz* **Acts:** Phosphate binder **Dose:** 750–1500 mg PO daily in ÷ doses, w/ or immediately after meal; titrate q2–3wk based on PO_4^{2-} levels **W/P:** [C, ?/–]

No data in GI Dz; not for peds **CI:** Bowel obstruction, fecal impaction, ileus **Disp:** Chew tabs 500, 750, 1000 mg; oral powder 750, 1000 mg **SE:** N/V, graft occlusion, HA, ↓ BP **Notes:** Chew tabs before swallowing; separate from meds that interact w/ antacids by 2 h

Lapatinib (Tykerb) BOX: Hepatotox has been reported (severe or fatal) **Uses:** *Advanced breast CA w/ capecitabine w/ tumors that over-express HER2 and failed w/ anthracycline, taxane, & trastuzumab* and in combo w/ letrozole in postmenopausal women **Acts:** TKI **Dose:** Per protocol, 1250 mg PO d 1–21 w/ capecitabine 2000 mg/m²/d ÷ 2 doses/d on d 1–14; 1500 mg PO daily in combo w/ letrozole; ↓ w/ severe cardiac or hepatic impair **W/P:** [D, ?/+] Avoid CYP3A4 inhib/inducers **CI:** Component hypersens **Disp:** Tabs 250 mg **SE:** N/V/D, anemia, ↓ plt, neutropenia, ↑ QT interval, hand-foot synd, ↑ LFTs, rash, ↓ left ventricular ejection fraction, interstitial lung Dz and pneumonitis **Notes:** Consider baseline LVEF & periodic ECG & LFTs at baseline & during Tx

Latanoprost (Xalatan) **Uses:** *Open-angle glaucoma, ocular HTN* **Acts:** Prostaglandin, ↑ outflow of aqueous humor **Dose:** 1 gtt eye(s) hs **W/P:** [C, M] **Disp:** 0.005% soln **SE:** May darken light irides; blurred vision, ocular stinging, & itching, ↑ number & length of eyelashes **Notes:** Wait 15 min before using contacts; separate from other eye products by 5 min

Ledipasvir/Sofosbuvir (Harvoni) **Uses:** *Chronic hep C genotype 1* **Acts:** Direct hep C antiviral **Dose:** 90 mg/400 mg PO qd × 12 wk (Tx-naïve w/ or w/o cirrhosis & tx-experienced w/o cirrhosis) or × 24 wk (Tx-experienced w/ cirrhosis) **W/P:** [B, ?/–] Avoid w/ amiodarone & P-gp inducers **CI:** Ø **Disp:** Tabs (ledipasvir/sofosbuvir) 90/400 mg **SE:** HA, fatigue, N/D, insomnia, ↑ lipase, ↑ bili

Leflunomide (Arava) BOX: PRG must be excluded prior to start of Rx; hepatotox; Tx should not be initiated in pts w/ acute or chronic liver Dz **Uses:** *Active RA, orphan drug for organ rejection* **Acts:** DMARD, ↓ pyrimidine synth **Dose:** Initial 100 mg/d PO for 3 d, then 10–20 mg/d **W/P:** [X, –] w/ Bile acid sequestrants, warfarin, rifampin, MTX; not rec in pts w/ preexisting liver Dz **CI:** PRG **Disp:** Tabs 10, 20 mg **SE:** D, Infxn, HTN, alopecia, rash, N, jt pain, hep, interstitial lung Dz, immunosuppressive peripheral neuropathy **Notes:** Monitor monthly & at baseline LFTs, D/C therapy if ALT > 3 × ULN & begin drug elimination procedure, CBC, PO₋₃⁴ during initial Rx; vaccine should be up-to-date, do not give w/ live vaccines

Lenalidomide (Revlimid) BOX: Significant teratogen; pt must be enrolled in RevAssist risk-reduction program; hematologic tox; DVT & PE risk **Uses:** *MDS, combo w/ dexamethasone in multiple myeloma in pt failing one prior Rx* **Acts:** Thalidomide analog, immune modulator **Dose:** **Adults.** MDS: 10 mg PO qd; swallow whole w/ water; multiple myeloma 25 mg/d d 1–21 of 28-d cycle w/ protocol dose of dexamethasone **W/P:** [X, –] w/ Renal impair **CI:** PRG **Disp:** Caps 2.5, 5, 10, 15, 20, 25 mg **SE:** D, pruritus, rash, fatigue, night sweats, edema, nasopharyngitis, ↓ BM (plt, WBC), ↑ K⁺, ↑ LFTs, thromboembolism **Notes:** Monitor

CBC and for thromboembolism, hepatotox; routine PRG tests required; Rx only in 1-mo increments; limited distribution network; males must use condom and not donate sperm; use at least 2 forms contraception > 4 wk beyond D/C; see PI for dose adjustments based on nonhematologic & hematologic tox

Lenvatinib (Lenvima) Uses: *Locally recurrent/met radioactive iodine-refractory thyroid CA* Acts: Kinase inhib Dose: 24 mg PO qd; ↓ to 14 mg PO qd w/CrCl < 30 mL/min or w/ severe hepatic impair W/P: [D, −] see PI for dose modifications based on tox; ↑ BP, cardiac failure, arterial thromboembolic events, hepatotox, ✓ LFT/UA baseline and periodically, renal impair/failure, GI perf/fistula, ↑ QT interval, ↓ Ca⁺² (✓ Ca⁺² qmo), RPLS, bleeding, TSH suppression (✓ TSH qmo), embryo-fetal tox CI: Ø Disp: Caps 4, 10 mg SE: N/V/D, Abd pain, stomatitis, dry mouth, ↓ appetite, ↓ Wt, HA, ↑ BP, fatigue, arthralgia, myalgia, dysphonia, cough, proteinuria, palmar–plantar erythrodysesthesia synd, rash, alopecia

Lepirudin (Refludan) Uses: *HIT* Acts: Direct thrombin inhib Dose: *Bolus:* 0.4 mg/kg IV push, then 0.15 mg/kg/h Inf; if > 110 kg, 44 mg of Inf 16.5 mg/h max; ↓ dose & Inf rate if CrCl < 60 mL/min or if used w/ thrombolytics W/P: [B, ?/−] Hemorrhagic event or severe HTN CI: Active bleeding Disp: Inj 50 mg SE: Bleeding, anemia, hematoma, anaphylaxis Notes: Adjust based on aPTT ratio, maintain aPTT 1.5–2.5 × control; S/Sxs of bleeding

Letrozole (Femara) Uses: *Breast CA: Adjuvant w/postmenopausal hormone receptor-positive early Dz; adjuvant in postmenopausal women w/ early breast CA w/ prior adjuvant tamoxifen therapy; 1st/2nd line in postmenopausal w/ hormone receptor-positive or unknown* Dz Acts: Nonsteroidal aromatase inhib Dose: 2.5 mg/d PO; q other day w/ severe liver Dz or cirrhosis W/P: [D, ?] [X, ?/−] CI: PRG, women who may become pregnant Disp: Tabs 2.5 mg SE: Anemia, N, hot flashes, arthralgia, hypercholesterolemia, decreased BMD, CNS depression Notes: Monitor CBC, TFT, lytes, LFTs, SCr, BP, bone density, cholesterol

Leucovorin (Generic) Uses: *OD of folic acid antag; megaloblastic anemia, augment 5-FU, impaired MTX elimination; w/ 5-FU in colon CA* Acts: Reduced folate source; circumvents action of folate reductase inhib (eg, MTX) Dose: *Leucovorin rescue:* 10 mg/m² PO/IM/IV q6h; start w/in 24 h after dose or 15 mg PO/IM/IV q6h, for 10 doses until MTX level < 0.05 micromole/L *Folate antagonist OD (eg, Pemetrexed):* 100 mg/m² IM/IV × 1, then 50 mg/m² IM/IV q6h × 8 d; 5-FU adjuvant Tx, colon CA per protocol; low dose: 20 mg/m²/d IV × 5 d w/ 5-FU 425 mg/m²/d IV × 5 d, repeat q4–5wk × 6; high dose: 200 mg/m² in combo w/ 5-FU 370 mg/m² *Megaloblastic anemia:* 1 mg IM/IV daily W/P: [C, ?/−] CI: Pernicious anemia or vit B₁₂-deficient megaloblastic anemias Disp: Tabs 5, 10, 15, 25 mg; Inj 50, 100, 200, 350, 500 mg SE: Allergic Rxn, N/V/D, fatigue, wheezing, ↑ plt Notes: Monitor Cr, methotrexate levels q24h w/ leucovorin rescue; do not use intrathecally/intraventricularly; w/ 5-FU CBC w/ diff, plt, LFTs, lytes

Leuprolide (Eligard, Lupron, Lupron DEPOT, Lupron DEPOT-Ped, Generic) Uses: *Advanced PCa (all except Depot-Ped), endometriosis

(*Lupron*), uterine fibroids (*Lupron*), & precocious puberty (*Lupron-Ped*)* **Acts:** LHRH agonist; paradoxically ↓ release of GnRH w/ ↓ LH from anterior pituitary; in ♂ ↓ testosterone; in ♀ ↓ estrogen **Dose:** *Adults.* PCa: *Lupron DEPOT:* 7.5 mg IM q28d or 22.5 mg IM q3mo or 30 mg IM q4mo or 45 mg IM q6mo) *Eligard:* 7.5 mg SQ q28d or 22.5 mg SQ q3mo or 30 mg SQ q4mo or 45 mg SQ 6 mo *Endometriosis (Lupron DEPOT):* 3.75 mg IM qmo × 6 or 11.25 IM q3mo × 2 *Fibroids:* 3.75 mg IM qmo × 3 or 11.25 mg IM × 1. *Peds.* CPP (*Lupron DEPOT-Ped*): 50 mcg/kg/d SQ Inj; ↑ by 10 mcg/kg/d until total downregulation achieved *Lupron DEPOT:* < **25 kg:** 7.5 mg IM q4wk; > **25–37.5 kg:** 11.25 mg IM q4wk; > **37.5 kg:** 15 mg IM q4wk, ↑ by 3.75 mg q4wk until response **W/P:** [X, –] w/ Impending cord compression in PCa, ↑ QT w/ meds or preexisting CV Dz **CI:** AUB, implant in women/peds; PRG **Disp:** Inj 5 mg/mL; *Lupron DEPOT:* 3.75 mg (1 mo for fibroids, endometriosis); *Lupron DEPOT* for PCa: 7.5 mg (1 mo), 11.25 (3 mo), 22.5 (3 mo), 30 (4 mo), 45 mg (6 mo); *Eligard depot* for PCA: 7.5 (1 mo); 22.5 (3 mo), 30 (4 mo), 45 mg (6 mo); *Lupron DEPOT-Ped:* 7.5, 11.25, 15, 30 mg **SE:** Hot flashes, gynecomastia, N/V, alopecia, anorexia, dizziness, HA, insomnia, paresthesias, depression exacerbation, peripheral edema, & bone pain (transient "flare Rxn" at 7–14 d after the 1st dose [LH/testosterone surge before suppression]); ↓ BMD w/ > 6 mo use, bone loss possible, abnormal menses, hyperglycemia **Notes:** Nonsteroidal antiandrogen (eg, bicalutamide) may block flare in men w/ PCa; *Viadur* implant no new Rx

Leuprolide Acetate/Norethindrone Acetate Kit (Lupaneta Pack) **Uses:** *Painful endometriosis* **Acts:** GnRH agonist w/ a progestin **Dose:** Leuprolide 11.25 mg IM q3mo × 2 w/ norethindrone 5 mg PO daily, 6 mo total; if symptoms recur, consider another 6 mo Tx **W/P:** [B, ?/–] Assess BMD before; monitor for depression; D/C w/ vision loss/changes **CI:** Component sens; AUB, PRG, breast-feeding, Hx breast/hormonally sens Ca, thrombosis, liver tumor or Dz **Disp:** Co-packaged leuprolide 11.25-mg depot w/ 90 norethindrone 5-mg tabs **SE:** *Leuprolide:* hot flashes/sweats, HA/migraine, depression/emotional lability, N/V, nervousness/anxiety, insomnia, pain, acne, asthenia, vaginitis, ↑ Wt, constipation/diarrhea; *norethindrone:* breakthrough bleeding/spotting **Notes:** Use non-hormonal methods of contraception

Levalbuterol (Xopenex, Xopenex HFA) **Uses:** *Asthma (Rx & Px of bronchospasm)* **Acts:** Sympathomimetic bronchodilator; *R*-isomer of albuterol β_2-agonist **Dose:** Based on NIH Guidelines 2007 *Adults.* Acute–severe exacerbation Xopenex HFA 4–8 puffs q20min up to 4 h, the q1–4h PRN or nebulizer 1.25–2.5 mg q20min × 3, then 1.25–5 mg q1–4h PRN *Peds* < **5 y.** Quick relief: 0.31–1.25 mg q4–6h PRN; severe: 1.25 mg q20min × 3, then 0.075–0.15 mg/kg q1–4h PRN, 5 mg max **5–11 y.** Acute–severe exacerbation: 1.25 mg q20min × 3, then 0.075–0.15 mg/kg q1–4h PRN, 5 mg max; quick relief: 0.31–0.63 q8h PRN > **12 y.** 0.63–1.25 mg nebulizer q8h **W/P:** [C, M] w/ Non–K⁺-sparing diuretics, CAD, HTN, arrhythmias, ↓ K⁺, hyperthyroidism, glaucoma, diabetes **CI:** Component hypersens **Disp:** MDI

(*Xopenex HFA*) 45 mcg/puff (15 g); soln nebulizer Inh 0.31, 0.63, 1.25 mg/3 mL; concentrate 1.25 mg/0.5 mL **SE:** Paradoxical bronchospasm, anaphylaxis, angioedema, tachycardia, nervousness, V, ↓ K+ **Notes:** May ↑ CV SEs compared w/ albuterol; do not mix w/ other nebs or dilute

Levetiracetam (Elepsia XR, Keppra, Keppra XR, Generic) Uses:
Adjunctive PO Rx in partial-onset Sz (adults & peds ≥ 4 y), myoclonic Szs (adults & peds ≥ 12 y) w/ JME, PGTC Szs (adults & peds ≥ 6 y) w/ idiopathic generalized epilepsy; adjunctive Inj Rx partial-onset Szs in adults w/ epilepsy; myoclonic Szs in adults w/ JME; Inj alternative for adults (≥ 16 y) when PO not possible **Acts:** Unknown **Dose:** *Adults & Peds > 16 y.* 500 mg PO bid, titrate q2wk, may ↑ 3000 mg/d max *Peds 4–15 y.* 10 mg/kg/dose ÷ bid to max 60 mg/kg/d (↓ in renal Insuff) **W/P:** [C, ?/–] Elderly, w/ renal impair, psychological disorders; ↑ suicidality risk for antiepileptic drugs, higher for those w/ epilepsy vs those using drug for psychological indications; Inj not for < 16 y **CI:** Component allergy **Disp:** Tabs 250, 500, 750, 1000 mg; tabs ER 500, 750 mg; soln 100 mg/mL; Inj 100 mg/mL **SE:** Dizziness, somnolence, HA, N/V, hostility, aggression, hallucinations, hematologic abnormalities, impaired coordination **Notes:** Do not D/C abruptly; postmarket hepatic failure and pancytopenia reported

Levobunolol (A-K Beta, Betagan) Uses:
Open-angle glaucoma, ocular HTN **Acts:** β-Adrenergic blocker **Dose:** 1 gtt daily-bid **W/P:** [C, M] w/ Verapamil or systemic β-blockers **CI:** Asthma, COPD, sinus bradycardia, heart block (2nd-, 3rd-degree) CHF **Disp:** Soln 0.25, 0.5% **SE:** Ocular stinging/burning, ↓ HR, ↓ BP **Notes:** Possible systemic effects if absorbed

Levocetirizine (Xyzal) Uses:
Perennial/seasonal allergic rhinitis, chronic urticaria **Acts:** Antihistamine **Dose:** *Adults.* 5 mg qd *Peds 6 mo–5 y.* 1.25 mg qd *6–11 y.* 2.5 mg qd **W/P:** [B, ?/–] ↓ Adult dose w/ renal impair, CrCl 50–80 mL/min: 2.5 mg qd, 30–50 mL/min: 2.5 mg q other day, 10–30 mL/min: 2.5 mg 2×/wk **CI:** Peds 6–11 y. w/ renal impair, adults w/ ESRD **Disp:** Tabs 5 mg, soln 0.5 mL/mL (150 mL) **SE:** CNS depression, drowsiness, fatigue, xerostomia **Notes:** Take in evening

Levofloxacin (Levaquin, Generic) BOX:
↑ Risk Achilles tendon rupture and tendonitis, may exacerbate muscle weakness related to myastheria gravis **Uses:** *SSSI, UTI, chronic bacterial prostatitis, acute pyelo, acute bacterial sinusitis, acute bacterial exacerbation of chronic bronchitis, CAP, including multidrug-resistant S. pneumoniae, nosocomial pneumonia; Rx Inh anthrax in adults & peds ≥ 6 mo* **Acts:** Quinolone, ↓ DNA gyrase. Spectrum: Excellent gram(+) except MRSA & *E. faecium*; excellent gram(–) except Stenotrophomonas maltophilia & Acinetobacter sp; poor anaerobic **Dose:** *Adults ≥ 18 y.* IV/PO: *Bronchitis:* 500 mg qd × 7 d *CAP:* 500 mg qd × 7–14 d or 750 mg qd × 5 d *Sinusitis:* 500 mg qd × 10–14 d or 750 mg qd × 5 d *Prostatitis:* 500 mg qd × 28 d *Uncomp SSSI:* 500 mg qd × 7–10 d *Comp SSSI/nosocomial pneumonia:* 750 mg qd × 7–14 d *Anthrax:* 500 mg qd × 60 d *Uncomp UTI:* 250 mg qd × 3 d *Comp UTI/acute pyelo:* 250 mg

qd × 10 d or 750 mg qd × 5 d; CrCl 10–19 mL/min: 500 mg, then 250 mg q other day or 750 mg, then 500 mg q48h *Hemodialysis:* 750 mg, then 500 mg q48h *Peds ≥ 6 mo. Anthrax > 50 kg:* 500 mg q24h × 60 d, < 50 kg 8 mg/kg (250 mg/dose max) q12h for 60 d, ↓ w/ renal impair, avoid antacids w/ PO; oral soln 1 h before, 2 h after meals *CAP:* ≥ 6 mo–≤ 4 y 8 mg/kg/dose q12h (max 750 mg/d), 5–16 y 8 mg/kg/dose qd (750 mg max) **W/P:** [C, −] w/ Cation-containing products (eg, antacids), w/ drugs that ↑ QT interval **CI:** Quinolone sens **Disp:** Tabs 250, 500, 750 mg; premixed IV 250, 500, 750 mg; Inj 25 mg/mL; *Leva-Pak* 750 mg × 5 d **SE:** N/D, dizziness, rash, GI upset, photosens, CNS stimulant w/ IV use, *C. difficile* enterocolitis; rare fatal hepatox, peripheral neuropathy, delirium, tendon rupture **Notes:** Use w/ steroids ↑ tendon rupture risk; only for anthrax in peds

Levofloxacin Ophthalmic (Iquix, Quixin) Uses: *Bacterial conjunctivitis* Acts: See Levofloxacin Dose: 1–2 gtt in eye(s) q2h while awake up to 8×/d × 2 d, then q4h while awake × 5 d **W/P:** [C, −] **CI:** Quinolone sens **Disp:** 25 mg/mL ophthal soln 0.5% (Quixin), 1.5% (Iquix) **SE:** Ocular burning/ pain, ↓ vision, fever, foreign body sensation, HA, pharyngitis, photophobia

Levomilnacipran (Fetzima) BOX: Risk of suicidal thoughts/behavior in children, adolescents, and young adults; monitor for worsening depression and emergence of suicidal thoughts/behaviors Uses: *Depression in adults* Acts: SNRI Dose: *Adults.* 20 mg qd for 2 d, then 40 mg qd; may ↑ by 40 mg every 2 days to 120 mg max; usual 40–120 mg/d; ↓ w/ CrCl < 60 mL/min *Peds.* Not approved **W/P:** [C, ?/-] CDC rec: HIV-infected mothers not breast-feed (transmission risk); see PI; serotonin synd w/ certain meds: tricyclics, lithium, triptans, fentanyl, tramadol, buspirone, St John's Wort; SSRIs & SNRIs may cause ↓ Na+; ↑ BP, ↑ HR; ↑ risk of bleeding w/ASA, NSAIDs, warfarin; urinary retention/hesitancy; may elicit mania in bipolar pts presenting w/ depression **Disp:** ER caps, 20, 40, 80, 120 mg **CI:** Hypersens; do not use w/MAOI, linezolid, or methylene blue (serotonin synd risk); uncontrolled NAG, ESRD **SE:** N/V, ED, testicular pain, ejaculation disorder, hyperhidrosis **Notes:** 80 mg/d max w/strong CYP3A4 inhib; with abrupt D/C confusion, dysphoria, irritability, agitation, anxiety, insomnia, paresthesias, HA & insomnia can occur; taper dose and monitor w/ D/C; EtOH may accelerate drug release

Levonorgestrel (Next Choice, Plan B One-Step [OTC], Generic [OTC]) Uses: *Emergency contraceptive ("morning-after pill")* Acts: Prevents PRG if taken < 72 h after unprotected sex/contraceptive failure; progestin, alters tubal transport & endometrium Dose: *Adults & Peds (postmenarche ♀)* w/in 72 h of unprotected intercourse: *Next Choice* 0.75 mg q12h × 2 ♀ ≤ 17 y. *Plan B One-Step* 1.5 mg × 1 (OTC) **W/P:** [X, M] w/ AUB; may ↑ ectopic PRG risk **CI:** Known/suspected PRG **Disp:** *Next Choice* tab, 0.75 mg, 2 blister packs; *Plan B One-Step* tab, 1.5 mg, 1 blister pack **SE:** N/V/D, Abd pain, fatigue, HA, menstrual changes, dizziness, breast changes **Notes:** Will not induce Ab w/ PRG; federal court ruling in 2013 made these emergency contraceptives OTC w/o age or point-of-sale restrictions; Plan B open purchase; next choice behind counter; no Rx

Levonorgestrel IUD (Liletta, Mirena) Uses: *Contraception, long-term (3–5 y)* **Acts:** Progestin, alters endometrium, thicken cervical mucus, inhibits ovulation and implantation **Dose:** *Liletta:* up to 3 y; *Mirena:* up to 5 y; insert w/in 7 d menses onset or immediately after 1st-tri Ab; wait 6 wk if postpartum; replace any time during menstrual cycle **W/P:** [X, M] **CI:** PRG, w/ active hepatic Dz or tumor, uterine anomaly, breast Ca, acute/Hx of PID, postpartum endometriosis, infected Ab last 3 mo, gynecological neoplasia, abnormal Pap, AUB, untreated cervicitis/vaginitis, multiple sex partners, ↑ susceptibility to Infxn **Disp:** 52 mg IUD **SE:** Failed insertion, ectopic PRG, sepsis, PID, infertility, PRG comps w/ IUD left in place, Ab, embedment, ovarian cysts, perforation uterus/cervix, intestinal obst/perforation, peritonitis, N, Abd pain, ↑ BP, acne, HA **Notes:** Inform pt does not protect against STD/HIV; see PI for insertion instructions; reexamine placement after 1st menses; 80% PRG w/in 12 mo of removal; *Liletta:* evaluate pt 4–6 wk after insertion, then annually

Levorphanol (Levo-Dromoran) [C-II] Uses: *Mod–severe pain; chronic pain* **Acts:** Narcotic analgesic, morphine derivative **Dose:** 2–4 mg PO PRN q6–8h; ↓ in hepatic impair **W/P:** [B/D (prolonged use/high doses at term), ?/–] w/ ↑ ICP, head trauma, adrenal Insuff **CI:** Component allergy, PRG **Disp:** Tabs 2 mg **SE:** Tachycardia, ↓ BP, drowsiness, GI upset, constipation, resp depression, pruritus

Levothyroxine (Levoxyl, Synthroid, Others) BOX: Not for obesity or Wt loss; tox w/ high doses, especially when combined w/ sympathomimetic amines Uses: *Hypothyroidism, pituitary TSH suppression, myxedema coma* **Acts:** T$_4$ supl l-thyroxine **Dose:** *Adults. Hypothyroid:* titrate until euthyroid; > 50 y w/o heart Dz or < 50 w/ heart Dz 25–50 mcg/d, ↑ q6–8wk; > 50 y w/ heart Dz 12.5–25 mcg/d, ↑ q6–8wk; usual 100–200 mcg/d *Myxedema:* 200–500 mcg IV, then 100–300 mcg/d *Peds. Hypothyroid: 1–3 mo:* 10–15 mcg/kg/24 h PO; *3–6 mo:* 8–10 mcg/kg/d PO; *6–12 mo:* 6–8 mcg/kg/d PO; *1–5 y:* 5–6 mcg/kg/d PO; *6–12 y:* 4–5 mcg/kg/d PO; > *12 y:* 2–3 mcg/kg/d PO; if growth and puberty complete 1.7 mcg/kg/d; ↓ dose by 50% if IV; titrate based on response & thyroid tests; dose can ↑ rapidly in young/middle-aged; best on empty stomach **W/P:** [A, M] Many drug interactions; in elderly w/ CV Dz; thyrotoxicosis; w/ warfarin monitor INR **CI:** Recent MI, uncorrected adrenal Insuff **Disp:** Tabs 25, 50, 75, 88, 100, 112, 125, 137, 150, 175, 200, 300 mcg; Inj 100, 500 mcg **SE:** Insomnia, Wt loss, N/V/D, ↑ LFTs, irregular periods, ↓ BMD, alopecia, arrhythmia **Notes:** Take w/ full glass of water (prevents choking); PRG may ↑ need for higher doses; takes 6 wk to see effect on TSH; wait 6 wk before checking TSH after dose change

Lidocaine, Systemic (Xylocaine, Others) Uses: *Rx cardiac arrhythmias* **Acts:** Class IB antiarrhythmic **Dose:** *Adults. Antiarrhythmic, ET:* 5 mg/kg; follow w/ 0.5 mg/kg in 10 min if effective *IV load:* 1 mg/kg/dose bolus over 2–3 min; repeat in 5–10 min; 200–300 mg/h max; cont Inf 20–50 mcg/kg/min or 1–4 mg/min *ECC 2010. Cardiac arrest from VF/VT refractory VF: Initial:* 1–1.5 mg/kg IV/IO, additional 0.5–0.75 mg/kg IV push, repeat in 5–10 min, max total

3 mg/kg *ET:* 2–4 mg/kg as last resort *Reperfusing stable VT, wide complex tachycardia, or ectopy:* Doses of 0.5–0.75 mg/kg to 1–1.5 mg/kg may be used initially; repeat 0.5–0.75 mg/kg q5–10min; max dose 3 mg/kg **Peds. ECC 2010.** *VF/pulseless VT, wide-complex tach (w/ pulses):* 1 mg/kg IV/IO, then maint 20–50 mcg/kg/min (repeat bolus if Inf started > 15 min after initial dose); RSI: 1–2 mg/kg IV/IO **W/P:** [B, M] ↓ Dose in severe hepatic impair **CI:** Adams-Stokes synd; heart block; corn allergy **Disp:** Inj IV: 1% (10 mg/mL), 2% (20 mg/mL); admixture 4, 10, 20%; IV Inf: 0.2, 0.4% **SE:** Dizziness, paresthesias, & convulsions associated w/ tox **Notes:** 2nd line to amiodarone in ECC; dilute ET dose 1–2 mL w/ NS; for IV forms, or CHF; *Systemic levels:* steady state 6–12 h; *Therapeutic:* 1.2–5 mcg/mL; *Toxic:* > 6 mcg/mL; *half-life:* 1.5 h; constant ECG monitoring is necessary during IV admin

Lidocaine, Lidocaine/Epinephrine (Anestacon Topical, Xylocaine, Xylocaine MPF, Xylocaine Viscous, Others)

BOX: Lidocaine gel should not be used for infant teething **Uses:** *Local anesthetic, epidural/caudal anesthesia, regional nerve block, topical on mucous membranes (mouth/pharynx/urethra)* **Acts:** Anesthetic; stabilizes neuronal membranes; inhibits ionic fluxes required for initiation and conduction **Dose:** *Adults. Local Inj anesthetic:* 4.5 mg/kg max total dose or 300 mg; w/ epi 7 mg/kg or total 500 mg max dose *Oral:* 15 mL viscous swish and spit or *pharyngeal:* gargle and swallow; do not use < 3-h intervals or > 8 × in 24 h *Urethra:* Jelly 5–30 mL (200–300 mg) jelly in men, 3–5 mL female urethra; 600 mg/24 h max *Peds. Topical:* Apply max 3 mg/kg/dose *Local Inj anesthetic:* Max 4.5 mg/kg (Table 1, p 334) **W/P:** [B, +] Epi-containing soln may interact w/ TCA or MAOI and cause severe ↑ BP **CI:** Do not use lidocaine w/ epi on digits, ears, or nose (vasoconstriction & necrosis) **Disp:** Inj local: 0.5, 1, 1.5, 2, 4, 10, 20%; Inj w/ epi 0.5%/1:200,000, 1%/1:100,000, 2%/1:100,000; (MPF) 1%/1:200,000, 1.5%/1:200,000, 2%/1:200,000; Dental formulations: 2%/1:50,000, 2%/1:100,000; cream 2, 3, 4%; lotion 30%; jelly 2%, gel 2, 2.5, 4, 5%; oint 5%; liq 2.5%; soln 2, 4%; viscous 2% topical spray 9.6% **SE:** Dizziness, paresthesias, & convulsions associated w/ tox **Notes:** See Table 1, p 334

Lidocaine/Prilocaine (EMLA, ORAQIX)

Uses: *Topical anesthetic for intact skin or genital mucous membranes*; adjunct to phlebotomy or dermal procedures **Acts:** Amide local anesthetics **Dose:** *Adults. EMLA cream:* thick layer 2–2.5 g to intact skin over 20–25 cm² of skin surface, cover w/ occlusive dressing (eg, Tegaderm) for at least 1 h *Anesthetic disc:* 1 g/10 cm² for at least 1 h *Peds. Max dose:* < **3 mo or < 5 kg:** 1 g/10 cm² for 1 h **3–12 mo & > 5 kg:** 2 g/20 cm² for 4 h **1–6 y & > 10 kg:** 10 g/100 cm² for 4 h **7–12 y & > 20 kg:** 20 g/200 cm² for 4 h **W/P:** [B, +] **CI:** Methemoglobinemia use on mucous membranes, broken skin, eyes; allergy to amide-type anesthetics **Disp:** Cream 2.5% lidocaine/2.5% prilocaine; anesthetic disc (1 g); *Oraqix* periodontal gel 2.5/2.5% **SE:** Burning, stinging, methemoglobinemia **Notes:** Longer contact time ↑ effect

Lidocaine/Tetracaine, Transdermal Patch (Synera), Cream (Pliaglis) Uses: *Topical anesthesia for venipuncture and dermatologic procedures (Synera); dermatologic procedures (Pliaglis)* Acts: Combo amide and ester local anesthetic Dose: *Adults & Peds. Synera:* Apply patch 20–30 min before procedure *Adults. Pliaglis:* Apply cream 20–60 min before procedure, vol based on site surface (see PI) W/P: [B, ?/–] Use on intact skin only; avoid eyes; not for mucous membranes; do not use w/ Hx methemoglobinemia, anaphylaxis reported; caution w/ Class I antiarrhythmic drugs; remove before MRI CI: Component sens (PABA or local anesthetics) Disp: *Synera:* 70 mg lidocaine/70 mg tetracaine in 50-cm^2 patch; *Pliaglis:* 70 mg lidocaine/70 mg tetracaine/gm (7%/7%) cream, 30-, 60-, 100-gm tube SE: Erythema, blanching, edema

Linaclotide (Linzess) BOX: CI peds < 6 y; avoid in peds 6–17 y; death in juvenile mice Uses: *IBS w/ constipation, chronic idiopathic constipation* Acts: Guanylate cyclase-C agonist Dose: *IBS-C:* 290 mcg PO daily *CIC:* 145 mcg PO daily; on empty stomach 30 min prior to 1st meal of the day; swallow whole W/P: [C, ?/–] CI: Pts < 6 y; GI obstruction Disp: Caps 145, 290 mcg SE: D, Abd pain/distention, flatulence

Linagliptin (Tradjenta) Uses: *Type 2 DM* Acts: DPP-4 inhib; ↑ active incretin hormones (↑ insulin release, ↓ glucagon) Dose: 5 mg qd W/P: [B, ?/–] CI: Hypersens Disp: Tabs 5 mg SE: Hypoglycemia w/ sulfonylurea; nasopharyngitis, pancreatitis Notes: CYP3A4 inhib

Linagliptin/Metformin (Jentadueto) BOX: Lactic acidosis w/ metformin accumulation; ↑ risk w/ sepsis, vol depletion, CHF, renal/hepatic impair, excess alcohol; w/ lactic acidosis suspected D/C and hospitalize Uses: *Combo type 2 DM* Acts: DDP-4 inhib; ↑ insulin synth/release w/ biguanide; ↓ hepatic glu prod & absorption; ↑ insulin sens Dose: Titrate as needed; give bid w/ meals, gradual ↑ dose due to GI SE (metformin), max 2.5/1000 mg bid W/P: [X, –] May cause lactic acidosis, pancreatitis, hepatic failure, hypersens Rxn; vit B$_{12}$ def CI: Component hypersens, renal impair, metabolic acidosis Disp: Tabs (linagliptin mg/metformin mg) 2.5/500, 2.5/850, 2.5/1000 SE: ↓ Glu, nasopharyngitis, D joint pain (linagliptin) Notes: Warn against excessive EtOH intake, may ↑ metformin lactate effect; temp D/C w/ surgery or w/ iodinated contrast studies

Lindane (Generic) BOX: Only for pts intolerant/failed 1st-line Rx w/ safer agents; szs and deaths reported w/ repeated/prolonged use; caution d/t increased risk of neurotox in infants, children, elderly, w/ other skin conditions, and if < 50 kg; instruct pts on proper use and inform that itching occurs after successful killing of scabies or lice Uses: *Head lice, pubic "crab" lice, body lice, scabies* Acts: Ectoparasiticide & ovicide Dose: *Adults & Peds. Cream or lotion:* Thin layer to dry skin after bathing, leave for 8–12 h, rinse; also use on laundry *Shampoo:* Apply 30 mL to dry hair, develop a lather w/ warm water for 4 min, comb out nits W/P: [C, –] CI: Premature infants, uncontrolled Sz disorders, Norwegian scabies, open wounds

Disp: Lotion 1%; shampoo 1% **SE:** Arrhythmias, Szs, local irritation, GI upset, ataxia, alopecia, N/V, aplastic anemia **Notes:** Caution w/ overuse (may be absorbed); caution w/ hepatic Dz in pts, may repeat Rx in 7 d; try OTC first w/ pyrethrins (*Pronto, Rid*, others)

Linezolid (Zyvox) **Uses:** *Infxns caused by gram(+) bacteria (including VRE), pneumonia, skin Infxns* **Acts:** Unique, binds ribosomal bacterial RNA; bacteriocidal for streptococci, bacteriostatic for enterococci & staphylococci. *Spectrum:* Excellent gram(+), including VRE & MRSA **Dose:** *Adults.* 600 mg IV or PO q12h *Peds ≤ 11 y.* 10 mg/kg IV or PO q8h (q12h in preterm neonates) **W/P:** [C, ?/–] **CI:** Concurrent MAOI use or w/in 2 wk, uncontrolled HTN, thyrotoxicosis, vasopressive agents, carcinoid tumor, SSRIs, tricyclics, w/ MAOI (may cause serotonin syndrome when used w/ these psych meds), avoid foods w/ tyramine & cough/cold products w/ pseudoephedrine; w/ ↓ BM **Disp:** Inj 200, 600 mg; tabs 600 mg; susp 100 mg/5 mL **SE:** Lactic acidosis, peripheral/optic neuropathy, HTN, N/D, HA, insomnia, GI upset, ↓ BM, tongue discoloration, prolonged use: *C. difficile* Infxn **Notes:** ✓ Weekly CBC; not for gram(–) Infxn, ↑ deaths in catheter-related Infxns; MAOI activity

Liothyronine [T₃] (Cytomel, Triostat) **BOX:** Not for obesity or Wt loss **Uses:** *Hypothyroidism, nontoxic goiter, myxedema coma* **Acts:** T₃ replacement **Dose:** *Adults.* Initial 25 mcg/24 h, titrate q1–2wk to response & TFT; maint of 25–100 mcg/d PO *Myxedema coma:* 25–50 mcg IV *Myxedema:* 5 mcg/d, PO ↑ 5–10 mcg/d q1–2wk; maint 50–100 mcg/d *Nontoxic goiter:* 5 mcg/d PO, ↑ 5–10 mcg/d q1–2wk, usual dose 75 mcg/d *T₃ suppression test:* 75–100 mcg/d × 7d; ↓ in elderly & CV Dz *Peds.* Initial 5 mcg/24 h, titrate by 50-mcg/24-h increments at q3–4d intervals; Maint: *Infants–12 mo:* 20 mcg/24 h *Peds 1–3 y:* 50 mcg/d *>3 y:* Adult dose **W/P:** [A, +] **CI:** Recent MI, uncorrected adrenal Insuff, uncontrolled HTN, thyrotoxicosis, artificial rewarming **Disp:** Tabs 5, 25, 50 mcg; Inj 10 mcg/mL **SE:** Alopecia, arrhythmias, CP, HA, sweating, twitching, ↑ HR, ↑ BP, MI, CHF, fever **Notes:** Monitor TFT; separate antacids by 4 h; monitor glu w/ DM meds; when switching from IV to PO, taper IV slowly

Liraglutide, Recombinant (Saxenda, Victoza) **BOX:** CI w/ personal or fam Hx of MTC or w/ MEN2 **Uses:** *Type 2 DM (Victoza),* adjunct to ↓ caloric & ↑ activity; chronic Wt management w/ BMI > 30 kg/m² or BMI > 27 kg/m² w/ comorbidity (ie, DM, ↑ BP) *(Saxenda)* * **Acts:** GLP-1 receptor agonist **Dose:** *Victoza:* 1.8 mg/d; begin 0.6 mg/d any time of day SQ (Abd/thigh/upper arm), ↑ to 1.2 mg after 1 wk, may ↑ to 1.8 mg after *Saxenda:* 0.6 mg wk 1, 1.2 mg wk 2, 1.8 mg wk 3, 2.4 mg wk 4, 3 mg wk 5 onward SQ qd **W/P:** [X, ?/–] Do not use *Saxenda* and *Victoza* together or w/ GLP-1 receptor antag **CI:** Personal/fam Hx MTC or MEN 2; component hypersens **Disp:** Multidose pens 0.6, 1.2, 1.8 mg/dose, 6 mg/mL **SE:** Pancreatitis, MTC, ↓ glucose w/ sulfonylurea, HA, N/D, Wt loss **Notes:** ↓ Gastric emptying

Lisdexamfetamine Dimesylate (Vyvanse) [C-II] **BOX:** Amphetamines have ↑ potential for abuse; prolonged administration may lead to dependence; may cause sudden death and serious CV events in pts w/ preexisting structure cardiac abnormalities **Uses:** *ADHD, binge eating disorder* **Acts:** CNS stimulant **Dose: Adults & Peds 6–12 y.** 30 mg qd, ↑ qwk 10–20 mg/d, 70 mg/d max **W/P:** [C, ?/–] w/ Potential for drug dependency in pt w/ psychological or Sz disorder, Tourette synd, HTN **CI:** Severe arteriosclerotic CV Dz, mod–severe ↑ BP, ↑ thyroid, sens to sympathomimetic amines, NAG, agitated states, Hx drug abuse, w/ or w/in 14 d of MAOI **Disp:** Caps 10, 20, 30, 40, 50, 60, 70 mg **SE:** HA, insomnia, decreased appetite **Notes:** AHA statement April 2008: All children diagnosed w/ ADHD who are candidates for stimulant meds should undergo CV assessment prior to use; may be inappropriate for geriatric use

Lisinopril (Prinivil, Zestril) **BOX:** ACE inhib can cause fetal injury/death in 2nd/3rd tri; D/C w/ PRG **Uses:** *HTN, CHF, prevent DN & AMI* **Acts:** ACE inhib **Dose:** 5–40 mg/24 h PO daily-bid, CHF target 40 mg/d **AMI:** 5 mg w/in 24 h of MI, then 5 mg after 24 h, 10 mg after 48 h, then 10 mg/d; ↓ in renal Insuff; use low dose; ↑ slowly in elderly **W/P:** [C (1st tri) D (2nd, 3rd tri), –] w/ Aortic stenosis/cardiomyopathy **CI:** PRG, ACE inhib sens, idiopathic or hereditary angioedema **Disp:** Tabs 2.5, 5, 10, 20, 30, 40 mg **SE:** Dizziness, HA, cough, ↓ BP, angioedema, ↑ K+, Cr, rare ↓ BM **Notes:** To prevent DN, start when urinary microalbuminuria begins; ✓ BUN, Cr, K+, WBC

Lisinopril/Hydrochlorothiazide (Prinzide, Zestoretic, Generic) **BOX:** ACE inhib can cause fetal injury/death in 2nd/3rd tri; D/C w/ PRG **Uses:** *HTN* **Acts:** ACE inhib w/ diuretic (HCTZ) **Dose:** Initial 10 mg lisinopril/12.5mg HCTZ, titrate upward to effect; > 80 mg/d lisinopril or > 50 mg/day HCTZ are not recommended; ↓ in renal Insuff; use low dose; ↑ slowly in elderly **W/P:** [C 1st tri, D after, –] w/ Aortic stenosis/cardiomyopathy, bilateral RAS **CI:** PRG, ACE inhib, idiopathic or hereditary angioedema, sens (angioedema) **Disp:** Tabs (mg lisinopril/mg HCTZ) 10/12.5, 20/12.5; **Zestoretic** also available as 20/25 **SE:** Anaphylactoid Rxn (rare), dizziness, HA, cough, fatigue, ↑ BP, angioedema, ↑/↓ K+, ↑Cr, rare ↓ BM/cholestatic jaundice **Notes:** Use only when monotherapy fails; ✓ BUN, Cr, K+, WBC

Lithium Carbonate, Citrate (Generic) **BOX:** Li tox related to serum levels and can be seen at close to therapeutic levels **Uses:** *Manic episodes of bipolar Dz*, augment antidepressants, aggression, PTSD **Acts:** ?, Effects shift toward intraneuronal metabolism of catecholamines **Dose: Adults & Peds ≥ 12 y. Bipolar, acute mania:** 1800 mg/d PO in 2–3 ÷ doses (target serum 1–1.5 mEq/L ✓ 2×/wk until stable) **Bipolar maint:** 900–1800/d PO in 2–3 ÷ doses (target serum 0.6–1.2 mEq/L); ↓ in renal Insuff, elderly **W/P:** [D, –] Many drug interactions; avoid ACE inhib & diuretics; thyroid Dz, caution in pts at risk of suicide **CI:** Severe renal impair or CV Dz, severe debilitation, dehydration, PRG, sodium depletion **Disp:** Carbonate: caps 150, 300, 600 mg; tabs 300, 600 mg; SR tabs 300 mg; CR tabs 450 mg; citrate: syrup 300 mg/5 mL **SE:** Polyuria, polydipsia, nephrogenic DI, long-term may affect renal conc ability and cause fibrosis; tremor; Na+ retention or diuretic use may ↑ tox; arrhythmias, dizziness, alopecia, goiter ↓ thyroid, N/V/D, ataxia, nystagmus, ↓ BP **Notes:** Levels: *Trough:* Just before next dose: *Therapeutic:* 0.8–1.2 mEq/mL; *Toxic:* > 1.5 mEq/mL; *half-life:* 18–20 h. Follow levels q1–2mo on maint, draw concentrations 8–12 h postdose

Lodoxamide (Alomide) **Uses:** *Vernal conjunctivitis/keratitis* **Acts:** Stabilizes mast cells **Dose:** *Adults & Peds > 2 y.* 1–2 gtt in eye(s) qid × 3 mo **W/P:** [B, ?] **Disp:** Soln 0.1% **SE:** Ocular burning, stinging, HA **Notes:** Do not use soft contacts during use

Lomitapide (Juxtapid) **BOX:** May cause ↑ transaminases and/or hepatic steatosis. Monitor ALT/AST & bili at baseline & regularly; adjust dose if ALT/AST > 3× ULN (see PI); D/C w/ significant liver tox **Uses:** *Homozygous familial hypercholesterolemia* **Acts:** Microsomal triglyceride transfer protein inhib **Dose:** 5 mg PO daily; ↑ to 10 mg after 2 wk, then at 4-wk intervals to 20, 40 mg; 60 mg max based on safety/tolerability; swallow whole w/ water > 2 h after evening meal; 40 mg max w/ ESRD on dialysis or mild hepatic impair; 30 mg max w/ weak CYP3A4 inhib (see PI) **W/P:** [X, –] Avoid grapefruit; adjust w/ warfarin, P-glycoprotein substrates, simvastatin, lovastatin **CI:** PRG, w/ strong–mod CYP3A4 inhibitors, mod–severe hepatic impair **Disp:** Caps 5, 10, 20, 30, 40, 60 mg **SE:** N/V/D, hepatotox, dyspepsia, Abd pain, flatulence, CP, influenza, fatigue, ↓ Wt, ↓ abs fat-soluble vits **Notes:** Limited distribution Juxtapid REMS Program; PRG test before; use w/ low-fat diet (< 20% fat energy); take daily vit E, linoleic acid, ALA, EPA, DHA supl

Loperamide (Diamode, Imodium) [OTC] **Uses:** *D* **Acts:** Slows intestinal motility **Dose:** *Adults.* Initial 4 mg PO, then 2 mg after each loose stool, up to 16 mg/d *Peds 2–5 y, 13–20 kg.* 1 mg PO tid; *6–8 y, 20–30 kg.* 2 mg PO bid; *8–12 y, > 30 kg.* 2 mg PO tid **W/P:** [C, –] Not for acute D caused by *Salmonella, Shigella,* or *C. difficile;* w/ HIV may cause toxic megacolon **CI:** Pseudomembranous colitis, bloody D, Abd pain w/o D, < 2 y **Disp:** Caps 2 mg; tabs 2 mg; liq 1 mg/5 mL, 1 mg/7.5 mL (OTC) **SE:** Constipation, sedation, dizziness, Abd cramp, N

Lopinavir/Ritonavir (Kaletra) **Uses:** *HIV Infxn* **Acts:** Protease inhib **Dose:** *Adults. Tx naïve:* 800/200 mg PO qd or 400/100 mg PO bid; *Tx-experienced pt:* 400/100 mg PO bid (↑ dose if w/ amprenavir, efavirenz, fosamprenavir, nelfinavir, nevirapine); do not use qd dosing w/ concomitant Rx *Peds 7–15 kg.* 12/3 mg/kg PO bid *15–40 kg.* 10/2.5 mg/kg PO bid > *40 kg.* Adult dose; w/ food **W/P:** [C, ?/–] Numerous interactions; w/ hepatic impair; do not use w/ salmeterol, colchicine (w/ renal/hepatic failure); adjust dose w/ bosentan, tadalafil for PAH, ↑ QT w/ QT-prolonging drugs, hypokalemia, congenital long QT syn, immune reconstitution syn **CI:** w/ Drugs dependent on CYP3A/CYP2D6 (Table 10, p 356), lovastatin, rifampin, statins, St. John's wort, fluconazole; w/ alpha 1-adrenoreceptor antag (alfuzosin); w/ PDE5 inhi sildenafil **Disp:** (mg lopinavir/mg ritonavir) Tabs 100/25, 200/50; soln 400/100/5 mL **SE:** Avoid disulfiram (soln has EtOH), metronidazole; GI upset, asthenia, ↑ cholesterol/triglycerides, pancreatitis; protease metabolic synd

Loratadine (Alavert, Claritin, Generic) [OTC]) **Uses:** *Allergic rhinitis, chronic idiopathic urticaria* **Acts:** Nonsedating antihistamine **Dose:** *Adults.* 10 mg/d PO. *Peds 2–5 y.* 5 mg PO daily > *6 y.* Adult dose; on empty stomach; ↓ in hepatic

Insuff; q other day dose w/ CrCl < 30 mL/min **W/P:** [B, +/–] **CI:** Component allergy **Disp:** Tabs 10 mg (OTC); rapidly disintegrating RediTabs 5, 10 mg; chew tabs 5 mg; syrup 1 mg/mL **SE:** HA, somnolence, xerostomia, hyperkinesis in peds

Lorazepam (Ativan, Generic) [C-IV] Uses: *Anxiety & anxiety w/ depression; sedation; control status epilepticus*; EtOH withdrawal; antiemetic **Acts:** Benzodiazepine; antianxiety agent; works via postsynaptic GABA receptors **Dose:** *Adults.* Anxiety: 1–10 mg/d PO in 2–3 ÷ doses *Preop:* 0.05 mg/kg–4 mg max IM 2 h before or 0.044 mg/kg–2 mg max IV 15–20 min before surgery *Insomnia:* 2–4 mg PO hs *Status epilepticus:* 4 mg/dose slow over 2–5 min IV PRN q10–15min; usual total dose 8 mg *Antiemetic:* 0.5–2 mg IV or PO q4–6h PRN *EtOH withdrawal:* 1–4 mg IV or 2 mg PO initial depending on severity; titrate *Peds. Status epilepticus:* 0.05–0.1 mg/kg/dose IV over 2–5 min, max 4 mg/dose repeat at 10- to 15-min intervals × 2 PRN *Antiemetic, 2–15 y:* 0.05 mg/kg (to 2 mg/dose) prechemotherapy; ↓ in elderly; do not administer IV > 2 mg/min or 0.05 mg/kg/min **W/P:** [D, –] w/ Hepatic impair, other CNS depression, COPD; ↓ dose by 50% w/ valproic acid and probenecid **CI:** Severe pain, severe ↓ BP, sleep apnea, NAG, allergy to propylene glycol or benzyl alcohol, severe resp Insuff (except mechanically ventilated) **Disp:** Tabs 0.5, 1, 2 mg; soln, PO conc 2 mg/mL; Inj 2, 4 mg/mL **SE:** Sedation, memory impair, EPS, dizziness, ataxia, tachycardia, ↓ BP, constipation, resp depression, paradoxical reactions, fall risk, abuse potential, rebound/withdrawal after abrupt D/C **Notes:** ~10 min for effect if IV; IV Inf requires inline filter

Lorcaserin (Belviq) Uses: *Manage Wt w/ BMI ≥ 30 kg/m² or ≥ 27 kg/m² w/ Wt-related comorbidity* **Acts:** Serotonin 2C receptor agonist **Dose:** 10 mg PO bid; D/C if not 5% Wt loss by wk 12 **W/P:** [X, –] ✓ glu w/ diabetic meds; monitor for depression/suicidal thoughts, serotonin or neuroleptic malignant synd, cognitive impair, psych disorders, valvular disease Dz, priapism; risk of serotonin synd when used w/ other serotonergic drugs; caution w/ drugs that are CYP2D6 substrates **CI:** PRG **Disp:** Tabs 10 mg **SE:** HA, nausea, dizziness, fatigue, dry mouth, constipation, back pain, cough, hypoglycemia, euphoria, hallucination, dissociation, ↓ HR, ↑ prolactin

Losartan (Cozaar) BOX: Can cause fetal injury and death if used in 2nd & 3rd tri; D/C Rx if PRG detected Uses: *HTN, DN, Px CVA in HTN and LVH* **Acts:** Angiotensin II receptor antag **Dose:** *Adults.* 25–50 mg PO daily-bid, max 100 mg; ↓ in elderly/hepatic impair *Peds ≥ 6 y. HTN:* Initial 0.7 mg/kg qd, ↑ to 50 mg/d PRN; 1.4 mg/kg qd or 100 mg/d max **W/P:** [C (1st tri, D 2nd & 3rd tri), ?/–] w/ NSAIDs; w/ K⁺-sparing diuretics, supl may cause ↑ K⁺; w/ RAS, hepatic impair **CI:** PRG, component sens **Disp:** Tabs 25, 50, 100 mg **SE:** ↓ BP in pts on diuretics; ↑ K⁺; GI upset, facial/angioedema, dizziness, cough, weakness, ↓ renal Fxn

Loteprednol (Alrex, Lotemax) Uses: *Lotemax: Steroid-responsive inflam disorders of conjunctiva/cornea/anterior globe (keratitis, iritis, post-op); Alrex: seasonal allergic conjunctivitis* **Acts:** Anti-inflam/steroid **Dose:** *Adults. Lotemax:* 1 drop into conjunctival sac qid up to every h initially; *Alrex:* 1 drop qid **W/P:** [C, ?/–] Glaucoma

CI: Viral Dz corneal and conjunctiva, varicella, mycobacterial and fungal Infxns; hypersens **Disp:** *Lotemax* 0.5% susp, 2.5, 5, 10, 15 mL; *Alrex* 0.2% susp, 2.5, 5, 10 mL **SE:** Glaucoma; ↑ risk Infxn; cornea/sclera thinning; HA, rhinitis **Notes:** May delay cataract surgery healing; avoid use > 10 d; shake before use

Lovastatin (Altoprev, Mevacor, Generic) Uses: *Hypercholesterolemia to ↓ risk of MI, angina* **Acts:** HMG-CoA reductase inhib **Dose:** *Adults.* 20 mg/d PO w/ P.M. meal; may ↑ at 4-wk intervals to 80 mg/d max or 60 mg ER tab; take w/ meals; see PI for dose limits w/ concurrent therapy (amiodarone, verapamil, diltiazem) *Peds 10–17 y. (at least 1-y postmenarchal) Familial ↑ cholesterol:* 10 mg PO qd, ↑ q4wk PRN to 40 mg/d max (immediate release w/ P.M. meal) **W/P:** [X, –] Avoid w/ grapefruit juice, gemfibrozil; use caution, carefully consider doses > 20 mg/d w/ renal impair **CI:** Active liver Dz, PRG, lactation, w/ strong CYP3A4 inhib **Disp:** Tabs generic 10, 20, 40 mg; *Mevacor* 20, 40 mg; *Altoprev* ER tabs 20, 40, 60 mg **SE:** HA & GI intolerance common; promptly report any unexplained muscle pain, tenderness, or weakness (myopathy) **Notes:** Maintain cholesterol-lowering diet; LFTs q12wk × 1 y, then q6mo; may alter TFT

Loxapine (Adasuve) BOX: Can cause bronchospasm w/ resp distress/resp arrest; elderly w/ dementia related psychosis on antipsychotic drugs have ↑ risk of death; not for dementia-related psychosis. Uses: *Acute agitation w/ schizophrenia or bipolar disorder* **Acts:** ?; likely antag of central DAD₂ and 5-HT₂ₐ receptors **Dose:** 10 mg/Inh q 24h **W/P:** [C, –] Neuroleptic malignant synd w/ CV, cerebrovascular Dz, or Sz; driving; ↑ risk stroke/TIA **CI:** (varies by product) Hx asthma/COPD/bronchospasm; acute resp distress **Disp:** 10-mg single-use powder inhaler **SE:** EPS, dystonia, ↑ HR, ↑/↓ BP, syncope; dysgeusia; sedation; throat irritation **Notes:** Restricted distribution (Adasuve REMS); give only in registered facility with equipment/personnel trained to manage acute bronchospasm

Lubiprostone (Amitiza) Uses: *Chronic idiopathic constipation in adults, IBS w/ constipation in females > 18 y, opioid-induced constipation w/ non-CA pain* **Acts:** Selective Cl⁻ channel activator; ↑ intestinal motility **Dose:** *Constipation:* 24 mcg PO bid w/ food *IBS:* 8 mcg bid w/ food **CI:** Mechanical GI obst **W/P:** [C, ?/–] Severe D, ↓ dose mod–severe hepatic impair **Disp:** Gelcaps 8, 24 mcg **SE:** N/D, may adjust dose based on tox (N), HA, GI distention, Abd pain **Notes:** Not approved in males; requires (–) PRG test before; use contraception; periodically reassess drug need; not for chronic use; may experience severe dyspnea w/in 1 h of dose, usually resolves w/in 3 h

Lucinactant (Surfaxin) Uses: *Px of RDS* **Acts:** Pulmonary surfactant **Dose:** *Peds.* 5.8 mL/kg birth Wt intratracheally no more often than q6h; max 4 doses in first 48 h of life **W/P:** [N/A, N/A] Frequent clinical assessments; interrupt w/ adverse Rxns and assess/stabilize infant; not for ARDS **CI:** Ø **Disp:** Susp 30 mg/mL **SE:** ET tube reflux/obstruction, pallor, bradycardia, oxygen desaturation, anemia, jaundice, metabolic/respiratory acidosis, hyperglycemia, ↓ Na, pneumonia,

↓ BP **Notes:** Warm vial for 15 min; shake prior to use; discard if not used w/in 2 h of warming

Luliconazole (Luzu) **Uses:** *Tinea pedis, tinea cruris, tinea corporis* **Acts:** Azole antifungal, inhi ergosterol synthesis **Dose:** *Tinea pedis:* Apply qd for 2 wk; *tinea corporis, tinea cruris:* apply qd for 1 wk **W/P:** [C, ?/–] **CI:** Ø **Disp:** Cream, 1%; 30/60 gm **SE:** Site reaction, rare

Lurasidone (Latuda) **BOX:** Elderly w/ dementia-related psychosis at ↑ death risk; not approved for dementia-related psychosis; antidepressants ↑ risk of suicidal thoughts and behavior in peds, adolescents, and young adults in short-term studies; monitor all pts for suicidal thoughts when starting **Uses:** *Schizophrenia* **Acts:** Atypical antipsychotic; central D2 and 5HT2A receptor antag **Dose:** 40–80 mg/d PO w/ food; 40 mg max w/ CrCl 10–49 mL/min OR mod–severe hepatic impair **W/P:** [B, –] **CI:** w/ Strong CYP3A4 inhib/inducer **Disp:** Tabs 20, 40, 60, 80, 120 mg **SE:** Somnolence, agitation, tardive dyskinesia, akathisia, parkinsonism, stroke, TIAs, Sz, orthostatic hypotension, syncope, dysphagia, neuroleptic malignant syndrome, body temp dysregulation, N, ↑ Wt, type 2 DM, ↑ lipids, hyperprolactinemia, ↓ WBC **Notes:** w/ DM risk ✓ glu

Lymphocyte Immune Globulin [ATG] (Atgam) **BOX:** Should only be used by physician experienced in immunosuppressive therapy or management of solid-organ and/or BMT pts; adequate lab and supportive resources must be readily available **Uses:** *Allograft rejection in renal transplant pts; aplastic anemia if not candidates for BMT* **Acts:** ↓ Circulating antigen-reactive T lymphocytes; human, & equine product **Dose:** *Adults.* **Prevent rejection:** 15 mg/kg/d IV × 14 d, then q other day × 7 d for total 21 doses in 28 d; initial w/in 24 h before/after transplant *Rx rejection:* Same but use 10–15 mg/kg/d; max 21 doses in 28 d, qd first 14 d *Aplastic anemia:* 10–20 mg/kg/d × 8–14 d, then q other day × 7 doses for total 21 doses in 28 d *Peds.* **Prevent renal allograft rejection:** 5–25 mg/kg/d IV *Aplastic anemia:* 10–20 mg/kg/day IV 8–14 d then q other day for 7 more doses **W/P:** [C, ?/–] D/C if severe unremitting thrombocytopenia, leukopenia **CI:** Hx previous Rxn or Rxn to other equine γ-globulin prep, ↓ plt and WBC **Disp:** Inj 50 mg/mL **SE:** D/C w/ severe ↓ plt and WBC; rash, fever, chills, ↓ BP, HA, CP, edema, N/V/D, lightheadedness **Notes:** Test dose: 0.1 mL 1:1000 dilution in NS, a systemic Rxn precludes use; give via central line; pretreat w/ antipyretic, antihistamine, and steroids; monitor WBC, plt; plt counts usually return to nl w/o D/C Rx 4 h Inf

Macitentan (Opsumit) **BOX:** Do not use w/ PRG, may cause fetal harm; exclude PRG before and 1 mo after stopping; use contraception during and 1 mo past stopping; for females, only available through a restricted distribution program **Uses:** *Pulm hypertension to prevent progression* **Acts:** Endothelin receptor antag **Dose:** 10 mg qd **W/P:** [X, –] May cause hepatic failure/tox; ↓ Hct;

pulm edema w PE, ↓ sperm count **CI:** PRG **Disp:** Tabs 10 mg **SE:** ↓ Hct; HA, UTI, influenza, bronchitis, nasopharyngitis, pharyngitis **Notes:** ✓ LFTs before and monitor; w/ PE D/C, may cause pulm edema; avoid w/ CYP3A4 inducers/ inhibs

Magaldrate/Simethicone (Riopan-Plus) [OTC] **Uses:** *Hyperacidity associated w/ peptic ulcer, gastritis, & hiatal hernia* **Acts:** Low-Na⁺ antacid **Dose:** 5–10 mL PO between meals & hs, on empty stomach **W/P:** [C, ?/+] **CI:** UC, diverticulitis, appendicitis, ileostomy/colostomy, renal Insuff (d/t Mg²⁺ content) **Disp:** Susp magaldrate/simethicone 540/20 mg/5 mL (OTC) **SE:** ↑ Mg²⁺, ↓ PO₄, white-flecked feces, constipation, N/V/D **Notes:** < 0.3 mg Na¹⁺/tab or tsp

Magnesium Citrate (Citroma, Others) [OTC] **Uses:** *Vigorous bowel prep* *constipation **Acts:** Cathartic laxative **Dose:** *Adults & Peds > 12 y.* 150–300 mL PO PRN *Peds 2–6 y.* 60–90 mL × 1 or ÷ doses; max 90 mL/24 h *6–12 y.* 90–210 mL × 1 or ÷ doses **W/P:** [B, +] w/ Neuromuscular Dz & renal impair **CI:** Ø, but OTC: "Do not use if on low-salt diet" **Disp:** Soln 290 mg/5 mL (300 mL); tabs 100 mg **SE:** N/V/D, rare resp depression **Notes:** Only for occasional use w/ constipation

Magnesium Hydroxide (Milk of Magnesia) [OTC] **Uses:** *Constipation*, hyperacidity, Mg²⁺ replacement **Acts:** NS laxative **Dose:** *Adults. Antacid:* 5–15 mL (400 mg/5 mL) or 2–4 tabs (311 mg) PO PRN up to qid *Laxative:* 30–60 mL (400 mg/5 mL) or 15–30 mL (800 mg/5 mL) or 8 tabs (311 mg) PO qhs or ÷ doses *Peds. Antacid:* < 12 y not OK *Laxative:* < 2 y not OK *2–5 y.* 5–15 mL (400 mg/5 mL) PO qhs or ÷ doses *6–11 y.* 15–30 mL (400 mg/5 mL) or 7.5–15 mL (800 mg/5 mL) PO qhs or ÷ doses *3–5 y.* 2 311-mg tabs PO qhs or ÷ doses *6–11 y.* 4 311-mg tabs PO qhs or ÷ doses **W/P:** [B, +] w/ Neuromuscular Dz or renal impair **CI:** Component hypersens **Disp:** Chew tabs 311, 400; liq 400, 800 mg/5 mL (OTC) **SE:** D, Abd cramps **Notes:** For occasional use in constipation, different forms may contain Al²⁺

Magnesium Oxide (Mag-Ox, Maox, Uro-Mag, Others) [OTC] **Uses:** *Replace low Mg²⁺ levels, short-term relief of constipation* **Acts:** Mg²⁺ supl, cathartic **Dose:** 400–800 mg/d or ÷ w/ food in full glass of H₂O; ↓ w/ renal impair **W/P:** [B, +] Separate dose from tetracyclines, bisphosphonates, thyroid meds, quinolones **CI:** Component hypersens **Disp:** Caps 140 mg; tabs 200, 250, 400, 420 500 mg (OTC) **SE:** N/D

Magnesium Sulfate (Various) **Uses:** *Replace low Mg²⁺; preeclampsia, eclampsia, & premature labor; cardiac arrest; AMI arrhythmias; cerebral edema; barium poisoning; Szs; ped acute nephritis*; refractory ↓ K⁺ & ↓ Ca²⁺ **Acts:** Mg²⁺ supl, bowel evacuation, ↓ acetylcholine in nerve terminals, ↓ rate of sinoatrial node firing **Dose:** *Adults. Mild deficiency:* 1 g IV/IM q6h × 4 doses & PRN; *Moderate deficiency (serum 1–1.5 mg/dL):* 1–4 g, 1 g/h max, no more than 12 g over 12 h; *Severe deficiency (serum < 1.0 mg/dL):* Up to 250 mg/kg IM over 4 h or 4–8 g IV; 1 g/h if no Sx; if Sx, ≤ 4 g over 4–5 min, 2 g q3–6h IV, then PRN to correct deficiency *Preeclampsia/premature labor:* 4-g load, then 1–2 g/h IV Inf *ECC 2010.*

VF/pulseless VT arrest w/ torsade de pointes: 1–2 g IV push (2–4 mL 50% soln) in 10 mL D5W. If pulse present, then 1–2 g in 50–100 mL D5W over 5–60 min **Peds & Neonates.** 25–50 mg/kg/dose IV, repeat PRN; max 2-g single dose **ECC 2010.** *Pulseless VT w/ torsade de pointes:* 25–50 mg/kg IV/IO bolus; max dose 2 g; *Pulseless VT w/ torsades de pointe or hypomagnesemia:* 25–50 mg/kg IV/IO over 10–20 min; max dose 2 g; *Status asthmaticus:* 25–50 mg/kg IV/IO over 15–30 min **W/P:** [A/C (varies; manufacturer specific), +] w/ Neuromuscular Dz; interactions, see Magnesium Oxide & individual aminoglycoside entries **CI:** Heart block, myocardial damage; in pre-eclampsia/eclampsia, do not use w/in 2 hr of delivery **Disp:** Premix IV Inj 10, 20, 40, 80 mg/mL; Inj 125, 500 mg/mL; oral/topical powder 227, 454, 1810, 2720 g **SE:** CNS depression, D, flushing, heart block, ↓ BP, vasodilation **Notes:** Different formulation may contain Al²⁺, monitor Mg²⁺ levels

Mannitol, Inh (Aridol) BOX: Powder for Inh; use may result in severe bronchospasm; testing only done by trained professionals **Uses:** *Assess bronchial hyperresponsiveness in pts w/o clinically apparent asthma* **Acts:** Bronchoconstrictor, ? mechanism **Dose:** *Adults & Peds > 6 y.* Inhal caps ↑ dose (see Disp) until + test (15% ↓ FEV1 or 10% ↓ FEV1 between consecutive doses) or all caps inhaled **W/P:** [C, ?/M] Pt w/ comorbid cond that may ↑ effects **CI:** Mannitol/gelatin hypersens **Disp:** Dry powder caps graduated doses: 0, 5, 10, 20, 40 mg **SE:** HA, pharyngeal pain, irritation, N, cough, rhinorrhea, dyspnea, chest discomfort, wheezing, retching, dizziness **Notes:** Not a stand-alone test or screening test for asthma

Mannitol, IV (Generic) **Uses:** *Cerebral edema, ↑ IOP, renal impair, poisonings* **Acts:** Osmotic diuretic **Dose:** *Test dose:* 0.2 g/kg/dose IV over 3–5 min; if no diuresis w/in 2 h, D/C *Oliguria:* 50–100 g IV over 90 min ↑ *IOP:* 0.25–2 g/kg IV over 30 min *Cerebral edema:* 0.25–1.5 g/kg/dose IV q6–8h PRN, maintain serum osmolarity < 300–320 mOsm/kg **W/P:** [C, ?/M] w/ CHF or vol overload, w/ nephrotox drugs & lithium, vesicant, avoid extrav **CI:** Anuria, dehydration, heart failure, PE intracranial bleeding **Disp:** Inj 5, 10, 15, 20, 25% **SE:** May exacerbate CHF, HA, electrolyte imbalance, acidosis, N/V/D, ↓ / ↑ BP, ↑ HR **Notes:** Monitor for vol depletion

Maraviroc (Selzentry) BOX: Possible drug-induced hepatotox **Uses:** *Tx of CCR5-tropic HIV Infxn* **Acts:** Antiretroviral, CCR5 coreceptor antag **Dose:** 300 mg bid **W/P:** [B, –] w/ Concomitant CYP3A inducers/inhib and ↓ renal function, caution in mild–mod hepatic impair **CI:** Pts w/ severe renal impair/ESRD taking potent CXP3A4 inhib/inducer **Disp:** Tabs 150, 300 mg **SE:** Fever, URI, cough, rash; HIV attaches to the CCR5 receptor to infect CD4+ T cells

Measles/Mumps/Rubella Vaccine, Live [MMR] (M-M-R II) **Uses:** *Vaccination against measles, mumps, & rubella 12 mo and older* **Acts:** Active immunization, live attenuated viruses **Dose:** 1 (0.5-mL) SQ Inj, 1st dose 12 mo, 2nd dose 4–6 y, at least 3 mo between doses (28 d if > 12 y), adults born after 1957 unless CI, Hx measles & mumps or documented immunity and women of child-bearing age w/ rubella immunity documented **W/P:** [C, ?/M] Hx of cerebral injury, Szs, fam Hx Szs (febrile Rxn), ↓ plt; delay w/ severe illness **CI:** Component and gelatin sens, Hx anaphylaxis to neomycin, blood dyscrasia, lymphoma, leukemia, malignant neoplasias affecting BM, immunosuppression, fever, PRG, Hx of active untreated TB **Disp:** Inj, single dose **SE:** Fever, febrile Szs (5–12 d after vaccination), Inj site Rxn, rash, ↓ plt **Notes:** Per FDA, CDC ↑ of febrile Sz (2×) w/ MMRV vs MMR and varicella separately; preferable to use 2 separate vaccines; allow 1 mo between Inj & any other measles vaccine or 3 mo between any other varicella vaccine; limited avail of MMRV; avoid those who have not been exposed to varicella for 6 wk post-Inj; may contain albumin or trace egg antigen; avoid salicylates for 6 wk postvaccination; avoid PRG for 3 mo following vaccination; do not give w/in 3 mo of transfusion or immune globulin

Measles/Mumps/Rubella/Varicella Virus Vaccine, Live [MMRV] (ProQuad) **Uses:** *Vaccination against measles, mumps, rubella, & varicella* **Acts:** Active immunization, live attenuated viruses **Dose:** 1 (0.5-mL) vial SQ Inj 12 mo–12 y or for 2nd dose of MMR*, at least 3 mo between doses (28 d if > 12 y) **W/P:** [C, ?/M] Hx of cerebral injury or Szs or fam Hx Szs (febrile Rxn), ↓ plt; delay w/ severe illness **CI:** Component and gelatin sens, Hx anaphylaxis to neomycin, blood dyscrasia, lymphoma, leukemia, malignant neoplasias affecting BM, immunosuppression, fever, active untreated TB, PRG **Disp:** Inj **SE:** Fever, febrile Szs, (5–12 d after vaccination), Inj site Rxn, rash, ↓ plt, **Notes:** Per FDA, CDC ↑ of febrile Sz (2 × risk) w/ combo vaccine (MMRV) vs MMR and varicella separately; preferable to use 2 separate vaccines; allow 1 mo between Inj & any other measles vaccine or 3 mo between any other varicella vaccine; limited avail of MMRV; substitute MMR II and/or Varivax; avoid those not been exposed to varicella for 6 wk post-Inj; may contain albumin or trace egg antigen; avoid salicylates

Mecasermin (Increlex) **Uses:** *Growth failure in severe primary IGF-1 deficiency or HGH antibodies* **Acts:** Human IGF-1 (recombinant DNA origin) **Dose:** *Peds.* Increlex ≥ 2 y 0.04–0.08 mg/kg SQ bid; may ↑ by 0.04 mg/kg per dose to 0.12 mg/kg bid; take w/in 20 min of meal d/t insulin-like hypoglycemic effect; dose must be tolerated for 7 d before ↑ dose **W/P:** [C, ?/M] Contains benzyl alcohol **CI:** Closed epiphysis, neoplasia, not for IV **Disp:** Vial 10 mg/mL (40 mL) **SE:** Tonsillar hypertrophy, ↑ AST, ↑ LDH, HA, Inj site Rxn, V, hypoglycemia **Notes:** Rapid dose ↑ may cause hypoglycemia; initial funduscopic exam and during Tx; consider monitoring glucose until dose stable; limited distribution; rotate Inj site

Mechlorethamine (Mustargen) **BOX:** Highly toxic; avoid Inh of dust/vapors & skin contact; limit use to experienced physicians; avoid exposure during PRG; vesicant **Uses:** *Hodgkin Dz (stages III, IV), cutaneous T-cell lymphoma (mycosis fungoides), lung CA, CML, malignant pleural effusions, CLL, polycythemia vera*, **Acts:** Alkylating agent, nitrogen analog of sulfur mustard **Dose:** Per protocol; *MOPP:* 6 mg/m^2 IV on d 1 & 8 of 28-d cycle 6–8 cycles; Stanford regimen:

6 g/m² single dose d 1, wks 1, 5, 9; *Intracavitary:* 0.2–0.4 mg/kg × 1, may repeat PRN; *Topical:* 0.01–0.02% soln, lotion, oint **W/P:** [D, ?/–] Severe myleosuppression; tumor lysis synd **CI:** PRG, known infect Dz **Disp:** Inj 10 mg; topical soln, lotion, oint **SE:** ↓ BM, thrombosis, thrombophlebitis at site; tissue damage w/ extrav (Na thiosulfate used topically to Rx); N/V/D, skin rash/allergic dermatitis w/ contact, amenorrhea, sterility (especially in men), secondary leukemia if treated for Hodgkin Dz, chromosomal alterations, hepatotox, peripheral neuropathy **Notes:** Highly volatile and emetogenic; give w/in 30–60 min of prep

Mechlorethamine Gel (Valchlor) Uses: *Stage 1A and 1B mycosis fungoides-type cutaneous T-cell lymphoma* **Acts:** Alkylating agent **Dose:** Apply thin film daily, if skin ulceration/blistering or mod dermatitis, D/C; w/ improvement, restart w/ ↓ dose to q3d; must be refrigerated, apply w/in 30 min, apply to dry skin and no shower for 4 h or wait 30 min after shower to apply **W/P:** [D, –] Mucosal injury may be severe; w/ eye contact irrigate immediately × 15 min and seek consultation, may cause blindness; dermatitis including blisters, swelling, pruritus, redness, ulceration; caregivers/others must avoid skin contact w/ pt; non-melanoma skin Ca risk; flammable **CI:** Hypersens **Disp:** Gel 0.016% 60-gm tube **SE:** Dermatitis, pruritus, skin/ulceration/blistering/hyperpigmentation/skin Infxn **Notes:** Caregivers must wear disposable nitrile gloves and wash hands thoroughly

Meclizine (Antivert, Generic) (Dramamine, Univert) [OTC]) Uses: *Motion sickness, vertigo* **Acts:** Histamine-1 receptor antag **Dose:** *Adults & Peds > 12 y. Motion sickness:* 25–50 mg PO 1 h before travel, repeat PRN q24h; 24h. *Vertigo:* 25–100 mg/d ÷ doses **W/P:** [B, ?/–] NAG, BPH, BOO, elderly, asthma **Disp:** Tabs 12.5, 25, 50 mg; chew tabs 25 mg; caps 12.5 mg (OTC) **SE:** Drowsiness, xerostomia, blurred vision, thickens bronchial secretions, fatigue, HA

Medroxyprogesterone (Depo-Provera, Depo-Sub Q Provera, Provera, Generic) **BOX:** Do not use in the Px of CV Dz or dementia; ↑ risk MI, stroke, breast CA, PE, & DVT in postmenopausal women (50–79 y); ↑ dementia risk in postmenopausal women (≥ 65 y); risk of sig bone loss; does not prevent against STD or HIV; long-term use > 2 y should be limited to situations where other birth control methods are inadequate **Uses:** *Contraception; secondary amenorrhea; endometrial CA, ↓ endometrial hyperplasia, endometriosis pain,* AUB caused by hormonal imbalance **Acts:** Progestin suppl; ↓ estrogen effect on the endometrium **Dose:** *Contraception:* 150 mg IM q3mo depo or 104 mg SQ q3mo (depo SQ) *Secondary amenorrhea:* 5–10 mg/d PO for 5–10 d *AUB:* 5–10 mg/d PO for 5–10 d beginning on the 16th or 21st d of menstrual cycle *Endometrial CA:* 400–1000 mg/wk IM *Estrogen-induced endometrial hyperplasia:* 5–10 mg/d × 12–14 d on d 1 or 16 of cycle *Endometriosis pain:* 104 mg SQ q3mo (no longer than 2 y); ↓ in hepatic Insuff **W/P:** *Provera* [X, –] *Depo Provera* [X, +] **CI:** Thrombophlebitis/embolic disorders, cerebral apoplexy, severe hepatic dysfunction, CA breast/genital organs, undiagnosed Vag bleeding, missed Ab, PRG, as a diagnostic test for PRG, cerebrovascular

Dz **Disp:** *Provera* tabs 2.5, 5, 10 mg; depot Inj 150, 400 mg/mL; depo SQ Inj 104 mg/0.65 mL **SE:** Breakthrough bleeding, spotting, altered menstrual flow, breast tenderness, galactorrhea, depression, insomnia, N, Wt gain, acne, Abd pain, ↓ libido **Notes:** Perform breast exam & Pap smear before contraceptive Rx; obtain PRG test if last Inj > 3 mo

Megestrol Acetate (Megace, Megace-ES, Generic) Uses: *Breast/ endometrial CAs; appetite stimulant in cachexia (CA & HIV)* **Acts:** Hormone; antileutenizing; progesterone analog **Dose:** *Endometrial CA:* 40–320 mg/d PO in ÷ doses *Breast CA:* 160 mg/d ÷ doses for at least 2 mo *Appetite:* 800 mg/d PO ÷ dose or *Megace-ES* 625 mg/d **W/P:** [D (tablet)/X (suspension), –] Thromboembolism; handle w/ care **CI:** PRG **Disp:** Tabs 20, 40 mg; susp 40 mg/mL, Megace-ES 125 mg/mL **SE:** DVT, edema, menstrual bleeding, photosens, N/V/D, HA, mastodynia, ↑ Ca, ↑ glu, insomnia, rash, ↓ BM, ↑ BP, CP, palpitations, **Notes:** Do not D/C abruptly; *Megace-ES* not equivalent to others mg/mg; *Megace-ES* approved only for anorexia; monitor for thromboembolic events

Meloxicam (Mobic, Generic) BOX: May ↑ risk MI/CVA & GI bleeding; CI in postop CABG Uses: *OA, RA, JRA* **Acts:** NSAID w/ ↑ COX-2 activity **Dose:** *Adults.* 7.5–15 mg/d PO *Peds* ≥ 2 y. 0.125 mg/kg/d, max 7.5 mg; ↓ in renal Insuff; take w/ food **W/P:** [C, D (3rd tri), ?/–] w/ Severe renal Insuff, CHF, ACE inhib, diuretics, Li²⁺, MTX, warfarin, ↑ K⁺ **CI:** Peptic ulcer, NSAID, or ASA sens, PRG, postop CABG **Disp:** Tabs 7.5, 15 mg; susp. 7.5 mg/5 mL **SE:** HA, dizziness, GI upset, GI bleeding, edema, ↑ BP, renal impair, rash (SJS), ↑ LFTs

Melphalan [L-PAM] (Alkeran, Generic) BOX: Administer under the supervision of a qualified physician experienced in the use of chemotherapy; severe BM depression, leukemogenic, & mutagenic hypersens (including anaphylaxis in ~2%) Uses: *Multiple myeloma, ovarian CAs*, breast CA, Hodgkin lymphoma, amyloidosis, CML, melanoma; allogenic & ABMT (high dose), neuroblastoma, rhabdomyosarcoma **Acts:** Alkylating agent, nitrogen mustard **Dose:** *Adults. Multiple myeloma:* 16 mg/m² IV q2wk × 4 doses then at 4-wk intervals after tox resolves; w/ renal impair ↓ IV dose *Ovarian CA:* 0.2 mg/kg PO qd × 5 d, repeat q4–5wk based on counts, ↓ in renal Insuff **W/P:** [D, ?/–] w/ Cisplatin, digitalis, live vaccines extrav, need central line **CI:** Allergy **Disp:** Tabs 2 mg; Inj 50 mg **SE:** N/V, secondary malignancy, AF, ↓ LVEF, ↓ BM, secondary leukemia, alopecia, dermatitis, stomatitis, pulm fibrosis; rare allergic Rxns, thrombocytopenia **Notes:** Take PO on empty stomach, false(+) direct Coombs test

Memantine (Namenda) Uses: *Mod–severe Alzheimer Dz*, mild–mod vascular dementia, mild cognitive impair **Acts:** NMDA receptor antag **Dose:** *Namenda:* Target 20 mg/d, start 5 mg/d, ↑ 5–20 mg/d, wait > 1 wk before ↑ dose; use bid if > 5 mg/d *Vascular dementia:* 10 mg PO bid; *Namenda XR* (Alzheimer) 7 mg inital 1× qd, ↑ by 7 mg/wk each wk to maint 28 mg/d × 1; ↓ to 14 mg w/ severe renal impair **W/P:** [B, ?/m] Hepatic/mod renal impair; Sx disorders, cardiac Dz

Disp: *Namenda* tabs 5, 10 mg; combo pack 5 mg × 28 + 10 mg × 21; soln 2 mg/mL **CI:** Component hypersens **SE:** Dizziness, HA, D **Notes:** Renal clearance ↓ by alkaline urine (↓ 80% at pH 8)

Memantine/Donepezil (Namzaric)

Uses: *Mod–severe Alzheimer Dz in pts stabilized on memantine & donepezil as sole agents* **Acts:** NMDA receptor antag w/ acetylcholinesterase inhib **Dose:** Memantine/donepezil 28/10 mg PO qd q P.M. (stable on memantine 10 mg bid or 28 mg ER qd & donepezil 10 mg qd); Memantine/donepezil 14/10 mg PO qd q P.M. (w/CrCl 5–29 mL/min & stable on memantine 5 mg bid or 14 mg ER qd & donepezil 10 mg qd); swallow whole or sprinkle on applesauce **W/P:** [C, ?/–] ↓ HR/heart block w/ conduction abnormalities; may exaggerate succinylcholine-type muscle relaxation w/ anesthesia; GI bleeding w/ risk of PUD; w/ Hx asthma or COPD **CI:** Component hypersens, piperidine deriv **Disp:** Caps memantine/donepezil 14/10, 28/10 mg **SE:** HA, dizziness, N/V/D, anorexia, ecchymosis, BOO **Notes:** Renal clearance ↓ w/ alkaline urine

Meningococcal Cojnugate Vaccine [Quadrivalent, MCV4] (Menactra, Menomune)

Uses: *Immunize against N. meningitidis (meningococcus) high-risk 2–10 and 19–55 y and everyone 11–18 y* high-risk (college freshmen, military recruits, travel to endemic areas, terminal complement deficiencies, asplenia); if given age 11–12 y, give booster at 16, should have booster w/in 5 y of college **Acts:** Active immunization; N. meningitidis A, C, Y, W-135 polysaccharide conjugated to diphtheria toxoid (*Menactra*) or lyophilized conjugate component (*Menveo*) **Dose:** *Adults 18–55 y & Peds > 2 y.* 0.5 mL IM × 1 **W/P:** [B/C, (manufacturer dependent) ?/–] w/ Immunosuppression (↓ response) and bleeding disorders, Hx Guillain-Barré **CI:** Allergy to class/diphtheria toxoid/compound/latex **Disp:** Inj *Menactra* 4 mcg/0.5 mL; *Menveo* 10 mcg A/5 mcg C/ 5 mcg Y/5 mcg Y/5 mcg W/0.5 mL **SE:** Inj site Rxns, HA, N/V/D, anorexia, fatigue, irritability, arthralgia, Guillain-Barré synd **Notes:** IM only; keep epi available for Rxns; use polysaccharide *Menomune* (MPSV4) if > 55 y; do not confuse w/ *Menactra, Menveo*; ACIP rec: MCV4 for 2–55 y, ↑ local Rxn compared to *Menomune* (MPSV4); peds 2–10, Ab levels ↓ 3 y w/ MPSV4, revaccinate in 2–3 y, use MCV4 revaccination

Meningococcal Group B Vaccine (Bexsero, Trumenba)

Uses: Immunization against *N. meningitidis* serogroup B* **Acts:** Active immunization **Dose:** *Bexsero:* Two 0.5-mL IM doses at least 1 mo apart; *Trumenba:* 0.5 mL IM 0, 2, and 6 mo **W/P:** [C, ?] Latex on syringe caps; keep supplies for anaphylactic emergencies **CI:** Component sens **Disp:** 0.5-mL prefilled syringe **SE:** *Bexsero:* Inj site pain, myalgia, erythema, fatigue, HA, induration, N, arthralgia (≥ 13%); *Trumenba:* Inj site pain fatigue, HA, muscle pain, chills

Meningococcal Groups C and Y and Haemophilus b Tetanus Toxoid Conjugate Vaccine (Menhibrix)

Uses: *Px meningococcal Dz and Hib in infants/young children* **Acts:** Active immunization; antibodies specific to organisms **Dose:** *Peds 6 wk–18 mo.* 4 doses 0.5 mL IM at 2, 4, 6, and 12–15 mo **W/P:** [C, N/A] Apnea in some infants reported; w/ Hx Guillain Barré synd; fainting may occur **CI:** Severe allergy to similar vaccines **Disp:** Inj **SE:** Inj pain, redness; irritability; drowsiness; ↓ appetite; fever

Meningococcal Polysaccharide Vaccine [MPSV4] (Menomune A/C/Y/W-135)
Uses: *Immunize against N. meningitidis (meningococcus)* in highrisk (college freshmen, military recruits), travel to endemic areas, terminal complement deficiencies, asplenia) **Acts:** Active immunization **Dose:** *Adults & Peds > 2 y.* 0.5 mL SQ only; peds < 2 y not recommended; 2 doses 3 mo apart, may repeat in 3–5 y if high risk; repeat in 2–3 y if 1st dose given 2–4 y **W/P:** [C, ?/M] If immunocompromised (↓ response) **CI:** Thimerosal/latex sens; w/ pertussis or typhoid vaccine, < 2 y **Disp:** Inj **SE:** Inj site Rxns, drowsiness, irritability, chills, D **Notes:** Keep epi (1:1000) available for Rxns; recommended > 55 y, but also alternative to MCV4 in 2–55 y if no MCV4 available (MCV4 is preferred); active against serotypes A, C, Y, & W-135 but not group B; antibody levels ↓ 3 y; high risk: revaccination q3–5y (use MCV4)

Meperidine (Demerol, Meperitab, Generic) [C–II]
Uses: *Mod–severe pain*, postop shivering, rigors from amphotericin B **Acts:** Narcotic analgesic **Dose:** *Adults.* 50–150 mg PO or IM/SQ q3–4h PRN *Shivering:* 25–50 mg IV × 1 *Peds.* 1.1–1.8 mg/kg/dose PO or IM/SQ q3–4h PRN, up to 100 mg/dose; hepatic impair, avoid in renal impair, avoid use in elderly **W/P:** [C, –] ↓ Sz threshold, adrenal Insuff, head injury, ↑ ICP, hepatic impair, not OK in sickle cell Dz **CI:** w/ MAOIs, w/in 14 d, resp Insuff **Disp:** Tabs 50, 100 mg; syrup/soln 50 mg/5 mL; Inj 25, 50, 75, 100 mg/mL **SE:** Resp/CNS depression, Szs, sedation, constipation, ↓ BP, rash N/V, biliary and urethral spasms, dyspnea **Notes:** Analgesic effects potentiated w/ hydroxyzine; 75 mg IM = 10 mg morphine IM; not best in elderly; do not use oral for acute pain; not OK for repetitive use in ICU setting, naloxone does not reverse neurotox, used as analgesic, is not recommended, limit Tx to < 48 h

Meprobamate (Generic) [C–IV]
Uses: *Short-term relief of anxiety* muscle spasm, TMJ relief **Acts:** Mild tranquilizer; antianxiety **Dose:** *Adults.* 400 mg PO tid-qid, max 2400 mg/d *Peds 6–12 y.* 100–200 mg PO bid-tid; ↓ in renal impair **W/P:** [D, +/−] Elderly; Sz Dz; caution w/ depression or suicidal tendencies; avoid abrupt D/C; avoid use w/ EtOH, CNS depressants **CI:** Acute intermittent prophyria **Disp:** Tabs 200, 400 mg **SE:** Drowsiness, syncope, tachycardia, edema, rash (SJS), N/V/D, ↓ WBC, agranulocytosis **Notes:** Do not abruptly D/C

Mercaptopurine [6-MP] (Purinethol, Purixan, Generic)
Uses: *ALL* 2nd-line Rx for CML & NHL, maint ALL in children, immunosuppressant w/ autoimmune Dzs (Crohn Dz, UC) **Acts:** Antimetabolite, purine analog **Dose:** *Adults. ALL induction:* 1.5–2.5 mg/kg/d; *maint* 60 mg/m²/d w/ allopurinol use 67–75% ↓ dose of 6-MP (interference w/ xanthine oxidase metabolism) *Peds. ALL induction:* 1.5–2.5 mg/kg/d; *maint* 1.5–2.5 mg/kg/d PO or 60 mg/m²/d w/ renal/hepatic Insuff; take on empty stomach **W/P:** [D, ?] w/ Allopurinol, immunosuppression, TMP-SMX,

warfarin, salicylates, severe BM Dz, PRG **CI:** Prior resistance, PRG **Disp:** Tabs 50 mg **SE:** Mild hematotox, mucositis, stomatitis, D, rash, fever, eosinophilia, jaundice, hep, hyperuricemia, hyperpigmentation, alopecia, N/V, ↓ appetite, ↓ BM, pancreatitis **Notes:** Handle properly; limit use to experienced physicians; ensure adequate hydration; for ALL, evening dosing may ↓ risk of relapse; low emetogenicity, TPMT deficiency ↑ immunosuppressive effect

Meropenem (Merrem, Generic) **Uses:** *Intra-Abd Infxns, bacterial meningitis, skin Infxn* **Acts:** Carbapenem; ↓ cell wall synth. *Spectrum:* Excellent gram(+) (except MRSA, MRSE & *E. faecium*); excellent gram(−), including extended-spectrum β-lactamase producers; good anaerobic **Dose: Adults.** *Abd Infxn:* 1–2 g IV q8h *Skin Infxn:* 500 mg IV q8h *Meningitis:* 2 g IV q8h *Peds > 3 mo, < 50 kg. Abd Infxn:* 20 mg/kg IV q8–12 h. *Meningitis:* 40 mg/kg IV q8h *Peds > 50 kg.* Use adult dose; max 2 g IV q8h; ↓ in renal Insuff (see PI) **W/P:** [B, ?/M] w/ Probenecid, VPA, Szs reported **CI:** β-Lactam anaphylaxis **Disp:** Inj 1 g, 500 mg **SE:** Less Sz potential than imipenem; *C. difficile* enterocolitis, D, ↓ plt, rash, N **Notes:** Overuse ↑ bacterial resistance

Mesalamine (Apriso, Asacol, Asacol HD, Canasa, Lialda, Pentasa, Rowasa, Generic) **Uses:** *Rectal: mild–mod distal UC, proctosigmoiditis, proctitis; oral: treat/maint of mild–mod UC* **Acts:** 5-ASA derivative, may inhibit prostaglandins, may ↓ leukotrienes and TNF-α **Dose:** *Rectal:* 60 mL qhs, retain 8 h (enema); *PO:* Caps: 1 g PO qid; tab: 1.6–2.4 g/d ÷ doses (tid-qid) × 6 wk; DR 2.4–4.8 g PO qd, 8 wk max; do not cut/crush/chew w/ food; ↓ initial dose in elderly; maint: depends on formulation **W/P:** [B/C (product specific), M] w/ Digitalis, PUD, pyloric stenosis, renal Insuff, elderly **CI:** Salicylate sens **Disp:** Tabs ER (*Asacol*) 400, (*Asacol HD*) 800 mg; ER caps (*Pentasa*) 250, 500 mg, (*Apriso*) 375 mg; DR tabs (*Lialda*) 1.2 g; supp (*Canasa*) 1000 mg; (*Rowasa*) rectal susp 4 g/60 mL **SE:** Yellow-brown urine, HA, malaise, Abd pain, flatulence, rash, pancreatitis, pericarditis, dizziness, rectal pain, hair loss, intolerance synd (bloody D) **Notes:** Retain rectally 1–3 h; ✓ CBC, Cr, BUN; Sx may ↑ when starting

Mesna, Inf (Generic), Oral (Mesnex) **Uses:** *Px hemorrhagic cystitis d/t ifosfamide or cyclophosphamide* **Acts:** Antidote, reacts w/ acrolein and other metabolites to form stable compounds **Dose:** Per protocol; dose as % of ifosfamide or cyclophosphamide dose. *IV bolus:* 20% (eg, 10–12 mg/kg) IV at 0, 4, & 8 h; *IV Inf:* 20% prechemotherapy, 40% w/ chemotherapy for 12–24 h; *Oral:* 100% ifosfamide dose given as 20% IV at hour 0 then 40% PO at hours 4 & 8; if PO dose vomited repeat or give dose IV; mix PO w/ juice **W/P:** [B; ?/−] **CI:** Thiol sens **Disp:** Inj 100 mg/mL; (*Mesnex*) tabs 400 mg **SE:** ↓ BP, ↓ plt, ↑ HR, ↑ RR allergic Rxns, HA, GI upset, taste perversion, edema, ↑ K$^+$, asthenia, anemia **Notes:** Hydration helps ↓ hemorrhagic cystitis; higher dose for BMT; IV contains benzyl alcohol; PO *Mesna* used for one fosfamide dose < 2 g/m^2/d

Metaprotereonol (Generic) **Uses:** *Asthma & reversible bronchospasm, COPD* **Acts:** Sympathomimetic bronchodilator **Dose: Adults.** Nebulized: 5% 2.5 mL q4–6h or PRN *MDI:* 1–3 Inh q3–4h, 12 Inh max/24 h; wait 2 min between Inh *PO:* 20 mg q6–8h. *Peds ≥ 12 y. MDI:* 2–3 Inh q3–4h, 12 Inh/d max *Nebulizer:* 2.5 mL (soln 0.4, 0.6%) tid-qid, up to q4h *Peds > 9 y or ≥ 27 kg.* 20 mg PO tid-qid *6–9 y or < 27 kg.* 10 mg PO tid-qid; ↓ in elderly **W/P:** [C, ?/–] w/ MAOI, TCA, sympathomimetics; avoid w/ β-blockers **CI:** Tachycardia, other arrhythmias **Disp:** Aerosol 0.65 mg/Inh; soln for Inh 0.4%, 0.6%; tabs 10, 20 mg; syrup 10 mg/5 mL **SE:** Nervousness, tremor, tachycardia, HTN, ↑ glu, ↓ K^+, **Notes:** Fewer β_1 effects than isoproterenol & longer acting, but not a 1st-line β-agonist; use w/ face mask < 4 y; oral ↑ ADR; contains ozone-depleting CFCs; will be gradually removed from US market

Metaxalone (Skelaxin) Uses: *Painful musculoskeletal conditions* **Acts:** Centrally acting skeletal muscle relaxant **Dose:** 800 mg PO tid-qid **W/P:** [C, ?/–] w/ Elderly, EtOH & CNS depression, anemia **CI:** Severe hepatic/renal impair; drug-induced, hemolytic, or other anemias **Disp:** Tabs 800 mg **SE:** N/V, HA, drowsiness, hep

Metformin (Fortmet, Glucophage, Glucophage XR, Glumetza, Riomet, Generic) **BOX:** Associated w/ lactic acidosis, risk ↑ w/ sepsis, dehydration, renal/hepatic impair, ↑ alcohol, acute CHF; Sxs include myalgias, malaise, resp distress, Abd pain, somnolence; Labs: ↓ pH, ↑ anion gap, ↑ blood lactate; D/C immediately & hospitalize if suspected Uses: *Type 2 DM*, PCOS, HIV lipodystrophy **Acts:** Biguanide; ↓ hepatic glu production & intestinal absorption of glu; ↑ insulin sens **Dose:** *Adults.* Initial: 500 mg PO bid; or 850 mg daily, titrate 1- to 2-wk intervals may ↑ to 2550 mg/d max; take w/ A.M. & P.M. meals; can convert total daily dose to daily dose of XR *Peds 10–16 y.* 500 mg PO bid, ↑ 500 mg/d to 2000 mg/d max in ÷ doses; do not use XR formulation in peds **W/P:** [B, +/–] Avoid EtOH; hold dose before ÷ 48 h after ionic imaging contrast; hepatic impair, elderly **CI:** SCr ≥ 1.4 mg/dL in females or ≥ 1.5 mg/dL in males; hypoxemic conditions (eg, acute CHF/sepsis); metabolic acidosis; abnormal CrCl from any cause (AMI, shock); w/ IV contrast (DIC dose) **Disp:** Tabs 500, 850, 1000 mg; XR tabs 500, 750, 1000 mg; *(Riomet)* soln 100 mg/mL **SE:** Anorexia, N/V/D, flatulence, weakness, myalgia, rash

Methadone (Dolophine, Methadose, Generic) [C-II] **BOX:** Deaths reported during initiation and conversion of pain pts to methadone Rx from Rx w/ other opioids; for PO only; tabs contain excipient; resp depression and QT prolongation, arrhythmias observed; only dispensed by certified opioid Tx programs for addiction; analgesic use must outweigh risks Uses: *Severe pain not responsive to non-narcotics; detox w/ maint of narcotic addiction* **Acts:** Narcotic analgesic **Dose:** *Adults.* 2.5 mg IM/IV/SQ q8–12h or PO q8h; titrate as needed; see PI for conversion from other opioids Detoxification: 20–30 mg PO, titrate (usual 80–120 mg/d), ↓ dose < 10% every 10–14 d *Peds.* (Not FDA approved) 0.1 mg/kg q4–12h IV; ↑ slowly to avoid resp depression; ↓ in renal impair **W/P:** [C, –] Avoid w/ severe liver Dz **CI:** Resp depression, acute asthma, ileus w/, selegiline **Disp:** Tabs 5, 10 mg; tabs dispersible 40 mg; PO soln 5, 10 mg/5 mL; PO conc 10 mg/mL; Inj 10 mg/mL **SE:**

Resp depression, sedation, constipation, urinary retention, ↑ QT interval, arrhythmias, ↓ HR, syncope, ↓ K⁺, ↓ Mg²⁺ **Notes:** Parenteral:oral 1:2; equianalgesic w/ parenteral morphine; longer 1/2; resp depression occurs later and lasts longer than analgesic effect, use w/ caution to avoid iatrogenic OD

Methenamine Hippurate (Hiprex), Methenamine Mandelate (Urex, Uroquid-Acid No. 2) **Uses:** *Suppress recurrent UTI long-term; use only after Infxn cleared by antibiotics* **Acts:** Converted to formaldehyde & ammonia in acidic urine; nonspecific bactericidal action **Dose: Adults.** *Hippurate:* 1 g PO bid. *Mandelate:* initial 1 g qid PO pc & hs, maint 1–2 g/d **Peds 6–12 y.** *Hippurate:* 0.5–1 g PO ÷ bid >2 y. *Mandelate:* 50–75 mg/kg/d PO ÷ qid; take w/ food, ascorbic acid w/ hydration **W/P:** [C, +] **CI:** Renal Insuff, severe hepatic Dz, & severe dehydration w/ sulfonamides (may precipitate in urine) **Disp:** *Methenamine hippurate:* Tabs 1 g; *Methenamine mandelate:* 500 mg, 1 g EC tabs **SE:** Rash, GI upset, dysuria, ↑ LFTs, super Infxn w/ prolonged use, *C. difficile*-associated diarrhea. **Notes:** Hippurate not indicated in peds < 6 y; not for pts w/ indwelling catheters as dwell time in bladder required for action; "Urex" used internationally for many meds

Methenamine/Phenyl Salicylate/Methylene Blue/Benzoic Acid/ Hyoscyamine (Hyophen) **Uses:** *Lower urinary tract discomfort* **Acts:** Methenamine in acid urine releases formaldehyde (antiseptic), phenyl salicylate mild analgesic methylene blue/benzoic acid mild antiseptic, hyoscyamine parasympatholytic ↓ muscle spasm **Dose: Adults & Peds > 12 y.** 1 tab PO qid w/ liberal fluid intake **W/P:** [C, ?/–] Avoid w/ sulfonamides, NAG, pyloric/duodenal obst, BOO, coronary artery spasm **CI:** Component hypersens **Disp:** Tabs **SE:** Rash, dry mouth, flushing, ↑ pulse, dizziness, blurred vision, urine/feces discoloration, voiding difficulty/retention **Notes:** Take w/ plenty of fluid, can cause crystalluria; not rec in peds ≤ 6 y

Methimazole (Tapazole, Generic) **Uses:** *Hyperthyroidism, thyrotoxicosis*, prep for thyroid surgery or radiation **Acts:** Blocks T₃ & T₄ formation but does not inactivate circulating T₃, T₄ **Dose: Adults.** Initial based on severity: 15–60 mg/d PO q8h. Maint: 5–15 mg PO daily. **Peds. Initial:** 0.4–0.7 mg/kg/24 h PO q8h. **Maint:** 0.2 mg/kg/d ÷ in 3 doses; take w/ food **W/P:** [D, –] w/ Other meds **CI:** Breast-feeding **Disp:** Tabs 5, 10 mg **SE:** GI upset, dizziness, blood dyscrasias, dermatitis, fever, hepatic Rxns, lupus-like synd **Notes:** Follow clinically & w/ TFT, CBC w/ diff

Methocarbamol (Robaxin, Generic) **Uses:** *Relief of discomfort associated w/ painful musculoskeletal conditions* **Acts:** Centrally acting skeletal muscle relaxant **Dose: Adults & Peds ≥ 16 y.** 1.5 g PO qid for 2–3 d, then 1 g PO qid maint *Tetanus:* 1–2 g IV q6h × 3 d, then use PO, max dose 24 g/d < **16 y.** *Tetanus:* 15 mg/kg/dose or 500 mg/m²/dose IV, may repeat PRN, max 1.8 g/m²/d × 3 d **W/P:** Sz disorders, hepatic & renal impair [C, ?/M] **CI:** MyG, renal impair w/ IV **Disp:** Tabs 500, 750 mg; Inj 100 mg/mL **SE:** Can discolor urine, lightheadedness, drowsiness, GI upset, ↓ HR, ↓ BP **Notes:** Tabs can be crushed and added to NG, do not operate heavy machinery; max rate IV = 3 mL/min

Methotrexate (Otrexup, Rasuvo, Rheumatrex Dose Pack, Trexall, Generic) BOX: Administration only by experienced physician; do not use in women of childbearing age unless absolutely necessary (teratogenic); impaired elimination w/ impaired renal Fxn, ascites, pleural effusion; severe ↓ BM w/ NSAIDs; hepatotox, occasionally fatal; can induce life-threatening pneumonitis; D and ulcerative stomatitis require D/C; lymphoma risk; may cause tumor lysis synd; can cause severe skin Rxn, opportunistic Infxns; w/ RT can ↑ tissue necrosis risk; preservatives make this agent unsuitable for intrathecal IT or higher dose use Uses: *ALL, AML, leukemic meningitis, trophoblastic tumors (choriocarcinoma, hydatidiform mole), breast, lung, head, & neck CAs, Burkitt lymphoma, mycosis fungoides, osteosarcoma, Hodgkin Dz & NHL, psoriasis; RA, JRA, SLE* Acts: ↓ Dihydrofolate reductase-mediated prod of tetrahydrofolate, ↓ DNA synth Dose: *Adults. CA:* Per protocol. *RA:* 7.5 mg/wk PO 1/wk or 2.5 mg q12h PO for 3 doses/wk *Psoriasis:* 2.5–5 mg PO q12h × 3d/wk or 10–25 mg PO/IM qwk *Peds.* JIA: 10 mg/m² PO/IM qwk, then 5–14 mg/m² × 1 or as 3 divided doses 12 h apart; ↓ elderly, w/ renal/hepatic impair W/P: [X, –] w/ Other nephro-/hepatotoxic meds, multiple interactions, w/ Sz, profound ↓ BM other than CA related CI: Severe renal/hepatic impair, PRG/lactation Disp: Dose pack 2.5 mg in 8, 12, 16, 20, or 24 doses; tabs 2.5, 5, 7.5, 10, 15 mg; Inj 25 mg/mL; Inj powder 20 mg, 1 g; *Otrexup:* 10/15/20/25 mg per 0.4 mL weekly self-admin kit; *Rasuvo:* single-dose auto-injector for weekly SC Inj (mg/mL) 7.5/0.15; 10/0.2; 12.5/0.25; 15/0.3; 17.5/0.35; 20/0.4; 22.5/0.45; 25/0.5; 27.5/0.55; 30/0.6 SE: ↓ BM, N/V/D, anorexia, mucositis, hepatotox (transient & reversible; may progress to atrophy, necrosis, fibrosis, cirrhosis), rashes, dizziness, malaise, blurred vision, alopecia, photosens, renal failure, pneumonitis; rare pulm fibrosis; chemical arachnoiditis & HA w/ IT delivery Notes: Monitor CBC, LFTs, Cr, MTX levels & CXR; "high dose" > 500 mg/m² requires leucovorin rescue to ↓ tox; w/ IT, use preservative-/alcohol-free soln; systemic levels: *Therapeutic:* > 0.01 micromole; *Toxic:* > 10 micromole over 24 h; administer Otrexup in abdomen or thigh SQ

Methyldopa (Generic) Uses: *HTN* Acts: Centrally acting antihypertensive, ↓ sympathetic outflow Dose: *Adults.* 250–500 mg PO bid-tid (max 2–3 g/d) or 250 mg–1 g IV q6–8h. *Peds Neonates.* 2.5–5 mg/kg PO/IV q8h. *Other peds.* 10 mg/kg/24 h PO in 2–3 ÷ doses or 5–10 mg/kg/dose IV q6–8h to max 65 mg/kg/24 h; ↓ in renal Insuff/elderly W/P: [B, +] CI: Liver Dz, w/ MAOIs, bisulfate allergy Disp: Tabs 250, 500 mg; Inj 50 mg/mL SE: Initial transient sedation/drowsiness, edema, hemolytic anemia, hepatic disorders, fevers, nightmares, ED Notes: Tolerance may occur, false(+) Coombs test; often considered DOC during PRG

Methylene Blue (Urolene Blue, Various) Uses: *Methemoglobinemia, vasoplegic synd, ifosfamide-induced encephalopathy, cyanide poisoning, dye in therapeutics/diagnosis* Acts: Low IV dose converts methemoglobin to hemoglobin; excreted, appears in urine as green/green-blue color; MAOI activity Dose: 1–2 mg/kg or 25–50 mg/m² IV over 5–10 min, repeat q1h; direct instillation into fistulous tract **W/P:** [X, –] w/ Severe renal impair, w/ psych meds such as SSRI, SNRI, TCAs (may cause serotonin synd), w/ G6PD deficiency **CI:** Intra spinal Inj, severe renal Insuff, PRG **Disp:** 1, 10 mL Inj **SE:** *IV use:* N, Abd, CP, sweating, fecal/urine discoloration, hemolytic anemia, ↑ BP **Notes:** Component of other medications; stains tissue blue, limits repeat use in surgical visualization

Methylergonovine (Methergine) Uses: *Postpartum bleeding (atony, hemorrhage)* **Acts:** Ergotamine derivative, rapid and sustained uterotonic effect **Dose:** 0.2 mg IM after anterior shoulder delivery or puerperium, may repeat in 2- to 4-h intervals or 0.2–0.4 mg PO q6–12h for 2–7 d **W/P:** [C, ?] w/ Sepsis, obliterative vascular Dz, hepatic/renal impair, w/ CYP3A4 inhib (Table 10, p 356), not rec for IV use **CI:** HTN, PRG, toxemia **Disp:** Inj 0.2 mg/mL; tabs 0.2 mg **SE:** HTN, N/V, CP, ↓ BP, Sz, HA **Notes:** Give IV only if absolutely necessary over > 1 min w/ BP monitoring

Methylnaltrexone Bromide (Relistor) Uses: *Opioid-induced constipation in pt w/ advanced illness such as CA* **Acts:** Peripheral opioid antag **Dose:** *Adults. Wt-based < 38 kg:* 0.15 mg/kg SQ; *38–61 kg:* 8 mg SQ; *62–114 kg:* 12 mg SQ *>114 kg:* 0.15 mg/kg, round to nearest 0.1 mL, dose q other day PRN, max 1 dose q24h **W/P:** [B, ?/M] w/ CrCl < 30 mL/min ↓ dose 50%, GI perf reported **Disp:** Inj 12 mg/0.6 mL **CI:** GI obstr **SE:** N/D, Abd pain, dizziness **Notes:** Does not affect opioid analgesic effects or induce withdrawal

Methylphenidate, Oral (Concerta, Focalin, Focalin XR, Metadate CD, Metadate SR, Methylin, Quillivant XR, Ritalin, Ritalin LA, Ritalin SR) [C-II] **BOX:** w/ Hx of drug or alcohol dependence, avoid abrupt D/C; chronic use can lead to dependence or psychotic behavior; observe closely during withdrawal of drug Uses: *ADHD, narcolepsy, depression* **Acts:** CNS stimulant, blocks reuptake of norepinephrine and DA **Dose:** *Adults. Narcolepsy:* 10 mg PO bid–tid, 60 mg/d max *Depression:* 2.5 mg q A.M., ↑ slowly, 20 mg/d max, ÷ bid 7 A.M. & 12 P.M.; use regular release only *Adults & Peds > 6 y. ADHD: IR:* 5 mg PO bid, ↑ 5–10 mg to 60 mg/d, max (2 mg/kg/d); *ER/SR:* use total IR dose qd *CD/LA:* 20 mg PO qd, ↑ 10–20 mg qwk to 60 mg/d max *Concerta:* 18 mg PO qA.M. Rx naïve or already on 20 mg/d; 36 mg PO qA.M. if on 30–45 mg/d; 54 mg PO qA.M. if on 40–60 mg/d; 72 mg PO qA.M. **W/P:** [C, M] Serious CV events, ↑ BP, psych events, Szs, priapism, peripheral vasculopathy, visual disturbance, ↓ growth, GI obstr, ✓ CBC w/ long-term use **Disp:** Chew tabs 2.5, 5, 10 mg; scored ER tabs (*Ritalin*) 5, 10, 20 mg; ER caps (*Ritalin LA*) 10, 20, 30, 40 mg; ER caps (*Metadate CD*) 10, 20, 30, 40, 50, 60 mg; ER caps (*Methylin ER*) 10, 20 mg; SR tabs (*Metadate SR, Ritalin SR*) 20 mg; ER tabs (*Concerta*) 18, 27, 36, 54 mg; oral soln 5, 10 mg/5 mL; ER susp (*QuilliVant XR*) 5 mg/mL **SE:** ↑ appetite, HA, dry mouth, nausea, insomnia, anxiety, dizziness, ↑ Wt, irritability, hyperhidrosis **W/P:** Component hypersens, marked anxiety/agitation, glaucoma, tics or fam Hx Tourette synd, MAOI w/in 2 wk **Notes:** See also transdermal form; titrate dose; take 30–45 min ac; do not chew or crush; *Concerta* "ghost tablet" in stool, avoid w/ GI narrowing;

Metadate contains sucrose, avoid w/ lactose/galactose problems; do not use these meds w/ halogenated anesthetics; abuse and diversion concerns; AHA rec all ADHD peds need CV assessment/possible ECG before Rx

Methylphenidate, Transdermal (Daytrana) [C-II] **BOX:** w/ Hx of drug or alcohol dependence; chronic use can lead to dependence or psychotic behavior; observe closely during withdrawal of drug **Uses:** *ADHD in children 6–17 y* **Acts:** CNS stimulant, blocks reuptake of norepinephrine and DA **Dose:** *Adults & Peds 6–17 y.* Apply to hip in A.M. (2 h before desired effect), remove 9 h later; titrate 1st wk 10 mg/9 h, 2nd wk 15 mg/9 h, 3rd wk 20 mg/9 h, 4th wk 30 mg/9 h **W/P:** [C, +/–] See Methylphenidate, Oral; sensitization may preclude subsequent use of oral forms; abuse and diversion concerns **CI:** Significant anxiety, agitation; component allergy; glaucoma; w/ or w/in 14 d of MAOI; tics or family Hx Tourette synd **Disp:** Patches 10, 15, 20, 30 mg **SE:** Local Rxns, N/V, nasopharyngitis, ↓ Wt, ↓ appetite, lability, insomnia, tic, priapism **Notes:** Titrate dose weekly; effects last hours after removal; evaluate BP, HR at baseline and periodically; avoid heat exposure to patch, may cause OD, AHA rec: all ADHD peds need CV assessment and consideration for ECG before Rx

Methylprednisolone (A-Methapred, Depo-Medrol, Medrol, Medrol Dosepak, Solu-Medrol, Generic) [See Steroids, p 287 and Tables 2 & 3, pp 335 & 336] **Uses:** *Steroid-responsive conditions (endocrine, rheumatic, collagen, dermatologic, allergic, ophthalmic, respiratory, hematologic, neoplastic, edematous, GI, CNS, others)* **Acts:** Glucocorticoid **Dose:** See Steroids *Peds. ECC 2010.* Status asthmaticus, anaphylactic shock: 2 mg/kg IV/IO/ IM (max 60 mg). *Maint:* 0.5 mg/kg IV q6h or 1 mg/kg q12h to 120 mg/d **W/P:** [C, ?/M] May mask Infx, cataract w/ prolonged use; avoid vaccines **CI:** Fungal Infx, component allergy **Disp:** Oral (*Medrol*) 4, 8, 16, 32 mg, (*Medrol Dosepak*) 21 4-mg tabs taken over 6 d; Inj acetate (*Depo-Medrol*) 20, 40, 80 mg/mL; Inj succinate (*Solu-Medrol*) 40, 125, 500 mg, 1, 2 g **SE:** Fluid and electrolyte disturbances, muscle weakness/loss, ulcers, impaired wound healing, others (see PI) **Notes:** Taper dose to avoid adrenal Insuff

Metoclopramide (Metozolv ODT, Reglan, Generic) **BOX:** Chronic use may cause tardive dyskinesia; D/C if Sxs develop; avoid prolonged use (> 12 wk) **Uses:** *Diabetic gastroparesis, symptomatic GERD; chemo & postop N/V, facilitate small-bowel intubation & upper GI radiologic exam*, *GERD, diabetic gastroparesis (Metozolv)* stimulate gut in prolonged postop ileus* **Acts:** ↑ Upper GI motility; blocks DA in chemoreceptor trigger zone, sensitizes tissues to ACH **Dose:** *Adults. Gastroparesis (Reglan):* 10 mg PO 30 min ac & hs for 2–8 wk PRN, or same dose IM/IV for 10 d, then PO *Reflux:* 10–15 mg PO 30 min ac & hs *Chemo antiemetic:* 1–2 mg/kg/dose IV 30 min before chemo, then q2h × 2 doses, then q3h × 3 doses *Postop:* 10–20 mg IV/IM q4–6h PRN *Adults & Peds > 14 y. Intestinal intubation:* 10 mg IV × 1 over 1–2 min *Peds. Reflux:* 0.1–0.2 mg/kg/dose PO 30 min ac & hs *Chemo antiemetic:* 1–2 mg/kg/dose IV as adults *Postop:*

0.25 mg/kg IV q6–8h PRN *Peds. Intestinal intubation: 6–14 y.* 2.5–5 mg IV × 1 over 1–2 min *< 6 y.* Use 0.1 mg/kg IV × 1 **W/P:** [B, M] Drugs w/ extrapyramidal ADRs, MAOIs, TCAs, sympathomimetics; NMS reported IV w/ EPS meds, GI bleeding, pheochromocytoma, Sz disorders, GI obst **Disp:** Tabs 5, 10 mg; syrup 5 mg/5 mL; ODT *(Metozolv)* 5, 10 mg; Inj 5 mg/mL **SE:** Dystonic Rxns common w/ high doses (Rx w/ IV diphenhydramine), fluid retention, restlessness, D, drowsiness **Notes:** ↓ w/ Renal impair/elderly; ✓ baseline Cr

Metolazone (Zaroxolyn, Generic) Uses: *Mild–mod essential HTN & edema of renal Dz or cardiac failure* **Acts:** Thiazide-like diuretic; ↓ distal tubule Na reabsorption **Dose:** *HTN:* 2.5–5 mg/d PO qd *Edema:* 2.5–20 mg/d PO qd **W/P:** [B, –] Avoid w/ Li, gout, digitalis, SLE, many interactions **CI:** Anuria, hepatic coma or precoma **Disp:** Tabs 2.5, 5, 10 mg **SE:** Monitor fluid/lytes; dizziness, ↓ BP, ↓ K+, ↑ HR, ↑ uric acid, CP, photosens

Metoprolol Succinate (Toprol XL, Generic), Metoprolol Tartrate (Lopressor, Generic) BOX: Do not acutely stop Rx as marked worsening of angina can result; taper over 1–2 wk **Uses:** *HTN, angina, AMI, CHF (XL form)* **Acts:** β₁-Adrenergic receptor blocker **Dose:** *Adults. Angina:* 50–200 mg PO bid max 400 mg/d; ER form dose qd *HTN:* 50–200 mg PO bid, max 450 mg/d, ER form dose qd *AMI:* 5 mg IV q2min × 3 doses, then 50 mg PO q6h × 48 h, then 100 mg PO bid *CHF: (XL* form preferred) 12.5–25 mg/d PO × 2 wk, ↑ 2-wk intervals, target 200 mg max, use low dose w/ greatest severity *ECC 2010. AMI:* 5 mg slow IV q5min, total 15 mg; then 50 mg PO, titrate to effect *Peds 1–17 y. HTN* IR form 1–2 mg/kg/d PO, max 6 mg/kg/d (200 mg/d) *≥ 6 y. HTN* ER form 1 mg/kg/d PO, initial max 50 mg/d, ↑ PRN to 2 mg/kg/d max; ↓ w/ hepatic failure; take w/ meals **W/P:** [C, M] Uncompensated CHF, ↓ HR, heart block, hepatic impair, MyG, PVD, Raynaud, thyrotoxicosis **CI:** For HTN/angina: SSS (unless paced), severe PVD, cardiogenic shock, severe PAD, 2nd-, 3rd-H block, pheochromocytoma. For MI: sinus brady < 45 BPM, 1st-degree block (PR > 0.24 s), 2nd-, 3rd-degree block, SBP < 100 mm Hg, severe CHF, cardiogenic shock **Disp:** Tabs 25, 50, 100 mg; ER tabs 25, 50, 100, 200 mg; Inj 1 mg/mL **SE:** Drowsiness, insomnia, ED, ↓ HR, bronchospasm **Notes:** IR:ER 1:1 daily dose but ER/XL is qd; OK to split XL tab, but do not crush/chew; do not abruptly D/C, may see rebound ↑ HR

Metronidazole (Flagyl, Flagyl ER, MetroCream, MetroGel, MetroLotion) BOX: Carcinogenic in rats **Uses:** *Bone/jt, endocarditis, intra-Abd, meningitis, & skin Infxns; amebiasis & amebic liver abscess; trichomoniasis in pt and partner; bacterial vaginosis; PID; giardiasis; abx-associated pseudomembranous colitis (C. difficile), eradicate H. pylori w/ combo Rx, rosacea, prophylactic in postop colorectal surgery* **Acts:** Interferes w/ DNA synth. **Spectrum:** Excellent anaerobic, *C. difficile* **Dose:** *Adults. Anaerobic Infxns:* 500 mg IV q6–8h. *Amebic dysentery:* 500–750 mg/d PO q8h × 5–10 d *Trichomonas:* 250 mg PO tid for 7 d or 2 g PO × 1 (Rx partner) *C. difficile:* 500 mg PO or IV q8h for 7–10 d (PO preferred; IV only if pt NPO), if no response, change to PO vancomycin

Vaginosis: 1 applicator intravag qd or bid × 5 d, or 500 mg PO bid × 7 d or 750 mg PO qd × 7 d *Acne rosacea/skin:* Apply bid *Giardia:* 500 mg PO bid × 5–7 d. *H. pylori:* 250–500 mg PO w/ meals & hs × 14 d, combine w/ other antibiotic & a PPI or H_2 antag **Peds.** *Anaerobic Infxns:* PO: 15–35 mg/kg/d ÷ q8h *IV:* 30 mg/kg IV/d ÷ q6H, 4 g/d max ÷ dose *Amebic dysentery:* 35–50 mg/kg/24 h PO in 3 ÷ doses for 5–10 d *Trichomonias:* 15–30 mg/kg/d PO ÷ q8h × 7 d *C. difficile:* 30 mg/kg/d PO ÷ q6h × 10 d, max 2 g/d; ↓ w/ severe hepatic/renal impair **W/P:** [B, –] Avoid EtOH, w/ warfarin, CYP3A4 substrates (Table 10, p 356), ↑ Li levels **CI:** Oral/topical: Component hypersens; oral w/ disulfram, w/ EtOH, 1st tri PRG **Disp:** Tabs 250, 500 mg; ER tabs 750 mg; caps 375 mg; IV 500 mg/100 mL; lotion 0.75%; gel 0.75, 1%; intravag gel 0.75% (5 g/applicator 37.5 mg in 70-g tube); cream 0.75, 1% **SE:** Disulfiram-like Rxn; dizziness, HA, GI upset, anorexia, urine discoloration, flushing, metallic taste **Notes:** For trichomoniasis, Rx pt's partner; no aerobic bacteria activity; use in combo w/ serious mixed Infxns; wait 24 h after 1st dose to breast-feed or 48 h if extended Rx, take ER on empty stomach

Mexiletine (Generic) BOX: Mortality risks noted for flecainide and/or encainide (class I antiarrhythmics); reserve for use in pts w/ life-threatening ventricular arrhythmias **Uses:** *Suppress symptomatic ventricular arrhythmias* DN **Acts:** Class Ib antiarrhythmic (Table 9, p 355) **Dose:** *Adults.* 200–300 mg PO q8h; initial 200 mg q8h, can load w/ 400 mg if needed, ↑ q2–3d, 1200 mg/d max, ↓ dose w/ hepatic impairment or CHF, administer ATC w/ food **W/P:** [C, +] CHF; may worsen severe arrhythmias; interacts w/ hepatic inducers & suppressors; blood dyscrasias **CI:** Cardiogenic shock or 2nd-/3rd-degree AV block w/o pacemaker **Disp:** Caps 150, 200, 250 mg **SE:** Lightheadedness, dizziness, anxiety, incoordination, GI upset, ataxia, hepatic damage, blood dyscrasias, PVCs, N/V, tremor **Notes:** ✓ LFTs, CBC, false(+) ANA

Micafungin (Mycamine) Uses: *Candidemia, acute dissem and esophageal candidiasis, Candida peritonitis & abscesses; prophylaxis Candida Infxn w/ HSCT* **Acts:** Echinocandin; ↓ fungal cell wall synth **Dose:** *Candidemia, acute disseminated candidiasis, Candida peritonitis & abscesses:* 100 mg IV daily; *Esophageal candidiasis:* 150 mg IV daily; *Prophylaxis of Candida Infxn:* 50 mg IV daily over 1 h **W/P:** [C, ?/–] Sirolimus, nifedipine, itraconazole dosage adjustment may be necessary **CI:** Component or other echinocandin allergy **Disp:** Inj 50, 100 mg vials **SE:** N/V/D, HA, pyrexia, Abd pain, ↓ K^+, ↓ plt, histamine Sxs (rash, pruritus, facial swelling, vasodilatation), anaphylaxis, anaphylactoid Rxn, hemolysis, hemolytic anemia, ↑ LFTs, hepatotox, renal impair

Miconazole (Monistat 1 Combination Pack, Monistat 3, Monistat 7) [OTC] (Monistat-Derm) Uses: *Candidal Infxns, dermatomycoses (tinea pedis/tinea cruris/tinea corporis/tinea versicolor/candidiasis)* **Acts:** Azole antifungal, alters fungal membrane permeability **Dose:** *Intravag:* 100 mg supp or 2% cream intravag qhs × 7 d or 200 mg supp or 4% cream intravag qhs × 3 d *Derm:* Apply bid, A.M./P.M. *Tinea versicolor:* Apply qd. Treat tinea pedis and tinea corporis for 1 mo and other Infxns for 2 wk **Peds ≥12 y.** 100 mg supp or 2% cream intravag qhs × 7 d or 200 mg supp or 4% cream intravag qhs × 3 d. Not for OTC use in children < 2 y **W/P:** [C, ?] Azole sens **Disp:** *Monistat-Derm:* (Rx) Cream 2%; *Monistat 1 Combination Pack:* 2% cream w/ 1200 mg supp, *Monistat 3:* Vag cream 4%, supp 200 mg; *Monistat 7:* cream 2%, supp 100 mg; lotion 2%; powder 2%; effervescent tab 2%, oint 2%, spray 2%; Vag supp 100, 200, 1200 mg; Vag cream 2%, 4%; [OTC] **SE:** Vag burning; on skin, contact dermatitis, irritation, burning **Notes:** May interfere w/ condom and diaphragm, do not use w/ tampons

Miconazole/Zinc Oxide/Petrolatum (Vusion) **Uses:** *Candidal diaper rash* **Acts:** Combo antifungal **Dose:** *Peds ≥ 4 wk.* Apply at each diaper change × 7 d **W/P:** [C, ?] **CI:** Ø **Disp:** Miconazole zinc oxide/petrolatum oint 0.25/15/81.35%, 50-, 90-g tube **SE:** Ø **Notes:** Keep diaper dry, not for Px

Midazolam (Generic) [C-IV] **BOX:** Associated w/ resp depression and resp arrest, especially when used for sedation in noncritical care settings; reports of airway obst, desaturation, hypoxia, and apnea w/ other CNS depressants; cont monitoring required; initial doses in elderly & debilitated should be conservative **Uses:** *Preop sedation, conscious sedation for short procedures & mechanically ventilated pts, induction of general anesthesia* **Acts:** Short-acting benzodiazepine **Dose:** *Adults.* 1–5 mg IV or IM or 0.02–0.35 mg/kg based on indication; titrate to effect *Peds. Preop:* > 6 mo: 0.25–0.5 mg/kg PO × 1 (max 20 mg) or 0.05–0.1 mg/kg IV over 2–3 min (max 6 mg); > 12 y: 1–2.5 mg over 2 min (max 10 mg) *General anesthesia:* 0.025–0.1 mg/kg IV q2min for 1–3 doses PRN to induce anesthesia; ↓ in elderly, w/ narcotics or CNS depressants **W/P:** [D, M] w/ CYP3A4 substrate (Table 10, p 356), multiple drug interactions **CI:** Component hypersens, NAG, intrathecal/epidural Inj of parenteral forms. **Disp:** Inj 1, 5 mg/mL; syrup 2 mg/mL **SE:** Resp depression; ↓ BP w/ conscious sedation, N **Notes:** Reversal w/ flumazenil; monitor for resp depression

Midodrine (Proamatine) **BOX:** Indicated for pts for whom orthohypotension significantly impairs daily life despite standard care **Uses:** *Tx orthostatic hypotension* **Acts:** Vasopressor/antihypotensive; α₁-agonist **Dose:** 10 mg PO tid when pt plans to be upright **W/P:** [C, ?] **CI:** Pheochromocytoma, renal Dz, thyrotoxicosis, severe heart Dz, urinary retention, supine HTN **Disp:** Tabs 2.5, 5, 10 mg **SE:** BP, paresthesia, pruritis (mostly scalp), goosebumps, chills, urinary Sxs (urge/frequency/retention) **Notes:** SBP ≥ 200 mm Hg in ~13% pts given 10 mg

Mifepristone (Korlym, Mifeprex) **BOX:** Antiprogestational; can cause termination of PRG. Exclude PRG before use or Rx is interrupted for > 14 d in ♀ of reproductive potential **Uses:** *Control hyperglycemia w/ Cushing synd and type 2 DM in nonsurgical or failed surgical candidates (Korlym);* termination of PRG (≤ 49 d) *(Mifeprex)** **Acts:** Antiprogestin; glucocorticoid receptor blocker **Dose:** *Korlym:* Start 300 mg PO qd w/ meal, ↑ PRN to 1200 mg/d max (20 mg/kg/d); mod renal hepatic impair 600 mg/d max *Mifeprex:* 600 mg PO × 1 **W/P:** [X, –] Do not use w/ severe hepatic impair or w/ OCP; avoid w/ ↑ QT or drugs that ↑ QT; ✓ for adrenal Insuff; ✓ K⁺; ✓ Vag bleeding or w/ anticoagulants; caution w/ drugs metabolized by CYP3A, CYP2C8/2C9, CYP2B6 (eg, bupropion, efavirenz) **CI:** PRG, w/ simvastatin, lovastatin, CYP3A substrates, long-term steroids, unexplained uterine bleeding, endometrial hyperplasia/Ca **Disp:** *Korlym:* tabs 300 mg; *Mifeprex:* tabs 200 mg K⁺, arthralgia, edema, ↑ BP, dizziness, ↓ appetite, endometrial hypertrophy **Notes:** *Mifeprex* is RU486

Miglitol (Glyset)   **Uses:** *Type 2 DM* **Acts:** α-Glucosidase inhib; delays carbohydrate digestion **Dose:** Initial 25 mg PO tid; maint 50–100 mg tid (w/ 1st bite of each meal), titrate over 4–8 wk **W/P:** [B, –] w/ Digitalis & digestive enzymes, not rec w/ SCr > 2 mg/dL **CI:** DKA, obstructive/inflam GI disorders; colonic ulceration **Disp:** Tabs 25, 50, 100 mg **SE:** Flatulence, D, Abd pain **Notes:** Use alone or w/ sulfonylureas

Milnacipran (Savella)   **BOX:** Antidepressants associated w/ ↑ risk of suicide ideation in children and young adults **Uses:** *Fibromyalgia* **Acts:** Antidepressant, SNRI **Dose:** 50 mg PO bid; titrate: d 1 12.5 mg × 1, d 2–3 12.5 mg bid, d 4–7 25 mg bid, then 50 mg bid; may ↑ to 200 mg/d; ↓ to 25 mg bid w/ CrCl < 30 mL/min **W/P:** [C, /?] Caution w/ hepatic impair, hepatox, serotonin synd, ↑ bleeding risk, do not D/C abruptly **CI:** NAG, w/ recent MAOI **Disp:** Tab 12.5, 25, 50, 100 mg **SE:** HA, N/V, constipation, dizziness, ↑ HR, ↑ BP **Notes:** Monitor HR and BP

Milrinone (Primacor, Generic)   **Uses:** *CHF acutely decompensated*, Ca antag intoxication **Acts:** Phosphodiesterase inhib, (+) inotrope & vasodilator; little chronotropic activity **Dose:** 50 mcg/kg, IV over 10 min then 0.375–0.75 mcg/kg/min IV Inf; ↓ w/ renal impair **W/P:** [C, ?] **CI:** Allergy to drug; w/ inamrinone **Disp:** Inj 200 mcg/mL **SE:** Arrhythmias, ↓ BP, HA **Notes:** Monitor fluids, lytes, CBC, Mg²⁺, BP, HR; not for long-term use

Mineral Oil, Oral [OTC], Mineral Oil Enema (Fleet Mineral Oil) [OTC]   **Uses:** *Constipation, bowel irrigation, fecal impaction* **Acts:** Lubricant laxative **Dose:** *Adults. Constipation:* 15–45 mL PO/d PRN *Fecal impaction or after barium:* 118 mL rectally × 1 *Peds > 5 y. Constipation:* 5–15 mL PO qhs. *2–11 y. Fecal impaction:* 59 mL rectally × 1 **W/P:** [?, ?] w/ N/V, difficulty swallowing, bedridden pts; may ↓ absorption of vits A, D, E, K, warfarin **CI:** Colostomy/ileostomy, appendicitis, diverticulitis, UC **Disp:** All [OTC] liq, PO microemulsion 2.5 mL/5 mL, rectal enema 118 mL **SE:** Lipid pneumonia (aspiration of PO), N/V, temporary anal incontinence **Notes:** Take PO upright, do not use PO in peds < 6 y

Mineral Oil/Pramoxine HCl/Zinc Oxide (Tucks Ointment [OTC])   **Uses:** *Temporary relief of anorectal disorders (itching, etc)* **Acts:** Topical anesthetic **Dose:** *Adults & Peds ≥ 12 y.* Cleanse, rinse, & dry, apply externally or into anal canal w/ tip 5×/d × 7 d max **W/P:** [?, ?] Do not place into rectum **CI:** Ø **Disp:** Oint 1% 30-g tube **SE:** Local irritation **Notes:** D/C w/ or if rectal bleeding occurs or if condition worsens or does not improve w/in 7 d

Minocycline (Arestin, Dynacin, Minocin, Solodyn, Generic)   **Uses:** *Mod–severe nonnodular acne (Solodyn),* anthrax, rickettsiae, skin Infxn, URI, UTI, nongonococcal urethritis, amebic dysentery, asymptomatic meningococcal carrier, *M. marinum*, adjunct to dental scaling for periodontitis (*Arestin*)* **Acts:** Tetracycline, bacteriostatic, ↓ protein synth **Dose:** *Adults & Peds > 12 y. Usual:* 200 mg, then 100 mg q12h or 100–200 mg IV or PO, then 50 mg qid *Gonococcal urethritis, men:* 100 mg q12h × 5 d *Syphilis:* Usual dose × 10–15 d *Meningococcal carrier:* 100 mg q12h × 5 d *M. marinum:* 100 mg q12h × 6–8 wk *Uncomp urethral, endocervical, or rectal Infxn:* 100 mg q12h × 7 d minimum *Adults & Peds > 12 y.* Acne: (*Solodyn*) 1 mg/kg PO qd × 12 wk **> 8 y.** 4 mg/kg initially, then 2 mg/kg q12h w/ food to ↓ irritation, hydrate well, ↓ dose or extend interval w/ renal impair **W/P:** [D, –] Associated w/ pseudomembranous colitis, w/ renal impair, may ↓ OCP, or w/ warfarin may ↑ INR **CI:** Allergy, children < 8 y **Disp:** Tabs 50, 75, 100 mg; tabs ER (*Solodyn*) 45, 55, 65, 80, 90, 105, 115, 135 mg; caps (*Minocin*) 50, 75, 100 mg; *Minocin* inj 100 mg/vial susp 50 mg/mL (*Arestin*); topical power **SE:** D, HA, fever, rash, joint pain, fatigue, dizziness, photosens, hyperpigmentation, SLE synd, pseudotumor cerebri **Notes:** Do not cut/crush/chew; keep away from children, tooth discoloration in < 8 y or w/ use last half of PRG

Minoxidil, Oral (Generic) **BOX:** May cause pericardial effusion, occasional tamponade, and angina pectoris may be exacerbated; only for nonresponders to max doses of 2 other antihypertensives and a diuretic; administer under supervision w/ a β-blocker and diuretic; monitor for ↓ BP in those receiving guanethidine w/ malignant HTN **Uses:** *Severe HTN* **Acts:** Peripheral vasodilator **Dose:** *Adults & Peds > 12 y.* 5 mg PO qd, titrate q3d, 100 mg/d max usual range 2.5–80 mg/d in 1–2 ÷ doses *Peds.* 0.2–1 mg/kg/24 h ÷ PO q12–24h, titrate q3d, max 50 mg/d; ↓ w/ elderly, renal Insuff **W/P:** [C, –] Caution in renal impair, CHF **CI:** Pheochromocytoma, component allergy **Disp:** Tabs 2.5, 10 mg **SE:** Pericardial effusion & vol overload w/ PO use; hypertrichosis w/ chronic use, edema, ECG changes, Wt gain **Notes:** Avoid for 1 mo after MI

Minoxidil, Topical (Theroxidil, Rogaine) [OTC] **Uses:** *Male & female pattern baldness* **Acts:** Stimulates vertex hair growth **Dose:** Apply 1 mL soln bid to area, or 1/2 capful of foam bid ♂/qd ♀ **D/C** if no growth in 4 mo **W/P:** [?, ?] **CI:** Component allergy **Disp:** Soln & aerosol foam 2, 5%; ♂ and ♀ products differ in dosing **SE:** Changes in hair color/texture **Notes:** Requires chronic use to maintain hair

Mipomersen (Kynamro) **BOX:** May cause hepatotox; ✓ AST, ALT, bili, alk phos before and during; hold if ALT/AST > 3 × ULM; D/C w/ hepatotox; may cause ↑ hepatic fat w or w/o ↑ ALT/AST **Uses:** *Adjunct to lipid-lowering meds to ↓ LDL* **Acts:** Inhib apolipoprotein B-100 synth **Dose:** *Adults.* 200 mg SQ, 1 × wk **W/P:** [B, –] Inj site reactions (pain, redness, etc); flu-like Sxs w/in 48 h **CI:** Mod/severe liver Dz, unexplained ↑ ALT/AST **Disp:** Single-use vial or prefilled syringe, 1 mL, 200 mg/mL **SE:** HA, palpitations, N/V, pain in extremities, ↑ ALT/AST

Mirabegron (Myrbetriq) **Uses:** *OAB* **Acts:** β-3 adrenergic agonist; relaxes smooth muscle **Dose:** *Adults.* 25 mg PO daily; ↑ to 50 mg daily after 8 wk PRN; 25 mg max daily w/ severe renal or mod hepatic impair; swallow whole **W/P:** [C, –] w/ Severe uncontrolled HTN; can cause angioedema; urinary retention w/

BOO & antimuscarinic drugs; w/ drugs metabolized by CYP2D6; do not use w/ ESRD or severe hepatic impair **CI:** Component hypersens **Disp:** Tabs ER 25, 50 mg **SE:** HTN, HA, UTI, nasopharyngitis, N/D, constipation, Abd pain, dizziness, tachycardia, URI, arthralgia, fatigue

Mirtazapine (Remeron, Remeron SolTab, Generic) **BOX:** ↑ Risk of suicidal thinking and behavior in children, adolescents, and young adults w/ MDD and other psychological disorders; not for peds **Uses:** *Depression* **Acts:** $α_2$-Antag antidepressant, ↑ norepinephrine & 5-HT **Dose:** 15 mg PO hs, up to 45 mg/d hs **W/P:** [C, M] Has anticholesterol effects, w/ Sz, clonidine, CNS depressant use, CYP1A2, CYP3A4 inducers/inhib w/ hepatic & renal impair **CI:** MAOIs w/in 14 d **Disp:** Tabs 7.5, 15, 30, 45 mg; rapid dispersion tabs (SolTab) 15, 30, 45 mg **SE:** Somnolence, ↑ cholesterol, constipation, xerostomia, ↑ Wt, dizziness, asthenia, agranulocytosis, ↓ BP, edema, musculoskeletal pain **Notes:** Do not ↑ dose < q1–2wk; handle rapid tabs w/ dry hands, do not cut or chew; not FDA approved for Rx of bipolar depression; do not D/C abruptly

Misoprostol (Cytotec, Generic) **BOX:** Use in PRG can cause Ab, premature birth, or birth defects; do not use to ↓ decrease ulcer risk in women of childbearing age; must comply w/ birth control measures **Uses:** *Px NSAID-induced gastric ulcers; medical termination of PRG < 49 d w/ mifepristone*; induce labor (cervical ripening); incomplete & therapeutic Ab **Acts:** Prostaglandin (PGE-1); antisecretory & mucosal protection; induces uterine contractions **Dose:** *Ulcer prevention:* 100–200 mcg PO qid w/ meals; in females, start 2nd/3rd d of next nl period *Induction of labor (term):* 25–200 mcg intravag or 50–100 mcg PO q4h (max 5 doses). *PRG termination:* 400 mcg PO on d 3 of mifepristone or 800 mcg intravag × 1; take w/ food **W/P:** [X, −] **CI:** PRG, component allergy **Disp:** Tabs 100, 200 mcg **SE:** Miscarriage w/ severe bleeding; HA, D, Abd pain, constipation **Notes:** Not used for induction of labor w/ previous C-section or major uterine surgery

Mitomycin (Mitosol [Topical], Generic) **BOX:** Administer only by physician experienced in chemotherapy; myelosuppressive; can induce hemolytic uremic synd w/ irreversible renal failure **Uses:** *Stomach, pancreas*, breast, colon CA; SCC of the anus; NSCLC, head & neck, cervical; bladder CA (intravesically), *Mitosol* for glaucoma surgery **Acts:** Alkylating agent; generates oxygen-free radicals w/ DNA strand breaks **Dose:** (Per protocol) 20 mg/m² q6–8wk IV or 10 mg/m² combo w/ other myelosuppressive drugs q6–8wk *Bladder CA:* 20–40 mg in 40 mL NS via a urethral catheter once/wk; ↓ in renal/hepatic impair **W/P:** [X, −] w/ Cr > 1.7 mg/dL/ ↑ cardiac tox w/ vinca alkaloids/doxorubicin **CI:** ↓ Plt, coagulation disorders, ↑ bleeding tendency, PRG **Disp:** Inj 5, 20, 40 mg; *Mitosol* 0.2 mg/vial **SE:** ↓ BM (persists for 3–8 wk, may be cumulative; minimize w/ lifetime dose < 50–60 mg/m²), N/V, anorexia, stomatitis, renal tox, microangiopathic hemolytic anemia w/ renal failure (hemolytic–uremic synd), venoocclusive liver Dz, interstitial pneumonia, alopecia, extrav Rxns, contact dermatitis; CHF w/ doses > 30 mg/m²

Mitoxantrone (Generic) BOX: Administer only by physician experienced in chemotherapy; except for acute leukemia, do not use w/ ANC count of < 1500 cells/mm[3]; severe neutropenia can result in Infxn, follow CBC; cardiotox (CHF), secondary AML reported Uses: *AML (w/ cytarabine), ALL, CML, PCA, MS, lung CA*, breast CA, & NHL Acts: DNA-intercalating agent; ↓ DNA synth by interacting w/ topoisomerase II Dose: Per protocol; ↓ w/ hepatic impair, leukopenia, thrombocytopenia W/P: [D, –] Reports of secondary AML, w/ MS ↑ CV risk, do not treat MS pt w/ low LVEF CI: PRG, sig ↓ in LVEF Disp: Inj 2 mg/mL SE: ↓ BM, N/V, stomatitis, alopecia (infrequent), cardiotox, urine discoloration, secretions & scleras may be blue-green Notes: Maintain hydration; baseline CV evaluation w/ ECG & LVEF; cardiac monitoring prior to each dose; not for intrathecal use

Modafinil (Provigil, Generic) [C-IV] BOX: Controlled substance; can be abused or lead to dependence; Px misuse & abuse Uses: *Improve wakefulness in pts w/ excess daytime sleepiness (narcolepsy, sleep apnea, shift work sleep disorder)* Acts: Alters DA & norepinephrine release, ↓ GABA-mediated neurotransmission Dose: 200 mg PO q A.M.; max 400 mg/dose; ↓ dose 50% w/ elderly/hepatic impair W/P: [C, M] CV Dz; ↑ effects of warfarin, diazepam, phenytoin; ↓ OCP, cyclosporine, & theophylline effects CI: Component allergy Disp: Tabs 100, 200 mg SE: Serious rash, including SJS, HA, N/D, paresthesias, rhinitis, agitation, psychological Sx Notes: CV assessment before using

Moexipril (Univasc, Generic) BOX: ACE inhib can cause fetal injury/death in 2nd/3rd tri; D/C w/ PRG Uses: *HTN, post-MI*, DN Acts: ACE inhib Dose: 7.5–30 mg in 1–2 ÷ doses 1 h ac; ↓ in renal impair W/P: [C (1st tri, D 2nd & 3rd tri), ?] CI: ACE inhib sens, w/ aliskiren Disp: Tabs 7.5, 15 mg SE: ↓ BP, edema, angioedema, HA, dizziness, cough, ↑ K⁺

Mometasone, Inh (Asmanex, Asmanex HFA) Uses: *Maint Rx for asthma* Acts: Corticosteroid Dose: *Adults & Peds > 11 y.* On bronchodilators alone or inhaled steroids: 220 mcg × 1 q P.M. or in ÷ doses (max 440 mcg/d). On oral steroids: 440 mcg bid (max 880 mcg/d) w/ slow oral taper Peds 4–11 y. 110 mcg × 1 q P.M. (max 110 mcg/d) W/P: [C, ?/M] Candida Infxn of mouth/throat; hypersens Rxns possible; may worsen certain Infxn (TB, fungal, etc); monitor for ↑/↓ cortisol Sxs; ↓ bone density; ↓ growth in peds; monitor for NAG or cataracts; may ↑ glu CI: Acute asthma attack; component hypersens/milk proteins Disp: MDI 100, 200 mcg/actuation SE: HA, allergic rhinitis, pharyngitis, URI, sinusitis, oral candidiasis, dysmenorrhea, musculoskeletal/back pain, dyspepsia Notes: Rinse mouth after use; treat paradoxical bronchospasm w/ Inh bronchodilator

Mometasone, Nasal (Nasonex) Uses: *Nasal Sx allergic/seasonal rhinitis; prophylaxis of seasonal allergic rhinitis; nasal polyps in adults* Acts: Corticosteroid Dose: *Adults & Peds ≥ 12 y. Rhinitis:* 2 sprays/each nostril qd Adults. *Nasal polyps:* 2 sprays/each nostril bid Peds 2–11 y. 1 spray/each nostril qd W/P: [C, M] Monitor for adverse effects on nasal mucosa (bleeding, candidal Infxn, ulceration, perf); may worsen existing Infxns; monitor for NAG, cataracts; monitor for ↑/↓ cortisol Sxs; ↓ growth in peds **CI:** Component hypersens **Disp:** 50 mcg mometasone/spray **SE:** Viral Infxn, pharyngitis, epistaxis, HA

Mometasone/Formoterol (Dulera) **BOX:** Increased risk of worsening wheezing or asthma-related death in pediatric/adolescent pts w/ long-acting β₂-adrenergic agonists; use only if asthma not controlled on agent such as Inh steroid **Uses:** *Maint Rx for asthma* **Acts:** Corticosteroid (mometasone) w/ LA bronchodilator β₂ agonist (formoterol) **Dose:** *Adults & Peds > 12 y.* 2 Inh q12h **W/P:** [C, ?/M] w/ P450 3A4 inhib (eg, ritonavir), adrenergic/beta blockers, meds that ↑ QT interval; candida Infxn of mouth/throat, immunosuppression, adrenal suppression, ↓ bone density, w/ glaucoma/cataracts, may ↑ glu, ↓ K; other LABA should not be used **CI:** Acute asthma attack; component hypersens **Disp:** MDI 120 Inh/canister (mcg mometasone/mcg formoterol) 100/5, 200/5 **SE:** Nasopharyngitis, sinusitis, HA, palpitations, CP, rapid heart rate, tremor or nervousness, oral candidiasis **Notes:** For pts not controlled on other meds (eg, low-medium dose Inh steroids) or whose Dz severity warrants 2 maint therapies

Montelukast (Singulair, Generic) **Uses:** *Px/chronic Rx asthma ≥ 12 mo; seasonal allergic rhinitis ≥ 2 y; perennial allergic rhinitis ≥ 6 mo; Px EIB ≥ 15 y; prophylaxis & Rx of chronic asthma, seasonal allergic rhinitis* **Acts:** Leukotriene receptor antag **Dose:** *Adults & Peds > 15 y. Asthma:* 10 mg/d PO in P.M.; EIB: 10 mg × 1 2 h pre-exercise *6–23 mo:* 4-mg pack granules qd. *2–5 y.* 4 mg/d PO q P.M. *6–14 y.* 5 mg/d PO q P.M. **W/P:** [B, M] **CI:** Component allergy **Disp:** Tabs 10 mg; chew tabs 4, 5 mg; granules 4 mg/pack **SE:** HA, dizziness, fatigue, rash, GI upset, Churg-Strauss synd, flu, cough, neuropsych events (agitation, restlessness, suicidal ideation) **Notes:** Not for acute asthma; use w/in 15 min of opening package

Morphine (Astramorph/PF, Duramorph, Infumorph, Kadian SR, MS Contin, Oramorph SR, Roxanol) [C-II] **BOX:** Do not crush/chew SR/CR forms; swallow whole or sprinkle on applesauce; 100 and 200 mg for opioid-tolerant pt only for mod–severe pain when pain control needed for an extended period and not PRN; be aware of misuse, abuse, diversion; no alcoholic beverages while on therapy **Uses:** *Rx severe pain*, AMI, acute pulmonary edema **Acts:** Narcotic analgesic; SR/CR forms for chronic use **Dose:** *Adults. Short-term use PO:* 5–30 mg q4h PRN; *IV/IM:* 2.5–15 mg q2–6h; *Supp:* 10–30 mg q4h PRN; *SR formulations* 15–60 mg q8–12h (do not chew/crush); *IT/ epidural* (Duramorph, Infumorph, Astramorph/PF): Per protocol in Inf device *ECC 2010. STEMI:* 2–4 mg IV (over 1–5 min), then give 2–8 mg IV q5–15min as needed. *NSTEMI:* 1–5 mg slow IV if Sxs unrelieved by nitrates or nitrate; use w/ caution; can be reversed w/ 0.4–2 mg IV naloxone *Peds > 6 mo.* 0.1–0.2 mg/kg/ dose IM/IV q2–4h PRN; 0.15–0.2 mg/kg PO q3–4h PRN **W/P:** [C, +/–] Severe resp depression possible; w/ head injury; chewing DR forms can cause severe rapid release of morphine; administer *Duramorph* in staffed environment d/t cardiopulmonary effects; IT doses 1/10 of epidural dose **CI:** (many product specific)

Severe asthma, resp depression, GI obst/ileus; *Oral soln:* CHF d/t lung Dz, head injury, arrhythmias, brain tumor, acute alcoholism, DTs, Sz disorders; *MS Contin and Kadian* CI include hypercarbia **Disp:** IR tabs 15, 30 mg; soln 10, 20, 100 mg/5 mL; supp 5, 10, 20, 30 mg; Inj 2, 4, 5, 8, 10, 15, 25, 50 mg/mL; *MS Contin CR* tabs 15, 30, 60, 100, 200 mg; *Oramorph SR* tabs 15, 30, 60, 100 mg; *Kadian SR* caps 10, 20, 30, 40, 50, 60, 70, 80, 100, 130, 150, 200 mg; *Duramorph/Astramorph PF:* Inj 0.5, 1 mg/mL; *Infumorph* 10, 25 mg/mL **SE:** Narcotic SE (resp depression, sedation, constipation, N/V, pruritus, diaphoresis, urinary retention, biliary colic), granulomas w/ IT **Notes:** May require scheduled dosing to relieve severe chronic pain

Morphine/Naltrexone (Embeda) [C-II] **BOX:** For mod–severe chronic pain; do not use as PRN analgesic; swallow whole or sprinkle contents of cap on applesauce; do not crush/dissolve, chew caps—rapid release & absorption of morphine may be fatal & of naltrexone may lead to withdrawal in opioid-tolerant pts; do not consume EtOH or EtOH-containing products; 100/4 mg caps for use in opioid-tolerant pts only, may cause fatal resp depression; high potential for abuse **Uses:** *Chronic mod–severe pain* **Acts:** Mu-opioid receptor agonist & antag **Dose:** *Adults.* Individualize PO q12–24h; if opioid naïve start 20/0.8 mg q24h; titrate q48h; ↓ start dose in elderly, w/ hepatic/renal Insuff; taper to D/C **W/P:** [C, –] w/ EtOH, CNS depression, muscle relaxants, use w/in 14 d of D/C of MAOI, do not D/C abruptly **CI:** Resp depression, acute/severe asthma/hypercarbia, ileus, hypersens **Disp:** Caps ER (morphine mg/naltrexone mg) 20/0.8, 30/1.2, 50/2, 60/2.4, 80/3.2, 100/4 **SE:** N/V/D, constipation, somnolence, dizziness, HA, ↓ BP, pruritus, insomnia, anxiety, resp depression, Sz, MI, apnea, withdrawal w/ abrupt D/C, anaphylaxis, biliary spasm

Moxifloxacin (Avelox) **BOX:** ↑ Risk of tendon rupture and tendonitis; ↑ risk w/ age > 60, transplant pts; may ↑ Sx of MG **Uses:** *Acute sinusitis & bronchitis, skin/soft-tissue/intra-Abd Infxns, conjunctivitis, CAP*, TB, anthrax, endocarditis* **Acts:** 4th-gen quinolone; ↓ DNA gyrase. *Spectrum:* Excellent gram(+) except MRSA & *E. faecium*; good gram(−) except *P. aeruginosa, Stenotrophomonas maltophilia,* & *Acinetobacter* sp; good anaerobic **Dose:** 400 mg/d PO/IV daily; avoid cation products, antacids tid **W/P:** [C, −] Quinolone sens; interactions w/ Mg^{2+}, Ca^{2+}, Al^{2+}, Fe^{2+} -containing products, & class IA & III antiarrhythmic agents (Table 9, p 355) **CI:** Quinolone/component sens **Disp:** Tabs 400 mg, ABC Pak 5 tabs, Inj 400 mg **SE:** Dizziness, N, QT prolongation, Szs, photosens, peripheral neuropathy risk

Moxifloxacin, Ophthalmic (Moxeza, Vigamox) **Uses:** *Bacterial conjunctivitis** **Acts:** See Moxifloxacin **Dose:** Instill into affected eye(s): *Moxeza* 1 gtt bid × 7 d; *Vigamox* 1 gtt tid × 7 d **W/P:** [C, M] Not well studied in peds < 12 mo **CI:** Quinolone/component sens **Disp:** Ophthal soln 0.5% **SE:** ↓ Visual acuity, ocular pain, itching, tearing, conjunctivitis; prolonged use may result in fungal overgrowth; do not wear contacts w/ conjunctivitis

Multivitamins, Oral [OTC] (See Table 12, p 359)

Mupirocin (Bactroban, Bactroban Nasal) Uses: *Impetigo (oint); skin lesion infect w/ *S. aureus* or *S. pyogenes*; eradicate MRSA in nasal carriers* Acts: ↓ Bacterial protein synth Dose: *Topical:* Apply small amount tid × 5–14 d *Nasal:* Apply 1/2 single-use tube bid in nostrils × 5 d W/P: [B, ?/M] CI: Do not use w/ other nasal products Disp: Oint 2%; cream 2%; nasal oint 2% 1-g single-use tubes SE: Local irritation, rash Notes: Pt to contact healthcare provider if no improvement in 3–5 d

Mycophenolate Mofetil (CellCept, Generic) BOX: ↑ Risk of Infxns, lymphoma, other CAs, PML; risk of PRG loss and malformation; female of childbearing potential must use contraception Uses: *Px organ rejection after transplant* Acts: Cytostatic to lymphocytes Dose: *Adults.* 1 g PO bid; doses differ based on transplant *Peds. BSA 1.2–1.5 m²:* 750 mg PO bid *BSA > 1.5 m²:* 1 g PO bid; used w/ steroids & cyclosporine or tacrolimus; ↓ in renal Insuff or neutropenia *IV:* Infuse over > 2 h *PO:* Take on empty stomach, do not open caps W/P: [D, –] CI: Component allergy; IV use in polysorbate 80 allergy Disp: Caps 250, 500 mg; susp 200 mg/mL; Inj 500 mg SE: N/V/D, pain, fever, HA, Infxn, HTN, anemia, leukopenia, edema Notes: Cellcept & Myfortic not interchangeable

Mycophenolic Acid (Myfortic, Generic) BOX: ↑ Risk of Infxns, lymphoma, other CAs, PML; risk of PRG loss and malformation, female of childbearing potential must use contraception Uses: *Px rejection after renal transplant* Acts: Cytostatic to lymphocytes Dose: *Adults.* 720 mg PO bid; doses differ based on transplant *Peds. BSA 1.19–1.58 m²:* 540 mg bid *BSA > 1.58 m²:* Adult dose; used w/ steroids or tacrolimus; ↓ w/ renal Insuff/neutropenia; take on empty stomach W/P: [D, –] CI: Component allergy Disp: DR tabs 180, 360 mg SE: N/V/D, GI bleeding, pain, fever, HA, Infxn, HTN, anemia, leukopenia, pure red cell aplasia, edema Notes: Cellcept & Myfortic not interchangeable

Nabilone (Cesamet) [C-II] Uses: *Refractory chemotherapy-induced emesis* Acts: Synthetic cannabinoid Dose: *Adults.* 1–2 mg PO bid 1–3 h before chemotherapy, 6 mg/d max; may continue for 48 h beyond final chemotherapy dose *Peds.* ↑ Per protocol: < 18 kg 0.5 mg bid; 18–30 kg 1 mg bid; > 30 kg 1 mg tid W/P: [C, –] Elderly, HTN, heart failure, w/ psychological illness, substance abuse; high protein binding w/ 1st-pass metabolism may lead to drug interactions CI: Hypersens to cannabinoids/marijuana Disp: Caps 1 mg SE: Drowsiness, vertigo, xerostomia, euphoria, ataxia, HA, difficulty concentrating, tachycardia, ↓ BP Notes: May require initial dose evening before chemotherapy; Rx only quantity for single Tx cycle

Nabumetone (Relafen, Generic) BOX: May ↑ risk of MI/CVA & GI bleeding, perf; CI w/ postop CABG Uses: *OA and RA*, pain Acts: NSAID; ↓ prostaglandins Dose: 1000–2000 mg/d ÷ qd-bid w/ food W/P: [C, –] Severe hepatic Dz, peptic ulcer Dz, anaphylaxis w/ "ASA triad" CI: NSAID sensitivity, perioperative pain, after CABG surgery Disp: Tabs 500, 750 mg SE: Dizziness, rash, GI upset, edema, peptic ulcer, ↑ BP, photosens

Nadolol (Corgard, Generic) BOX: Do not abruptly withdraw Uses: *HTN & angina migraine prophylaxis*, prophylaxis of variceal hemorrhage Acts: Competitively blocks β-adrenergic receptors (β₁, β₂) Dose: 40–80 mg/d; ↑ to 240 mg/d (angina) or 320 mg/d (HTN) at 3- to 7-d intervals; ↓ in renal Insuff & elderly W/P: [C +/M] CI: Uncompensated CHF, shock, heart block, asthma Disp: Tabs 20, 40, 80, 160 mg SE: Nightmares, paresthesias, ↓ BP, ↓ HR, fatigue, ↓ sex function

Nafarelin, Metered Spray (Synarel) Uses: *Endometriosis, CPP* Acts: GnRH agonist; ↓ gonadal steroids w/ use > 4 wk Dose: Adults. Endometriosis: 400 mcg/d (1 spray q A.M./P.M. alternate nostril; if no amenorrhea ↑ 2 sprays bid, start d 2–4 of menstrual cycle Peds. CPP: 1600 mcg/d (2 sprays each nostril q A.M./P.M.), can ↑ to 1800 mcg/d W/P: [X, –] CI: Component hypersens, undiagnosed uterine bleeding, PRG, breast-feeding Disp: 0.5-oz bottle 60 sprays (200 mcg/spray) SE: ♀: hot flashes, headaches, emotional lability, ↓ libido, vaginal dryness, acne, myalgia, ↓ breast size, ↓ BMD; Peds: drug sensitivity Rxn, acne, transient ↑ breast enlargement/pubic hair, Vag bleeding, emotional lability, body odor, seborrhea Notes: ✓ PRG test before use; for endometriosis only if > 18 y, and no more than 6 mo; no sig effect w/ rhinitis, if needed, use decongestant 2 h before dose

Nafcillin (Nallpen, Generic) Uses: *Infxns d/t susceptible strains of Staphylococcus & Streptococcus* Acts: Bactericidal; antistaphylococcal PCN; ↓ cell wall synth. Spectrum: Good gram(+) except MRSA & enterococcus, no gram(−), poor anaerobe Dose: Adults. 500 mg IM/IV q4–6 h; 1 g if severe Infxn Peds < 40 kg. 25 mg/kg IM bid Neonates. 10 mg/kg bid W/P: [B, ?] CI: PCN allergy, allergy to corn-related products Disp: Inj powder l, 2 g SE: Interstitial nephritis, N/D, fever, rash, allergic Rxn Notes: In setting of both hepatic & renal impair, modification of dose may be necessary

Naftifine (Naftin) Uses: *Tinea pedis, cruris, & corporis* Acts: Allylamine antifungal, ↓ cell membrane ergosterol synth Dose: Apply qd (cream) or bid (gel) W/P: [B, ?] CI: Component sens Disp: 1% cream; gel SE: Local irritation, dry skin

Nalbuphine (Generic) Uses: *Mod–severe pain; preop & obstetric analgesia* Acts: Narcotic agonist–antag; ↓ ascending pain pathways Dose: Adults. Pain: 10 mg/70 kg IV/IM/SQ q3–6h; adjust PRN; 20 mg/dose or 160 mg/d max Anesthesia: Induction: 0.3–3 mg/kg IV over 10–15 min; maint 0.25–0.5 mg/kg IV Peds. 0.2 mg/kg IV or IM, 20 mg/dose or 160 mg/d max; ↓ w/ renal/hepatic impair W/P: [B, M] w/ Opiate use CI: Component sens Disp: Inj 10, 20 mg/mL SE: CNS depression, drowsiness; caution, ↓ BP, diaphoresis

Naloxegol (Movantik) Uses: * Opioid-induced constipation* Acts: Opioid antag Dose: 25 mg PO qd; if intolerant or CrCl < 60 mL/min: 12.5mg qd 1 h ac or 2 h pc; swallow whole; avoid grapefruit W/P: [C (may precipitate opioid withdrawal in fetus), –] GI perf, opioid withdrawal CI: GI obst; use w/ strong CYP3A4 inhib; component hypersens Disp: Tabs 12.5, 25 mg SE: N/V/D, Abd pain, flatulence, HA Notes: D/C maint laxative before, may resume PRN after 3 d; w/ mod CYP3A4 inhib, ↓ dose; avoid w/ strong CYP3A4 inducers and other opioid antags

Naloxone (Evzio, Generic) Uses: *Opioid addiction (diagnosis) & OD* Acts: Competitive opioid antag Dose: *Adults.* 0.4–2 mg IV, IM, or SQ q2–3min; via ET tube, dilute in 1-2 mL NS; may be given intranasal; total dose 10 mg max; *Evzio:* 0.4 mg IM or SQ *Peds.* 0.01–0.1 mg/kg/dose IV, IM, or SQ; repeat IV q3min × 3 doses PRN *ECC 2010. Reverse narcotic effects:* 0.1 mg/kg q2min PRN; max dose 2 mg; smaller doses (1–5 mcg/kg may be used); cont Inf 2–160 mcg/kg/h W/P: [C, ?], *Evzio* [B, ?/–], may precipitate withdrawal in addicts CI: Component hypersens Disp: Inj 0.4, 1 mg/mL; *Evzio* 0.4 mg/0.4mL prefilled auto-injector w/ electronic voice instructions SE: ↓ BP, ↑ BP, fever, tachycardia, VT, VF, irritability, agitation, coma, GI upset, pulm edema, tremor, piloerection, sweating Notes: If no response after 10 mg, suspect nonnarcotic cause; w/ *Evzio* use in the field, seek emergent care immediately; duration of action less than most opioids, may need repeat dosing; for bystander use, administer in anterolateral thigh

Naltrexone (ReVia, Vivitrol, Generic) BOX: Can cause hepatic injury, CI w/ active liver Dz Uses: *EtOH & narcotic addiction* Acts: Antagonizes opioid receptors Dose: *EtOH/narcotic addiction:* 50 mg/d PO; must be opioid-free for 7–10 d; *EtOH dependence:* 380 mg IM q4wk (*Vivitrol*) W/P: [C, M] Monitor for Inj site reactions (*Vivitrol*); w/ hepatic/renal impair CI: Opioid use Disp: Tabs 50 mg; Inj 380 mg (*Vivitrol*) SE: Hepatotox; insomnia, GI upset, jt pain, HA, fatigue

Naphazoline (Albalon, Naphcon, Generic), Naphazoline/ Pheniramine (Naphcon A, Visine A, Generic) Uses: *Relieve ocular redness & itching caused by allergy* Acts: Sympathomimetic (α-adrenergic vasoconstrictor) & antihistamine (pheniramine) Dose: 1–2 gtt up to q6h, 3 d max W/P: [C, +] CI: NAG, in children < 6 y, w/ contact lenses, component allergy SE: CV stimulation, dizziness, local irritation Disp: Ophthal 0.012, 0.025, 0.1%/15 mL; naphazoline & pheniramine 0.025%/0.3% soln

Naproxen (Aleve [OTC], Anaprox, Anaprox DS, EC-Naprosyn, Naprelan, Naprosyn, Generic) BOX: May ↑ risk of MI/CVA & GI bleeding Uses: *Arthritis & pain* Acts: NSAID; ↓ prostaglandins Dose: *Adults & Peds > 12 y.* 200–500 mg bid-tid to 1500 mg/d max *> 2 y.* JRA: 5 mg/kg/dose bid; ↓ in hepatic impair W/P: [C, (D 3rd tri), –] CI: NSAID or ASA triad sensitivity, peptic ulcer, post-CABG pain, 3rd-tri PRG Disp: *Tabs:* 250, 375, 500 mg; *DR:* 375, 500, 750 mg; *CR:* 375, 550 mg; susp 25 mg/5 mL; *Aleve:* tabs 200 mg; multiple OTC forms SE: Dizziness, pruritus, GI upset, peptic ulcer, edema Notes: Take w/ food to ↓ GI upset; 220 mg naproxen sodium = 200 mg naproxen base

Naproxen/Esomeprazole (Vimovo) BOX: ↑ Risk MI/CVA, PE; CI, CABG surgery pain; ↑ risk GI bleeding, gastric ulcer, gastric/duodenal perf Uses: *Pain and/or swelling, RA, OA, ankylosing spondylitis, w/ risk NSAID-assoc gastric ulcers* Acts: NSAID; ↓ prostaglandins & PPI ↓ gastric acid Dose: (naproxen/ esomeprazole) 375/20 mg to 500/20 mg PO bid W/P: [C 1st, 2nd tri; D 3rd; –] CI: PRG 3rd tri; asthma, urticaria from ASA or NSAID; mod–severe hepatic/renal Insuff; post-CABG pain Disp: Tabs (naproxen/esomeprazole) DR 375/20 mg;

500/20 mg **SE:** N/D, Abd pain, gastritis, ulcer, ↑ BP, CHF, edema, serious skin rash (eg, SJS, etc), ↓ renal Fxn, papillary necrosis **Notes:** Risk of GI adverse events in elderly; atrophic gastritis w/ long-term PPI use; possible ↑ risk of fractures w/ all PPI; may ↑ Li levels; may cause MTX tox; may ↑ INR on warfarin; may ↓ effect BP meds; may ↓ absorption drugs requiring acid environment

Naratriptan (Amerge, Generic) **Uses:** *Acute migraine* **Acts:** Serotonin 5-HT₁ receptor agonist **Dose:** 1–2.5 mg PO × 1; repeat PRN in 4 h; 5 mg/24 h max; ↓ in mild renal/hepatic Insuff, take w/ fluids **W/P:** [C, M] **CI:** CAD, WPW, other cardiac disorder; Hx CVA/TIA, PVD, IBD, ↑ uncontrolled BP; recent use of another triptan or ergotamine; component hypersens; severe renal/hepatic impair **Disp:** Tabs 1, 2.5 mg **SE:** Dizziness, sedation, GI upset, paresthesias, ECG changes, coronary vasospasm, arrhythmias

Natalizumab (Tysabri) **BOX:** PML reported **Uses:** *Relapsing MS to delay disability and ↓ recurrences, Crohn Dz* **Acts:** Integrin receptor antag **Dose:** 300 mg IV q4wk; 2nd-line Tx only **CI:** PML; immune compromise or w/ immunosuppressant **W/P:** [C, ?/–] Baseline MRI to rule out PML **Disp:** Vial 300 mg **SE:** Infxn, immunosuppression; Inf Rxn precluding subsequent use; HA, fatigue, arthralgia **Notes:** Give slowly to ↓ Rxns; limited distribution (TOUCH Prescribing program); D/C immediately w/ signs of PML (weakness, paralysis, vision loss, impaired speech, cognitive ↓); evaluate at 3 and 6 mo, then q6mo thereafter

Nateglinide (Starlix, Generic) **Uses:** *Type 2 DM* **Acts:** ↑ Pancreatic insulin release **Dose:** 120 mg PO tid 1–30 min ac; ↓ to 60 mg tid if near target HbA₁c **W/P:** [C, –] w/ CYP2C9 metabolized drug (Table 10, p 356) **CI:** DKA, type 1 DM **Disp:** Tabs 60, 120 mg **SE:** Hypoglycemia, URI; salicylates, nonselective β-blockers may enhance hypoglycemia **Notes:** If a meal is skipped, the dose should be held

Nebivolol (Bystolic) **Uses:** *HTN* **Acts:** β₁-Selective blocker **Dose:** *Adults.* 5 mg PO daily, ↑ q2wk to 40 mg/d max, ↓ w/ CrCl < 30 mL/min **W/P:** [C, +/–] w/ Bronchospastic Dz, DM, heart failure, pheochromocytoma, w/ CYP2D6 inhib **CI:** Bradycardia, 2nd/3rd-degree heart block, cardiogenic shock, decompensated cardiac failure, SSS (unless paced), severe hepatic impair, component hypersens **Disp:** Tabs 2.5, 5, 10, 20 mg **SE:** HA, fatigue, dizziness

Nefazodone (Generic) **BOX:** Fatal hep & liver failure possible, D/C if LFTs > 3× ULN, do not retreat; closely monitor for worsening depression or suicidality, particularly in ped pts **Uses:** *Depression* **Acts:** ↑ Neuronal uptake of serotonin & norepinephrine **Dose:** Initial 100 mg PO bid; usual 300–600 mg/d in 2 ÷ doses **W/P:** [C, M] **CI:** w/ terfenadine, astemizole, cisapride, pimozide, carbamazepine, triazolam; Hx of nefazodone liver injury **Disp:** Tabs 50, 100, 150, 200, 250 mg **SE:** Postural ↓ BP & allergic Rxns; HA, drowsiness, xerostomia, constipation, GI upset, liver failure **Notes:** Monitor LFTs, HR, BP

Nelarabine (Arranon) **BOX:** Fatal neurotox possible **Uses:** *T-cell ALL or T-cell lymphoblastic lymphoma unresponsive > 2 other regimens* **Acts:** Nucleoside (deoxyguanosine) analog **Dose:** *Adults.* 1500 mg/m² IV over 2 h d 1, 3, 5 of 21-d cycle **Peds.** 650 mg/m² IV over 1 h d 1–5 of 21-d cycle **W/P:** [D, ?/–] **Disp:** Vial 5 mg/mL **SE:** Fatigue, N/V/D, constipation, heme disorders, cough, dyspnea, somnolence, dizziness, pyrexia **Notes:** Prehydration, urinary alkalinization, allopurinol before dose; monitor CBC

Nelfinavir (Viracept) **Uses:** *HIV Infxn, other agents* **Acts:** Protease inhib causes immature, noninfectious virion production **Dose:** *Adults.* 750 mg PO tid or 1250 mg PO bid. **Peds.** 25–35 mg/kg PO tid or 45–55 mg/kg bid; take w/ food **W/P:** [B, –] Many drug interactions; do not use w/salmeterol, colchicine (w/ renal/hepatic failure); adjust dose w/ bosentan, tadalafil for PAH; do not use tid dose w/ PRG **CI:** Phenylketonuria, w/ triazolam/midazolam use or drug dependent on CYP3A4 (Table 10, p 356); w/ alpha 1-adrenoreceptor antag (alfuzosin), PDE5 inhib sildenafil **Disp:** Tabs 250, 625 mg; powder 50 mg/g **SE:** Food ↑ absorption; interacts w/ St. John's wort; dyslipidemia, lipodystrophy, D, rash, ↑ QT interval **Notes:** PRG registry; tabs can be dissolved in water; monitor LFTs

Neomycin (Neo-Fradin, Generic) **BOX:** Systemic absorption of oral route may cause neuro-/oto-/nephrotox; resp paralysis possible w/ any route of administration **Uses:** *Hepatic coma, bowel prep* **Acts:** Aminoglycoside, poorly absorbed PO; ↓ GI bacterial flora **Dose:** *Adults.* 4–12 g/24 h PO in 3–4 ÷ doses; 12 g/d max; not > 2 wk **Peds.** 50–100 mg/kg/24 h PO in 3–4 ÷ doses **W/P:** [D, ?/–] Renal failure, neuromuscular disorders, hearing impair **CI:** Intestinal obst, GI inflam/ulcerative Dz **Disp:** Tabs 500 mg; PO soln 125 mg/5 mL **SE:** Hearing loss w/ long-term use; rash, N/V **Notes:** Do not use parenterally (↑ tox); part of the Condom bowel prep; also topical form

Neomycin/Bacitracin/Polymyxin B, Topical (Neosporin Ointment) (See Bacitracin/Neomycin/Polymyxin B, Topical [Neosporin Ointment], p 67); Neomycin/Colistin/Hydrocortisone (Cortisporin-TC Otic Drops); Neomycin/Colistin/Hydrocortisone/Thonzonium (Cortisporin-TC Otic Suspension) **Uses:** *Otitis externa*, Infxns of mastoid/fenestration cavities **Acts:** Abx w/ anti-inflam **Dose:** *Adults.* 5 gtt in ear(s) q6–8h **Peds.** 3–4 gtt in ear(s) q6–8h **CI:** Component allergy; HSV, vaccinia, varicella **W/P:** [B, ?] **Disp:** Otic gtt & susp **SE:** Local irritation, rash **Notes:** Shake well limit use to 10 d to minimize ototox

Neomycin/Dexamethasone (AK-Neo-Dex Ophthalmic, NeoDecadron Ophthalmic) **Uses:** *Steroid-responsive inflam conditions of the cornea, conjunctiva, lid, & anterior segment* **Acts:** Abx w/ anti-inflam corticosteroid **Dose:** 1–2 gtt in eye(s) q3–4h or thin coat q6–8h until response, then ↓ to daily **W/P:** [C, ?] **Disp:** Cream: neomycin 0.5%/dexamethasone 0.1%; oint: neomycin 0.35%/dexamethasone 0.05%; soln: neomycin 0.35%/dexamethasone 0.1% **SE:** Local irritation **Notes:** Use under ophthalmologist's supervision; no contacts w/ use

Neomycin/Polymyxin B (Neosporin Cream) [OTC] **Uses:** *Infxn in minor cuts, scrapes, & burns* **Acts:** Bactericidal **Dose:** Apply bid-qid **W/P:** [C, ?]

CI: Component allergy **Disp:** Cream: neomycin 3.5 mg/polymyxin B 10,000 units/g **SE:** Local irritation **Notes:** Different from *Neosporin oint*

Neomycin/Polymyxin B Bladder Irrigant (Neosporin GU Irrigant) **Uses:** *Cont irrigant prevent bacteriuria & gram(−) bacteremia associated w/ indwelling catheter* **Acts:** Bactericidal; not for *Serratia* sp or streptococci **Dose:** 1 mL irrigant in 1 L of 0.9% NaCl; cont bladder irrigation w/ 1 L of soln/24 h 10 d max **W/P:** [D] **CI:** Component allergy **Disp:** Soln neomycin sulfate 40 mg & polymyxin B 200,000 units/mL; amp 1, 20 mL **SE:** Rash, neomycin ototox or nephrotox (rare) **Notes:** Potential for bacterial/fungal super-Infxn; not for Inj; use only 3-way catheter for irrigation

Neomycin/Polymyxin B/Hydrocortisone, (Cortisporin Ophthalmic, Generic) **Uses:** *Ocular bacterial Infxns* **Acts:** Abx w/ anti-inflam **Dose:** Apply a thin layer to the eye(s) or 1 gtt qd-qid **W/P:** [C, ?] **Disp:** Ophthal soln; ophthal oint **SE:** Local irritation **Notes:** Do not wear contacts during Tx

Neomycin/Polymyxin B/Hydrocortisone, Otic (Cortisporin Otic Solution, Generic Suspension) **Uses:** *Otitis externa and infected mastoidectomy and fenestration cavities* **Acts:** Abx & anti-inflam **Dose:** *Adults.* 3–4 gtt in the ear(s) q6–8 h *Peds > 2 y.* 3 gtt in the ear(s) q6–8 h **CI:** Viral Infxn, component hypersens **W/P:** [C, ?] **Disp:** Otic susp (generic); otic soln (Cortisporin) **SE:** Local irritation

Neomycin/Polymyxin B/Dexamethasone, Ophthalmic (Maxitrol) **Uses:** *Steroid-responsive ocular conditions w/ bacterial Infxn* **Acts:** Abx w/ anti-inflam corticosteroid **Dose:** 1–2 gtt in eye(s) q3–4h; apply oint in eye(s) q6–8 h **CI:** Component allergy; viral, fungal, TB eye Dz **W/P:** [C, ?] **Disp:** Oint: neomycin sulfate 3.5 mg/polymyxin B sulfate 10,000 units/dexamethasone 0.1%/g; susp: identical/1 mL, 5 mL bottle **SE:** Local irritation **Notes:** Use under supervision of ophthalmologist; contacts should not be worn during therapy

Neomycin/Polymyxin B/Prednisolone (Poly-Pred Ophthalmic) **Uses:** *Steroid-responsive ocular conditions w/ bacterial Infxn* **Acts:** Abx & anti-inflam **Dose:** 1–2 gtt in eye(s) q4–6h; apply oint in eye(s) q6–8 h **W/P:** [C, ?] **Disp:** Susp neomycin/polymyxin B/prednisolone 0.5%/mL **SE:** Irritation **Notes:** Use under supervision of ophthalmologist; do not wear contacts during Tx

Nepafenac (Nevanac) **Uses:** *Inflam postcataract surgery* **Acts:** NSAID **Dose:** 1 gtt 0.03% qd or 1 gtt 0.1% tid 1 d preop; continue 14 d postop **CI:** NSAID/ASA sens **W/P:** [C, ?/−] May ↑ bleeding time, delay healing, causes keratitis **Disp:** Susp 0.1, 0.3% **SE:** Capsular opacity, visual changes, foreign-body sensation, ↑ IOP **Notes:** Prolonged use ↑ risk of corneal damage; shake well before use; separate from other drops by > 5 min

Nesiritide (Natrecor) **Uses:** *Acutely decompensated CHF* **Acts:** Human B-type natriuretic peptide **Dose:** 2 mcg/kg IV bolus, then 0.01 mcg/kg/min IV, max 0.03 mcg/kg/min **W/P:** [C, ?/−] When vasodilators are not appropriate **CI:** SBP < 100 mm Hg, cardiogenic shock **Disp:** Vials 1.5 mg **SE:** ↓ BP, HA, GI upset, arrhythmias, ↑ Cr **Notes:** Requires cont BP monitoring; some studies indicate ↑ i mortality; 175 kg max dose Wt studied

Netupitant/Palonosetron (Akynzeo) **Uses:** *Px N/V w/chemo* **Acts** Substance P/NK₁ and 5-HT₃ receptor antag **Dose:** Emetogenic chemo (ie, cispla tin) 1 cap PO 1 h pre-chemo w/ dexamethasone 12 mg 30 min pre-chemo d 1, 8 m d 2–4; other chemo as above, dexamethasone not needed d 2–4; w or w/o foo **W/P:** [C, +] –HA, dyspepsia, fatigue, constipation, erythema, asthenia **CI:** Ø Disp **Caps** 300 mg netupitant/0.5 mg palonosetron **SE:** Serotonin synd **Notes:** Avoid w severe hepatic/renal Dz

Nevirapine (Viramune, Viramune XR, Generic) **BOX:** Reports o fatal hepatotox even w/ short-term use; severe life-threatening skin Rxns (SJS TEN, & allergic Rxns); monitor closely during first 18 wk of Rx **Uses:** *HIV Infxn* **Acts:** Nonnucleoside RT inhib **Dose:** *Adults.* Initial 200 mg/d PO × 14 d then 200 mg bid, 400 mg qd (XR) *Peds > 15 d.* 150 mg/m² PO qd × 14 d, then 15 mg/m² bid; max 400 mg/d for any pt (w/o regard to food) **W/P:** [B, –] OPC **CI** Mod–severe hepatic impair or PEP use **Disp:** Tabs 200 mg; (*Viramune XR*) tabs E 100, 400 mg; susp 50 mg/5 mL **SE:** Life-threatening rash; HA, fever, D, neutrope nia, hep **Notes:** HIV resistance when used as monotherapy; use in combo w/ a least 2 additional antiretroviral agents; restart once daily dosing ×14 d if stoppe > 7 d; not recommended if CD4 > 250 mcL in women or > 400 mcL in men unles benefit > risk of hepatotox; always perform lead-in trial w/ IR formulation

Nicotinic Acid (Niacor, Niaspan, Nicolar, Slo-Niacin) [OT Forms] **Uses:** *Sig hyperlipidemia/hypercholesteremia, nutritional supl* **Acts** Vit B₃; ↓ lipolysis; ↓ esterification of triglycerides; ↑ lipoprotein lipase **Dose** *Hypercholesterolemia:* Start 500 mg PO qhs, ↑ 500 mg q4wk, maint 1–2 g/d; 2 g max; qhs w/ low-fat snack; do not crush/chew; niacin supl 1 ER tab PO qd or 10 mg PO qd; *Pellagra:* Up to 500 mg/d PO **W/P:** [C, +] CI: Liver Dz, peptic ulcer, arteria hemorrhage **Disp:** ER tabs (*Niaspan*) 500, 750, 1000 mg & (*Slo-Niacin*) 250, 50 750 mg; tabs 500 mg (*Niacor*); many OTC: tabs 50, 100, 250, 500 mg; ER cap 125, 250, 400 mg; ER tabs 250, 500, 750, 1000 mg; elixir 50 mg/5 mL **SE:** Uppe body/facial flushing & warmth; hepatox; GI upset, flatulence, exacerbate pepti ulcer, HA, paresthesias, liver damage, gout, altered glu control in DM **Notes:** ASA NSAID 30–60 min prior to ↓ flushing; ✓ cholesterol, LFTs, if on statins (eg, Lipito etc) also ✓ CPK and K⁺; *RDA adults:* male 16 mg/d, female 14 mg/d

Niacin/Lovastatin (Advicor) **Uses:** *Hypercholesterolemia* **Acts:** Comb antilipemic agent, w/ HMG-CoA reductase inhib **Dose:** *Adults.* Niacin 500 m lovastatin 20 mg, titrate q4wk, max niacin 2000 mg/lovastatin 40 mg **W/P:** [X, – See individual agents, D/C w/ LFTs > 3× ULN **CI:** Component hypersens, liver D ↑ LFT, PUD, arterial bleeding w/ CYP3A4 inhib (eg, itraconazole, ketoconazol HIV protease inhib, erythromycin, etc), PRG, lactation **Disp:** Niacin mg/lovastati mg: 500/20, 750/20, 1000/20, 1000/40 tabs **SE:** Flushing, myopathy/rhabdomyolysi N, Abd pain, ↑ LFTs **Notes:** ↓ Flushing by taking ASA or NSAID 30 min before

Niacin/Simvastatin (Simcor) Uses: *Hypercholesterolemia* Acts: Combo antilipemic agent w/ HMG-CoA reductase inhib Dose: *Adults* Niacin 500 mg/simvastatin 20 mg, titrate q4wk not to exceed niacin 2000 mg/simvastatin 40 mg; max 1000 mg/20 mg/d w/ amlodipine and ranolazine W/P: [X, –] See individual agents, discontinue Rx if LFTs > 3× ULN CI: PRG, active liver Dz, PUD, arterial bleeding, w/ strong CYP3A4 inhib, w/ gemfibrozil, cyclosporine, danazol, verapamil, or diliazem, component hypersens Disp: Niacin mg/simvastatin mg: 500/20, 500/40, 750/20, 1000/20, 1000/40 tabs SE: Flushing, myopathy/rhabdomyolysis, N, Abd pain, ↑ LFTs Notes: ↓ Flushing by taking ASA or NSAID 30 min before

Nicardipine (Cardene, Cardene SR, Generic) Uses: *Chronic stable angina & HTN*; prophylaxis of migraine Acts: CCB Dose: *Adults.* PO: 20–40 mg PO tid SR: 30–60 mg PO bid IV: 5 mg/h IV cont Inf; ↑ by 2.5 mg/h q15min to max 15 mg/h Peds. (Not established) PO: 20–30 mg PO q8h IV: 0.5–5 mcg/kg/min; ↓ in renal/hepatic impair W/P: [C, ?/–] Heart block, CAD CI: Cardiogenic shock, aortic stenosis Disp: Caps 20, 30 mg; SR caps 30, 45, 60 mg; Inj 2.5 mg/mL SE: Flushing, tachycardia, ↓ BP, edema, HA Notes: *PO-to-IV conversion:* 20 mg tid = 0.5 mg/h, 30 mg tid = 1.2 mg/h, 40 mg tid = 2.2 mg/h; take w/ food (not high fat)

Nicotine, Gum (Nicorette, Others) [OTC] Uses: *Aid to smoking cessation, relieve nicotine withdrawal* Acts: Systemic delivery of nicotine Dose: Wk 1–6 one piece q1–2h PRN; wk 7–9 one piece q2–4h PRN; wk 10–12 one piece q4–8h PRN; max 24 pieces/d W/P: [C, ?] CI: Life-threatening arrhythmias, unstable angina Disp: 2 mg, 4 mg/piece; mint, orange, original flavors SE: Tachycardia, HA, GI upset, hiccups Notes: Must stop smoking & perform behavior modification for max effect; use at least 9 pieces first 6 wk; > 25 cigarettes/d use 4 mg; < 25 cigarettes/d use 2 mg

Nicotine, Nasal Spray (Nicotrol NS) Uses: *Aid to smoking cessation, relieve nicotine withdrawal* Acts: Systemic delivery of nicotine Dose: 0.5 mg/actuation; 1–2 doses/h, 5 doses/h max; 40 doses/d max W/P: [D, M] CI: Life-threatening arrhythmias, unstable angina Disp: Nasal inhaler 10 mg/mL SE: Local irritation, tachycardia, HA, taste perversion Notes: Must stop smoking & perform behavior modification for max effect; 1 dose = 1 spray each nostril = 1 mg

Nicotine, Transdermal (Habitrol, NicoDerm CQ [OTC], Others) Uses: *Aid to smoking cessation; relief of nicotine withdrawal* Acts: Systemic delivery of nicotine Dose: Individualized; 1 patch (14–21 mg/d) & taper over 6 wk W/P: [D, M] CI: Life-threatening arrhythmias, unstable angina, adhesive allergy Disp: Habitrol & NicoDerm CQ: 7, 14, 21 mg of nicotine/24 h SE: Insomnia, pruritus, erythema, local site Rxn, tachycardia, vivid dreams Notes: Wear patch 16–24 h; must stop smoking & perform behavior modification for max effect; > 10 cigarettes/d start w/ 21-mg patch; < 10 cigarettes/d 14-mg patch; do not cut patch; rotate site

Nifedipine (Adalat CC, Afeditab CR, Procardia, Procardia XL, Generic) Uses: *Vasospastic or chronic stable angina & HTN*; tocolytic Acts: CCB Dose: *Adults.* SR tabs 30–90 mg/d. *Tocolysis:* per local protocol Peds. 0.6–0.9

mg/kg/d PO ÷ 3–4 doses **W/P:** [C, +] Heart block, aortic stenosis, cirrhosis **CI:** Component hypersens **Disp:** Caps 10, 20 mg; SR tabs 30, 60, 90 mg **SE:** HA common on initial Rx; reflex tachycardia may occur w/ regular-release dosage forms; peripheral edema, ↓ BP, flushing, dizziness **Notes:** Adalat CC & Procardia XL not interchangeable; SL administration not OK

Nilotinib (Tasigna) **BOX:** May ↑ QT interval; sudden deaths reported, use w/ caution in hepatic failure; administer on empty stomach **Uses:** *Ph(+) CML, refractory or at 1st diagnosis* **Acts:** TKI **Dose:** *Adults.* 300 mg bid—newly diagnosed; 400 mg bid—resistant/intolerant on empty stomach 1 h prior or 2 h post meal. **W/P:** [D, ?/–] Avoid w/ CYP3A4 inhib/inducers (Table 10, p 356), adjust w/ hepatic impair, heme tox, avoid QT-prolonging agents, w/ Hx pancreatitis, ↓ absorption w/ gastrectomy **CI:** ↓ K+, ↓ Mg2+, long QT synd **Disp:** 200 mg caps **SE:** ↓ BM, ↑ QT, sudden death, cardiac/vascular occlusions, pancreatitis, ↑ lipase, hepatotox, electrolyte abn, hemorrhage, fluid retention **Notes:** Use chemotherapy precautions when handling

Nilutamide (Nilandron) **BOX:** Interstitial pneumonitis possible; most cases in first 3 mo; ✓ CXR before and during Rx **Uses:** *Combo w/ surgical castration for metastatic PCa* **Acts:** Nonsteroidal antiandrogen **Dose:** 300 mg/d PO × 30 d then 150 mg/d **W/P:** [Not used in females] Avoid w/ EtOH **CI:** Severe hepatic impair, resp Insuff **Disp:** Tabs 150 mg **SE:** Interstitial pneumonitis, hot flashes, ↓ libido, impotence, N/V/D, gynecomastia, hepatic dysfunction **Notes:** May cause Rxn when taken w/ EtOH, follow LFTs

Nimodipine (Nymalize, Generic) **BOX:** Not for parenteral administration **Uses:** *Improve outcome following subarachnoid hemorrhage* **Acts:** CCB; prevent vasospasm **Dose:** 20 mL (60 mg) q4h × 21 d; start w/in 96 h of subarachnoid hemorrhage; if given via NG flush w/ 20 mL NS after administration; ↓ in hepatic failure **W/P:** [C, –] Not for peripheral use **CI:** Component allergy, w/ strong CYP3A4 inhib **Disp:** Caps 30 mg; *Nymalize:* 60 mg per 20 mL **SE:** ↓ BP, HA, N bradycardia, constipation, rash

Nintedanib (Ofev) **Uses:** *Idiopathic pulmonary fibrosis* **Acts:** Kinase inhib **Dose:** 150 mg PO q12h; w/ food; do not chew/crush **W/P:** [D, ±] May ↑ GI perf/bleeding risk **CI:** Ø **Disp:** Caps 100,150 mg **SE:** N/V/D, ↓ appetite, ↓W **Notes:** ✓ LFTs before; temporary ↓ to 100 mg may be needed w/ adverse Rxns

Nisoldipine (Sular, Generic) **Uses:** *HTN* **Acts:** CCB **Dose:** 8.5–34 mg/d PO; take on empty stomach; ↓ start doses w/ elderly or hepatic impair **W/P:** [C, –] **Disp:** ER tabs 8.5, 10, 17, 20, 25.5, 30, 34, 40 mg **SE:** Edema, HA, flushing, ↓ BP **Notes:** Nisoldipine Geomatrix (Sular) formulation not equivalent to original formulation (ER)

Nitazoxanide (Alinia) **Uses:** *Cryptosporidium, Giardia lamblia, C. difficile-associated D* **Acts:** Antiprotozoal interferes w/ pyruvate ferredoxin oxidoreductase. *Spectrum: Cryptosporidium, Giardia* **Dose:** *Adults.* 500 mg PO q12h × 3 d; for *C. difficile* × 10 d *Peds 1–3 y.* 100 mg PO q12h × 3 d *4–11 y.* 200 mg PO q12h

3 d > *12 y.* 500 mg q12h × 3 d; take w/ food **W/P:** [B, ?] Not effective in HIV or immunocompromised **Disp:** 100 mg/5 mL PO susp, 500 tab **SE:** Abd pain N/V/D **Notes:** Susp contains sucrose, interacts w/ highly protein-bound drugs

Nitrofurantoin (Furadantin, Macrobid, Macrodantin, Generic)
Uses: *Prophylaxis & Rx UTI* **Act:** Interferes w/ metabolism & cell wall synth. *Spectrum:* Some gram(+) & (−) bacteria; *Pseudomonas, Serratia,* & most *Proteus* resistant **Dose:** *Adults.* *Prophylaxis:* 50–100 mg/d PO *Rx:* 50–100 mg PO qid × 7 d; *Macrobid* 100 mg PO bid × 7 d **Peds.** *Prophylaxis:* 1–2 mg/kg/d ÷ in 1–2 doses, max 100 mg/d *Rx:* 5–7 mg/kg/24 h in 4 ÷ doses (w/ food/milk/antacid) **W/P:** [B, +/ not OK if child < 1 mo] Avoid w/ CrCl < 60 mL/min **CI:** Anuria, oliguria, CrCl < 60 mL/min, PRG at term, neonates < 1 mo, Hx hepatic Dz due to nitrofurantoin, component hypersens **Disp:** Caps 25, 50, 100 mg; (*Furadantin*) susp 25 mg/5 mL **SE:** GI effects, dyspnea, various acute/chronic pulm Rxns, peripheral neuropathy, hemolytic anemia w/ G6PD deficiency, rare aplastic anemia **Notes:** Macrocrystals (*Macrodantin*) < N than other forms; not for comp UTI; may turn urine brown; ineffective for pyelonephritis or cystitis

Nitroglycerin (Nitro-Bid IV, Nitro-Bid Ointment, Nitrodisc, Nitrolin-gual, NitroMist, Nitrostat, Transderm-Nitro, Others) **Uses:** *Angina pectoris, acute & prophylactic Rx, CHF, BP control* **Acts:** Relaxes vascular smooth muscle, dilates coronary arteries **Dose:** *Adults.* *SL:* 1 tab q5min SL PRN for 3 doses *Translingual:* 1–2 metered doses sprayed onto PO mucosa q3–5min, max 3 doses *PO:* 2.5–9 mg tid *IV:* 5–20 mcg/min, titrated to effect *Topical:* Apply 1/2 in of oint to chest wall tid, wipe off at night *Transdermal:* 0.2–0.4 mg/h/patch daily *Aerosol:* 1 spray at 5-min intervals, max 3 doses *ECC 2010. IV bolus:* 12.5–25 mcg (if no spray or SL dose given) *Inf:* Start 10 mcg/min, ↑ by 10 mcg/min q3–5min until desired effect; ceiling dose typically 200 mcg/min *SL:* 0.3–0.4 mg, repeat q5min *Aerosol:* Spray 0.5–1 s at 5-min intervals **Peds.** 0.25–0.5 mcg/kg/min IV, titrate *ECC 2010.* *Heart failure, HTN emergency, pulm HTN:* Cont Inf 0.25–0.5 mcg/kg/min initial, titrate 1 mcg/kg/min q15–20min (typical dose 1–5 mcg/kg/min) **W/P:** [C, ?] Restrictive cardiomyopathy **CI:** w/ Sildenafil, tadalafil, vardenafil, head trauma, NAG, pericardial tamponade, constrictive pericarditis, severe anemia **Disp:** SL tabs 0.3, 0.4, 0.6 mg; translingual spray 0.4 mg/dose; SR caps 2.5, 6.5, 9 mg; Inj 0.1, 0.2, 0.4 mg/mL (premixed); 5 mg/mL Inj soln; oint 2%; transdermal patches 0.1, 0.2, 0.4, 0.6 mg/h; aerosol (*NitroMist*) 0.4 mg/spray; (*Rectiv*) intra-anal 0.4% **SE:** HA, ↓ BP, lightheadedness, GI upset **Notes:** Nitrate tolerance w/ chronic use after 1–2 wk; minimize by providing 10–12 h nitrate-free period daily, using shorter-acting nitrates tid, & removing LA patches & oint before sleep to ↓ tolerance

Nitroprusside (Nitropress) **BOX:** Warning: Cyanide tox & excessive hypotension **Uses:** *Hypertensive crisis, acute decompensated heart failure, controlled ↓ BP periop (↓ bleeding)*, aortic dissection, pulm edema **Acts:** ↓ Systemic vascular resistance **Dose:** *Adults & Peds.* 0.25–10 mcg/kg/min IV Inf, titrate; usual dose 3 mcg/kg/min *ECC 2010.* 0.1 mcg/kg/min start, titrate (max dose 5–10 mcg/kg/min) *Peds. ECC 2010. Cardiogenic shock, severe HTN:* 0.3–1 mcg/kg/min, titrate to 8 mcg/kg/min PRN **W/P:** [C, ?] ↓ Cerebral perfusion **CI:** Compensatory ↑ BP due to coarctation or AV shunt, in surgery pt w/ ↑ cerebral circulation or moribund, Leber's optic atrophy, CHF w/ ↑ PVR (ie, sepsis) **Disp:** Inj 25 mg/mL **SE:** Excessive hypotensive effects, palpitations, HA **Notes:** Thiocyanate (metabolite w/ renal excretion) w/ tox at 5–10 mg/dL, more likely if used for > 2–3 d; w/ aortic dissection use w/ β-blocker; continuous BP monitoring essential

Nivolumab (Opdivo) Uses: *Unresectable/met melanoma following ipilimumab & BRAF inhib (if BRAF V600 mutation(+)); met squamous NSCLC w/ progression on/after platinum* **Acts:** MoAb against PD-1; ↑ anti-tumor immune response **Dose:** 3 mg/kg IV Inf over 60 min q2wk until progression or tox **W/P:** [X, –] Pneumonitis, colitis, hep, renal/thyroid effects **CI:** Ø **Disp:** Single-use vial 40 mg/4 mL or 100 mg/10 mL **SE:** Melanoma: rash; NSCLC: fatigue, dyspnea, MS pain, ↓ appetite, cough, N, constipation **Notes:** Women of reproductive potential to use contraception during and least 5 mo after final dose; ✓ Cr, TFTs, LFTs before & periodically

Nizatidine (Axid, Axid AR [OTC], Generic) Uses: *Duodenal ulcers, GERD, heartburn* **Acts:** H_2-receptor antag **Dose:** *Adults.* Active ulcer: 150 mg PO bid or 300 mg PO hs; maint 150 mg PO hs *GERD:* 150 mg PO bid *Heartburn:* 75 mg PO bid *Peds. GERD:* 10 mg/kg PO bid, 150 mg bid max; ↓ in renal impair **W/P:** [B, ?] **CI:** H_2-receptor antag sensitivity **Disp:** Tabs 75 mg [OTC]; caps 150, 300 mg; soln 15 mg/mL **SE:** Dizziness, HA, constipation, D **Notes:** Contains bisulfites

Norepinephrine (Levophed) Uses: *Acute ↓ BP, cardiac arrest (adjunct)* **Acts:** Peripheral vasoconstrictor of arterial/venous beds **Dose:** *Adults.* 8–30 mcg/min IV, titrate *Peds.* 0.05–0.1 mcg/kg/min IV, titrate **W/P:** [C, ?] **CI:** ↓ BP d/t hypovolemia, vascular thrombosis, do not use w/ cyclopropane/halothane anesthetics **Disp:** Inj 1 mg/mL **SE:** ↓ HR, arrhythmia **Notes:** Correct vol depletion as much as possible before vasopressors; interaction w/ TCAs leads to severe HTN; use large vein to avoid extrav; phentolamine 5–10 mg/10 mL NS injected locally for extrav

Norethindrone Acetate/Ethinyl Estradiol Tablets (FemHRT) (See Estradiol/Norethindrone Acetate)

Nortriptyline (Aventyl, Pamelor) BOX: ↑ Suicide risk in pts < 24 y w/ MDD/other psychological disorders especially during 1st month of Tx; risk ↓ pts > 65 y; observe all pts for clinical Sxs; not recommended for ped use Uses: *Endogenous depression* **Acts:** TCA; ↑ synaptic CNS levels of serotonin &/or norepinephrine **Dose:** *Adults.* 25 mg PO tid-qid; > 150 mg/d not OK; *Elderly:* 10–25 mg hs **W/P:** [C, –] NAG, CV Dz **CI:** TCA allergy, use w/ MAOI **Disp:** Caps 10, 25, 50, 75 mg; (*Aventyl*); soln 10 mg/5 mL **SE:** Anticholinergic (blurred vision, retention, xerostomia, sedation) **Notes:** Max effect may take > 2–3 wk

Nystatin (Mycostatin, Nilstat, Nystop) Uses: *Mucocutaneous Candida* Infxns (oral, skin, Vag)* **Acts:** Alters membrane permeability. *Spectrum:* Susceptible

Candida sp **Dose: *Adults & Peds.*** *PO:* 400,000–600,000 units PO "swish & swallow" qid *Vag:* 1 tab Vag hs × 2 wk *Topical:* Apply bid-tid to area *Peds Infants.* 200,000 units PO q6h **W/P:** [B (C PO), +] **Disp:** PO susp 100,000 units/mL; PO tabs 500,000 units; troches 200,000 units; Vag tabs 100,000 units; topical cream/oint 100,000 units/g; powder 100,000 units/g **SE:** GI upset, SJS **Notes:** Not absorbed through mucus membranes/intact skin, poorly absorbed through GI; not for systemic Infxns; see also Triamcinolone/Nystatin

Obinutuzumab (Gazyva) **BOX:** May reactivate hep B and cause progressive multifocal leukoencephalopathy w/ death **Uses:** *CLL* **Acts:** Cytolytic anti-CD20 antibody **Dose:** Six 28-day cycles; 100 mg d 1, 900 mg d 2, 1000 mg d 8 & 15, then 1000 mg d 1 cycle 2–6 **W/P:** [C, −] Tumor lysis synd, give fluids, premedicate for ↑ uric acid, monitor renal Fxn; Inf reactions, premedicate w/ glucocorticoid, acetaminophen, and antihistamine; ↓ WBC, ↓ plts; do not give live vaccines before or during Tx **CI:** Ø **Disp:** 1000 mg/40 mL; single-use vial **SE:** Fever; cough; ↑ Cr; ↑ ALT/AST, alk phos; ↓ alb, ↓ Ca⁺⁺, ↓ Na⁺, ↓ plt **Notes:** Do not use if CrCl < 30 mg/mL

Octreotide (Sandostatin, Sandostatin LAR, Generic) **Uses:** *↓ Severe D associated w/ carcinoid & neuroendocrine GI tumors (eg, VIPoma, ZE synd), acromegaly*; bleeding esophageal varices **Acts:** LA peptide; mimics natural somatostatin **Dose: *Adults.*** 100–600 mcg/d SQ/IV in 2–4 ÷ doses; start 50 mcg daily-bid *Sandostatin LAR (depot):* 10–30 mg IM q4wk *Peds.* 1–10 mcg/kg/24 h SQ in 2–4 ÷ doses **W/P:** [B, +] Hepatic/renal impair **Disp:** Inj 0.05, 0.1, 0.2, 0.5, 1 mg/mL; 10, 20, 30 mg/5 mL LAR depot **SE:** N/V, Abd discomfort, flushing, edema, fatigue, cholelithiasis, hyper-/hypoglycemia, hep, hypothyroidism **Notes:** Stabilize for at least 2 wk before changing to LAR form

Ofatumumab (Arzerra) **BOX:** Reactivation of hep B/hepatic failure/death and PML **Uses:** *Rx refractory CLL* **Acts:** MoAb, binds CD20 molecule on nl & abn B-lymphocytes w/ cell lysis **Dose:** 300 mg (0.3 mg/mL) IV wk 1, then 2000 mg (2 mg/mL) qwk × 7 doses, then 2000 mg q4wk × 4 doses; titrate Inf; start 12 mL/h × 30 min, ↑ 25 mL/h for 30 min, ↑ to 50 mL/h × 30 min, ↑ to 100 mL/h × 30 min, then titrate to max Inf 200 mL/h **W/P:** [C, ?] ✓ WBC, screen high risk for hep B, can reactivate, D/C immediately **Disp:** Inj 20 mg/mL (5 mL) **SE:** Inf Rxns (bronchospasm, pulmonary edema, ↑/↓ BP, syncope, cardiac ischemia, angioedema), ↓ WBC, anemia, fever, fatigue, rash, N/D, pneumonia, Infxns, PML **Notes:** Premed w/ acetaminophen, antihistamine, and IV steroid

Ofloxacin (Generic) **BOX:** Use associated w/ tendon rupture and tendonitis **Uses:** *Lower resp tract, skin, & skin structure, & UTI, prostatitis, uncomp gonorrhea, & Chlamydia Infxns* **Acts:** Bactericidal; ↓ DNA gyrase. *Broad spectrum gram(+) & (−):* S. pneumoniae, S. aureus, S. pyogenes, H. influenzae, P. mirabilis, N. gonorrhoeae, C. trachomatis, E. coli **Dose:** 200–400 mg PO bid or IV q12h, ↓ in renal impair, take on empty stomach **W/P:** [C, −] ↓ Absorption w/ antacids, sucralfate, Al²⁺, Ca²⁺, Mg²⁺, Fe²⁺, Zn⁺ -containing drugs, Hx Szs **CI:** Quinolone

allergy **Disp:** Tabs 200, 300, 400 mg; Inj 20, 40 mg/mL; ophthal & otic 0.3% **SE:** N/V/D, photosens, insomnia, HA, local irritation, ↑ QTc interval, peripheral neuropathy risks **Notes:** *Floxin* brand D/C

Ofloxacin, Ophthalmic (Ocuflox) Uses: *Bacterial conjunctivitis, corneal ulcer* **Acts:** See Ofloxacin **Dose:** *Adults & Peds > 1 y.* 1–2 gtt in eye(s) q2–4h × 2 d, then qid × 5 more d **W/P:** [C, +/–] **CI:** Quinolone allergy **Disp:** Ophthal 0.3% soln **SE:** Burning, hyperemia, bitter taste, chemosis, photophobia

Ofloxacin, Otic (Floxin Otic, Floxin Otic Singles) Uses: *Otitis externa; chronic suppurative otitis media w/ perf drums; otitis media in peds w/ tubes* **Acts:** See Ofloxacin **Dose:** *Adults & Peds > 13 y. Otitis externa:* 10 gtt in ear(s) daily × 7 d *Peds 1–12 y. Otitis media* 5 gtt in ear(s) bid × 10 d **W/P:** [C, –] **CI:** Quinolone allergy **Disp:** Otic 0.3% soln 5/10 mL bottles; singles 0.25 mL foil pack **SE:** Local irritation **Notes:** OK w/ tubes/perforated drums; 10 gtt = 0.5 mL

Olanzapine (Zyprexa, Zyprexa Zydis, Generic) BOX: ↑ Mortality in elderly w/ dementia-related psychosis Uses: *Bipolar mania, schizophrenia*, psychotic disorders, acute agitation in schizophrenia* **Acts:** DA & serotonin antag; atypical antipsychotic **Dose:** *Bipolar/schizophrenia:* 5–10 mg/d qwk PRN, 20 mg/d max *Agitation;* atypical antipsychotic 5–10 mg IM q2–4h PRN, 30 mg d/max **W/P:** [C, –] **Disp:** Tabs 2.5, 5, 7.5, 10, 15, 20 mg; ODT (*Zyprexa Zydis*) 5, 10, 15, 20 mg; Inj 10 mg **SE:** HA, somnolence, orthostatic ↓ BP, tachycardia, dystonia, xerostomia, constipation, hyperglycemia; ↑ Wt, ↑ prolactin levels; sedation may be ↑ in peds **Notes:** Takes wk to titrate dose; smoking ↓ levels; may be confused w/ *Zyrtec* or *Zyprexa Relprevv*

Olanzapine, LA Parenteral (Zyprexa Relprevv) BOX: ↑ Risk for severe sedation/coma following parenteral Inj, observe closely for 3 h in appropriate facility; restricted distribution; ↑ mortality in elderly w/ dementia-related psychosis; not approved for dementia-related psychosis Uses: *Schizophrenia* **Acts:** See Olanzapine **Dose:** IM: 150 mg/q2 wk, 300 mg/q4wk, 210 mg/q2wk, 405 mg/q4 wk, or 300 mg/q2wk **W/P:** [C, –] IM only, do not confuse w/ *Zyprexa* IM; can cause neuroleptic malignant synd, ↑ glu/lipids/prolactin, ↓ BP, tardive dyskinesia, cognitive impair, ↓ CBC **CI:** Ø **Disp:** Vials 210, 300, 405 mg **SE:** HA, sedation, ↑ Wt, cough, N/V/D, ↑ appetite, dry mouth, nasopharyngitis, somnolence **Notes:** ✓ Glu/lipids/CBC baseline and periodically: establish PO tolerance before Δ to IM

Olaparib (Lynparza) Uses: *Deleterious/suspected deleterious germline BRCA-mutated advanced ovarian CA after Tx w/ ≥ 3 lines of chemo* **Acts:** PARP inhib **Dose:** 400 mg PO bid until progression or tox; swallow whole; hold/↓ to manage tox **W/P:** [D, –] MDS/AML (✓ CBC baseline & qmo); pneumonitis; embryo-fetal tox **CI:** Ø **Disp:** Caps 50 mg **SE:** N/V/D, dyspepsia, dysgeusia, ↓ appetite, HA, cough, anemia, fatigue, URI, pharyngitis, nasopharyngitis, arthralgia, myalgia, Abd/back/musculoskeletal pain, rash, dermatitis, ↑ Cr, ↑ MCV, ↓ Hgb, ↓ plt, ↓ ANC **Notes:** Avoid w/ mod–strong CYP3A inhib, ↓ dose if used together; avoid w/ mod–strong CYP3A inducers

Olmesartan (Benicar); Olmesartan/Hydrochlorothiazide (Benicar HCT) BOX: Use in PRG 2nd/3rd tri can harm fetus; D/C when PRG detected Uses: *Hypertension, alone or in combo* Acts: *Benicar ARB; Benicar HCT ARB w/ diuretic HCTZ* Dose: *Adults. Benicar:* 20–40 mg qd; *Benicar HCT:* 20–40 mg olmesartan w/ 12.5–25 mg HCTZ based on effect *Peds 6–16 y. Benicar:* < 35 kg start 10 mg PO, range 10–20 mg qd; ≥ 35 kg start 20 mg PO qd, target 20–40 mg qd W/P: [C 1st tri, D 2nd, 3rd, ?/–] *Benicar HCT* not rec w/ CrCl < 30 mL/min; follow closely if vol depleted w/ start of med; sprue-like enteropathy reported CI: Component allergy; w/ aliskiren Disp: *(Benicar)* Tabs 5, 20, 40 mg; *(Benicar HCT)* mg olmesartan/mg HCTZ: 20/12.5, 40/12.5, 40/25 SE: Dizziness, ↓ K+ w/ HCTZ product (may require replacement) Notes: If *Benicar* does not control BP a diuretic can be added or *Benicar HCT* used; ? ↑ sprue-like entropathy

Olmesartan/Amlodipine/Hydrochlorothiazide (Tribenzor) Uses: *Hypertension* Acts: Combo ARB, CCB, thiazide diuretic Dose: Begin w/ 20/5/12.5 olmesartan/amlodipine/HCTZ, ↑ to max 40/10/25 mg W/P: [C 1st tri, D 2nd, 3rd; –]; sprue-like enteropathy reported CI: Anuria; sulfa allergy; PRG, neonate exposure, CrCl < 30 mg/min, age > 75 y, w/ aliskiren, severe liver Dz Disp: Tabs: (olmesartan mg/amlodipine mg/HCTZ mg) 20/5/12.5, 40/5/12.5, 40/5/25, 40/10/12.5, 40/10/25 SE: Edema, HA, fatigue, N/D, muscle spasms, jt swelling, URI, syncope Notes: Avoid w/ vol depletion; thiazide diuretics may exacerbate SLE, associated NA glaucoma; ? ↑ sprue-like entropathy

Olodaterol (Striverdi Respimat) BOX: LABA ↑ risk for asthma-related deaths Uses: *Maint bronchodilator Tx for COPD (chronic bronchitis/emphysema)* Acts: LABA, bronchodilation Dose: 2 Inh qd (2 Inh/d max) W/P: D/C w/ paradoxical bronchospasm or w/ deterioration; hypersens Rxn, including angioedema; caution w/ CV diseases, DM, hyperthyroid ↓ K+, Szs CI: Monotherapy for asthma Disp: Inh spray 2.5 mcg olodaterol, 2 actuations = 1 dose SE: Nasopharyngitis, skin rash, UTI, back pain, arthralgia, bronchitis Notes: Not for acute COPD; must use w/ Inh short-acting beta₂ agonist; beta-blockers may ↓ effectiveness

Olopatadine, Nasal (Patanase) Uses: *Seasonal allergic rhinitis* Acts: H₁-receptor antag Dose: 2 sprays each nostril bid W/P: [C, ?] Disp: 0.6% 240-Spray bottle SE: Epistaxis, bitter taste somnolence, HA, rhinitis

Olopatadine, Ophthalmic (Pataday, Patanol, Pazeo) Uses: *Allergic conjunctivitis* Acts: H₁-receptor antag Dose: *Patanol:* 1 gtt in eye(s) bid; *Pataday & Pazeo:* 1 gtt in eye(s) qd W/P: [C, ?] Disp: *Patanol:* soln 0.1% 5 mL; *Pataday:* 0.2% 2.5 mL; *Pazeo:* 0.7% 2.5 mL SE: Local irritation, HA, rhinitis, blurred vision Notes: Wait 10 min after to insert contacts

Olsalazine (Dipentum) Uses: *Maint remission in UC* Acts: Topical antiinflam Dose: 500 mg PO bid (w/ food) W/P: [C, –] w/ Renal/liver impair CI: Salicylate sensitivity Disp: Caps 250 mg SE: D, HA, blood dyscrasias, hep

Omacetaxine (Synribo) Uses: *CML w/ resistance &/or intolerant to ≥ 2 TKI* Acts: Inhib protein synthesis Dose: *Induct:* 1.25 mg/m² SQ bid × 14 consecutive d 28-d cycle, repeat until hematologic response achieved; *Maint:* 1.25 mg/m² SQ twice daily × 7 consecutive d 28-d cycle, continue as long as beneficial; adjust based on tox (see PI) **W/P:** [D, –] Severe myelosuppression (✓ CBC q1–2wk); severe bleeding (✓ plt); glu intolerance (✓ glu); embryo-fetal tox **CI:** Ø **Disp:** Inj powder 3.5 mg/vial **SE:** Anemia, neutropenia, ↓ plts/WBC, N/V/D, fatigue, asthenia, Inj site Rxn, pyrexia, Infxn, bleeding, ↑ glu, constipation, Abd pain, edema, HA, arthralgia, insomnia, cough, epistaxis, alopecia, rash

Omalizumab (Xolair)   **BOX:** Reports of anaphylaxis 2–24 h after administration, even in previously treated pts **Uses:** *Mod–severe asthma in ≥ 12 y w/ reactivity to an allergen & when Sxs inadequately controlled w/ Inh steroids* **Acts:** Anti-IgE Ab **Dose:** 150–375 mg SQ q2–4wk (dose/frequency based on serum IgE level & body Wt; see PI) **W/P:** [B, ?/–] **CI:** Component allergy, acute bronchospasm **Disp:** 150-mg single-use 5-mL vial **SE:** Inj Site Rxn, sinusitis, HA, anaphylaxis reported in 3 pts **Notes:** Continue other asthma meds as indicated

Ombitasvir/Paritaprevir/Ritonavir w/ Dasabuvir (Viekira Pak) **Uses:** *Chronic HCV, genotype 1* **Acts:** Antiretroviral; (O) ↓ HCV NS5A; (P) ↓ HCV NS 3/4A protease; (R) CYP3A inhib to ↑ paritaprevir levels; (D) non-nucleoside ↓ HCV RNA polymerase **Dose:** 2 tabs ombitasvir/paritaprevir/ritonavir q A.M. × 12 wk w/ 1 tab dasabuvir bid × 12 wk; given w/ ribavirin (except genotype 1b w/o cirrhosis); for pts w/ cirrhosis or liver transplant, use × 24 wk; genotype 1b w/o cirrhosis, use × 12 wk, no ribavirin **W/P:** [B, ?] ↑ ALT severe liver injury reported; many drug interactions; not rec w/ mod/decompensated hep impair; w/ estrogens ✓ LFTs 1st 4 wk; risk of HIV-1 protease inhib resistance in HCV/HIV co-infected pts **CI:** Component hypersens, severe hepatic impair, w/ estradiol products (use non-estrogen contraception); inducers of CYP3A/CYP2C8/CYP2C8 (see drug label) **Disp:** Oral combo 28-d package: Tabs ombitasvir 12.5 mg/paritaprevir 75 mg/ritonavir 50 mg (fixed dose) plus tabs dasabuvir 250 mg **SE:** Fatigue, HA, insomnia, derm Rxns, D, ↑ bili, weakness, cough, w/ liver transplant or HCV/HIV ↑ incidence of some SEs **Notes:** Take w/ food, ✓ LFTs, HCV RNA at baseline & end of Tx

Omega-3 Fatty Acid [Fish Oil] (Epanova, Lovaza, Omtryg) **Uses:** *Rx hypertriglyceridemia* **Acts:** Omega-3 acid ethyl esters, ↓ thrombus inflam & triglycerides **Dose:** *Hypertriglyceridemia:* 4 g/d ÷ in 1–2 doses **W/P:** [C, –], Fish hypersens; PRG, risk factor w/ anticoagulant use, w/ bleeding risk **CI:** Component hypersens **Disp:** *Epanova & Lovaza:* 1000-mg caps; *Omtryg:* 1200-mg caps **SE:** Dyspepsia, N, GI pain, rash, flu-like synd **Notes:** Only FDA-approved fish oil supl; not for exogenous hypertriglyceridemia (type 1 hyperchylomicronemia); many OTC products; D/C after 2 mo if triglyceride levels do not ↓; previously called "Omacor"

Omeprazole (Prilosec, Prilosec [OTC, Generic]) **Uses:** *Duodenal/gastric ulcers (adults), GERD, and erosive gastritis (adults and children)*, prevent NSAID ulcers, ZE synd, *H. pylori* Infxns **Acts:** PPI **Dose:** *Adults.* 20–40 mg

PO qd-bid × 4–8 wk; *H. pylori* 20 mg PO bid × 10 d w/ amoxicillin & clarithromycin or 40 mg PO × 14 d w/ clarithromycin; pathologic hypersecretory cond 60 mg/d (varies); 80 mg/d max *Peds 1–16 y & 5–10 kg.* 5 mg/d *10–20 kg.* 10 mg PO qd > *20 kg.* 20 mg PO qd; 40 mg/d max **W/P:** [C, –/+] w/ Drugs that rely on gastric acid (eg, ampicillin); avoid w/ atazanavir and nelfinavir; caution w/ warfarin, diazepam, phenytoin; do not use w/ clopidogrel (controversial ↓ effect); response does not R/O malignancy **Disp:** OTC tabs 20 mg; *Prilosec* DR caps 10, 20, 40 mg; *Prilosec* DR susp 2.5, 10 mg **SE:** HA, Abd pain, N/V/D, flatulence **Notes:** Combo w/ Abx Rx for *H. pylori*; ? ↑ risk of fractures, *C. difficile*, CAP w/ all PPI; risk of hypomagnesemia w/ long-term use

Omeprazole/Sodium Bicarbonate (Zegerid, Zegerid OTC) **Uses:** *Duodenal/gastric ulcers, GERD and erosive gastritis (↓ GI bleeding in critically ill pts)*, prevent NSAID ulcers, ZE synd, *H. pylori* Infxns **Acts:** PPI w/ sodium bicarbonate **Dose:** *Duodenal ulcer:* 20 mg PO qd-bid × 4–8 wk; *Gastric ulcer:* 40 mg PO qd-bid × 4–8 wk; *GERD w/ no erosions:* 20 mg PO daily × 4 wk, w/ erosions treat 4–6 wk; *UGI bleed prevention:* 40 mg q6–8h then 40 mg/d × 14 d **W/P:** [C, –/+] w/ drugs that rely on gastric acid (eg, ampicillin); avoid w/ atazanavir and nelfinavir; w/ warfarin, diazepam, phenytoin; do not use w/ clopidogrel (controversial ↓ effect); response does not R/O malignancy **Disp:** Omeprazole mg/sodium bicarb mg: *Zegerid* OTC caps 20/1100; *Zegerid* 20/1100, mg 40/1100; *Zegerid* powder packet for oral susp 20/1680, 40/1680 **SE:** HA, Abd pain, N/V/D, flatulence **Notes:** Not approved in peds; take 1 h ac; mix powder in small cup w/ 2 tbsp water (not food or other liq), refill and drink; do not open caps; possible ↑ risk of fractures, *C. difficile*, CAP w/ all PPI; risk of hypomagnesemia w/ long-term use, monitor

Omeprazole/Sodium Bicarbonate/Magnesium Hydroxide (Zegerid w/ Magnesium Hydroxide) **Uses:** *Duodenal or gastric ulcer, GERD, maint esophagitis* **Acts:** PPI w/ acid buffering **Dose:** 20–40 mg empty stomach 1 h pc; *Duodenal ulcer, GERD:* 20 mg 4–8 wk; *Gastric ulcer:* 40 mg 4–8 wk; *Esophagitis maint:* 20 mg **W/P:** [C, ?/–] w/ Resp alkalosis, ↓ K$^+$, ↓ Ca^{+2}; ↑ drug levels metabolized by CYP450; may ↑ INR w/ warfarin; may ↓ absorption drugs requiring acid environment **CI:** ↓ Renal Fxn **Disp:** Chew tabs 20, 40 mg omeprazole; w/ 600 mg NaHCO$_3$; 700 mg MgOH$_2$ **SE:** N/V/D, Abd pain, HA **Notes:** Atrophic gastritis w/ long-term PPI; ? ↑ risk of fractures, *C. difficile*, CAP w/ all PPI; long-term use + Ca^{2+} → milk-alkali synd

Ondansetron (Zofran, Zofran ODT, Generic) **Uses:** *Px chemotherapy-associated & postop N/V* **Acts:** Serotonin receptor (5-HT$_3$) antag **Dose:** *Adults & Peds 6 mo–18 y. Emetogenic chemo:* three 0.15-mg/kg doses IV over 15 min (max 16 mg/dose), 1st dose 30 min before chemo, other doses 4 & 8 h after 1st dose. *Adults & Peds 1 mo–12 y > 40 kg. Postop N/V:* 4 mg × 1 IV over 2–5 min; w/ hepatic impair max 8 mg/d *Adults & Peds > 12 y.* 24 mg PO 30 min before chemo *Peds 4–11 y.* 4 mg PO tid, 1st dose 30 min before chemo *Adults.* 16 mg PO 1 h before anesthesia **W/P:** [B, +/−] Arrhythmia risk, may ↑ QT interval **Disp:** Tabs 4, 8, 24 mg; soln 4 mg/5 mL; Inj 2 mg/mL; *Zofran* ODT tabs 4, 8 mg; **SE:** D, HA, constipation, dizziness **Notes:** ODT contains phenylalanine. No single IV dose > 16 mg

Ondansetron, Oral Soluble Film (Zuplenz) Uses: *Px chemotherapy/ RT-associated & postop N/V* Acts: Serotonin receptor (5-HT₃) antag **Dose:** *Adults.* Highly emetogenic chemo: 24 mg (8 mg film × 3) 30 min pre-chemo; *RT N/V:* 8 mg film tid *Adults & Peds > 12 y.* Mod emetogenic chemo: 8 mg film 30 min pre-chemo, then 8 mg in 8 h; 8 mg film bid × 1–2 d after chemo *Adults. Postop:* 16 mg (8 mg film × 2) 1 h preop; ↓ w/ hepatic impair **W/P:** [B, +/−] **CI:** w/ Apomorphine (↓ BP, LOC) **Disp:** Oral soluble film 4, 8 mg **SE:** HA, malaise/ fatigue, constipation, D **Notes:** Use w/ dry hands, do not chew/swallow; place on tongue, dissolves in 4–20 s; peppermint flavored

Oprelvekin (Neumega) BOX: Allergic Rxn w/ anaphylaxis reported; D/C w/ any allergic Rxn Uses: *Px ↑ plt w/ chemotherapy* Acts: ↑ Proliferation & maturation of megakaryocytes (IL-11) **Dose:** *Adults.* 50 mcg/kg/d SQ for 10–21 d *Peds > 12 y.* 75–100 mcg/kg/d SQ for 10–21 d < 12 y. Use only in clinical trials; ↓ w/ CrCl < 30 mL/min 25 mcg/kg **W/P:** [C, ?/−] **Disp:** 5 mg powder for Inj **SE:** Tachycardia, palpitations, arrhythmias, edema, HA, dizziness, visual disturbances, papilledema, insomnia, fatigue, fever, N, anemia, dyspnea, allergic Rxns, including anaphylaxis **Notes:** D/C 48 h before chemo

Oral Contraceptives (See Table 5, p 341) BOX: Cigarette smoking ↑ risk of serious CV SEs; ↑ risk w/ > 15 cigarettes/d, > 35 y; strongly advise women on OCP to not smoke; pts should be counseled that these products do not protect against HIV or other STDs Uses: *Birth control; regulation of anovulatory bleeding; dysmenorrhea; endometriosis; polycystic ovaries; acne* (Note: FDA approvals vary widely, see PI) Acts: *Birth control:* Suppresses LH surge, Px ovulation; progestins thicken cervical mucus; ↓ fallopian tubule cilia, ↓ endometrial thickness to ↓ chances of fertilization *Anovulatory bleeding:* Cyclic hormones mimic body's natural cycle & regulate endometrial lining, results in regular bleeding q28d; may ↓ uterine bleeding & dysmenorrhea **Dose:** Start d 1 menstrual cycle or 1st Sunday after onset of menses; 28-d cycle pills take daily; 21-d cycle pills take daily, no pills during last 7 d of cycle (during menses); some available as transdermal patch or intrauterine ring **W/P:** [X, +] Migraine, HTN, DM, sickle cell Dz, gallbladder Dz; monitor for breast Dz; w/ drospirenone containing OCP; ✓ K⁺ if taking drugs w/ ↑ K⁺ risk; drospirenone implicated in ↑ VTE risk **CI:** AUB, PRG, estrogen-dependent malignancy, ↑ hypercoagulation/liver Dz, hemiplegic migraine, smokers > 35 y; drospirenone has mineralocorticoid effect; do not use w/ renal/liver/adrenal problems **Disp:** See Table 5, p 341; 28-d cycle pills (21 active pills + 7 placebo or Fe or folate supl); 21-d cycle pills (21 active pills) **SE:** Intramenstrual bleeding, oligomenorrhea, amenorrhea, ↑ appetite/Wt gain, ↓ libido, fatigue, depression, mood swings, mastalgia, HA, melasma, ↑ Vag discharge, acne/greasy skin, corneal edema, N; drospirenone-containing pills have ↑ blood clots compared to other progestins

Notes: Taken correctly, up to 99.9% effective for contraception; no STD Px; instruct in use of condoms; to reduce STD risk, use additional barrier contraceptive; long-term, can ↓ risk of ectopic PRG, benign breast Dz, ovarian & uterine CA. Suggestions for OCP prescribing and/or regimen changes are noted below. Listing of other forms of Rx birth control on p 28.

- *Rx menstrual cycle control:* Start w/ monophasic × 3 mo before switching to another brand; w/ continued bleeding change to pill w/ ↑ estrogen
- *Rx birth control:* Choose pill w/ lowest SE profile for particular pt; SEs numerous; d/t estrogenic excess or progesterone deficiency; each pill's SE profile can be unique (see PI); newer extended-cycle combos have shorter/fewer hormone-free intervals, ? ↓ PRG risk; OCP troubleshooting SE w/ suggested OCP
  - *Absent menstrual flow:* ↑ Estrogen, ↓ progestin: Brevicon, Necon 1/35, Norinyl 1/35, Modicon, Necon 1/50, Norinyl 1/50, Ortho-Cyclen, Ortho-Novum 1/35, Ovcon 35
  - *Acne:* Use ↑ estrogen, ↓ androgenic: Brevicon, Ortho-Cyclen, Estrostep, Ortho Tri-Cyclen, Mircette, Modicon, Necon, Ortho Evra, Yasmin, Yaz
  - *Break-through bleeding:* ↑ Estrogen, ↑ progestin, ↓ androgenic: Desogen, Estrostep, Loestrin 1/20, Ortho-Cept, Yasmin, Zovia 1/50
  - *Breast tenderness or ↑ Wt:* ↓ Estrogen, ↓ progestin: Use ↓ estrogen pill rather than current; Alesse, Levlite, Loestrin 1/20 Fe, Ortho Evra, Yasmin, Yaz
  - *Depression:* ↓ Progestin: Alesse, Brevicon, Modicon, Necon, Ortho Evra, Ovcon 35, Ortho-Cyclen, Ortho Tri-Cyclen Tri-Levlen, Triphasil, Trivora
  - *Endometriosis:* ↓ Estrogen, ↑ progestin: Loestrin 1.5/30, Loestrin 1/20 Fe, Lo Ovral, Levlen, Levora, Nordette, Zovia 1/35; cont w/o placebo pills or w/ 4 d of placebo pills
  - *HA:* ↓ Estrogen, ↓ progestin: Alesse, Ortho Evra
  - *Moodiness &/or irritability:* ↓ Progestin: Alesse, Brevicon, Levlite, Modicon, Necon 1/35, Ortho Evra, Ortho-Cyclen, Ortho Tri-Cyclen, Ovcon 35, Tri-Levlen, Triphasil, Trivora
  - *Severe menstrual cramping:* ↑ Progestin: Desogen, Loestrin 1.5/30, Mircette, Ortho-Cept, Yasmin, Yaz, Zovia 1/50E, Zovia 1/35E

Oritavancin (Orbactiv) Uses: *ABSSSI; use only in confirmed Infxn to ↓ resistance* Acts: Lipoglycopeptide; bactericidal spectrum: includes methicillin-susceptible/resistant strains and *S. pyogenes*, enterococcus Dose: 1200 mg IV 3 h × 1 dose W/P: [C, ?/–] w/ Warfarin, may ↑ PT/PTT; hypersens Rxn reported; avoid rapid Inf CDAD; use alternative w/ osteomyelitis CI: Component hypersens; IV heparin 48 h after oritavancin Disp: 400 mg powder to recons SE: N/V/D, SQ abscesses HA Notes: Not approved in peds

Orphenadrine (Norflex, Generic) Uses: *Discomfort associated w/ painful musculoskeletal conds* Acts: Central atropine-like effect; indirect skeletal muscle relaxation, euphoria, analgesia Dose: 100 mg PO bid, 60 mg IM/IV q12h W/P: [C, +/–] CI: NAG, GI or bladder obst, cardiospasm, MyG Disp: SR tabs

100 mg; Inj 30 mg/mL **SE:** Drowsiness, dizziness, blurred vision, flushing, tachycardia, constipation

Oseltamivir (Tamiflu) **Uses:** *Px & Rx influenza A & B* **Acts:** ↓ Viral neuraminidase **Dose:** *Adults. Tx:* 75 mg PO bid for 5 d w/in 48 h of Sx onset; *Prophylaxis:* 75 mg PO qd × 10 d w/in 48 h of contact **Peds.** *Tx:* Dose bid × 5 d < *15 kg.* 30 mg *15–23 kg.* 45 mg *23–40 kg.* 60 mg > *40 kg.* Adult dose *Prophylaxis:* Same dosing but qd for 10 d; ↓ w/ renal impair **W/P:** [C, ?/–] **CI:** Component allergy **Disp:** Caps 30, 45, 75 mg, powder 6 mg/mL for susp (Note: 12 mg/mL dose is being phased out due to dosing concerns) **SE:** N/V, insomnia, reports of neuropsychological events in children (self-injury, confusion, delirium) **Notes:** Start w/in 48 h of Sx onset or exposure; H1N1 strains susceptible; ✓ CDC updates http://www.cdc.gov/h1n1flu/guidance/

Ospemifene (Osphena): **BOX:** ↑ Risk endometrial Ca; ↑ risk of CVA, DVT/PE **Uses:** *Mod–severe dyspareunia* **Acts:** Estrogen agonist/antag **Dose:** *Adults.* 1 tab qd **W/P:** [X, –] Severe liver Dz **CI:** Undiagnosed genital bleeding/ estrogen-dependent neoplasia; active or Hx DVT, PE, CVA, or MI; component hypersens; PRG **Disp:** Tab 60 mg **SE:** Hot flashes, Vag discharge, hyperhidrosis, muscle cramps **Notes:** Metabolized by CYP3A4, CYP2C9, and CYP2C9; highly protein bound, may be displaced by other highly protein-bound drugs

Oxacillin (Generic) **Uses:** *Infxns d/t susceptible S. aureus, Streptococcus & other organisms* **Acts:** Bactericidal; ↓ cell wall synth. *Spectrum:* Excellent gram(+), poor gram(–) **Dose:** *Adults.* 250–500 mg (2 g severe) IM/ IV q4–6h **Peds.** 150–200 mg/kg/d IV ÷ q4–6h **W/P:** [B, M] **CI:** PCN sensitivity **Disp:** Powder for Inj 500 mg, 1, 2, 10 g **SE:** GI upset, interstitial nephritis, blood dyscrasias, may ↓ OCP effectiveness

Oxaliplatin (Eloxatin, Generic) **BOX:** Administer w/ supervision of physician experienced in chemotherapy; appropriate management is possible only w/ adequate diagnostic & Rx facilities; anaphylactic-like Rxns reported **Uses:** *Adjuvant Rx stage III colon CA (primary resected) & met colon CA w/ 5-FU* **Acts:** Metabolized to platinum derivatives, crosslinks DNA **Dose:** Per protocol; see PI *Premedicate:* Antiemetic w/ or w/o dexamethasone **W/P:** [D, –] see PI **CI:** Allergy to components or platinum **Disp:** Inj 50, 100 mg **SE:** Anaphylaxis, granulocytopenia, paresthesia, N/V/D, stomatitis, fatigue, neuropathy, hepatotox, pulm tox **Notes:** 5-FU & leucovorin are given in combo; epi, corticosteroids, & antihistamines alleviate severe Rxns

Oxandrolone (Oxandrin, Generic) [C-III] **BOX:** Risk of peliosis hep, liver cell tumors, may ↑ risk atherosclerosis **Uses:** *Wt ↑ after Wt ↓ from severe trauma, extensive surgery* **Acts:** Anabolic steroid; ↑ lean body mass **Dose:** *Adults.* 2.5–20 mg/d PO ÷ bid–qid **Peds.** ≤ 0.1 mg/kg/d ÷ bid–qid **W/P:** [X, ?/–] ↑ INR w/ warfarin **CI:** PRG, PCa, breast CA, breast CA w/ hypercalcemia, nephrosis **Disp:** Tabs 2.5, 10 mg **SE:** Acne, hepatotox, dyslipidemia **Notes:** ✓ lipids & LFTs; use intermittently, 2–4 wk typical

Oxaprozin (Daypro, Generic) BOX: May ↑ risk of MI/CVA & GI bleeding Uses: *Arthritis & pain* Acts: NSAID; ↓ prostaglandin synth Dose: *Adults.* 600–1200 mg/d (÷ dose helps GI tolerance); ↓ w/ renal/hepatic impair *Peds. JRA (Daypro): 22–31 kg:* 600 mg/d. *32–54 kg:* 900 mg/d; max 1800 mg/d or 26 mg/kg/d W/P: [C (D 3rd tri), ?] Peptic ulcer, bleeding disorders CI: ASA/NSAID sensitivity, perioperative pain w/ CABG Disp: Tabs 600 mg SE: CNS inhib, sleep disturbance, rash, GI upset, peptic ulcer, edema, renal failure, anaphylactoid Rxn w/ "ASA triad" (asthmatic w/ rhinitis, nasal polyps, and bronchospasm w/ NSAID use)

Oxazepam (Generic) [C-IV] Uses: *Anxiety, acute EtOH withdrawal*, anxiety w/ depressive Sxs Acts: Benzodiazepine; diazepam metabolite Dose: *Adults.* 10–15 mg PO tid-qid; severe anxiety & EtOH withdrawal may require up to 30 mg qid *Peds > 6 y.* 1 mg/kg/d ÷ doses W/P: [C, ?/–] CI: Component allergy, NAG, psychosis Disp: Caps 10, 15, 30 mg; tabs 15 mg SE: Sedation, ataxia, dizziness, rash, blood dyscrasias, dependence Notes: Avoid abrupt D/C

Oxcarbazepine (Oxtellar XR, Trileptal, Generic) Uses: *Partial Szs*, bipolar disorders Acts: Blocks voltage-sensitive Na+ channels, stabilization of hyperexcited neural membranes Dose: *Adults.* 300 mg PO bid, ↑ weekly to target maint 1200–2400 mg/d *Peds.* 8–10 mg/kg bid, 600 mg/d max, ↑ weekly to target maint dose; ↓ w/ renal Insuff W/P: [C, –] Carbamazepine sensitivity CI: Component sensitivity Disp: Tabs 150, 300, 600 mg; (*Oxtellar XR*) ER tabs 150, 300, 600 mg; susp 300 mg/5 mL SE: ↓ Na+, HA, dizziness, fatigue, somnolence, GI upset, diplopia, concentration difficulties, fatal skin/multiorgan hypersens Rxns Notes: Do not abruptly D/C, ✓ Na+ if fatigued; advise about SJS and topic epidermal necrolysis

Oxiconazole (Oxistat) Uses: *Tinea cruris, tinea corporis, tinea pedis, tinea versicolor* Acts: ? ↓ Ergosterols in fungal cell membrane. *Spectrum:* Most *Epidermophyton floccosum, Trichophyton mentagrophytes, Trichophyton rubrum, Malassezia furfur* Dose: Apply thin layer qd-bid W/P: [B, M] CI: Component allergy Disp: Cream, lotion 1% SE: Local irritation

Oxybutynin (Ditropan, Ditropan XL, Generic) Uses: *Symptomatic relief of urgency, nocturia, incontinence w/ neurogenic or reflex neurogenic bladder* Acts: Anticholinergic, relaxes bladder smooth muscle, ↑ bladder capacity Dose: *Adults.* 5 mg bid-tid, 5 mg 4×/d max. XL 5–10 mg/d, 30 mg/d max *Peds > 5 y.* 5 mg PO bid-tid; 15 mg/d max *Peds 1–5 y.* 0.2 mg/kg/dose bid-qid (syrup 5 mg/5 mL); 15 mg/d max; ↓ in elderly; periodic drug holidays OK W/P: [B, ?] CI: NAG, MyG, GI/GU obst, UC, megacolon Disp: Gel 5 mg; XL tabs 5, 10, 15 mg; syrup 5 mg/5 mL SE: Anticholinergic (drowsiness, xerostomia, constipation, tachycardia), ↑ QT interval, memory impair; ER form empty shell expelled in stool

Oxybutynin, Topical (Gelnique) Uses: *OAB* Acts: Anticholinergic, relaxes bladder smooth muscle, ↑ bladder capacity Dose: 1 g sachet qd to dry skin (Abd/shoulders/thighs/upper arms) W/P: [B, ?/–] CI: Gastric or urinary retention; NAG Disp: Gel 10%, 1-g sachets (100 mg oxybutynin) SE: Anticholinergic (lethargy, xerostomia, constipation, blurred vision, ↑ HR); rash, pruritus, redness, pain at site; UTI **Notes:** Cover w/ clothing, skin-to-skin transfer can occur; gel is flammable; after applying wait 1 h before showering

Oxybutynin Transdermal System (Oxytrol) **Uses:** *Rx OAB* **Acts:** Anticholinergic, relaxes bladder smooth muscle, ↑ bladder capacity **Dose:** One 3.9 mg/d system apply 2×/wk (q3–4d) to Abd, hip, or buttock **W/P:** [B, ?/–] **CI:** GI/GU obst, NAG **Disp:** 3.9 mg/d transdermal patch **SE:** Anticholinergic, itching/redness at site **Notes:** Do not apply to same site w/in 7 d

Oxycodone (OxyContin, Roxicodone, Generic) [C-II] **BOX:** High abuse potential; CR only for extended chronic pain, not for PRN use; 60-, 80-mg tab for opioid-tolerant pts; do not crush, break, or chew **Uses:** *Mod–severe pain, usually in combo w/ nonnarcotic analgesics* **Acts:** Narcotic analgesic **Dose:** *Adults.* 5 mg PO q6h PRN (IR). *Mod–severe chronic pain:* 10–160 mg PO q12h (ER); can give ER q8h if effect does not last 12 h *Peds* > 11 yr see package insert for conversion from other narcotics; ↓ w/ severe liver/renal Dz, elderly; w/ food **W/P:** [C (D if prolonged use/near term), M] **CI:** Allergy, resp depression, acute asthma, ileus w/ microsomal morphine **Disp:** IR caps (*OxyIR*) 5 mg; CR tabs (*Roxicodone*) 15, 30 mg; ER tabs (*OxyContin*) 10, 15, 20, 30, 40, 60, 80 mg; liq 5 mg/5 mL; soln conc 20 mg/mL **SE:** ↓ BP, sedation, resp depression, dizziness, GI upset, constipation, risk of abuse **Notes:** *OxyContin* for chronic CA pain; do not crush/chew/cut ER product; sought after as drug of abuse; reformulated *OxyContin* is intended to prevent the opioid medication from being cut, broken, chewed, crushed, or dissolved to release more medication

Oxycodone/Acetaminophen (Percocet, Primlev, Tylox) [C-II] **BOX:** Acetaminophen hepatotox (acute liver failure, liver transplant, death) reported; often d/t acetaminophen > 4000 mg/d or more than one acetaminophen product **Uses:** *Mod–severe pain* **Acts:** Narcotic analgesic **Dose:** *Adults.* 1–2 tabs/caps PO q4–6h PRN (acetaminophen max dose 4 g/d) *Peds.* Oxycodone 0.05–0.15 mg/kg/dose q4–6h PRN, 5 mg/dose max **W/P:** [C (D prolonged use or near term), M] **CI:** Allergy, paralytic ileus, resp depression **Disp:** *Percocet* tabs, mg oxycodone/mg APAP: 2.5/325, 5/325, 7.5/325, 10/325, 7.5/500, 10/650; *Tylox* caps 5 mg oxycodone, 500 mg APAP; *Primlev:* 5/300, 7.5/300, 10/300 mg, soln 5 mg oxycodone & 325 mg APAP/5 mL **SE:** ↓ BP, sedation, dizziness, GI upset, constipation

Oxycodone/Acetaminophen, Extended Release (Xartemis XR) [CII] **BOX:** Addiction risk; risk of resp depression; accidental consumption, esp. peds, can be fatal; use during PRG can cause neonatal opioid withdrawal; contains acetaminophen, associated with liver failure, transplant, and death **Uses:** *Acute pain that requires opioids where alternatives are inadequate* **Acts:** Opioid agonist and acetaminophen **Dose:** 2 tabs q12h w/o regard to food; do not crush/chew **W/P:** [C, –] Do not use before delivery; not equivalent to other combo products; caution w/ other CNS depressants, MAOI, neuromuscular blockers, elderly, debilitated, w/ hepatitic impair; may ↑ ICP (examine pupils); assoc w/ skin reactions; may ↓ BP; acetaminophen hepato tox

> 4000 mg, avoid w/ other acetaminophen products; impairs mental/physical abilities; drugs that ↓ CYP3A4 may ↓ oxycodone clearance **CI:** Component hypersens; resp dep, severe asthma/hypercarbia, ileus **Disp:** Tabs oxycodone/acetaminophen: 7.5/325 mg **SE:** ↓ resp, ↓ BP, sedation, coma

Oxycodone/Aspirin (Percodan) [C-II] Uses: *Mod–severe pain* Acts: Narcotic analgesic w/ NSAID **Dose:** *Adults.* 1–2 tabs/caps PO q4–6h PRN *Peds.* Oxycodone 0.05–0.15 mg/kg/dose q4–6h PRN, up to 5 mg/dose; ↓ in severe hepatic failure **W/P:** [D, –] w/ Peptic ulcer, CNS depression, elderly, Hx Szs **CI:** Component allergy, children (< 16 y) w/ viral Infxn (Reyes synd), resp depression, ileus, hemophilia **Disp:** *Generics:* 4.83 mg oxycodone hydrochloride, 0.38 mg oxycodone terephthalate, 325 mg ASA; *Percodan* 4.83 mg oxycodone hydrochloride, 325 mg ASA **SE:** Sedation, dizziness, GI upset/ulcer, constipation, allergy **Notes:** Monitor for possible drug abuse; max 4 g ASA/d

Oxycodone/Ibuprofen (Combunox) [C-II] **BOX:** May ↑ risk of serious CV events; CI in perioperative CABG pain; ↑ risk of GI events such as bleeding Uses: *Short-term (not > 7 d) management of acute mod–severe pain* Acts: Narcotic w/ NSAID **Dose:** 1 tab q6h PRN 4 tab max/24 h; 7 d max **W/P:** [C, –] w/ Impaired renal/hepatic Fxn; COPD; CNS depression; avoid in PRG **CI:** Paralytic ileus, 3rd-tri PRG, allergy to ASA or NSAIDs, where opioids are CI **Disp:** Tabs 5 mg oxycodone/400 mg ibuprofen **SE:** N/V, somnolence, dizziness, sweating, flatulence, ↑ LFTs **Notes:** ✓ Renal Fxn; abuse potential w/ oxycodone

Oxycodone/Naloxone (Targiniq ER) [C-II] **BOX:** Addiction, abuse, and misuse potential; life-threatening resp depression; accidental ingestion; neonatal opioid withdrawal synd; CYP450/3A4 interaction Uses: *Long-term, daily mod–severe pain* Acts: Opioid w/ opioid antag **Dose:** 1 tab 40 mgoxycodone/20 mg naloxone PO only in opioid-tolerant pts (max 80 mg oxycodone/40 mg naloxone/d); *Opioid naïve or not opioid tolerant:* Initial: 1 tab 10 mg oxycodone/5 mg naloxone PO q12h; *Rescue medication:* IR for breakthrough pain; *Conversion from other PO narcotics:* see PI; *Geriatrics:* Start low dose; ↓ dose 50% w /renal impair; ↓ 33–50% w/ hepatic impair; swallow whole **W/P:** CNS depression; severe D (> 3 d); severe D (> 3 d); ↓ BP; caution w/ elderly, cachectic, debilitated, chronic pulm Dz, head injury/↑ ICP; ↑ opioid effects w/ CYP3A4 inhib **CI:** Component hypersns **Disp:** ER tabs (mg oxycodone/mg naloxone) 10/5, 20/10, 40/20 **SE:** Edema, withdrawal synd, fatigue, HA, depression, dizziness, hyperhidrosis, ↑ serum glu, N/V/D, Abd pain, anorexia, constipation, gastroenteritis, UTI, ↓ Hgb, viral Infxn, weakness, bronchitis **Notes:** Monitor for ↓ resp, mental status Δ, S/Sxs of addiction, hypogonadism, or hypoadrenalism; C-II; take only tab at one time; may cause fetal harm in pregnancy

Oxymorphone (Opana, Opana ER) [C-II] **BOX:** *(Opana ER)* Abuse potential, CR only for chronic pain; do not consume EtOH-containing beverages, may cause fatal OD Uses: *Mod–severe pain, sedative* Acts: Narcotic analgesic **Dose:** 10–20 mg PO q4–6h PRN if opioid-naïve or 1–1.5 mg SQ/IM q4–6h PRN or 0.5 mg IV q4–6h PRN; starting 20 mg/dose max PO; *Chronic pain:* ER 5 mg PO q12h; if opioid-naïve ↑ PRN 5–10 mg PO q12h q3–7d; take 1 h pc or 2 h ac; ↓ dose w/ elderly, renal/hepatic impair **W/P:** [C, ?] **CI:** Component hypersens, resp depression, acute asthma, hypercarbia, paralytic ileus, mod–severe hepatic impair **Disp:** Tabs 5, 10 mg; ER tabs 5, 10, 20, 30, 40 mg **SE:** ↓ BP, sedation, GI upset, constipation, histamine release **Notes:** Related to hydromorphone

Oxytocin (Pitocin, Generic) BOX: Not rec for elective induction of labor **Uses:** *Induce labor, control postpartum hemorrhage* **Acts:** Stimulate muscular contractions of the uterus **Dose:** 0.0005–0.001 units/min IV Inf; titrate 0.001–0.002 units/min q30–60min **W/P:** [C, +/–] **CI:** Where Vag delivery not favorable, fetal distress **Disp:** Inj 10 units/mL **SE:** Uterine rupture, fetal death; arrhythmias, anaphylaxis, H_2O intoxication **Notes:** Monitor vital signs; nasal form for breast-feeding only; postpartum bleeding 10–40 units in 1000 mL at sufficient rate to stop bleeding

Paclitaxel (Abraxane, Taxol, Generic) BOX: Administration only by physician experienced in chemotherapy; fatal anaphylaxis and hypersens possible; severe myelosuppression possible **Uses:** *Ovarian & breast CA, PCa*, Kaposi sarcoma, NSCLC* **Acts:** Mitotic spindle poison; promotes microtubule assembly & stabilization against depolymerization **Dose:** Per protocols; use glass or polyolefin containers (eg, nitroglycerin tubing set); PVC sets leach plasticizer; ↓ in hepatic failure **W/P:** [D, –] **CI:** Neutropenia ANC < 1500 cells/mm^3, < 1000 cells/mm^3 in w/ AIDS-related Kaposi's syndrome; solid tumors, component allergy **Disp:** Inj 6 mg/mL, vial 5, 16.7, 25, 50 mL; (*Abraxane*) 100 mg/vial **SE:** ↓ BM, peripheral neuropathy, transient ileus, myalgia, ↓ HR, ↓ BP, mucositis, N/V/D, fever, rash, HA, phlebitis; hematologic tox schedule-dependent; leukopenia dose-limiting by 24-h Inf; neurotox limited w/ short (1–3 h) Inf; allergic Rxns (dyspnea, ↓ BP, urticaria, rash); alopecia **Notes:** Maint hydration; allergic Rxn usually w/in 10 min of Inf; minimize w/ corticosteroid, antihistamine pretreatment

Palbociclib (Ibrance) Uses: *Postmenopausal, ER(+), HER2(–), advanced breast CA w/ letrozole* **Acts:** Kinase inhib **Dose:** 125 mg PO qd w/ food × 21 d, off × 7 d (28-d cycle) w/ letrozole 2.5 mg PO qd through 28-d cycle; adjust dose based on SEs **W/P:** [X (contraception during & 2 wk after final dose), –] Infxn; ✓ WBC (✓ CBC at start of each cycle & d 14 of first 2 cycles); avoid w/ strong CYP3A inhib and mod–strong CYP3A inducers **CI:** Ø **Disp:** Caps 75, 100, 125 mg **SE:** Fatigue, N/V/D, stomatitis, ↓ appetite, ↓ WBC/Hbg/plts, URI, alopecia, asthenia, epistaxis, peripheral neuropathy

Palifermin (Kepivance) Uses: *Oral mucositis w/ BMT* **Acts:** Synthetic keratinocyte GF **Dose:** *Phase 1:* 60 mcg/kg IV qd × 3, 3rd dose 24–48 h before chemotherapy. *Phase 2:* 60 mcg/kg IV qd × 3, after stem cell Inf (at least 4 d from last dose) **W/P:** [C, ?/–] **CI:** Hypersen to palifermin, *E. coli*–derived proteins, or any component or formulation **Disp:** Inj 6.25 mg **SE:** Unusual mouth sensations, tongue thickening, rash, ↑ amylase & lipase, edema, erythema, arthralgia **Notes:** *E. coli*–derived; separate phases by 4 d; safety unknown w/ nonhematologic malignancies

Paliperidone (Invega, Invega Sustenna, Invega Trinza) BOX: Not for dementia-related psychosis Uses: *Schizophrenia* Acts: Risperidone metabolite, DA & serotonin receptor antag Dose: *Invega:* 6 mg PO q A.M., 12 mg/d max; CrCl 50–79 mL/min: 6 mg/d max; CrCl 10–49 mL/min: 3 mg/d max. *Invega Sustenna:* 234 mg day 1, 156 mg 1 week later IM (deltoid), then 117 mg monthly (deltoid or gluteal); range 39–234 mg/mo IM [C, ?/–] w/ ↓ HR, ↓ K+/Mg²⁺, renal/hepatic impair; w/ phenothiazines, ranolazine, ziprasidone, prolonged QT, Hx arrhythmia CI: Risperidone/paliperidone hypersens Disp: *Invega:* ER tabs 1.5, 3, 6, 9 mg; *Invega Sustenna:* Prefilled syringes 39, 78, 117, 156, 234 mg; *Invega Trinza:* IM ER susp 273, 410, 819 mg SE: Impaired temperature regulation, ↑ QT & HR, HA, anxiety, dizziness, N, dry mouth, fatigue, EPS hyperprolactinemia, tremor Notes: Do not chew/cut/crush pill; determine tolerability to oral risperidone or paliperidone before using injectable; convert to Trinza after adequate response to 4 mo Sustenna

Palivizumab (Synagis) Uses: *Px RSV Infxn* Acts: MoAb Dose: *Peds.* 15 mg/kg IM monthly, typically Nov–Apr; AAP rec max 3 doses for those born 32–34 6/7 wk w/o significant congenital heart/lung Dz W/P: [C, ?] Renal/hepatic dysfunction CI: Component allergy Disp: Vials 50 mg/0.5 mL, 100 mg/mL SE: Hypersens Rxn, URI, rhinitis, cough, ↑ LFTs, local irritation, fever, ↓ plts

Palonosetron (Aloxi) Uses: *Px acute & delayed N/V w/ emetogenic chemotherapy; prevent postoperative N/V up to 24 h* Acts: 5-HT₃-receptor antag Dose: *Adults. Chemotherapy:* 0.25 mg IV 30 min pre-chemo; 0.5 mg PO 1 h pre-chemo w/o regard to food *Postoperative N/V:* 0.075 mg immediately before induction *Peds 1 mo to 17 y.* 20 mcg/kg (max 1.5 mg) × 1 IV over 15 min 30 min pre-chemo W/P: [B, ?] May ↑ QTc interval CI: Component allergy Disp: 0.05 mg/mL (1.5 & 5 mL vials); 0.5-mg caps SE: HA, constipation, dizziness, Abd pain, anxiety ↑ QT interval, Szs

Pamidronate (Generic) Uses: *Hypercalcemia of malignancy, Paget Dz, palliate symptomatic bone mets* Acts: Bisphosphonate; ↓ nl & abn bone resorption Dose: *Hypercalcemia:* 60–90 mg IV over 2–24 h or 90 mg IV over 24 h if severe; may repeat in 7 d *Paget Dz:* 30 mg/d IV slow Inf over 4 h × 3 d *Osteolytic bone mets in myeloma:* 90 mg IV over 4 h qmo *Osteolytic bone mets breast CA:* 90 mg IV over 2 h q3–4wk; 90 mg/max single dose W/P: [D, ?/–] Avoid invasive dental procedures w/ use CI: PRG, bisphosphonate sensitivity Disp: Inj 30, 60, 90 mg SE: Fever, malaise, convulsions, Inj site Rxn, uveitis, fluid overload, HTN, Abd pain, N/V, constipation, UTI, bone pain, ↓ K⁺, ↓ Ca²⁺, ↓ Mg²⁺, hypophosphatemia; ONJ (mostly CA pts; avoid dental work), renal tox Notes: Perform dental exam pretherapy; follow Cr, hold dose if Cr ↑ by 0.5 mg/dL w/ nl baseline or by 1 mg/dL w/ abn baseline; restart when Cr returns w/in 10% of baseline; may ↑ atypical subtrochanteric femur fractures

Pancrelipase (Creon, Panakare Plus, Pancreaze, Pertzye, Ultresa, Voikace, Zenpep, Generic) Uses: *Exocrine pancreatic secretion deficiency (eg, CF, chronic pancreatitis, pancreatic Insuff), steatorrhea of malabsorption*

Acts: Pancreatic enzyme supl; amylase, lipase, protease **Dose:** 1–3 caps (tabs) w/ meals & snacks; ↑ to 8 caps (tabs); do not crush or chew EC products; dose dependent on digestive requirements of pt; avoid antacids **W/P:** [C, ?/–] Rare fibrosing colonopathy, oral irritation, ↑ uric acid, viral exposure from animal products **CI:** Ø **Disp:** Caps, tabs **SE:** N/V, Abd cramps, apnea **Notes:** Individualize Rx; dosing based on lipase component, food, nasal congestion

Pancuronium (Generic)   BOX: Should only be administered by adequately trained individuals **Uses:** *Paralysis w/ mechanical ventilation* **Acts:** Nondepolarizing neuromuscular blocker **Dose:** *Adults & Peds > 1 mo.* Initial 0.06–0.1 mg/kg; maint 0.01 mg/kg 60–100 min after, then 0.01 mg/kg q25–60min PRN; ↓ w/ renal/hepatic impair; intubate pt & keep on controlled ventilation; use adequate sedation and analgesia **W/P:** [C, ?/–] **CI:** Component or bromide sensitivity **Disp:** Inj 1, 2 mg/mL **SE:** Tachycardia, HTN, pruritus, other histamine/hypersens Rxns, apnea **Notes:** Crossreactivity w/ other neuromuscular blocker possible

Panitumumab (Vectibix)   BOX: Derm tox common (89%) and severe in 12%; can associated w/ Infxn (sepsis, abscesses requiring I&D; w/ severe derm tox, hold or D/C and monitor for Infxn; severe Inf Rxns (anaphylactic Rxn, bronchospasm, fever, chills, hypotension) in 1%; w/ severe Rxns, immediately D/C Inf and possibly permanent D/C **Uses:** *Rx EGFR-expressing met colon CA* **Acts:** Anti-EGFR MoAb **Dose:** 6 mg/kg IV Inf over 60 min q14d; doses > 1000 mg over 90 min ↓ Inf rate by 50% w/ grade 1–2 Inf Rxn, D/C permanently w/ grade 3–4 Rxn. For derm tox, hold until < grade 2 tox. If improves < 1 mo, restart 50% original dose. If tox recurs or resolution > 1 mo permanently D/C. If ↓ dose tolerated, ↑ dose by 25% **W/P:** [C, –] D/C nursing during, 2 mo after **Disp:** 20 mg/mL vial (5, 10 mL) **SE:** Rash, acneiform dermatitis, pruritus, paronychia, ↓ Mg^{2+}, Abd pain, N/V/D, constipation, fatigue, dehydration, photosens, conjunctivitis, ocular hyperemia, ↑ lacrimation, stomatitis, mucositis, pulm fibrosis, severe derm tox, Inf Rxns **Notes:** May impair female fertility; ✓ lytes; wear sunscreen/ hats, limit sun exposure

Panobinostat (Farydak)   BOX: Severe D in 25%; w/ D, start anti-D meds and ↓ dose of D/C; severe/fatal cardiac events, arrhythmias, ECG changes **Uses:** *Multiple myeloma in combo w/ bortezomib & dexamethasone after at least 2 prior regimens* **Acts:** Histone deacetylase inhib **Dose:** 20 mg PO q other day × 3 doses/wk of wk 1 & 2 of each 21-d cycle for 8 cycles (d 1, 3, 5, 8, 10, 12) **W/P:** [X, –] Embryo-fetal tox, hepatotox, fatal GI & pulm hemorrhage **Disp:** Caps 10, 15, 20 mg **SE:** N/V/D, anorexia, fever, fatigue, edema; ↓ Na+, ↓ K+, ↓ PO_4^{-}, ↑ Cr, ↓ plts, ↓ RBC, ↓ WBC, ↓ lymphocytes, ↓ neutrophils **Notes:** ✓ LFTs; avoid w/ severe hepatic impair; ✓ CBC/plts/lytes; CYP3A4 inhib ↓ dose; avoid w/ CYP3A4 inducers or w/ CYP2D6 substrates; avoid QT-prolonging drugs ✓

Pantoprazole (Protonix, Generic)   Uses: *GERD, erosive gastritis*, ZE synd, PUD **Acts:** PPI **Dose:** *Adults.* 40 mg/d PO; do not crush/chew tabs; 40 mg IV/d (not > 3 mg/min); max 80 mg/d **Peds.** 0.5–1 mg/kg/d ages **Peds** 6–13 y, limited data

W/P: [B, ?/–] Do not use w/ clopidogrel (↓ effect) **Disp:** DR tabs 20, 40 mg; powder for oral susp 40 mg (mix in applesauce or juice, give immediately); Inj 40 mg **SE:** CP, anxiety, GI upset, ↑ LFTs **Notes:** ? ↑ Risk of fractures w/ all PPI; risk of hypomagnesemia w/ long-term use, monitor; ↑ *C. difficile* risk

Parathyroid Hormone (Natpara) **BOX:** ↑ Osteosarcoma in animal model; only available through restricted Natpara REMS (www.natapararems.com) **Uses:** *Adjunct to Ca⁺² & vit D supl in hypoparathyroidism* **Acts:** ↑ Serum Ca⁺² by ↑ renal tubular reabsorption, ↑ intestinal Ca⁺² absorption & ↑ bone turnover **Dose:** Start 50 mcg qd SQ, ↑ 25mcg q4wk to max 100 mcg; goal Ca⁺² in lower half of nl (8–9 mg/dL); ✓ 25-hydroxyvitamin D & Ca⁺² before, then q3–7 d after dose change **W/P:** [C, ?] Osteosarcoma risk; avoid w/ Paget Dz, w/ open epiphyses, Hx skeletal XRT, unexplained ↑ alk phos; ✓ Ca⁺² levels, especially w/ digoxin (tox ↑ w/ ↑ Ca⁺²) **CI:** Ø **Disp:** Multidose cartridge 25, 50, 75, 100 mcg **SE:** Paresthesia, ↑/↓ Ca⁺², N/V/D, hypercalciuria, extremity pain **Notes:** Peds safety not established; no dose adjustment if ≥ 65 y or w/ mild–mod renal or hepatic impair

Paregoric [Camphorated Tincture of Opium] [C-III] **Uses:** *D*, pain & neonatal opiate withdrawal synd **Acts:** Narcotic **Dose:** *Adults.* 5–10 mL PO qd-qid PRN **Peds.** 0.25–0.5 mL/kg qd-qid **W/P:** [B (D w/ prolonged use/high dose near term, +] **CI:** Toxic D; convulsive disorder, morphine sensitivity **Disp:** Liq 2 mg morphine = 20 mg opium/5 mL **SE:** ↓ BP, sedation, constipation **Notes:** Contains anhydrous morphine from opium; do not confuse w/ opium tincture; short-term use only; contains benzoic acid (benzyl alcohol metabolite)

Paroxetine (Brisdelle) **BOX:** Potential for suicidal thinking/behavior; monitor closely **Uses:** *Mod–severe menopause vasomotor Sx (not for psych use)* **Acts:** SSRI, nonhormonal Rx for condition **Dose:** 7.5 mg PO qhs **W/P:** [X, ?/M] Serotonin synd, bleeding w/ NSAID, ↓ Na⁺, ↓ tamoxifen effect, fractures, mania/hypomania activation, Szs, akathisia, NAG, cognitive/motor impair, w/ strong CYP2D6 inhib **CI:** w/ or w/in 14 d of MAOI, w/ thioridazine/pimozide/PRG **Disp:** Caps 7.5 mg **SE:** HA, fatigue, N/V **Notes:** See other paroxetine listings

Paroxetine (Paxil, Paxil CR, Pexeva, Generic) **BOX:** Closely monitor for worsening depression or emergence of suicidality, particularly in children, adolescents, and young adults; not for use in peds **Uses:** *Depression, OCD, panic disorder, social anxiety disorder*, PMDD **Acts:** SSRI **Dose:** 10–60 mg PO qd in A.M.; CR 25 mg PO; ↑ 12.5 mg/d wk (max range 26–62.5 mg/d) **W/P:** [X, ?/] ↑ Bleeding risk **CI:** w/ MAOI, thioridazine, pimozide, linezolid, methylthioninium chloride (methylene blue) **Disp:** Tabs 10, 20, 30, 40 mg; susp 10 mg/5 mL; CR tabs 12.5, 25, 37.5 mg **SE:** HA, somnolence, dizziness, GI upset, N/D, ↓ appetite, sweating, xerostomia, tachycardia, ↓ libido, ED, anorgasmia, palpitations, diaphoresis

Pasireotide (Signifor) **Uses:** *Cushing Dz* **Acts:** Somatostatin analog, inhib ACTH secretion **Dose:** 0.6–0.9 mg SQ bid; titrate on response/ tolerability; hepatic impair (Child-Pugh B): 0.3–0.6 mg SQ bid, (Child-Pugh C): avoid; pancreatic fistula: 0.9 mg SQ bid × 7 d, start A.M. of procedure **W/P:** [C, –]

w/ Risk for ↓ HR or ↑ QT; w/ drugs that ↓ HR, ↑ QT, cyclosporine, bromocriptine **CI:** Ø **Disp:** Inj single-dose 0.3, 0.6, 0.9 mg/mL **SE:** N/V/D, hyperglycemia, HA, Abd pain, cholelithiasis, fatigue, DM, hypocortisolism, ↓ HR, QT prolongation, ↑ glu, ↑ LFTs, ↓ pituitary hormones, Inj site Rxn, edema, alopecia, asthenia, myalgia, arthralgia **Notes:** Prior to and periodically (see PI), ✓ FPG, HbA1c, LFTs, ECG, gallbladder US

Pazopanib (Votrient) **BOX:** Administer only by physician experienced in chemotherapy; severe and fatal hepatotox observed **Uses:** *Rx advanced RCC* met soft-tissue sarcoma after chemotherapy **Acts:** TKI **Dose:** 800 mg PO qd, ↓ to 200 mg qd if mod hepatic impair, not rec in severe hepatic Dz (bili > 3× ULN) **W/P:** [D, –] Avoid w/ CYP3A4 inducers/inhib and QTc-prolonging drugs, all SSRI **CI:** Severe hepatic Dz **Disp:** Tabs 200 mg **SE:** ↑ BP, N/V/D, GI perf, anorexia, hair depigmentation, ↓ WBC, ↓ plt, ↑ bleeding, ↑ AST/ALT/bili, ↓ Na, CP, ↑ QT, impaired wound healing **Notes:** Hold for surgical procedures; take 1 h ac or 2 h pc

Pegfilgrastim (Neulasta) **Uses:** *↓ Frequency of Infxn in pts w/ nonmyeloid malignancies receiving myelosuppressive chemotherapy associated w/ febrile neutropenia* **Acts:** Granulocyte and macrophage-stimulating factor **Dose:** 6 mg SQ × 1/chemotherapy cycle **W/P:** [C, M] w/ Sickle cell **CI:** Allergy to *E. coli*-derived proteins or filgrastim **Disp:** *Syringes:* 6 mg/0.6 mL **SE:** Splenic rupture, HA, fever, weakness, fatigue, dizziness, insomnia, edema, N/V/D, stomatitis, anorexia, constipation, taste perversion, dyspepsia, Abd pain, granulocytopenia, neutropenic fever, ↑ LFTs & uric acid, arthralgia, myalgia, bone pain, ARDS, alopecia, worsen sickle cell Dz **Notes:** Never give between 14 d before & 24 h after dose of cytotoxic chemotherapy

Peginterferon Alpha-2a [Pegylated Interferon] (Pegasys) **BOX:** Can cause or aggravate fatal or life-threatening neuropsychological, autoimmune, ischemic, and infectious disorders. Monitor pts closely **Uses:** *Chronic hep C w/ compensated liver Dz* **Acts:** Immune modulator **Dose:** 180 mcg (1 mL) SQ weekly; see PI; SQ dosing; ↓ in renal impair **W/P:** [C, ?–] **CI:** Autoimmune hep, decompensated liver Dz **Disp:** 180 mcg/mL Inj **SE:** Depression, insomnia, suicidal behavior, GI upset, ↓ WBC and plt, alopecia, pruritus; do not confuse w/ peginterferon alpha-2b

Peginterferon Alpha-2b [Pegylated Interferon] (PegIntron) **BOX:** Can cause or aggravate fatal or life-threatening neuropsychological, autoimmune, ischemic, and infectious disorders; monitor pts closely **Uses:** *Rx hep C* **Acts:** Immune modulator **Dose:** Typical dose (see PI) 1 mcg/kg/wk SQ; 1.5 mcg/kg/wk combo w/ ribavirin **W/P:** [C, ?/–] w/ Psychological disorder Hx **CI:** Autoimmune hep, decompensated liver Dz, hemoglobinopathy **Disp:** Vials 50, 80, 120, 150 mcg/0.5 mL; reconstitute w/ 0.7 mL w/ sterile water **SE:** Depression, insomnia, suicidal behavior, GI upset, neutropenia, thrombocytopenia, alopecia, pruritus **Notes:** Give hs or w/ APAP to ↓ flu-like Sxs; monitor CBC/plt; use immediately or store in refrigerator × 24 h; do not freeze

Peginterferon Beta-1a (Plegridy) Uses: *Relapsing forms of MS* Acts: ? Dose: *Adults.* 125 mcg SQ; titrate; start 63 mcg SQ d 1, 94 mcg SQ d 15, 125 mcg SQ d 29 onward W/P: [C, ?/–]Monitor LFT; ↑ risk of depression/suicidal ideation; can cause Szs CI: Component hypersens Disp: Single-dose pen or syringe 125 mcg/0.5 mL; starter pack (pen or syringe) 63 mcg/0.5 mL, 94 mcg/0.5 mL SE: Inj site erythema/rash/pruritus, influenza-like illness, pyrexia, chills, HA, myalgia, arthralgia Notes: ✓ CBC and LFTs; D/C if new autoimmune disorder diagnosed

Pegloticase (Krystexxa) BOX: Anaphylaxis/Inf Rxn reported; administer in settings prepared to manage these Rxns; premed w/ antihistamines and corticosteroids Uses: *Refractory gout* Acts: PEGylated recombinant urate-oxidase enzyme Dose: 8 mg IV q2wk (in 250 mL NS/½NS over 120 min) premed w/ antihistamines and corticosteroids W/P: [C, –] CI: G6PD deficiency Disp: Inj 8 mg/mL in 1-mL vial SE: Inf Rxn (anaphylaxis, urticaria, pruritis, erythema, CP, dyspnea); may cause gout flare, N Notes: ✓ Uric acid level before each Inf, consider D/C if 2 consecutive levels > 6 mg/dL; do not IV push

Pembrolizumab (Keytruda) Uses: *Unresectable/met melanoma w/ progression after ipilimumab and a BRAF inhib (if BRAF V600 +); NSCLC* Acts: Anti-PD-1 MoAb Dose: 2 mg/kg IV Inf over 30 min q3wk; see PI for dose modifications w/ tox W/P: [D, –] Immune Rxns (pneumonitis, colitis, hep, hypophysitis, nephritis, ↑/↓ thyroid), hold or D/C steroids based on severity of Rxn (see PI); embryo-fetal tox CI: Ø Disp: Inj soln 100 mg/4 mL; powder 50 mg/ vial SE: N/V/D, constipation, ↓ appetite, rash, pruritus, fatigue, cough, arthralgia, fever, edema, HA, insomnia, dizziness, ↑ AST, anemia, NSCLC w/PD-L1 IHC 22C3 pharmDx test

Pemetrexed (Alimta) Uses: *w/ Cisplatin in nonresectable mesothelioma*, NSCLC Acts: Antifolate antineoplastic Dose: 500 mg/m² IV over 10 min q21d; hold if CrCl < 45 mL/min; give w/ vit B₁₂ (1000 mcg IM q9wk) & folic acid (350–1000 mcg PO qd); start 1 wk before; dexamethasone 4 mg PO bid × 3, start 1 d before each Rx W/P: [D, –] w/ Renal/hepatic/BM impair CI: Component sens Disp: 500-mg vial SE: Neutropenia, thrombocytopenia, N/V/D, anorexia, stomatitis, renal failure, neuropathy, fever, fatigue, mood changes, dyspnea, anaphylactic Rxns Notes: Avoid NSAIDs, follow CBC/plt; ↓ dose w/ grade 3–4 mucositis

Pemirolast (Alamast) Uses: *Allergic conjunctivitis* Acts: Mast cell stabilizer Dose: 1–2 gtt in each eye qid W/P: [C, ?/–] Disp: 0.1% (1 mg/mL) in 10-mL bottles SE: HA, rhinitis, cold/flu Sxs, local irritation Notes: Wait 10 min before inserting contacts

Penbutolol (Levatol) Uses: *HTN* Acts: β-Adrenergic receptor blocker, β₁, β₂ Dose: 20–40 mg/d; ↓ in hepatic Insuff W/P: [C 1st tri; D 2nd/3rd tri, M] CI: Asthma, cardiogenic shock, cardiac failure, heart block, ↓ HR, COPD, pulm edema Disp: Tabs 20 mg SE: Flushing, ↓ BP, fatigue, hyperglycemia, GI upset, sexual dysfunction, bronchospasm Notes: ISA

Penciclovir (Denavir) Uses: *Herpes simplex (herpes labialis/cold sores)* Acts: Competitive inhib of DNA polymerase Dose: Apply at 1st sign of lesions, then q2h while awake × 4 d **W/P:** [B, ?/–] **CI:** Allergy, previous Rxn to famciclovir **Disp:** Cream 1% **SE:** Erythema, HA **Notes:** Do not apply to mucous membranes

Penicillin G, Aqueous (Potassium or Sodium) (Pfizerpen, Pentids) **Uses:** *Bacteremia, endocarditis, pericarditis, resp tract Infxns, meningitis, neurosyphilis, skin/skin structure Infxns* **Acts:** Bactericidal; ↓ cell wall synth. *Spectrum:* Most gram(+) (not staphylococci), streptococci, *N. meningitidis*, syphilis, clostridia, & anaerobes (not *Bacteroides*) **Dose:** *Adults.* Based on indication range 0.6–24 mill units/d in ÷ doses q4h. *Peds Newborns < 1 wk.* 25,000–50,000 units/kg/dose IV q12h *Infants 1 wk–< 1 mo.* 25,000–50,000 units/kg/dose IV q8h *Children.* 100,000–400,000 units/kg/24h IV ÷ q4h; ↓ in renal impair **W/P:** [B, M] **CI:** Allergy **Disp:** Powder for Inj **SE:** Allergic Rxns; interstitial nephritis, D, Szs **Notes:** Contains 1.7 mEq of K⁺/mill units

Penicillin G Benzathine (Bicillin) **Uses:** *Single-dose regimen for streptococcal pharyngitis, rheumatic fever, glomerulonephritis prophylaxis, & syphilis* **Acts:** Bactericidal; ↓ cell wall synth. *Spectrum:* See Penicillin G **Dose:** *Adults.* 1.2–2.4 mill units deep IM Inj q2–4wk *Peds.* 50,000 units/kg/dose, 2.4 mill units/dose max; deep IM Inj q2–4 wk **W/P:** [B, M] **Disp:** Inj 300,000, 600,000 units/mL; Bicillin L-A benzathine salt only; Bicillin C-R combo of benzathine & procaine (300,000 units procaine w/ 300,000 units benzathine/mL or 900,000 units benzathine w/ 300,000 units procaine/2 mL) **SE:** Inj site pain, acute interstitial nephritis, anaphylaxis **Notes:** IM use only; sustained action, w/ levels up to 4 wk; drug of choice for noncongenital syphilis

Penicillin G Procaine (Wycillin, Others) **Uses:** *Infxns of resp tract, skin/soft tissue, scarlet fever, syphilis* **Acts:** Bactericidal; ↓ cell wall synth. *Spectrum:* PCN G–sensitive organisms that respond to low, persistent serum levels **Dose:** *Adults.* 0.6–4.8 mill units/d in ÷ doses q12–24h; give probenecid at least 30 min prior to PCN to prolong action *Peds.* 25,000–50,000 units/kg/d IM ÷ qd-bid **W/P:** [B, M] **CI:** Allergy **Disp:** Inj 300,000, 500,000, 600,000 units **SE:** Pain at Inj site, interstitial nephritis, anaphylaxis **Notes:** LA parenteral PCN; levels up to 15 h

Penicillin V (Pen-Vee K, Veetids, Others) **Uses:** Susceptible streptococcal Infxns, otitis media, URIs, skin/soft-tissue Infxns (PCN-sensitive staphylococci) **Acts:** Bactericidal; ↓ cell wall synth. *Spectrum:* Most gram(+), including streptococci **Dose:** *Adults.* 250–500 mg PO q6h, q8h, q12h *Peds.* 25–50 mg/kg/24 h PO in 3–4 ÷ dose above the age of 12 y, dose can be standardized vs Wt based; ↓ in renal impair; take on empty stomach **W/P:** [B, M] **CI:** Allergy **Disp:** Tabs 125, 250, 500 mg; susp 125, 250 mg/5 mL **SE:** GI upset, interstitial nephritis, anaphylaxis, convulsions **Notes:** Well tolerated PO PCN; 250 mg = 400,000 units of PCN G

Pentamidine (NebuPent, Pentam 300) **Uses:** *Rx & Px of PCP* **Acts:** ↓ DNA, RNA, phospholipid, & protein synth **Dose:** *Rx: Adults & Peds.* 4 mg/kg/24 h IV qd × 14–21 d. *Prevention: Adults & Peds > 5 y.* 300 mg once q4wk, give via Respirgard II nebulizer; ↓ IV w/ renal impair **W/P:** [C, ?] **CI:** Component allergy, use w/ didanosine **Disp:** Inj 300 mg/vial; aerosol 300 mg **SE:** Pancreatic cell necrosis w/ hyperglycemia; pancreatitis, CP, fatigue, dizziness, rash, GI upset, renal impair, ↓ WBC, ↓ plt, ↑ QT, ↓ BP **Notes:** Follow CBC, glu, pancreatic Fxn monthly for first 3 mo; monitor for ↓ BP following IV dose; prolonged use may ↑ Infxn risk

Pentazocine (Talwin) [C-IV] **Uses:** *Mod–severe pain; preanesthetic* **Acts:** Partial narcotic agonist–antag **Dose:** *Adults.* 30 mg IM or IV q3–4h PRN; max 360 mg/24 h *Labor:* 20–30 mg *Peds > 1 y.* Sedation 0/5 mg/kg IM; ↓ in renal/hepatic impair **W/P:** [C (1st tri, D w/ prolonged use/high dose near term), +/–] **CI:** Component allergy **Disp:** Inj 30 mg/mL **SE:** Dysphoria; drowsiness, GI upset, xerostomia, Szs **Notes:** 30 mg IM = 10 mg of morphine = 75–100 mg meperidine

Pentobarbital (Nembutal) [C-II] **Uses:** *Insomnia (short-term), convulsions*, sedation, induce coma w/ severe head injury* **Acts:** Barbiturate **Dose:** *Adults. Sedative:* 150–200 mg IM, 100 mg IV, may repeat up to 500 mg max *Hypnotic:* 100–200 mg PO or PR hs PRN *Induced coma:* Load 5–10 mg/kg IV, w/ maint 1–3 mg/kg/h IV *Peds. Induced coma:* As adult **W/P:** [D, +/–] Severe hepatic impair **CI:** Allergy **Disp:** Caps 50, 100 mg; elixir 18.2 mg/5 mL (= 20 mg pentobarbital); supp 30, 60, 120, 200 mg; Inj 50 mg/mL **SE:** Resp depression, ↓ BP w/ aggressive IV use for cerebral edema; ↓ HR, ↓ BP, sedation, lethargy, resp ↓, hangover, rash, SJS, blood dyscrasias **Notes:** Tolerance to sedative–hypnotic effect w/in 1–2 wk

Pentosan Polysulfate Sodium (Elmiron) **Uses:** *Relieve pain/discomfort w/ interstitial cystitis* **Acts:** Bladder wall buffer **Dose:** 100 mg PO tid; on empty stomach w/ H_2O 1 h ac or 2 h pc **W/P:** [B, ?/–] **CI:** Hypersens to pentosan or related compounds (LMWH, heparin) **Disp:** Caps 100 mg **SE:** Alopecia, N/D, HA, ↑ LFTs, anticoagulant effects, ↓ plts, rectal bleeding **Notes:** Reassess after 3 mo; related to LMWH, heparin

Pentoxifylline (Trental, Generic) **Uses:** *Rx Sxs of PVD* **Acts:** ↓ Blood cell viscosity, restores RBC flexibility **Dose:** 400 mg PO tid pc; Rx min 8 wk for effect; ↓ to bid w/ GI/CNS SEs **W/P:** [C, +/–] **CI:** Cerebral/retinal hemorrhage, methylxanthine (caffeine) intolerance **Disp:** Tabs CR 400 mg; tabs ER 400 mg **SE:** Dizziness, HA, GI upset

Perampanel (Fycompa) **BOX:** Serious/life-threatening psychiatric & behavioral Rxns (aggression, hostility, irritability, anger, homicidal threats/ideation) reported; monitor, or D/C if Sxs severe/worsen **Uses:** *Adjunct in partial-onset Sz w/ or w/o secondarily generalized Szs* **Acts:** Noncompetitive AMPA glutamate receptor antag **Dose:** *Adults & Peds ≥ 12 y.* 2 mg PO qhs if not on enzyme-inducing AEDs; 4 mg PO qhs if on enzyme-inducing AEDs; ↑ 2 mg qhs weekly; 12 mg qhs max, titrate ↑ at 2-wk intervals; mild–mod hepatic impair 6 mg max & 4 mg w/ ↑ dose q 2wk; severe hepatic/renal impair or dialysis: avoid **W/P:** [C, –] ✓ For suicidal behavior; avoid strong CYP3A inducers; monitor/dose adjust w/ CYP450 inducers; 12-mg daily dose may ↓ effect of OCP w/ levonorgestrel **CI:** Ø **Disp:** Tabs 2, 4, 6, 8, 10, 12 mg **SE:** N, dizziness, vertigo, ataxia, gait balance/disturb, falls, somnolence, fatigue, irritability, ↑ Wt, anxiety, aggression, anger, blurred vision

Perindopril Erbumine (Aceon, Generic) BOX: ACE inhib can cause death to developing fetus; D/C immediately w/ PRG Uses: *HTN*, CHF, DN, post-MI Acts: ACE inhib Dose: 2–8 mg/d ÷ dose; 16 mg/d max; avoid w/ food; ↓ w/ elderly/renal impair W/P: [C (1st tri, D 2nd & 3rd tri), ?/–] ACE inhib-induced angioedema CI: Bilateral RAS, primary hyperaldosteronism Disp: Tabs 2, 4, 8 mg SE: Weakness, HA, ↓ BP, dizziness, GI upset, cough Notes: OK w/ diuretics

Perinodopril/Amlodipine (Prestalia) BOX: Do not use in PRG Uses: *HTN* Acts: ACE inhib w/ CCB Dose: Start 3.5/2.5 mg PO qd; adjust q1–2wk to BP goal W/P: [D,?/ –] ACE inhib edema CI: w/ Aliskiren DM Disp: Tabs, 3.5/2.5, 7/5, 14/10 mg SE: Edema, cough, HA, dizziness Notes: Monitor for worsening of angina/CP

Permethrin (Elimite, Nix, Generic [OTC]) Uses: *Rx lice/scabies* Acts: Pediculicide Dose: Adults & Peds > 2 y. Lice: Saturate hair & scalp; allow 10 min before rinsing Scabies: Apply cream head to toe; leave for 8–14 h, wash w/ H₂O W/P: [B, ?/–] CI: Allergy > 2 mo Disp: Topical lotion 1%; cream 5% SE: Local irritation Notes: Sprays available (Rid, A200, Nix) to disinfect clothing, bedding, combs, & brushes; lotion not OK in peds < 2 mo; may repeat after 7 d

Perphenazine (Generic) BOX: Elderly pts w/ dementia-related psychosis treated w/ antipsychotic drugs are at ↑ risk of death Uses: *Psychotic disorders, severe N* Acts: Phenothiazine, blocks brain dopaminergic receptors Dose: Adults. Antipsychotic: 4–16 mg PO tid; max 64 mg/d; starting doses for schizophrenia lower in nonhospitalized pts N/V: 8–16 mg/d in ÷ doses Peds 1–6 y. 4–16 mg/d PO in ÷ doses 6–12 y. 6 mg/d PO in ÷ doses > 12 y. 4–16 mg PO bid-tid; ↓ in hepatic Insuff W/P: [C, ?/–] NAG, severe ↑/↓ BP CI: Phenothiazine sensitivity, BM depression, severe liver or cardiac Dz, subcortical brain damage Disp: Tabs 2, 4, 8, 16 mg SE: ↓ BP, ↑/↓ HR, EPS, drowsiness, Szs, photosens, skin discoloration, blood dyscrasias, constipation

Pertuzumab (Perjeta) BOX: Embryo-fetal death & birth defects; animal studies: oligohydramnios, delayed renal development, & death; advise pt of risk & need for effective contraception Uses: *HER2(+) met breast CA w/ trastuzumab & docetaxel in pts who have not received prior anti-HER2 therapy or chemo* Acts: HER2 dimerization inhib Dose: 840 mg 60 min IV Inf × 1; then 420 mg 30–60 min IV Inf q3wk; see PI for tox dose adjust W/P: [D, –] LV dysfunction (monitor LVEF); Inf Rxn CI: Ø Disp: Inj vial 420 mg/14 mL SE: N/V/D, alopecia, ↓ RBC/WBC, fatigue, rash, peripheral neuropathy, hypersens, anaphylaxis, pyrexia, asthenia, stomatitis, pruritus, dry skin, paronychia, HA, dysgeusia, dizziness, myalgia, arthralgia, URI, insomnia, CHF

Phenazopyridine (Azo-Standard, Pyridium, Urogesic, Many Others) [OTC] Uses: *Lower urinary tract irritation* Acts: Anesthetic on urinary tract mucosa Dose: 100–200 mg PO tid; 2 d max w/ Abx for UTI; ↓ w/ renal Insuff W/P:

[B, ?] Hepatic Dz **CI:** Renal failure, CrCl < 50 mL/min **Disp:** Tabs (*Pyridium*) 100, 200 mg [OTC] 45, 97.2, 97.5 mg **SE:** GI disturbances, red-orange urine color (can stain clothing, contacts), HA, dizziness, acute renal failure, methemoglobinemia, tinting of sclera/skin **Notes:** Take w/ food

Phenelzine (Nardil, Generic) **BOX:** Antidepressants ↑ risk of suicidal thinking and behavior in children and adolescents w/ MDD and other psychological disorders; not for peds use **Uses:** *Depression*, bulimia **Acts:** MAOI **Dose:** *Adults.* 15 mg PO tid, ↑ to 60–90 mg/d ÷ doses *Elderly.* 17.5–60 mg/d ÷ doses **W/P:** [C, –] Interacts w/ SSRI, ergots, triptans **CI:** CHF, Hx liver Dz, pheochromocytoma **Disp:** Tabs 15 mg **SE:** Postural ↓ BP; edema, dizziness, sedation, rash, sexual dysfunction, xerostomia, constipation, urinary retention **Notes:** 2–4 wk for effect; avoid tyramine foods (eg, cheeses) rarely primary Rx

Phenobarbital (Generic) [C-IV] **Uses:** *Sz disorders*, insomnia, anxiety **Acts:** Barbiturate **Dose:** *Adults.* Sedative–hypnotic: 30–120 mg/d PO or IM PRN Anticonvulsant: Load 10–20 mg/kg × 1 IV, then 1–3 mg/kg/24 h PO or IV *Peds.* Sedative–hypnotic: 2–3 mg/kg/24 h PO or IM hs PRN Anticonvulsant: Load 15–20 mg/kg × 1 IV, then 3–5 mg/kg/24 h PO ÷ in 2–3 doses; ↓ w/ CrCl < 10 mL/min **W/P:** [D, M] **CI:** Porphyria, hepatic impair, dyspnea, airway obst **Disp:** Tabs 15, 30, 60, 100 mg; elixir 20 mg/5 mL; Inj 60, 65, 130 mg/mL **SE:** ↓ HR, ↓ BP, hangover, SJS, blood dyscrasias, resp depression **Notes:** Tolerance develops to sedation; paradoxic hyperactivity seen in ped pts; long half-life allows single daily dosing. Levels: *Trough:* Just before next dose. *Therapeutic: Trough:* 15–40 mcg/mL; *Toxic: Trough:* > 40 mcg/mL *half-life:* 40–120 h

Phentermine (Adipex-P, Suprenza, Generic) **Uses:** *Wt loss in exogenous obesity* **Acts:** Anorectic/sympathomimetic amine **Dose:** 1 daily in A.M., lowest dose possible; place on tongue, allow to dissolve, then swallow **W/P:** [X, –] **CI:** CV Dz, hyperthyroidism, glaucoma, PRG, nursing, w/in 14 d of MAOI **Disp:** Tabs 15, 30, 37.5 mg; (*Suprenza*) ODT 15, 30, 37.5 mg **SE:** Pulm hypertension, aortic/mitral/tricuspid regurgitation valve Dz, dependence, ↑ HR, ↑ BP, palpitations, insomnia, HA, psychosis, restlessness, mood change, impotence, dry mouth, taste disturbance **Notes:** Avoid use at night

Phentermine/Topiramate (Qsymia) [C-IV] **Uses:** *Wt management w/ BMI ≥ 30 kg/m² or ≥ 27 kg/m² w/ Wt-related comorbidity* **Acts:** Anorectic (sympathomimetic amine w/ anticonvulsant) **Dose:** 3.75/23 mg PO qd × 14 d, then 7.5/46 mg PO qd; max dose 15/92 mg qd or 7.5/46 mg w/ mod–severe renal impair or mod hepatic impair; D/C if not > 3% Wt loss on 7.5/46 mg dose or 5% Wt loss on 15/92 mg dose by week 12; D/C max dose gradually to prevent Szs **W/P:** [X, –] **CI:** PRG, glaucoma, hyperthyroidism, use w/ or w/in 14 d of MAOI **Disp:** Caps (phentermine/topiramate ER) 3.75/23, 7.5/46, 11.25/69, 15/92 mg **SE:** Paresthesia, dizziness, dysgeusia, insomnia, constipation, dry mouth, ↑ HR, ↑ BP, palpitations, HA, restlessness, mood change, memory impair, metabolic acidosis, kidney stones, ↑ Cr, acute myopia, glaucoma, depression, suicidal behavior/ideation **Notes:** ✓

PRG baseline & qmo; effective contraception necessary, ✓ HR/BP/electrolytes REMS restricted distribution

Phenylephrine, Nasal (Neo-Synephrine Nasal) [OTC]
BOX: Not for use in peds < 2 y **Uses:** *Nasal congestion* **Acts:** α-Adrenergic agonist **Dose:** *Adults.* 0.25–1% 2–3 sprays/drops in each nostril 94 h PRN *Peds 2–6 y.* 0.125% 1 drop/nostril q2–4h *6–12 y.* 1–2 sprays/nostril q4h 0.25% 2–3 drops **W/P:** [C, +/–] HTN, acute pancreatitis, hep, coronary Dz, NAG, hyperthyroidism **CI:** ↓ HR, arrhythmias **Disp:** Nasal spray 0.25, 0.5, 1%; drops: 0.125, 0.25 mg/mL **SE:** Arrhythmias, HTN, nasal irritation, dryness, sneezing, rebound congestion w/ prolonged use, HA **Notes:** Do not use > 3 d

Phenylephrine, Ophthalmic (AK-Dilate, Neo-Synephrine Ophthalmic, Zincfrin [OTC])
Uses: *Mydriasis, ocular redness [OTC], perioperative mydriasis, posterior synechiae, uveitis w/ posterior synechiae* **Acts:** α-Adrenergic agonist **Dose:** *Adults. Redness:* 1 gtt 0.12% q3–4h PRN up to qid *Exam mydriasis:* 1 gtt 2.5% (15 min–1 h for effect) *Preop:* 1 gtt 2.5–10% 30–60 min preop *Peds.* As adult, only use 2.5% for exam, preop, and ocular conds **W/P:** [C, May cause late-term fetal anoxia/↓ HR, +/–] HTN, w/ elderly w/ CAD **CI:** NAG **Disp:** Ophthal soln 0.12% (Zincfrin OTC), 2.5, 10% **SE:** Tearing, HA, irritation, eye pain, photophobia, arrhythmia, tremor

Phenylephrine, Oral (Sudafed, Others) [OTC]
BOX: Not for use in peds < 2 y **Uses:** *Nasal congestion* **Acts:** α-Adrenergic agonist **Dose:** *Adults.* 10–20 mg PO q4h PRN, max 60 mg/d *Peds.* 4–5 y: 2.5 mg q4h max 6 doses/d; > 6–12: 5 mg q4h, max 30 mg/d ≥ 12: adult dosing **W/P:** [C, +/–] HTN, acute pancreatitis, hep, coronary Dz, NAG, hyperthyroidism **CI:** MAOI w/in 14 d, NAG, severe ↑ BP or CAD, urinary retention **Disp:** Liq 7.5 mg/5 mL; drops: 1.25/0.8 mL, 2.5 mg/5 mL; tabs 5, 10 mg; chew tabs 10 mg; tabs qd 10 mg; strips: 1.25, 2.5, 10 mg; many combo OTC products **SE:** Arrhythmias, HTN, HA, agitation, anxiety, tremor, palpitations; can be chemically processed into methamphetamine; products now sold behind pharmacy counter w/o prescription

Phenylephrine, Systemic (Generic)
BOX: Prescribers should be aware of full prescribing information before use **Uses:** *Vascular failure in shock, allergy, or drug-induced ↓ BP* **Acts:** α-Adrenergic agonist ↓ BP **Dose:** *Adults. Mild–mod* ↓ BP: 2–5 mg IM or SQ ↑ BP for 2 h; 0.1–0.5 mg IV elevates BP for 15 min. *Severe ↓ BP/ shock:* Cont Inf at 100–180 mcg/min; after BP stable *Peds.* ↓ BP: 5–20 mcg/kg/ dose IV q10–15min or 0.1–0.5 mcg/kg/min IV Inf, titrate to effect **W/P:** [C, +/–] HTN, acute pancreatitis, hep, coronary Dz, NAG, hyperthyroidism **CI:** ↓ HR, arrhythmias **Disp:** Inj 10 mg/mL **SE:** Arrhythmias, HTN, peripheral vasoconstriction ↑ w/ oxytocin, MAOIs, & TCAs; HA, weakness, necrosis, ↓ renal perfusion **Notes:** Restore blood vol if loss has occurred; use large veins to avoid extrav; phentolamine 10 mg in 10–15 mL of NS for local Inj to Rx extrav

Phenytoin (Dilantin, Generic)
Uses: *Tonic-clonic (grand mal) & psychomotor (temporal lobe) Szs, Szs w/ neurosurgery+* **Acts:** ↓ Sz spread in the motor

cortex **Dose:** **Adults & Peds.** *Load:* 15–20 mg/kg IV, 50 mg/min max or PO in 400-mg doses at 4-h intervals **Adults.** *Maint:* Initial 200 mg PO or IV bid or 300 mg tis, then follow levels; alternatively 5–7 mg/kg/d based on IBW ÷ daily-tid **Peds.** *Maint:* 4–7 mg/kg/24h PO or IV ÷ daily-bid; avoid PO susp (erratic absorption) **W/P:** [D, +] **CI:** Heart block, sinus bradycardia **Disp:** *Dilantin Infatab:* chew 50 mg. *Dilantin/Phenytek:* caps 100 mg; caps ER 30, 100, 200, 300 mg; susp 125 mg/5 mL; Inj 50 mg/mL **SE:** Nystagmus/ataxia early signs of tox; gum hyperplasia w/ long-term use. *IV:* ↓ BP, ↓ HR, arrhythmias, phlebitis; peripheral neuropathy, rash, blood dyscrasias, SJS **Notes:** Levels: *Trough:* Just before next dose. *Therapeutic:* 10–20 mcg/mL. *Toxic:* > 20 mcg/mL. Phenytoin albumin bound, levels = bound & free phenytoin; w/ ↓ albumin & azotemia, low levels may be therapeutic (nl free levels); do not change dosage at intervals < 7–10 d; hold tube feeds 1 h before and after dosing if using oral susp; avoid large dose ↑

Physostigmine (Generic) **Uses:** *Reverse tox CNS effects of atropine & scopolamine OD* **Acts:** Reversible cholinesterase inhib **Dose:** *Adults.* 0.5–2 mg IV or IM q20 min *Peds.* 0.01–0.03 mg/kg/dose IV q5–10 min up to 2 mg total PRN **W/P:** [C, ?] **CI:** GI/GU obst, CV Dz, asthma **Disp:** Inj 1 mg/mL **SE:** Rapid IV administration associated w/ Szs; cholinergic SEs; sweating, salivation, lacrimation, GI upset, asystole, changes in HR **Notes:** Excessive readministration can result in cholinergic crisis; crisis reversed w/ atropine; contains bisulfite (allergy possible)

Phytonadione [Vitamin K₁] (Mephyton, Generic) **BOX:** Hypersens Rxns associated w/ or immediately following Inf **Uses:** *Coagulation disorders d/t faulty formation of factors II, VII, IX, X*; hyperalimentation **Acts:** Cofactor for production of factors II, VII, IX, & X **Dose:** *Adults & Peds.* *Anticoagulant-induced prothrombin deficiency:* 1–10 mg PO or IV slowly *Hyperalimentation:* 10 mg IM or IV qwk *Infants.* 0.5–1 mg/dose; IM w/in 1 h of birth or PO **W/P:** [C, +] **CI:** Allergy Rxn **Disp:** Tabs 5 mg; Inj 2, 10 mg/mL **SE:** Anaphylaxis from IV dosage; give IV slowly; GI upset (PO), Inj site Rxns **Notes:** w/ Parenteral Rx, 1st change in PT/INR usually seen in 12–24 h; makes anticoagulation difficult; see PI for dosing algorithm based on INR of S/Sx of bleeding

Pimecrolimus (Elidel) **BOX:** Associated w/ rare skin malignancies and lymphoma, limit to area, not for age < 2 y **Uses:** *Atopic dermatitis* refractory, severe perianal itching **Acts:** Inhibits T lymphocytes **Dose:** *Adults & Peds > 2 y.* Apply bid **W/P:** [C, ?/–] w/ Local Infxn, lymphadenopathy; immunocompromised; avoid in pts < 2 y **CI:** Allergy component, < 2 y **Disp:** Cream 1% **SE:** Phototox, local irritation/burning, flu-like Sxs, may ↑ malignancy **Notes:** Use on dry skin only; wash hands after; 2nd-line/short-term use only

Pimozide (Orap) **BOX:** ↑ Mortality in elderly w/ dementia-related psychosis **Uses:** * Tourette Dz* agitation, psychosis **Acts:** Typical antipsychotic, DA antag **Dose:** Inital 1–2 mg/d to max of 10 mg/d or 0.2 mg/kg/d (whichever is less); ↓ w/ hepatic impair **W/P:** [C/–] NAG, elderly, hepatic impair, neurologic Dz, **CI:** Compound hypersens, CNS depression, coma, dysrhythmia, ↑ QT syndrome, w/ QT prolonging drugs, ↓ K, ↓ Mg, w/ CYP3A4 inhib (Table 10, p 356) **Disp:** Tabs 1, 2 mg **SE:** CNS (somnolence, agitation, others), rash, xerostomia, weakness, rigidity, visual changes, constipation, ↑ salivation, akathisia, tardive dyskinesia, neuroleptic malignant syndrome, ↑ QT **Notes:** ✓ ECG

Pindolol (Generic) **Uses:** *HTN* **Acts:** β-Adrenergic receptor blocker, β₁, β₂, ISA **Dose:** 5–10 mg bid, 60 mg/d max; ↓ in hepatic/renal failure **W/P:** [B (1st tri; D 2nd/3rd tri), +/–] **CI:** Uncompensated CHF, cardiogenic shock, ↓ HR, heart block, asthma, COPD **Disp:** Tabs 5, 10 mg **SE:** Insomnia, dizziness, fatigue, edema, GI upset, dyspnea; fluid retention may exacerbate CHF

Pioglitazone (Actos, Generic) **BOX:** May cause or worsen CHF **Uses:** *Type 2 DM* **Acts:** ↑ Insulin sensitivity, a thiazolidinedione **Dose:** 15–45 mg/d PO **W/P:** [C, –] w/ Hx bladder CA **CI:** CHF, hepatic impair **Disp:** Tabs 15, 30, 45 mg **SE:** Wt gain, myalgia, URI, HA, hypoglycemia, edema, ↑ fracture risk in women; may ↑ bladder CA risk **Notes:** Not 1st-line agent

Pioglitazone/Metformin (ACTOplus Met, ACTOplus MET XR, Generic) **BOX:** Metformin can cause lactic acidosis, fatal in 50% of cases; pioglitazone may cause or worsen CHF **Uses:** *Type 2 DM as adjunct to diet and exercise* **Acts:** Combined ↑ insulin sensitivity w/ ↓ hepatic glu release **Dose:** Initial 1 tab PO qd-bid, titrate; max daily pioglitazone 45 mg & metformin 2550 mg; XR: 1 tab PO qd w/ evening meal; max daily pioglitazone 45 mg & metformin IR 2550 mg, metformin ER 2000 mg; give w/ meals **W/P:** [C, –] Stop w/ radiologic IV contrast agents; w/ Hx bladder CA; do not use w/ active bladder CA **CI:** CHF, renal impair, acidosis **Disp:** Tabs (pioglitazone mg/metformin mg) 15/500, 15/850; tabs XR (pioglitazone mg/metformin ER mg) 15/1000, 30/1000 mg **SE:** Lactic acidosis, CHF, ↓ glu, edema, Wt gain, myalgia, URI, HA, GI upset, liver damage **Notes:** Follow LFTs; ↑ fracture risk in women receiving pioglitazone; pioglitazone may ↑ bladder CA risk

Piperacillin/Tazobactam (Zosyn, Generic) **Uses:** *Infxns of skin, bone, resp & urinary tract, Abd, sepsis* **Acts:** 4th-gen PCN plus β-lactamase inhib; bactericidal; ↓ cell wall synth. *Spectrum:* Good gram(+), excellent gram(–); anaerobes & β-lactamase producers **Dose:** 3.375–4.5 g IV q6h; ↓ in renal Insuff **W/P:** [B, M] **CI:** PCN or β-lactam sensitivity **Disp:** Frozen and powder for Inj: 2.25, 3.375, 4.5 g **SE:** D, HA, insomnia, GI upset, serum sickness-like Rxn, pseudomembranous colitis **Notes:** Often used in combo w/ aminoglycoside

Pirbuterol (Maxair, Generic) **Uses:** *Px & Rx reversible bronchospasm* **Acts:** β₂-Adrenergic agonist **Dose:** 2 Inh q4–6h; max 12 Inh/d **W/P:** [C, ?/–] **Disp:** Aerosol 0.2 mg/actuation (contains ozone-depleting CFCs; will be gradually removed from US market) **SE:** Nervousness, restlessness, trembling, HA, taste changes, tachycardia **Notes:** Teach pt proper inhaler technique

Pirfenidone (Esbriet) **Uses:** *Idiopathic pulm fibrosis* **Acts:** Unknown **Dose:** 801 mg tid w/ food; d 1–7, 1 cap tid; d 8–14, 2 caps tid; d 15 onward, 3 caps tid; w/food **W/P:** [C, –] Do NOT use w/ severe hepatic/renal impair **Disp:** Caps 267 mg **SE:** N/V/D, HA, fatigue, insomnia, dizziness, arthralgia, Abd pain, GERD, dyspepsia, anorexia, ↓ Wt, URI, sinusitis **Notes:** Avoid sun, wear sunscreen; CYP1A2 inhib (ie, ciprofloxacin, fluvoxamine) may ↑ adverse Rxns; ✓ hepatic/ renal Fxn; smoking ↓ efficacy

Piroxicam (Feldene, Generic) **BOX:** May ↑ risk of MI/CVA & GI bleeding **Uses:** *Arthritis & pain* **Acts:** NSAID; ↓ prostaglandins **Dose:** 10–20 mg/d **W/P:** [C/D if 3rd tri, –] GI bleeding **CI:** ASA/NSAID sensitivity **Disp:** Caps 10, 20 mg **SE:** Dizziness, rash, GI upset, edema, acute renal failure, peptic ulcer

Pitavastatin (Livalo) **Uses:** *Reduce elevated total cholesterol* **Acts:** Statin, HMG-CoA reductase inhib **Dose:** 1–4 mg qd w/o regard to meals; CrCl < 60 mL/ min: start 1 mg w/ 2 mg max **W/P:** [X, /–] May cause myopathy and rhabdomyolysis **CI:** Active liver Dz, w/ lopinavir/ritonavir/cyclosporine, severe renal impair not on dialysis **Disp:** Tabs 1, 2, 4 mg **SE:** Muscle pain, back pain, jt pain, and constipation, ↑ LFTs **Notes:** ✓ LFTs; OK w/ grapefruit

Plasma Protein Fraction (Plasmanate) **Uses:** *Shock & ↓ BP* **Acts:** Plasma vol expander **Dose:** *Adults. Initial:* 250–500 mL IV (not > 10 mL/min); subsequent Inf based on response *Peds.* 10–15 mL/kg/dose IV; subsequent Inf based on response; safety & efficacy in children not established **W/P:** [C, +] **CI:** Renal Insuff, CHF, cardiopulmonary bypass **Disp:** Inj 5% **SE:** ↓ BP w/ rapid Inf; hypocoagulability, metabolic acidosis, PE **Notes:** 0.25 mEq K/L & 145 mEq Na/L; not substitute for RBC

Plerixafor (Mozobil) **Uses:** *Mobilize stem cells for ABMT in lymphoma and myeloma in combo w/ G-CSF* **Acts:** Hematopoietic stem cell mobilizer **Dose:** 0.24 mg/kg SQ qd; max 40 mg/d; CrCl < 50 mL/min: 0.16 mg/kg, max 27 mg/d **W/P:** [D, /?] **CI:** **Disp:** IV: 20 mg/mL (1.2 mL) **SE:** HA, N/V/D, Inj site Rxns, ↑ WBC, ↓ plt **Notes:** Give w/ filgrastim 10 mcg/kg

Pneumococcal 13-Valent Conjugate Vaccine (Prevnar 13) **Uses:** *Immunization against pneumococcal Infxns in infants & children* **Acts:** Active immunization **Dose:** 0.5 mL IM/dose; series of 4 doses; 1st dose age 2 mo; then 4 mo, 6 mo, and 12–15 mo; if previous Prevnar switch to Prevnar 13; if completed Prevnar series, supplemental dose Prevnar 13 at least 8 wk after last Prevnar dose **W/P:** [C, +] w/ ↓ plt **CI:** Sensitivity to components/diphtheria toxoid, febrile illness **Disp:** Inj **SE:** Local Rxns, anorexia, fever, irritability, ↑/↓ sleep, V/D **Notes:** Keep epi (1:1000) available for Rxns; replaces *Prevnar* (has additional spectrum); does not replace *Pneumovax-23* in age > 24 mo w/ immunosuppression; inactivated capsular antigens

Pneumococcal Vaccine, Polyvalent (Pneumovax 23) **Uses:** *Immunization against pneumococcal Infxns in pts at high risk (all pts > 65 y, also asplenia, sickle cell Dz, HIV, and other immunocompromised and w/ chronic illnesses)* **Acts:** Active immunization **Dose:** 0.5 mL IM or SQ **W/P:** [C, ?] **CI:** Do not vaccinate during immunosuppressive Rx **Disp:** Inj 0.5 mL **SE:** Fever, Inj site Rxn also hemolytic anemia w/ other heme conditions, ↓ plt w/

stable ITP, anaphylaxis, Guillain-Barré synd **Notes:** Keep epi (1:1000) available for Rxns. Revaccinate q3–5 y if very high risk (eg, asplenia, nephrotic synd), consider revaccination if > 6 y since initial or if previously vaccinated w/ 14-valent vaccine; inactivated capsular antigens

Podophyllin (Condylox, Condylox Gel 0.5%, Podocon-25) **Uses:** *Topical Rx of benign growths (genital & perianal warts [condylomata acuminata]*, papillomas, fibromas) **Acts:** Direct antimitotic effect; exact mechanism unknown **Dose:** *Condylox gel & Condylox:* Apply bid for 3 consecutive d/wk, then hold for 4 d, may repeat 4 × 0.5 mL/d max; *Podocon-25:* Use sparingly on the lesion, leave on for only 30–40 min for 1st application, then 1–4 h on subsequent applications, thoroughly wash off; limit < 5 mL or < 10 cm²/Rx **W/P:** [X, ?] Immunosuppression **CI:** DM, bleeding lesions **Disp:** *Podocon-25* (w/ benzoin) 15-mL bottles; *Condylox gel* 0.5% 3.5-g gel; *Condylox soln* 0.5% 3.5-g clear soln **SE:** Local Rxns, sig absorption; anemias, tachycardia, paresthesias, GI upset, renal/hepatic damage **Notes:** *Podocon-25* applied by the clinician; do not dispense directly to pt

Polyethylene Glycol [PEG] 3350 (MiraLAX) [OTC] **Uses:** *Occasional constipation* **Acts:** Osmotic laxative **Dose:** 17-g powder (1 heaping tsp) in 8 oz (1 cup) of H_2O & drink; max 14 d **W/P:** [C, ?] Rule out bowel obst before use **CI:** GI obst, allergy to PEG **Disp:** Powder for reconstitution; bottle cap holds 17 g **SE:** Upset stomach, bloating, cramping, gas, severe D, hives **Notes:** Can add to H_2O, juice, soda, coffee, or tea

Polyethylene Glycol Electrolyte Soln [PEG-ES] (Colyte, GoLYTELY) **Uses:** *Bowel prep prior to examination or surgery* **Acts:** Osmotic cathartic **Dose:** *Adults.* Following 3- to 4-h fast, drink 240 mL of soln q10min until 4 L consumed or until BMs are clear *Peds.* 25–40 mL/kg/h for 4–10 h until BM clear; max dose 4 L? **W/P:** [C, ?] **CI:** GI obst, bowel perforation, megacolon, UC **Disp:** Powder for recons to 4 L **SE:** Cramping or N, bloating **Notes:** 1st BM should occur in approximately 1 h; chilled soln more palatable; flavor packets available

Pomalidomide (Pomalyst) **BOX:** Contraindicated in PRG; a thalidomide analog, a known human teratogen; exclude PRG before/during Tx; use 2 forms of contraception; available only through a restricted program; DVT/PE w/ multiple myeloma treated w/ pomalidomide **Uses:** *Multiple myeloma previously treated w/ at least 2 regimens, including lenalidomide and bortezomib w/ progression w/in 60 days of last therapy* **Acts:** Immunomodulatory drug w/ antineoplastic action **Dose:** 4 mg qd, d 1–21 in a 28-d cycle, until Dz prog; hold/reduce dose w/ ↓ WBC/plts **W/P:** [X, −] Hematologic tox, especially w/ ↓ WBC **CI:** PRG **Disp:** Caps 1, 2, 3, 4 mg **SE:** Birth defects; ↓ WBC/plts/Hgb; DVT/PE; neuropathy; confusion, dizziness, HA; fever, fatigue, N/V/D, constipation; rash **Notes:** Avoid w/ CYP1A2 inhibs; cannot donate blood/sperm; male condoms w/ intercourse

Ponatinib (Iclusig) **BOX:** Venous/arterial occlusion (27%); DVT/PE, MI, CVA, PVD, often need revascularization; heart failure & hepatotox w/ liver failure and death, (monitor cardiac & hepatic Fxn) **Uses:** *T315I+ CML; Ph+ ALL; CML or Ph+ ALL w/ no other TKI indicated* **Acts:** TKI **Dose:** 45 mg qd, DC and then reduce dose for tox [D, −] ↓ WBC; vascular occlusion; heart failure; hepato-tox; pancreatitis; ↑ BP; neuropathy; ocular tox, including blindness; arrhythmias, bradycardia & SVT; edema; tumor lysis; poor wound healing; GI perf **CI:** Ø **Disp:** Tabs 15, 45 mg **SE:** ↑ BP, fever, rash, HA, fatigue, arthralgias, N, Abd pain, consti-pation, pneumonia; sepsis; ↑ QT interval; anemia, ↓ plts, ↓ WBC, ↓ neutrophils, ↓ lymphs; ↑ AST, ↑ ALT, ↑ alk phos, ↑ bili, ↑ lipase, ↓ glu, ↑/↓ K+, ↓ Na+, ↓ HCO3−, ↑ creat, ↑ Ca++, ↓ phos, ↓ albumin **Notes:** CBC q 2 wk × 3 mos; ✓ following base-line and periodically. Eye exam, LFTs; BP; lipase q2wk × 2 mo; monitor BP; w/ CYP3A4 inhib ↓ dose; avoid w/ CYP3A inducers & meds that ↑ gastric pH

Posaconazole (Noxafil) Uses: *Px *Aspergillus* and *Candida* Infxns in severely immunocompromised; Rx oropharyngeal candida* **Acts:** ↓ Cell membrane ergosterol synth **Dose:** *Adults & Peds > 13 y. Px Aspergillus/Candida Infxn:* 300 mg IV bid d1, maint 300 mg qd; or 300 mg PO bid d 1, maint 300 mg qd; or susp 200 mg (5 mL) tid *Oropharyngeal Candidiasis:* 100 mg (2.5 mL) bid qd, maint 100 mg (2.5 mL) qd × 13 d **W/P:** [C, ?] Multiple drug interactions; ↑ QT, cardiac Dzs, severe renal/liver impair **CI:** Component hypersens; w/ many drugs, including alfu-zosin, astemizole, alprazolam, phenothiazines, terfenadine, triazolam, others **Disp:** Soln 300 mg/16.7 mL; DR tabs 100 mg **SE:** ↑ QT, ↑ LFTs, hepatic failure, fever, N/V/D, HA, Abd pain, anemia, ↓ plt, ↓ K+ rash, dyspnea, cough, anorexia, fatigue **Notes:** Monitor LFTs, CBC, lytes; administer w/ meal or nutritional supplement

Potassium Citrate (Urocit-K, Generic) Uses: *Alkalinize urine; Px uri-nary stones (uric acid, Ca stones if hypocitraturic)* **Acts:** ↓ Urinary alkalinizer **Dose:** 30–60 mEq/d based on severity of hypocitraturia; max 100 mEq/d **W/P:** [A, +] **CI:** Severe renal impair, dehydration, ↑ K+, peptic ulcer; w/ K+-sparing diuretics, salt substitutes **Disp:** Tabs 5, 10, 15 mEq/d **SE:** GI upset, ↓ Ca2+, ↑ K+, metabolic alkalosis

Potassium Iodide (Iosat, Lugol's Solution, SSKI, Thyro-Block, ThyroSafe, ThyroShield) [OTC] Uses: *Thyroid storm*, ↓ vascularity before thyroid surgery, block thyroid uptake of radioactive iodine (nuclear scans or nuclear emergency), thin bronchial secretions **Acts:** Iodine supl **Dose:** *Adults & Peds > 2 y. Preop thyroidectomy:* 50–100 mg PO tid (1–2 gtts or 0.05–0.1 mL SSKI); give 10 d preop *Protection:* 130 mg/d **Peds.** *Protection: < 1 y.* 16.25 mg qd *d 1 mo–3y.* 32.5 mg qd *3–18 y.* 65 mg qd **W/P:** [D, +] K+, TB, PE, bronchitis, renal impair **CI:** Iodine sensitivity **Disp:** Tabs 65, 130 mg; soln (SSKI) 1 g/mL; Lugol soln, strong iodine 100 mg/mL; syrup 325 mg/5 mL **SE:** Fever, HA, urticaria, angioedema, goiter, GI upset, eosinophilia **Notes:** w/ Nuclear radiation emergency, give until radiation exposure no longer exists

Potassium Supplements (Kaochlor, Kaon, K-Lor, Klorvess, Micro-K, Generic) Uses: *Px or Rx of ↓ K+* (eg, diuretic use)* **Acts:** K+ supl **Dose:** *Adults.* 20–100 mEq/d PO ÷ qd-qid; IV 10–20 mEq/h, max 40 mEq/h & 150 mEq/d (monitor K+ levels frequently and in presence of continuous ECG monitoring w/ high-dose IV)

Peds. Calculate K⁺ deficit; 1–3 mEq/kg/d PO ÷ qd-qid; IV max dose 0.5–1 mEq/kg × 1–2 h **W/P:** [A, +] Renal Insuff; w/ NSAIDs & ACE inhib **CI:** ↑ K⁺ **Disp:** PO forms (Table 6, p 351) Inj **SE:** GI irritation; ↓ HR, ↑ K⁺, heart block **Notes:** Mix powder & liq w/ beverage (unsalted tomato juice, etc); SR tabs must be swallowed whole; follow/monitor K⁺; Cl⁻ salt OK w/ alkalosis; w/ acidosis use acetate, bicarbonate, citrate, or gluconate salt; do not administer IV K⁺ undiluted

Pralatrexate (Folotyn) Uses: *Tx refractory T-cell lymphoma* **Acts:** Folate analog metabolic inhib; ↓ dihydrofolate reductase **Dose:** IV push over 3–5 min: 30 mg/m² once weekly for 6 wk **W/P:** [D, –] **Disp:** Inj 20 mg/mL (1 mL, 2 mL) **SE:** ↓ Plt, anemia, ↓ WBC, mucositis, N/V/D, edema, fever, fatigue, rash **Notes:** Give folic acid supplements prior to and after; ANC should be ≥ 1000/mm³

Pramipexole (Mirapex, Mirapex ER, Generic) Uses: *Parkinson Dz (Mirapex, Mirapex ER), RLS (Mirapex)* **Acts:** DA agonist **Dose:** *Mirapex:* 1.5–4.5 mg/d PO, initial 0.375 mg/d in 3 ÷ doses; titrate slowly *RLS:* 0.125–0.5 mg PO 2–3 h before bedtime *Mirapex ER:* Start 0.375 PO qd, ↑ dose every 5–7 d to 0.75, then by 0.75 mg to max 4.5 mg/d **W/P:** [C, ?/–] Daytime falling asleep; ↓ BP **CI:** Ø **Disp:** *Mirapex:* Tabs 0.125, 0.25, 0.5, 0.75, 1, 1.5 mg; *Mirapex ER:* 0.375, 0.75, 1.5, 2.25, 3, 3.75, 4.5 mg **SE:** Somnolence, N, constipation, dizziness, fatigue, hallucinations, dry mouth, muscle spasms, edema

Pramoxine (Anusol Ointment, Proctofoam NS, Others) Uses: *Relief of pain & itching from hemorrhoids, anorectal surgery*; topical for burns & dermatosis **Acts:** Topical anesthetic **Dose:** Apply freely to anal area 3–5×/d **W/P:** [C, ?] **Disp:** [OTC] All 1%; foam (*Proctofoam NS*), cream, oint, lotion, gel, pads, spray **SE:** Contact dermatitis, mucosal thinning w/ chronic use

Pramoxine/Hydrocortisone (Proctofoam-HC) Uses: *Relief of pain & itching from hemorrhoids* **Acts:** Topical anesthetic, anti-inflam **Dose:** Apply freely to anal area tid-qid **W/P:** [C, ?/–] **Disp:** *Cream:* pramoxine 1% acetate 1/2.5/2.35%; *foam:* pramoxine 1% hydrocortisone 1%; *lotion:* pramoxine 1% hydrocortisone 1/2.5%; ointment pramoxine 1% & hydrocortisone 1/2.5% **SE:** Contact dermatitis, mucosal thinning w/ chronic use

Prasugrel (Effient) **BOX:** Can cause sig, sometimes fatal, bleeding; do not use w/ planned CABG, w/ active bleeding, Hx TIA or stroke or pts > 75 y Uses: *↓ Thrombotic CV events (eg, stent thrombosis) post-PCI*, administer ASAP in ECC setting w/ high-risk ST depression or T-wave inversion w/ planned PCI **Acts:** ↓ Plt aggregation **Dose:** 10 mg/d; Wt < 60 kg, consider 5 mg/d; 60 mg PO loading dose in ECC; use at least 12 mo w/ cardiac stent (bare or drug eluting); consider > 15 mo w/ drug-eluting stent **W/P:** [B, ?] Active bleeding; ↑ bleed risk; w/ CYP3A4 substrates **CI:** Active bleeding, Hx TIA/stroke risk factors: ≥ 75 y, propensity to bleed, Wt < 60 kg, CABG, meds that ↑ bleeding **Disp:** Tabs 5, 10 mg **SE:** ↑ Bleeding time, ↑ BP, GI intolerance, HA, dizziness, rash, ↓ WBC **Notes:** Plt aggregation to baseline ~ 7 d after D/C, plt transfusion reverses acutely

Pravastatin (Pravachol, Generic) Uses: *↓ Cholesterol* Acts: HMG-CoA reductase inhib Dose: 10–80 mg PO hs; ↓ in sig renal/hepatic impair W/P: [X, –] w/ Gemfibrozil CI: Liver Dz or persistent LFTs ↑ Disp: Tabs 10, 20, 40, 80 mg SE: Use caution w/ concurrent gemfibrozil; HA, GI upset, hep, myopathy, renal failure Notes: OK w/ grapefruit juice

Prazosin (Minipress, Generic) Uses: *HTN*, BPH Acts: Peripherally acting α-adrenergic blocker Dose: *Adults.* 1 mg PO tid; can ↑ to 20 mg/d max PRN. *Peds.* 0.05–0.1 mg/kg/d in 3 ÷ doses; max 0.5 mg/kg/d W/P: [C, ?] Use w/ PDE5 inhib (eg, sildenafil) can cause ↓ BP CI: Component allergy, concurrent use of PDE5 inhib Disp: Caps 1, 2, 5 mg; tabs ER 2.5, 5 mg SE: Dizziness, edema, palpitations, fatigue, GI upset, IFIS Notes: Can cause orthostatic ↓ BP, take the 1st dose hs; tolerance develops to this effect; tachyphylaxis may result

Prednisolone (Flo-Pred, Omnipred, Orapred, Pediapred, Generic) (See Steroids, p 287 & Table 2, p 335)

Prednisone (Generic)(See Steroids, p 287 & Table 2, p 335)

Pregabalin (Lyrica, Generic) Uses: *DM neuropathy peripheral pain; postherpetic neuralgia; fibromyalgia; adjunct w/ adult partial onset Szs* Acts: Nerve transmission modulator, antinociceptive, antiseizure effect; mechanism ?; related to gabapentin Dose: *Neuropathic pain:* 50 mg PO tid, ↑ to 300 mg/d w/in 1 wk based on response, 300 mg/d max *Postherpetic neuralgia:* 75–150 mg tid or 50–100 mg tid; start 75 mg bid or 50 mg tid; ↑ to 300 mg/d w/in 1 wk PRN; if pain persists after 2–4 wk, ↑ to 600 mg/d *Partial onset Sz:* Start 150 mg/d (75 mg bid or 50 mg tid); may ↑ to max 600 mg/d ↓ w/ CrCl < 60; w/ or w/o food W/P: [C, –] w/ Sig renal impair (see PI), w/ elderly & severe CHF avoid abrupt D/C CI: Hypersens Disp: Caps 25, 50, 75, 100, 150, 200, 225, 300 mg; soln 20 mg/mL SE: Dizziness, drowsiness, xerostomia, edema, blurred vision, Wt gain, difficulty concentrating; suicidal ideation Notes: w/ D/C, taper over at least 1 wk

Probenecid (Probalan, Generic) Uses: *Px gout & hyperuricemia; extends levels of PCNs & cephalosporins* Acts: Uricosuric, renal tubular blocker of weak organic anions Dose: *Adults. Gout:* 250 mg bid × 1 wk, then 500 mg PO bid; can ↑ by 500 mg/mo up to 2–3 g/d *Antibiotic effect:* 1–2 g PO 30 min before dose *Peds > 2 y.* 25 mg/kg, then 40 mg/kg/d PO qid W/P: [B, ?] CI: Uric acid kidney stones, initiations during accute gout attack, coadministration of salicylates, age < 2 y, MDD, renal impair Disp: Tabs 500 mg SE: HA, GI upset, rash, pruritus, dizziness, blood dyscrasias

Procainamide (Generic) BOX: Positive ANA titer or SLE w/ prolonged use; only use in life-threatening arrhythmias; hematologic tox can be severe, follow low CBC Uses: *Supraventricular/ventricular arrhythmias* Acts: Class 1a antiarrhythmic (Table 9, p 355) Dose: *Adults. Recurrent VF/VT:* 20–50 mg/min IV (total 17 mg/kg max) *Maint:* 1–4 mg/min *Stable wide-complex tachycardia of unknown origin, AF w/ rapid rate in WPW:* 20 mg/min IV until arrhythmia suppression, ↓ BP, or QRS widens > 50%, then 1–4 mg/min *Recurrent VF/VT:*

20–50 mg/min IV; max total 17 mg/kg *ECC 2010*. Stable monomorphic VT, refractory reentry SVT, stable wide-complex tachycardia, AF w/ WPW: 20 mg/min IV until one of these: arrhythmia stopped, hypotension, QRS widens > 50%, total 17 mg/kg; then maint Inf of 1–4 mg/min *Peds. ECC 2010*. SVT, atrial flutter, VT (w/ pulses): 15 mg/kg IV/IO over 30–60 min **W/P:** [C, +] ↓ In renal/hepatic impair **CI:** Complete heart block, 2nd-/3rd-degree heart block w/o pacemaker, torsades de pointes, SLE **Disp:** Inj 100, 500 mg/mL **SE:** ↓ BP, lupus-like synd, GI upset, taste perversion, arrhythmias, tachycardia, heart block, angioneurotic edema, blood dyscrasias **Notes:** Levels: *Trough:* Just before next dose. *Therapeutic:* 4–10 mcg/mL; NAPA + procaine 10–30 mcg/mL; *Toxic* (procainamide only): > 10 mcg/mL; NAPA + procaine > 30 mcg/mL; *half-life:* procaine 3–5 h, NAPA 6–10 h

Procarbazine (Matulane)   BOX: Highly tox; handle w/ care; should be administard under the supervision of an experienced CA chemotherapy physician **Uses:** *Hodgkin Dz*, NHL, brain & lung tumors **Acts:** Alkylating agent; ↓ DNA & RNA synth **Dose:** Per protocol **W/P:** [D, ?] w/ EtOH ingestion **CI:** Inadequate BM reserve **Disp:** Caps 50 mg **SE:** ↓ BM, hemolytic Rxns (w/ G6PD deficiency), N/V/D; disulfiram-like Rxn; cutaneous & constitutional Sxs, myalgia, arthralgia, CNS effects, azoospermia, urination retention

Prochlorperazine (Compro, Procomp, Generic)   BOX: ↑ Mortality in elderly pts w/ dementia-related psychosis **Uses:** *N/V, agitation, & psychotic disorders* **Acts:** Phenothiazine; blocks postsynaptic dopaminergic CNS receptors **Dose:** *Adults. Antiemetic:* 5–10 mg PO tid-qid or 25 mg PR bid or 5–10 mg deep IM q4–6h *Antipsychotic:* 10–20 mg IM acutely or 5–10 mg PO tid-qid for maint; ↑ doses may be required for antipsychotic effect *Peds.* 0.1–0.15 mg/kg/dose IM q4–6h or 0.4 mg/kg/24 h PO/PR ÷ tid-qid **W/P:** [C, +/–] NAG, severe liver/cardiac Dz **CI:** Phenothiazine sensitivity, BM suppression; age < 2 y or Wt < 9 kg **Disp:** Tabs 5, 10 mg; syrup 5 mg/5 mL; supp 25 mg; Inj 5 mg/mL **SE:** EPS common; Rx w/ diphenhydramine or benztropine

Promethazine (Promethegan, Generic)   BOX: Do not use in pts < 2 y; resp depression risk; tissue damage, including gangrene w/ extravasation **Uses:** *N/V, motion sickness, adjunct to postop analgesics, sedation, rhinitis* **Acts:** Phenothiazine; blocks CNS dopaminergic mesolimbic dopaminergic receptors **Dose:** *Adults.* 12.5–50 mg PO, PR, or IM bid-qid PRN *Peds > 2 y.* 0.1–0.5 mg/kg/dose PO or IM 4–6h PRN **W/P:** [C, +/–] Use w/ agents w/ resp depressant effects **CI:** Component allergy, NAG, age < 2 y **Disp:** Tabs 12.5, 25, 50 mg; syrup 6.25 mg/5 mL; supp 12.5, 25, 50 mg; Inj 25, 50 mg/mL **SE:** Drowsiness, tardive dyskinesia, EPS, lowered Sz threshold, ↓ BP, GI upset, blood dyscrasias, photosens, resp depression in children **Notes:** IM/PO preferred route; not SQ or intra-arterial

Propafenone (Rythmol, Rythmol SR, Generic)   BOX: Excess mortality or nonfatal cardiac arrest rate possible; avoid use w/ asymptomatic and symptomatic non–life-threatening ventricular arrhythmias **Uses:** *Life-threatening ventricular arrhythmias, AF* **Acts:** Class Ic antiarrhythmic (Table 9, p 355) **Dose:** *Adults.* 150–300 mg PO q8h *Peds.* 8–10 mg/kg/d ÷ in 3–4 doses; may ↑ 2 mg/kg/d, 20 mg/kg/d max **W/P:** [C, ?] w/ Ritonavir, MI w/in 2 y, w/ liver/renal impair, safety in peds not established **CI:** Uncontrolled CHF, bronchospasm, cardiogenic shock, AV block w/o pacer **Disp:** Tabs 150, 225, 300 mg; SR caps 225, 325, 425 mg **SE:** Dizziness, unusual taste, 1st-degree heart block, arrhythmias, prolongs QRS & QT intervals; fatigue, GI upset, blood dyscrasias

Propantheline (Pro-Banthine, Generic) **Uses:** *PUD*, symptomatic Rx of small intestine hypermotility, spastic colon, ureteral spasm, bladder spasm, pyloro-spasm **Acts:** Antimuscarinic **Dose:** *Adults.* 15 mg PO ac & 30 mg PO hs; ↓ in elderly *Peds.* 2–3 mg/kg/24 h PO ÷ tid-qid **W/P:** [C, ?] **CI:** NAG, UC, toxic megacolon, GI atony in elderly, MG, GI/GU obst **Disp:** 15 mg **SE:** Anticholinergic (eg, xerostomia, blurred vision)

Propofol (Diprivan, Generic) **Uses:** *Induction & maint of anesthesia; sedation in intubated pts* **Acts:** Sedative–hypnotic; mechanism unknown; acts in 40 s **Dose:** *Adults. Anesthesia:* 2–2.5 mg/kg, then 100–200 mcg/kg/min IV *ICU sedation:* 5 mcg/kg/min IV, ↑ PRN 5–10 mcg/kg/min q5–10 min, 5–50 mcg/kg/min cont Inf *Peds. Anesthesia:* 2.5–3.5 mg/kg induction; then 125–300 mcg/kg/min; ↓ in elderly, debilitated, ASA II/IV pts **W/P:** [B, –] **CI:** If general anesthesia CI, sensitivity to egg, egg products, soybeans, soybean products **Disp:** Inj 10 mg/mL **SE:** May ↑ triglycerides w/ extended dosing; ↓ BP, pain at site, apnea, anaphylaxis **Notes:** 1 mL has 0.1-g fat; monitor during Inf for "propofol Inf synd" (eg, heart failure, rhabdomyolysis, renal failure) mostly peds

Propranolol (Hemangeol, Inderal LA, Innopran XL, Generic) **Uses:** *HTN, angina, MI, hyperthyroidism, essential tremor, hypertrophic subaortic stenosis, pheochromocytoma; Px migraines & atrial arrhythmias*, thyrotoxicosis **Acts:** β-Adrenergic receptor blocker, β₁, β₂; only β-blocker to block conversion of T₄ to T₃ **Dose:** *Adults. Angina:* 80–320 mg/d PO ÷ bid-qid or 80–320 mg/d SR *Arrhythmia:* 10–30 mg/dose PO q6–8h or 1 mg IV slowly, repeat q5min, 5 mg max *HTN:* 40 mg PO bid or 60–80 mg/d SR, weekly to max 640 mg/d *Hypertrophic subaortic stenosis:* 20–40 mg PO tid-qid. *MI:* 180–240 mg PO ÷ tid-qid. *Migraine prophylaxis:* 80 mg/d ÷ tid-qid, ↑ weekly 160–240 mg/d ÷ tid-qid max; wean if no response in 6 wk *Pheochromocytoma:* 30–60 mg/d ÷ tid-qid. *Thyrotoxicosis:* 1–3 mg IV × 1; 10–40 mg PO q6h *Tremor:* 40 mg PO bid, ↑ PRN 320 mg/d max *ECC 2010. SVT:* 0.5–1 mg IV given over 1 min; repeat PRN up to 0.1 mg/kg *Peds. Arrhythmia:* 0.5–1.0 mg/kg/d ÷ tid-qid, ↑ PRN q3–7d to 8 mg/kg max; 0.01–0.1 mg/kg IV over 10 min, 1 mg max infants, 3 mg max children *HTN:* 0.5–1.0 mg/kg ÷ tid-qid, PRN q3–7d to 8 mg/kg max; ↓ in renal impair **W/P:** [C (1st tri, D if 2nd or 3rd tri), +] **CI:** Uncompensated CHF, cardiogenic shock, HR, heart block, PE, severe resp Dz **Disp:** Tabs 10, 20, 40, 80 mg; SR caps 60, 80, 120, 160 mg; oral soln 4, 8, mg/mL; Inj 1 mg/mL **SE:** ↓ HR, ↓ BP, fatigue, GI upset, ED **Notes:** Hemangeol approved for proliferating infantile hemangioma (see PI)

Propylthiouracil (Generic) **BOX:** Severe liver failure reported; use only if pt cannot tolerate methimazole; d/t fetal anomalies w/ methimazole, PTU may be drug of choice in 1st tri **Uses:** *Hyperthyroidism* **Acts:** ↓ Production of T_3 & T_4 & conversion of T_4 to T_3 **Dose:** *Adults.* Initial: 100 mg PO q8h (may need up to 1200 mg/d); after pt euthyroid (6–8 wk), taper dose by 1/2 q4–6wk to maint, 50–150 mg/24 h; can usually D/C in 2–3 y; ↓ in elderly *Peds.* Initial: 5–7 mg/kg/24 h PO + q8h *Maint:* 1/3–2/3 of initial dose **W/P:** [D, –] See PI **CI:** Allergy **Disp:** Tabs 50 mg **SE:** Fever, rash, leukopenia, dizziness, GI upset, taste perversion, SLE-like synd, ↑ LFT, liver failure **Notes:** Monitor pt clinically; report any S/Sx of hepatic dysfunction, ✓ TFT and LFT

Protamine (Generic) **BOX:** Severe ↓ BP, CV collapse, noncardiogenic pulm edema, pulm vasoconstriction, and pulm HTN can occur; risk factors: high dose/ overdose, repeat doses, prior protamine use, current or use of prior protamine-containing product (eg, NPH or protamine zinc insulin, some beta-blockers), fish allergy, prior vasectomy, severe LV dysfunction, abnormal pulm testing; weigh risk/benefit in pts w/ 1 or more risk factors; resuscitation equipment must be available **Uses:** *Reverse heparin effect* **Acts:** Neutralize heparin by forming a stable complex **Dose:** Based on degree of heparin reversal; give IV slowly; 1 mg reverses ~ 100 units of heparin given in the preceding 30 min; 50 mg max **W/P:** [C, ?] Allergy **Disp:** Inj 10 mg/mL **SE:** Follow coagulation markers; anticoagulant effect if given w/o heparin; ↓ BP, ↓ HR, dyspnea, hemorrhage **Notes:** ✓ aPTT ~ 15 min after use to assess response

Prothrombin Complex Concentrate, Human (Kcentra) **BOX:** Risk VKA reversal w/ a TE event, must be weighed against the risk of NOT reversing VKA; this risk is higher in those who have had a prior TE; fatal and nonfatal arterial and venous TEs have occurred; monitor; may not be effective in pts w/ TEs in the prior 3 mo **Uses:** *Urgent reversal of acquired coagulation factor deficiencies caused by VKAs; only for acute major bleeding* **Acts:** Reverse VKA coagulopathy; replaces factor II, VII, IX, X & protein C & S **Dose:** Based on INR and Wt: *INR 2–4:* 25 units/kg, (max 2500 units); *INR 4–6:* 35 units/kg, (max 3500 units); *INR > 6:* 50 unit/kg, (max 5000 units); 100 mg/kg max; give w/ vit K **W/P:** [C, ?] Hypersens Rxn; arterial/venous thrombosis; risk of viral Infxn, including variant CJD **CI:** Anaphylaxis/reactions to heparin, albumin or coagulation factors (protein C & S, antithrombin III); known HIT **DIC Disp:** Single vial; to reconstitute, see PI; separate IV for inf **SE:** TE (stroke, DVT/PE); DIC; ↓ BP, HA, N/V, HA, arthralgia **Notes:** INR should be < 1.3 w/in 30 min; risk of transmitting variant CJD, viral Dz (human blood product), and other Infxn (Hep A, B & C, HIV, etc)

Pseudoephedrine (Many Mono and Combo Brands) [OTC] **Uses:** *Decongestant* **Acts:** Stimulates α-adrenergic receptors w/ vasoconstriction **Dose:** *Adults. IR:* 60 mg PO q4–6h PRN; *ER:* 120 mg PO q12h, 240 mg/d max *Peds 2–5 y.* 15 mg q4–6h, 60 mg/24 h max *6–12 y.* 30 mg q4–6h, 120 mg/24 h max; ↓ w/ renal Insuff **W/P:** [C, +] Not rec for use in peds < 2 y **CI:** Poorly controlled HTN or CAD, w/ MAOIs w/in 14 d, urinary retention **Disp:** IR tabs 30, 60 mg; ER caplets 60, 120 mg; ER tabs 120, 240 mg; liq 15, 30 mg/5 mL; syrup 15, 30 mg/5mL; multiple combo OTC products **SE:** HTN, insomnia, tachycardia, arrhythmias, nervousness, tremor **Notes:** Found in many OTC cough/cold preparations; OTC restricted distribution by state (illicit ingredient in methamphetamine production)

Psyllium (Konsyl, Metamucil, Generic) [OTC] **Uses:** *Constipation & colonic diverticular Dz* **Acts:** Bulk laxative **Dose:** 1.25–30 g/d varies w/ specific product **W/P:** [B, ?] *Effer-Sylium* (effervescent psyllium) usually contains K+, caution w/ renal failure; phenylketonuria (in products w/ aspartame) **CI:** Suspected bowel obst **Disp:** Large variety available: granules; powder, caps, wafers **SE:** D, Abd cramps, bowel obst, constipation, bronchospasm **Notes:** Maintain adequate hydration

Pyrazinamide (Generic) **Uses:** *Active TB in combo w/ other agents* **Acts:** Bacteriostatic; unknown mechanism **Dose:** *Adults.* Dose varies based on Tx option chosen daily 1×2 wk–3 × wk; dosing based on lean body Wt; ↓ dose in renal/hepatic impair **Peds.** 20–40 mg/kg/d PO ÷ qd-bid; ↓ W/ renal/hepatic impair **W/P:** [C, +/–] **CI:** Severe hepatic damage, acute gout **Disp:** Tabs 500 mg **SE:** Hepatotox, malaise, GI upset, arthralgia, myalgia, gout, photosens **Notes:** Use in combo w/ other anti-TB drugs; consult http://www.cdc.gov/tb/ for latest TB recommendations; dosage regimen differs for "directly observed" Rx

Pyridoxine [Vitamin B₆] (Generic) **Uses:** *Rx & Px of vit B₆ deficiency* **Acts:** Vit B₆ supl **Dose:** *Adults. Deficiency:* 10–20 mg/d PO *Drug-induced neuritis:* 100–200 mg/d; 25–100 mg/d prophylaxis **Peds.** 5–25 mg/d × 3 wk **W/P:** [A (C if doses exceed RDA), +] **CI:** Component allergy tabs 25, 50, 100, 250, 500 mg; tabs SR 500 mg; liq 15, 200 mg/mL; caps: 50, 250 mg

Quetiapine (Seroquel, Seroquel XR, Generic) **BOX:** Closely monitor pts for worsening depression or emergence of suicidality, particularly in ped pts; not for use in peds; ↑ mortality in elderly w/ dementia-related psychosis **Uses:** *Acute exacerbations of schizophrenia, bipolar Dz* **Acts:** Serotonin & DA antag **Dose:** 150–750 mg/d; initiate at 25–100 mg bid-tid; slowly ↑ dose; *XR:* 400–800 mg PO q P.M.; start ↑ 300 mg/d, 800 mg/d max; ↓ dose w/ hepatic & geriatric pts **W/P:** [C, –] **CI:** Component allergy **Disp:** Tabs 25, 50, 100, 200, 300, 400 mg; tabs XR: 50, 150, 200, 300, 400 mg **SE:** Confusion w/ nefazodone; HA, somnolence, ↑ Wt, ↓ BP, dizziness, cataracts, neuroleptic malignant synd, tardive dyskinesia, ↑ QT interval

Quinapril (Accupril, Generic) **BOX:** ACE inhib used during PRG can cause fetal injury & death **Uses:** *HTN, CHF, DN, post-MI* **Acts:** ACE inhib **Dose:** 10–80 mg PO qd; ↓ in renal impair **W/P:** [D, +] w/ RAS, vol depletion **CI:** ACE inhib sensitivity, angioedema, PRG **Disp:** Tabs 5, 10, 20, 40 mg **SE:** Dizziness, HA, ↓ BP, impaired renal Fxn, angioedema, taste perversion, cough

Quinidine (Generic) **BOX:** Mortality rates increased when used to treat non–life-threatening arrhythmias **Uses:** *Px of tachydysrhythmias, malaria* **Acts:** Class IA antiarrhythmic **Dose:** *Adults. Antiarrhythmic IR:* 200–400 mg/dose q6h; *ER:*

300 mg q8–12h (sulfate) 324 mg q8–12h (gluconate) **Peds.** 15–60 mg/kg/24 h PO in 4–5 ÷ doses; ↓ in renal impair **W/P:** [C, +] **CI:** TTP, thrombocytopenia, medications that prolong QT interval, digitalis tox & AV block; conduction disorders **Disp:** Sulfate: Tabs 200, 300 mg; SR tabs 300 mg. Gluconate: SR tabs 324 mg; Inj 80 mg/mL **SE:** Extreme ↓ BP w/ IV use; syncope, QT prolongation, GI upset, arrhythmias, fatigue, cinchonism (tinnitus, hearing loss, delirium, visual changes), fever, hemolytic anemia, thrombocytopenia, rash **Notes:** Levels: Trough: just before next dose. Therapeutic: 2–5 mcg/mL, some pts require higher levels; Toxic: > 10 mcg/mL; half-life: 6–8h; sulfate salt 83% quinidine; gluconate salt 62% quinidine; use w/ drug that slows AV conduction (eg, digoxin, diltiazem, β-blocker) 267 mg of quinidine gluconate = 200 mg of quinidine sulfate

Quinupristin/Dalfopristin (Synercid)   **Uses:** *Vancomycin-resistant Infxns d/t E. faecium & other gram(+)* **Acts:** ↓ Ribosomal protein synth. **Spectrum:** Vancomycin-resistant E. faecium, methicillin-susceptible S. aureus, S. pyogenes; not against E. faecalis **Dose: Adults & Peds.** 7.5 mg/kg IV q12h (central line preferred); incompatible w/ NS or heparin; flush IV w/ dextrose; ↓ w/ hepatic failure **W/P:** [B, M] Multiple drug interactions w/ drugs metabolized by CYP3A4 (eg, cyclosporine) **CI:** Component allergy **Disp:** Inj 500 mg (150 mg quinupristin/350 mg dalfopristin) **SE:** Hyperbilirubinemia, Inf site Rxns & pain, arthralgia, myalgia

Rabeprazole (AcipHex, Generic)   **Uses:** *PUD, GERD, ZE* H. pylori **Acts:** PPI **Dose:** 20 mg/d; may ↑ to 60 mg/d; H. pylori 20 mg PO bid × 7 d (w/ amoxicillin and clarithromycin); do not crush/chew tabs; do not use clopidogrel **W/P:** [B, ?/–] Do not use w/ clopidogrel, possible ↓ effect (controversial) **Disp:** Tabs 20 mg ER **SE:** HA, fatigue, GI upset **Notes:** ? ↑ Risk of fractures, C. difficile, CAP w/ all PPI; risk of hypomagnesemia w/ long-term use, monitor

Radium-223 Dichloride (Xofigo)   **Uses:** *CRPC w/ symptomatic bone mets w/o visceral Dz* **Acts:** Alpha-emitter, complexes in bone w/ ↑ turnover **Dose:** 50 kBq/kg IV q4wk × 6 doses; slow IV over 1 min **W/P:** [X, –] NOT for women; ↓ WBC, ✓ CBC before/during each Tx dose, D/C if no CBC recovery 6–8 wk post-Tx **CI:** PRG **Disp:** Single vial 1000 kBq/mL or 6000 kBq/vial **SE:** ↓ CBC; N/V/D, edema **Notes:** Follow radiation safety/pharma quality control requirements; use condoms during & 6 mos post-Tx and female partners should use 1 additional BC method

Raloxifene (Evista)   **BOX:** Increased risk of VTE and death from stroke **Uses:** *Px osteoporosis, breast CA* **Acts:** SERM **Dose:** 60 mg/d **W/P:** [X, –] **CI:** Thromboembolism, PRG **Disp:** Tabs 60 mg **SE:** CP, insomnia, rash, hot flashes, GI upset, hepatic dysfunction, leg cramps

Raltegravir (Isentress)   **Uses:** *HIV in combo w/ other antiretroviral agents* **Acts:** HIV-integrase strand transfer inhib **Dose:** 400 mg PO bid, 800 mg PO bid if w/ rifampin; w/ or w/o food **W/P:** [C, –] **CI:** Ø **Disp:** Tabs 400 mg; chew tabs 25, 100 mg; 100 mg single-use oral susp **SE:** Development of immune reconstitution synd: ↑ CK, myopathy, and rhabdomyolysis, insomnia, N/D, HA, fever, ↑ cholesterol, paranoia, and anxiety **Notes:** Monitor lipid profile; initial therapy may cause immune reconstitution synd (inflam response to residual opportunistic Infxns (eg, *M. avium, Pneumocystis jiroveci*)

Ramelteon (Rozerem) Uses: *Insomnia* **Acts:** Melatonin receptor agonist **Dose:** 8 mg PO 30 min before bedtime **W/P:** [C, ?/–] w/ CYP1A2 inhib **CI:** w/ Fluvoxamine; hypersens **Disp:** Tabs 8 mg **SE:** Somnolence, dizziness **Notes:** Avoid w/ high-fat meal, do not break

Ramipril (Altace, Generic) **BOX:** ACE inhib used during PRG can cause fetal injury & death **Uses:** *HTN, CHF, DN, post-MI* **Acts:** ACE inhib **Dose:** 1.25–20 mg/d PO ÷ qd-bid; ↓ in renal failure **W/P:** [C-1st tri/D-2nd & 3rd, +] **CI:** ACE inhib-induced angioedema **Disp:** Caps 1.25, 2.5, 5, 10 mg **SE:** Cough, HA, dizziness, ↓ BP, renal impair, angioedema **Notes:** OK in combo w/ diuretics

Ramucirumab (Cyramza) **BOX:** Risk of hemorrhage, D/C if severe bleeding; GI hemorrhage/perf; ↓ wound healing, D/C prior to surgery **Uses:** *Advanced gastric or GE junction adenocarcinoma w/ Dz progression after fluoropyrimidine or platinum chemo; w/ docetaxel for met NSCLC w/ Dz progression on or after platinum chemo; combo w/ FOLFIRI for met colorectal Ca w/ Dz progression on or after Tx w/ bevacizumab, oxaliplatin,& fluoropyrimidine* **Acts:** VEGF receptor 2 antag **Dose:** *Gastric Ca:* 8 mg/kg IV q2wk single agent or w/ paclitaxel; *NSCLC:* 10 mg/kg IV d 1 of 21-d cycle of docetaxel; *Colorectal Ca:* 8 mg/kg IV q2wk prior to FOLFIRI **W/P:** [X, –] Arterial TE; ↑ BP; Inf Rxn; ↓ wound healing; worsening w/ cirrhosis; posterior leukoencephalopathy; proteinuria/nephrotic synd; embryo-fetal tox; thyroid dysfunction **Disp:** Single-dose vial 100 mg/10 mL, 500 mg/50 mL **SE:** D, ↑ BP; w/ paclitaxel: D, ↓ WBC, fatigue, epistaxis; w/ docetaxel: stomatitis, fatigue, asthenia; w/ FOLFIRI: D, ↓ WBC, stomatitis, anorexia, epistaxis **Notes:** monitor BP; ✓ proteinuria, hold w/ urine protein > 2 g/24 h, D/C if > 3 g/24 h

Ranibizumab (Lucentis) Uses: *Neovascular "wet" macular degeneration* **Acts:** VEGF inhib **Dose:** 0.5 mg intravitreal Inj qmo **W/P:** [C, ?] Hx thromboembolism **CI:** Periocular Infxn **Disp:** Inj 10 mg/mL **SE:** Endophthalmitis, retinal detachment/hemorrhage, cataract, intraocular inflam, conjunctival hemorrhage, eye pain, floaters

Ranitidine (Zantac, Zantac EFFERDose [OTC], Generic) Uses: *Duodenal ulcer, active benign ulcers, hypersecretory conditions, & GERD* **Acts:** H₂-receptor antag **Dose:** *Adults.* Ulcer: 150 mg PO bid, 300 mg PO hs, or 50 mg IV q6–8h; or 400 mg IV/d cont Inf, then maint of 150 mg PO hs *Hypersecretion:* 150 mg PO bid, up to 600 mg/d *GERD:* 300 mg PO bid; maint 300 mg PO hs *Dyspepsia:* 75 mg PO qd-bid *Peds.* 1.5–2 mg/kg/dose IV q6–8h or 2 mg/kg/dose PO q12h; ↓ in renal Insuff/failure **W/P:** [B, +] Sedation risk w/ midazolam **CI:** Component allergy **Disp:** Tabs 75, 150 mg [OTC], 150, 300 mg; caps 150, 300 mg; effervescent tabs 25 mg (contains phenylalanine); syrup 15 mg/mL; Inj 25 mg/mL **SE:** Dizziness, sedation, rash, GI upset **Notes:** PO & parenteral doses differ

Ranolazine (Ranexa) Uses: *Chronic angina* Acts: ↓ Ischemia-related Na⁺ entry into myocardium Dose: 500 mg bid–1000 mg PO bid CI: w/ Cirrhosis, CYP3A inhib/inducers (Table 10, p 356) W/P: [C, ?/–] HTN may develop w/ renal impair, agents that ↑ QTc, ↓ K⁺ Disp: SR tabs 500, 1000 mg SE: Dizziness, HA, constipation, arrhythmias Notes: Not 1st line; use w/ amlodipine, nitrates, or β-blockers

Rapivab (Peramivir) Uses: *Influenza in ≥ 18 y w/ Sxs ≤ 2 d* Acts: ↓ Influenza virus neuraminidase enzyme Dose: *Adults/Geriatric.* 600 mg IV × 1 over 15–30 min W/P: Rare serious skin Rxns; hypersens Rxns; neuropsych events in pts w/ encephalitis; serious bacterial Infxn may begin w/ influenza-like Sxs CI: Ø Disp: Single-use vial 200 mg/20 mL (20 mL) SE: ↑ BP, insomnia, ↑ glu, D, constipation, ↓ WBC, ↑ ALT/AST/CPK Notes: CrCl 30–49 mL/min: 200 mg × 1; CrCl 10–29 mL/min: 100 mg × 1; ESRD: 100 mg after dialysis

Rasagiline Mesylate (Azilect) Uses: *Early Parkinson Dz monotherapy; levodopa adjunct w/ advanced Dz, including levodopa and DA agonists* Acts: MAO B inhib Dose: *Early Dz:* 1 mg PO qd, start 0.5 mg PO qd w/ levodopa; ↓ w/ CYP1A2 inhib or hepatic impair CI: MAOIs, sympathomimetic amines, meperidine, methadone, tramadol, propoxyphene, dextromethorphan, mirtazapine, cyclobenzaprine, St. John's wort, sympathomimetic vasoconstrictors, SSRIs W/P: [C, ?] Avoid tyramine-containing foods; mod–severe hepatic impair Disp: Tabs 0.5, 1 mg SE: Arthralgia, indigestion, dyskinesia, hallucinations, ↓ N/V, postural ↓ BP, N/V, constipation, xerostomia, rash, sedation, CV conduction disturbances Notes: Rare melanoma reported; periodic skin exams (skin CA risk); D/C 14 d prior to elective surgery; initial ↓ levodopa dose OK

Rasburicase (Elitek) BOX: Anaphylaxis possible; do not use in G6PD deficiency and hemolysis; can cause methemoglobinemia; can interfere w/ uric acid assays; collect blood samples and store on ice Uses: *Reduce ↑ uric acid d/t tumor lysis* Acts: Catalyzes uric acid Dose: *Adult & Peds.* 0.20 mg/kg IV over 30 min, qd × 5; do not bolus, redosing based on uric acid levels W/P: [C, ?/–] Falsely ↓ uric acid values CI: Anaphylaxis, screen for G6PD deficiency to avoid hemolysis, methemoglobinemia Disp: 1.5, 7.5 mg Powder for Inj SE: Fever, neutropenia, GI upset, HA, rash Notes: Place blood test tube for uric acid level on ice to stop enzymatic Rxn; removed by dialysis; doses as low as 0.05 mg/kg have been used effectively in clinical trials

Regorafenib (Stivarga) BOX: May cause severe/fatal hepatotox; monitor LFTs & dose adjust or D/C for ↑ LFTs or hepatocellular necrosis Uses: *Metastatic colorectal CA & GIST (see PI/institution protocol)* Acts: Kinase inhib Dose: 160 mg PO q A.M. on d 1–21 of 28-d cycle; w/ low-fat food, swallow whole; see PI for tox dose adjust W/P: [D, –] Fetal tox; avoid w/ strong CYP3A4 inhib/inducers CI: Ø Disp: Tabs 40 mg SE: Fatigue, asthenia, N/V/D, Abd pain, ↓ appetite, ↓ Wt, HTN, HFSR, mucositis, dysphonia, Infxn, pain, rash, fever, hemorrhage, wound healing complications, RPLS, cardiac ischemia/infarction, derm tox, GI perforation/fistula

Repaglinide (Prandin) **Uses:** *Type 2 DM* **Acts:** ↑ Pancreatic insulin release **Dose:** No fixed dosage; range 0.5–4 mg w/ each meal; adjust weekly PRN; w/o previous Rx or w/ HbA1c < 8%, 0.5 mg ac each meal; w/ previous Rx & w/ HbA1c > 8%, 1–2 mg PO ac; max 16 mg/d; can be used in combo w/ metformin or other agents **W/P:** [C, ?/–] **CI:** DKA, type 1 DM **Disp:** Tabs 0.5, 1, 2 mg **SE:** HA, hyper-/hypoglycemia, GI upset

Repaglinide/Metformin (PrandiMet) **BOX:** Associated w/ lactic acidosis, risk ↑ w/ sepsis, dehydration, renal/hepatic impair, ↑ alcohol, acute CHF; Sxs include myalgias, malaise, resp distress, Abd pain, somnolence; Labs: ↓ pH, ↑ anion gap, ↑ blood lactate; D/C immediately & hospitalize if suspected **Uses:** *Type 2 DM* **Acts:** Meglitinide & biguanide (see Metformin) **Dose:** 1/500 mg bid w/in 15 min pc (skip dose w/ skipped meal); max 10/2500 mg/d or 4/1000 mg/meal **W/P:** [C, –] Suspend use w/ iodinated contrast, do not use w/ NPH insulin, use w/ cationic drugs & CYP2C8 & CYP3A4 inhib **CI:** SCr > 1.4 mg/dL (females) or > 1.5 mg/dL (males); metabolic acidosis; w/ gemfibrozil **Disp:** Tabs (repaglinide mg/metformin mg) 1/500, 2/500 **SE:** Hypoglycemia, HA, N/V/D, anorexia, weakness, myalgia, rash, ↓ vit B₁₂

Retapamulin (Altabax) **Uses:** *Topical Rx impetigo in pts > 9 mo* **Acts:** Pleuromutilin Abx, bacteriostatic, ↓ bacteria protein synth; *Spectrum:* S. aureus (not MRSA), S. pyogenes **Dose:** Apply bid × 5 d **W/P:** [B, ?] **Disp:** 1% ointment **SE:** Local irritation **Notes:** Rx should not exceed 2% BSA in peds or 100 cm² BSA in adults

Reteplase (Retavase) **Uses:** *Post-AMI* **Acts:** Thrombolytic **Dose:** 10 units IV over 2 min, 2nd dose in 30 min, 10 units IV over 2 min; *ECC 2010.* 10 units IV bolus over 2 min; 30 min later, 10 units IV bolus over 2 min w/ NS flush before and after each dose **W/P:** [C, ?/–] **CI:** Internal bleeding, spinal surgery/trauma, Hx CNS AVM/CVA, bleeding diathesis, severe uncontrolled ↑ BP, sensitivity to thrombolytics **Disp:** Kit form w/10.4 units (18.1 mg) for one or two doses **SE:** Bleeding including CNS, allergic Rxns

Ribavirin (Copegus, Moderiba, Generic) **BOX:** Monotherapy for chronic hep C ineffective; hemolytic anemia possible, teratogenic and embryocidal; use 2 forms of birth control for up to 6 mo after D/C drug; decrease in resp Fxn when used in infants as Inh **Uses:** *RSV Infxn in infants [Virazole]; hep C (in combo w/ peg-interferon α-2b)* **Acts:** ↓ replication of RNA & DNA viruses **Dose:** *RSV:* 6 g in 300 mL sterile H₂O, Inh 18 h in *Hep C:* See individual PI for dosing based on Wt & genotype **W/P:** [X, ?] May accumulate on soft contacts lenses **CI:** PRG, autoimmune hep, CrCl < 50 mL/min **Disp:** Powder for aerosol 6 g; tabs 200, 400, 600 mg; caps 200 mg; soln 40 mg/mL **SE:** Fatigue, HA, GI upset, anemia, myalgia, alopecia, bronchospasm, ↓ HCT; pancytopenia reported **Notes:** Virazole aerosolized by a SPAG, monitor resp Fxn closely; ✓ Hgb/Hct; PRG test monthly; 2 forms birth control, hep C viral genotyping may modify dose

Rifabutin (Mycobutin) **Uses:** *Px MAC Infxn in AIDS pts w/ CD4 count < 100 mcL* **Acts:** ↓ DNA-dependent RNA polymerase activity **Dose:** *Adults.*

150–300 mg/d PO. *Peds ≤ 1 y.* 15–25 mg/kg/d PO *Others:* 5 mg/kg/d, max 800 mg/d **W/P:** [B, ?/−] WBC < 1000 cells/mm³ or plts < 50,000 cells/mm³; ritonavir **CI:** Allergy **Disp:** Caps 150 mg **SE:** Discolored urine, rash, neutropenia, leukopenia, myalgia, ↑ LFTs **Notes:** SE/interactions similar to rifampin

Rifampin (Rifadin, Rimactane, Generic) **Uses:** *TB & Rx & prophylaxis of *N. meningitidis*, *H. influenzae*, or *S. aureus* carriers*; adjunct w/ severe *S. aureus* **Acts:** ↓ DNA-dependent RNA polymerase **Dose:** *Adults.* *N. meningitidis & H. influenzae carrier:* 600 mg/d PO for 4 d *TB:* 600 mg PO or IV qd or 2×/wk w/ combo regimen *Peds.* 10–20 mg/kg/dose PO or IV qd-bid; ↓ in hepatic failure **W/P:** [C, +] w/ Fosamprenavir, multiple drug interactions **CI:** Allergy, active *N. meningitidis* Infxn w/ saquinavir/ritonavir **Disp:** Caps 150, 300 mg; Inj 600 mg **SE:** Red-orange–colored bodily fluids, ↑ LFTs, flushing, HA **Notes:** Never use as single agent w/ active TB

Rifapentine (Priftin) **Uses:** *Pulm TB (active & latent)* **Acts:** ↓ DNA-dependent RNA polymerase. *Spectrum: Mycobacterium tuberculosis* **Dose:** *Intensive phase:* 600 mg PO 2×/wk for 2 mo; separate doses by > 3 d *Continuation phase:* 600 mg/wk for 4 mo; part of 3–4-drug regimen **W/P:** [C, +/− red-orange breast milk] Strong CYP450 inducer, ↓ protease inhib efficacy, antiepileptics, β-blockers, CCBs **CI:** Rifamycins allergy **Disp:** Tabs 150 mg **SE:** Neutropenia, hyperuricemia, HTN, HA, dizziness, rash, GI upset, blood dyscrasias, ↑ LFTs, hematuria, discolored secretions **Notes:** Monitor LFTs

Rifaximin (Xifaxan) **Uses:** *Traveler's D (noninvasive strains of *E. coli* in pts > 12 y (*Xifaxan*); hepatic encephalopathy (*Xifaxan 550*) > 18 y* **Acts:** Not absorbed, derivative of rifamycin. *Spectrum: E. coli* **Dose:** D (*Xifaxan*): 1 tab PO, tid × 3 d; encephalopathy (*Xifaxan 550*) > 550 mg PO bid **W/P:** [C, ?/−] Hx allergy; pseudomembranous colitis; w/ severe (Child-Pugh C) hepatic impair **CI:** Allergy to rifamycins **Disp:** Tabs: *Xifaxan:* 200 mg; *Xifaxan 550:* 550 mg **SE:** *Xifaxan:* Flatulence, HA, Abd pain, fecal tenesmus and urgency, N; *Xifaxan 550:* Edema, N, dizziness, fatigue, ascites, flatulence, HA **Notes:** D/C if D Sx worsen or persist > 24–48 h, or w/ fever or blood in stool

Rilpivirine (Edurant) **Uses:** *HIV in combo w/ other antiretroviral agents* **Acts:** NRTI **Dose:** *Adults.* 25 mg qd **W/P:** [B, −] **CI:** Ø **Disp:** Tabs 25 mg **SE:** HA, depression, insomnia, rash, ↑ AST/ALT, ↑ cholesterol, ↑ SCr **Notes:** Take w/ food; metabolized via CYP3A; CYP3A inducers may ↓ virologic response, CYP3A inhib may ↑ levels; ↑ gastric pH ↓ absorption

Rimantadine (Flumadine, Generic) **Uses:** *Prophylaxis & Rx of influenza A viral Infxns* **Acts:** Antiviral **Dose:** *Adults & Peds > 9 y.* 100 mg PO bid *Peds 1–9 y.* 5 mg/kg/d PO, 150 mg/d max; daily w/ severe renal/hepatic impair & elderly; initiate w/in 48 h of Sx onset **W/P:** [C, −] w/ Cimetidine; avoid w/ PRG, breast-feeding **CI:** Component & amantadine allergy **Disp:** Tabs 100 mg **SE:** Orthostatic ↓ BP, edema, dizziness, GI upset, ↓ Sz threshold **Notes:** See CDC (*MMWR*) for current influenza A guidelines

Rimexolone (Vexol Ophthalmic) Uses: *Postop inflam & uveitis* **Acts:** Steroid **Dose:** *Adults & Peds > 2 y. Uveitis:* 1–2 gtt/h daytime & q2h at night, taper to 1 gtt q6h *Postop:* 1–2 gtt qid × 2 wk **W/P:** [C, ?/–] Ocular Infxns **Disp:** Susp 1% **SE:** Blurred vision, local irritation **Notes:** Taper dose

Riociguat (Adempas) BOX: Do not administer if PRG; R/O PRG before, monthly during and 1 mo after Tx; Px PRG with appropriate birth control during and 1 mo post-Tx for females only; available through a restricted program Uses: *Persistent pulm HTN due to chronic thromboembolic Dz; adults w/ pulm HTN* **Acts:** Guanylate cyclase stimulator; guanylate cyclase NO receptor, leads to ↑ cGMP **Dose:** 1 mg PO tid; start 0.5 mg tid if ↓ BP a concern; ↑ 0.5 mg/dose q 2wk PRN; 2.5 mg tid max **W/P:** [X, –] ↓ BP, pulm edema w/ pulm veno-occlusive Dz, D/C if confirmed; bleeding **CI:** PRG; use of nitrates or nitric oxide; use of PDE **Disp:** Tabs 0.5, 1, 1.5, 2, 2.5 mg **SE:** N/V/D, GERD, constipation, gastritis; HA, dizziness; anemia **Notes:** Start w/ CYP and P-gp/BCRP inhib; do not take w/ antacids, separate by 1 h; not rec w/ severe liver or kidney Dz; may need ↑ dose in smokers; may need to ↓ dose if quit smoking

Risedronate (Actonel, Actonel w/ Calcium, Generic) Uses: *Paget Dz; Rx/Px glucocorticoid-induced/postmenopausal osteoporosis, ↑ bone mass in osteoporotic men; w/ Ca only FDA approved for female osteoporosis* **Acts:** Bisphosphonate; ↓ osteoclast-mediated bone resorption **Dose:** *Paget Dz:* 30 mg/d PO for 2 mo *Osteoporosis Rx/Px:* 5 mg qd or 35 mg qwk or 150 mg qmo; 30 min before 1st food/drink of the d; stay upright for at least 30 min after dose **W/P:** [C, ?/–] Ca²⁺ supls & antacids ↓ absorption; ONJ, avoid dental work **CI:** Component allergy, ↓ Ca²⁺, esophageal abnormalities, unable to stand/sit for 30 min, CrCl < 30 mL/min **Disp:** Tabs 5, 30, 35, 150 mg; Risedronate 35 mg (4 tabs)/Ca carbonate 1250 mg (24 tabs) **SE:** Back pain, HA, Abd pain, dyspepsia, arthralgia; flu-like Sxs, hypersens (rash, etc), esophagitis, bone pain, eye inflam **Notes:** Monitor LFTs, Ca²⁺, PO³⁺, K⁺; may ↑ atypical subtrochanteric femur fractures

Risedronate, Delayed Release (Atelvia) Uses: *Postmenopausal osteoporosis* **Acts:** See Risedronate **Dose:** One 35-mg tab 1 × wk; in A.M. following breakfast w/ 4 oz water; do not lie down for 30 min **W/P:** [C, ?/–] Ca²⁺ & Fe²⁺ supls/antacids ↓ absorption; do not use w/ Actonel or CrCl < 30 mL/min; ONJ reported, avoid dental work; may ↑ subtrochanteric femur fractures; severe bone/jt pain **CI:** Component allergy, ↓ Ca²⁺, esophageal abnormalities, unable to stand/sit for 30 min **Disp:** DR tabs 35 mg **SE:** D, influenza, arthralgia, back/Abd pain; rare hypersens, eye inflam **Notes:** Correct ↓ Ca²⁺ before use; ✓ Ca²⁺

Risperidone, Oral (Risperdal, Risperdal M-Tab, Generic) BOX: ↑ Mortality in elderly w/ dementia-related psychosis Uses: *Psychotic disorders (schizophrenia)*, dementia of the elderly, bipolar disorder, mania, Tourette disorder, autism **Acts:** Benzisoxazole antipsychotic **Dose:** *Adults & Peds.* See PI for Dz-specific dosing, ↓ dose w/ elderly, renal/hepatic impair **W/P:** [C, –], ↑ BP w/ antihypertensives, clozapine **CI:** Component allergy **Disp:** Tabs 0.25, 0.5, 1, 2, 3,

4 mg; soln 1 mg/mL; *M-Tab* (ODT) tabs 0.5, 1, 2, 3, 4 mg **SE:** Orthostatic ↓ BP, EPS w/ high dose, tachycardia, arrhythmias, sedation, dystonias, neuroleptic malignant synd, sexual dysfunction, constipation, xerostomia, ↓ WBC, neutropenia and agranulocytosis, cholestatic jaundice **Notes:** Several weeks for effect

Risperidone, Parenteral (Risperdal Consta) **BOX:** Not approved for dementia-related psychosis; ↑ mortality risk in elderly dementia pts on atypical antipsychotics; most deaths d/t CV or infectious events **Uses:** Schizophrenia **Acts:** Benzisoxazole antipsychotic **Dose:** 25 mg q2wk IM, may ↑ to max 50 mg q2wk; w/ renal/hepatic impair, start PO Risperdal 0.5 mg PO bid × 1 wk, titrate weekly **W/P:** [C, −], ↑ BP w/ antihypertensives, clozapine **CI:** Component allergy **Disp:** Inj 25, 37.5, 50 mg/vial **SE:** See Risperidone, Oral **Notes:** Long-acting Inj; give PO dose w/ initial Inj & continue × 3 wk

Ritonavir (Norvir) **BOX:** Life-threatening adverse events when used w/ certain nonsedating antihistamines, sedative hypnotics, antiarrhythmics, or ergot alkaloids d/t inhibited drug metabolism **Uses:** *HIV* combo w/ other antiretrovirals **Acts:** Protease inhib; ↓ maturation of immature noninfectious virions to mature infectious virus **Dose:** *Adults.* Initial 300 mg PO bid, titrate over 1 wk to 600 mg PO bid (titration will ↓ GI SE) *Peds > 1 mo.* Initiate @ 250 mg/m², titrate by 50 mg/m² q2–3d, goal 350–400 mg/m², max 600 mg bid; adjust w/ fosamprenavir, indinavir, nelfinavir, & saquinavir; take w/ food **W/P:** [B, +] w/ Ergotamine, amiodarone, bepridil, bosentan, colchicine, PDE inhib, flecainide, propafenone, quinidine, pimozide, midazolam, triazolam **CI:** Component allergy **Disp:** Caps & tabs 100 mg; soln 80 mg/mL **SE:** ↑ Triglycerides, ↑ LFTs, N/V/D, constipation, Abd pain, taste perversion, anemia, weakness, HA, fever, malaise, rash, paresthesias **Notes:** Refrigerate

Rituximab (Rituxan) **BOX:** Fatal Inf and mucocutaneous reactions possible; reactivation of hep B/hepatic failure/death and PML possible **Uses:** *NHL, CLL, RA w/ MTX and poor response to TNF antagonists; Wegner's granulomatosis* **Acts:** CD20-directed cytolytic Ab **Dose:** *IV infusion (not push):* NHL: 375 mg/m²; CLL 375 mg/m² first cycle, 500 mg/m² in cycles 2–6; w/ FC, q28d; *w/ Ibritumomab regimen:* 250 mg/m²; RA w/ MTX two 1000-mg Inf separated by 2 wk (one course) q24wk but not less than q16 wk; methylprednisolone 100 mg IV 30 min before **W/P:** [limited data, ?] Tumor lysis synd; Infxn risk; arrhythmias; bowel obst/perf; do not give live virus vaccine; cytopenias; renal tox w/ cisplatin **CI:** Ø **Disp:** Vial 100 mg/10 mL, 500 mg/50 mL **SE:** *Malignancy* Rx: Inf Rxn, fever, ↓ WBC, chills, infection; *RA* Rx: URI, nasopharyngitis, UTI, bronchitis, Inf Rxn, Infxn, CV events

Rivaroxaban (Xarelto) **BOX:** May ↑ risk of spinal/epidural hematoma w/ paralysis & increase risk of stroke w/ premature D/C, monitor closely **Uses:** *↓ Risk of stroke/embolism w/ non-valve AF, Rx DVT/PE & ↓ recurrence risk, Px DVT in knee/hip replacement surgery* **Acts:** Factor Xa inhib **Dose:** *Non-valve AF:* CrCl > 50 mL/min, 20 mg PO qd w/ P.M. meal; w/ CrCl 15–50 mL/min, 15 mg PO qd w/ P.M. meal; *DVT/PE:* 15 mg PO bid w/ food × 21 d, then 20 mg qd long term; *Replacement surgery:* 10 mg PO qd × 35 d (hip) or 12 d (knee), stroke 20 mg qd;

w/ or w/o food **W/P:** [C, –] Bleeding risk, PRG-realted bleeding, not for prosthetic heart valves, avoid w/ CYP3A4 inhib/inducers, other anticoagulants, and plt inhib **CI:** Active bleeding; component hypersens **Disp:** Tabs 10, 15, 20 mg **SE:** Bleeding **Notes:** See PI for dosage in relation to other anticoagulants

Rivastigmine (Exelon, Generic) **Uses:** *Mild–mod dementia in Alzheimer Dz* **Acts:** Enhances cholinergic activity **Dose:** 1.5 mg bid; ↑ to 6 mg bid, w/ ↑ at 2-wk intervals (take w/ food) **W/P:** [B, ?] w/ β-Blockers, CCBs, smoking, neuromuscular blockade, digoxin **CI:** Rivastigmine or carbamate allergy **Disp:** Caps 1.5, 3, 4.5, 6 mg; soln 2 mg/mL **SE:** Dose-related GI effects, N/V/D, dizziness, insomnia, fatigue, tremor, diaphoresis, HA, Wt loss (in 18–26%) **Notes:** Swallow caps whole, do not break/chew/crush; avoid EtOH

Rivastigmine, Transdermal (Exelon Patch, Generic) **Uses:** *Mild–mod Alzheimer and Parkinson Dz dementia* **Acts:** Acetylcholinesterase inhib **Dose:** *Initial:* 4.6-mg patch/d applied to back, chest, upper arm, ↑ 9.5 mg after 4 wk if tolerated **W/P:** [?, ?] SSS, conduction defects, asthma, COPD, urinary obst, Szs; death from multiple patches at same time reported **CI:** Hypersens to rivastigmine, other carbamates **Disp:** Transdermal patch 5 cm^2 (4.6 mg/24 h), 10 cm^2 (9.5 mg/24 h) **SE:** N/V/D

Rizatriptan (Maxalt, Maxalt MLT, Generic) **Uses:** *Rx acute migraine* **Acts:** Vascular serotonin receptor agonist **Dose:** 5–10 mg PO, repeat in 2 h PRN, 30 mg/d max **W/P:** [C, M] **CI:** Angina, ischemic heart Dz, ischemic bowel Dz, hemiplegic/basilar migraine, uncontrolled HTN, ergot or serotonin 5-HT$_1$ agonist use w/in 24 h, MAOI use w/in 14 d **Disp:** Tabs 5, 10 mg; *Maxalt MLT:* OD tabs 5, 10 mg **SE:** CP, palpitations, N/V, asthenia, dizziness, somnolence, fatigue

Rocuronium (Zemuron, Generic) **Uses:** *Skeletal muscle relaxation during rapid-sequence intubation, surgery, or mechanical ventilation* **Acts:** Nondepolarizing neuromuscular blocker **Dose:** *Rapid sequence intubation:* 0.6–1.2 mg/kg IV *Continuous Inf:* 8–12 mcg/kg/min IV; adjust/titrate based on *train of four* monitoring; ↓ in hepatic impair **W/P:** [C, ?] Anaphylactoid reactions can occur; concomitant use of corticosteroids has been associated w/ myopathy **CI:** Component or omer neuromuscular blocker allergy **Disp:** Inj preservative-free 10 mg/mL **SE:** BP changes, tachycardia **Notes:** Cross-reactivity w/ other neuromuscular blocker possible

Roflumilast (Daliresp) **Uses:** *↓ Exacerbations severe COPD* **Acts:** Selective PDE4 inhib, ↑ cAMP w/ ↓ inflam **Dose:** 500 mcg qd **W/P:** [C, –] Metabolized by CYP3A4 and 1A2; CYP3A4 and 1A2 inhib (cimetidine, erythromycin) increase levels, inducers (rifampin, carbamazepine) can decrease blood levels **CI:** Mod–severe liver impair **Disp:** Tabs 500 mcg **SE:** Worsening depression/suicidal behavior/ideation; N/D, ↓ Wt, HA, insomnia, anxiety **Notes:** Not a bronchodilator, not for acute exacerbations

Romidepsin (Istodax) **Uses:** *Rx cutaneous T-cell lymphoma in pts who have received at least one prior systemic therapy * **Acts:** HDAC inhib **Dose:** 14 mg/m^2 IV over 4 h d 1, 8, and 15 of a 28-d cycle; repeat cycles every 28 d if tolerated; Tx

D/C or interruption w/ or w/o dose reduction to 10 mg/m^2 to manage adverse drug reactions **W/P:** [D, ?] Risk of ↑ QT, hematologic tox; strong CYP3A4 inhibs may ↑ conc **Disp:** Inj 10 mg **SE:** N/V, fatigue, Infxn, anorexia, ↓ plt **Notes:** Hazardous agent, precautions for handling and disposal

Romiplostim (Nplate) **BOX:** ↑ Risk for heme malignancies and thromboembolism; D/C may worsen ↓ plt **Uses:** *Rx ↓ plt d/t ITP w/ poor response to other therapies* **Acts:** Thrombopoietic, thrombopoietin receptor agonist **Dose:** 1 mcg/kg SQ weekly, adjust 1 mcg/kg/wk to plt count > 50,000/mm^3; max 10 mcg/kg/wk **W/P:** [C, /?] **CI:** Ø 500 mcg/mL (250-mcg vial) **SE:** HA, fatigue, dizziness, N/V/D, myalgia, epistaxis **Notes:** ✓ CBC/diff/plt weekly; plt ↑ 4–9 d, peak 12–16 d; D/C if no ↑ plt after 4 wk max dose; ↓ dose w/ plt count > 200,000/mm^3 for 2 wk

Ropinirole (Requip, Requip XL, Generic) **Uses:** *Rx of Parkinson Dz, RLS* **Acts:** DA agonist **Dose:** *Parkinson Dz:* IR initial 0.25 mg PO tid, weekly ↑ 0.25 mg/dose, to 1 mg PO tid (may continue to titrate weekly to max dose of 24 mg/d); ER: 2 mg PO qd, titrate qwk by 2 mg/d to max 24 mg/d *RLS:* initial 0.25 mg PO 1–3 h before bedtime **W/P:** [C, ?/–] Severe CV/renal/hepatic impair **CI:** Component allergy **Disp:** Tabs IR 0.25, 0.5, 1, 2, 3, 4, 5 mg; tabs ER 2, 4, 6, 8, 12 mg **SE:** Syncope, postural ↓ BP, N/V, HA, somnolence, dose-related hallucinations, dyskinesias, dizziness **Notes:** D/C w/ 7-d taper

Rosiglitazone (Avandia) **BOX:** May cause or worsen CHF; may increase myocardial ischemia **Uses:** *Type 2 DM* **Acts:** Thiazolidinedione; ↑ insulin sensitivity **Dose:** 4–8 mg/d PO or in 2 ÷ doses (w/o regard to meals) **W/P:** [C, –] w/ ESRD, CHF, edema, **CI:** Severe CHF (NYHA class III IV) **Disp:** Tabs 2, 4, 8 mg **SE:** May ↑ CV, CHF & ? CA risk; Wt gain, hyperlipidemia, HA, edema, fluid retention, worsen CHF, hyper/hypoglycemia, hepatic damage w/ ↑ LFTs **Notes:** Increased MI risk now requires REMS restricted distribution program

Rosuvastatin (Crestor) **Uses:** *Rx primary hypercholesterolemia & mixed dyslipidemia* **Acts:** HMG-CoA reductase inhib **Dose:** 5–40 mg PO qd; max 5 mg/d w/ cyclosporine, 10 mg/d w/ gemfibrozil or CrCl < 30 mL/min (avoid Al-/Mg-based antacids for 2 h after) **W/P:** [X, ?/–] **CI:** Active liver Dz, unexplained ↑ LFTs **Disp:** Tabs 5, 10, 20, 40 mg **SE:** Myalgia, constipation, asthenia, Abd pain, N, myopathy, rarely rhabdomyolysis **Notes:** May ↑ warfarin effect; monitor LFTs; consider ↓ dose in Asian pts; OK w/ grapefruit

Rotavirus Vaccine, Live, Oral, Monovalent (Rotarix) **Uses:** *Px rotavirus gastroenteritis in peds* **Acts:** Active immunization w/ live attenuated rotavirus **Dose:** *Peds 6–24 wk:* 1st dose PO at 6 wk of age, wait at least 4 wk, then a 2nd dose by 24 wk of age **W/P:** [C, ?] **CI:** Component sensitivity, uncorrected congenital GI malformation, SCID, intussusception **Disp:** Single-dose vial **SE:** Irritability, cough, runny nose, fever, anaphylactic Rxn, D, ↓ appetite, otitis media, V **Notes:** Conclude by age 24 wk; can be given to infant in house w/ immunosuppressed family member or mother who is breast-feeding; safety and effectiveness not studied in immunocompromised infants

Rotavirus Vaccine, Live, Oral, Pentavalent (RotaTeq) Uses: *Px rotavirus gastroenteritis* **Acts:** Active immunization w/ live attenuated rotavirus **Dose:** *Peds 6–24 wk.* Single dose PO at 2, 4, & 6 wk **W/P:** [?, ?] **CI:** Component sensitivity, uncorrected congenital GI malformation, SCID, intussusception **Disp:** Oral susp 2-mL single-use tubes **SE:** Irritability, cough, runny nose, fever, anaphylactic Rxn, D, ↓ appetite, otitis media, V **Notes:** Begin series by age 12 wk and conclude by age 32 wk; can be given to infant in house w/ immunosuppressed family member or mother who is breast-feeding; safety and effectiveness not studied in immunocompromised infants

Rotigotine (Neupro) Uses: *Parkinson Dz, RLS* **Acts:** DA agonist **Dose:** *Adults. Parkinson Dz:* 2 mg/24 h (early Dz) or 4 mg/24 h (advanced Dz); ↑ by 2 mg/ 24 h qwk PRN to max of 6 mg/24 h (early Dz) or 8 mg/24 h (advanced Dz); *RLS:* 1 mg/24 h; ↑ by 1 mg/24 h qwk PRN to max 3 mg/24 h; apply patch to dry, intact skin; ↓ gradually w/ D/C **W/P:** [C, ?/–] Allergic Rxns w/ sulfite sens **CI:** Hypersens **Disp:** Transdermal system 1, 2, 3, 4, 6, 8 mg/24 h **SE:** N/V, site Rxn, somnolence, dizziness, anorexia, hyperhidrosis, insomnia, peripheral edema, dyskinesia, HA, postural hypotension, syncope, ↑ HR, ↑ BP, hallucinations, psychotic-like/compulsive behavior **Notes:** Do not use same site more than once q14 d

Rufinamide (Banzel) Uses: *Adjunct Lennox-Gastaut Szs* **Acts:** Anticonvulsant **Dose:** *Adults. Initial:* 400–800 mg/d ÷ bid (max 3200 mg/d ÷ bid) *Peds ≥ 4 y. Initial:* 10 mg/kg/d ÷ bid, target 45 mg/kg/d ÷ bid; 3200 mg/d max **W/P:** [C, /–] **CI:** Familial short QT synd **Disp:** Tabs 200, 400 mg; susp 40 mg/mL (460 mL) **SE:** ↓ QT, HA, somnolence, N/V, ataxia, rash **Notes:** Monitor for rash; use w/ OCP may lead to contraceptive failure; dose adjust w/ valproate; initial dose not > 400 mg

Ruxolitinib (Jakafi) Uses: *Myelofibrosis, polycythemia vera* **Acts:** Inhib Janus-assoc kinases, mediators of hematologic and immunologic cytokines and growth factors **Dose:** 20 mg bid if plt > 200,000 × 10^9/L; 15 mg bid if plt 100,000–200,000 × 10^9/L; ↑ based on response, 25 mg bid max; stop Tx if plt < 50,000 × 10^9/L; restart when > 50,000 × 10^9/L; 20 mg bid if plt > 125,000 × 10^9/L; 15 mg bid if plt 100–125,000 × 109/L; 10 mg bid if plt 75–100,000 × 10^9/L × 2 wk, if stable ↑ to 15 mg bid; if plt 50–75,000 × 10^9/L, 5 mg bid × 2 wk; if stable ↑ to 10 mg bid; if no ↓ in spleen size or Sxs D/C after 6 mo **W/P:** [C, –] **Do not** use if ESRD **and not** on dialysis; ↓ dose w/ strong CYP3A4 inhib **CI:** Ø **Disp:** Tabs 5, 10, 15, 20, 25 mg **SE:** ↓ Plt, ↓ WBC, anemia, bruising, HA, dizziness, serious Infxns including zoster **Notes:** w/ D/C for reason other than ↓ plt, taper 5 mg bid each wk

Salmeterol (Serevent, Serevent Diskus) **BOX:** Long-acting β₂-agonists, such as salmeterol, may ↑ risk of asthma-related death; do not use alone, only as additional Rx for pts not controlled on other asthma meds; LABAs may ↑ risk of asthma-related hospitalization in pediatric and adolescent pts Uses: *Asthma, exercise-induced asthma, COPD* **Acts:** Sympathomimetic bronchodilator, long acting β₂-agonist **Dose:** *Adults & Peds > 12 y.* 1 Diskus-dose Inh bid **W/P:** [C, ?/–] **CI:** Acute asthma; monotherapy concomitant use of Inh steroid, status astheticus **Disp:** Dry powder diskus 50 mcg/dose, **SE:** HA, pharyngitis, tachycardia, arrhythmias, nervousness, GI upset, tremors **Notes:** Not for acute attacks; must use w/ steroid or short-acting β-agonist

Saquinavir (Invirase) **BOX:** Invirase and Fortovase not bioequivalent/interchangeable; must use Invirase in combo w/ ritonavir, which provides saquinavir plasma levels = those w/ Fortovase **Uses:** *HIV Infxn* **Acts:** HIV protease inhib **Dose:** 1000 mg PO bid w/in 2 h of a full meal (dose w/ ritonavir 100 mg PO bid) w/in 2 h pc (dose adjust w/ delavirdine, lopinavir, & nelfinavir) **W/P:** [B, ?] **CI:** Complete AV block w/o implanted pacemaker; concomitant use antiarrhythmics, ergot derivatives, sedatives/hypnotics, trazodone, sildenafil, statins, rifamins, congenital ↑ QT synd; severe hepatic impair; refractory ↓ K⁺/↓ Mg²⁺; anaphylaxis to component **Disp:** Caps 200 mg, tabs 500 mg **SE:** Dyslipidemia, lipodystrophy, rash, hyperglycemia, GI upset, weakness **Notes:** Take w/in 2 h of a meal, avoid direct sunlight

Sargramostim [GM-CSF] (Leukine) **Uses:** *Myeloid recovery following BMT or chemotherapy* **Acts:** Recombinant GF, activates mature granulocytes & macrophages **Dose:** *Adults & Peds.* 250 mcg/m²/d IV cont until ANC > 1500 cells/m² for 3 consecutive d **W/P:** [C, ?/–] Li, corticosteroids **CI:** > 10% blasts, allergy to yeast, concurrent chemotherapy/RT **Disp:** Inj 250, 500 mcg **SE:** Bone pain, fever, ↑ BP, tachycardia, flushing, GI upset, myalgia **Notes:** Rotate Inj sites; use APAP PRN for pain

Saxagliptin (Onglyza) **Uses:** *Monotherapy/combo type 2 DM* **Acts:** DDP-4 inhib, ↑ insulin synth/release **Dose:** 2.5 or 5 mg qd w/o regard to meals; 2.5 mg qd w/ CrCl < 50 mL/min or w/ strong CYP3A4/5 inhib (eg, atazanavir, clarithromycin, indinavir, itraconazole, ketoconazole, nefazodone, nelfinavir, ritonavir, saquinavir, telithromycin) **W/P:** [B, ?] May ↓ glu when used w/ insulin secretagogues (eg, sulfonylureas); w/ pancreatitis; ? heart failure link **CI:** Hypersens Rxn **Disp:** Tabs 2.5, 5 mg **SE:** Peripheral edema, hypoglycemia, UTI, HA, Abd pain, severe joint pain

Saxagliptin/Metformin (Kombiglyze XR) **BOX:** Lactic acidosis can occur w/ metformin accumulation; ↑ risk w/ sepsis, vol depletion, CHF, renal/hepatic impair, excess alcohol; if lactic acidosis suspected D/C med and hospitalize **Uses:** *Type 2 DM* **Acts:** DDP-4 inhib, ↑ insulin synth/release & biguanide; ↓ hepatic glu production & intestinal absorption of glu; ↑ insulin sens **Dose:** 5/500 mg–5/2000 mg saxagliptin/metformin HCl XR PO qd w/ evening meal **W/P:** [B, ?/–] w/ Contrast studies **CI:** SCr > 1.4 mg/dL (females) or > 1.5 mg/dL (males); met acidosis; ? heart failure link **Disp:** Tabs (mg saxagliptin/mg metformin XR) 5/500, 5/1000, 2.5/1000 **SE:** Lactic acidosis; ↓ vit B₁₂ levels; ↓ glu w/ insulin secretagogue; N/V/D, anorexia, HA, URI, UTI, urticaria, myalgia, severe joint pain **Notes:** Do not exceed 5 mg/2000 mg saxagliptin/metformin HCl XR; do not crush or chew; w/ strong CYP3A4/5 inhib do not exceed 2.5 mg saxagliptin/d

Scopolamine, Transdermal (Transderm-Scop) **Uses:** *Px N/V associated w/ motion sickness, anesthesia, opiates* **Acts:** Anticholinergic, antiemetic

Dose: 1 mg/72 h, 1 patch behind ear q3d; apply > 4 h before exposure **W/P:** [C, +] w/ APAP, levodopa, ketoconazole, digitalis, KCl **CI:** NAG, GI or GU obst, thyrotoxicosis, paralytic ileus **Disp:** Patch 1.5 mg (releases 1 mg over 72 h) **SE:** Xerostomia, drowsiness, blurred vision, tachycardia, constipation **Notes:** antiemetic activity w/ patch requires several hours

Secobarbital (Seconal) [C-II] Uses: *Insomnia, short-term use*, preanesthetic agent **Acts:** Rapid-acting barbiturate **Dose:** *Adults.* 100–200 mg hs, 100–300 mg preop *Peds.* 2–6 mg/kg/dose, 100 mg/max; ↓ in elderly **W/P:** [D, +] w/ CYP2C9, 3A3/4, 3A5/7 inducer (Table 10, p 356); ↑ w/ other CNS depressants **CI:** Hypersens to barbiturates, marked hepatic impair dyspnea or airway obst, porphyria, PRG **Disp:** Caps 100 mg **SE:** Tolerance in 1–2 wk; resp depression, CNS depression, porphyria, photosens

Secukinumab (Cosentyx) Uses: *Mod–severe plaque psoriasis in candidates for systemic Tx or phototherapy* **Acts:** Human IL-17antag **Dose:** 300 mg SQ wk 0, 1, 2, 3, & 4, then 300 mg q4wk; 150 mg may be acceptable dose **W/P:** [B, M] Infxn; TB; exacerbates Crohn Dz; hypersens Rxn **CI:** Component hypersens **Disp:** Single-use pen or prefilled syringe 150 mg/mL; single-use vial 150 mg lyophilized powder **SE:** D, URI, nasopharyngitis **Notes:** D/C if Infxn develops; evaluate for TB prior; no live vaccines should be given

Selegiline, Oral (Eldepryl, Zelapar, Generic) BOX: Closely monitor for worsening depression or emergence of suicidality, particularly in ped pts Uses: *Parkinson Dz* **Acts:** MAOI **Dose:** 5 mg PO bid; 1.25–2.5 qd ODT tabs PO q A.M. (before breakfast w/o liq), 2.5 mg/d max; ↓ in elderly **W/P:** [C, ?] w/ Drugs that induce CYP3A4 (Table 10, p 356) (eg, phenytoin, carbamazepine, nafcillin, phenobarbital, & rifampin); avoid w/ antidepressants **CI:** w/ Meperidine, MAOI, dextromethorphan, tramadol, methadone, general anesthesia w/in 10 d, pheochromocytoma **Disp:** Tabs/caps 5 mg; once-daily tabs 1.25 mg **SE:** HA, dizziness, orthostatic ↓ BP, arrhythmias, tachycardia, edema, confusion, xerostomia **Notes:** ↓ Carbidopa/levodopa if used in combo; see transdermal form

Selegiline, Transdermal (Emsam) BOX: May ↑ risk of suicidal thinking and behavior in children and adolescents w/ MDD Uses: *Depression* **Acts:** MAOI **Dose:** Apply patch qd to upper torso, upper thigh, or outer upper arm **CI:** Tyramine-containing foods w/ 9- or 12-mg doses; serotonin-sparing agents **W/P:** [C, –] ↑ Carbamazepine and oxcarbazepine levels **Disp:** ER patches 9, 12 mg **SE:** Local Rxns requiring topical steroids; HA, insomnia, orthostatic, ↓ BP, serotonin synd, suicide risk **Notes:** Rotate site; see oral form

Selenium Sulfide (Head & Shoulders Clinical Strength Dandruff Shampoo, Selsun, Selsun Blue Shampoo, Generic, Others) [OTC] Uses: *Scalp seborrheic dermatitis*, scalp itching & flaking d/t *dandruff*; tinea versicolor **Acts:** Antiseborrheic **Dose:** *Dandruff, seborrhea:* Massage 5–10 mL into wet scalp, leave on 2–3 min, rinse, repeat; use 2× wk, then once q1–4wk PRN *Tinea versicolor:* Apply 2.5% qd on area & lather w/ small amounts of water; leave on 10 min, then rinse **W/P:** [C, ?] Avoid contact w/ open wounds or mucus membranes **CI:** Component allergy **Disp:** Shampoo 1% [OTC]; 2.5% shampoo, lotion [Rx] lotion **SE:** Dry or oily scalp, lethargy, hair discoloration, local irritation **Notes:** Do not use more than 2×/wk

Sertaconazole (Ertaczo) **Uses:** *Topical Rx interdigital tinea pedis* **Acts:** Imidazole antifungal. **Spectrum:** *Trichophyton rubrum, Trichophyton mentagrophytes, Epidermophyton floccosum* **Dose:** *Adults & Peds > 12.* Apply between toes & immediate surrounding healthy skin bid × 4 wk **W/P:** [C, ?] Avoid occlusive dressing **CI:** Component allergy **Disp:** 2% Cream **SE:** Contact dermatitis, dry/burning skin, tenderness **Notes:** Use in immunocompetent pts; not for oral, intravag, ophthal use

Sertraline (Zoloft, Generic) **BOX:** Closely monitor pts for worsening depression or emergence of suicidality, particularly in ped pts **Uses:** *Depression, panic disorders, PMDD, OCD, PTSD*, social anxiety disorder, eating disorders, premenstrual disorders **Acts:** ↓ Neuronal uptake of serotonin **Dose:** *Adults.* *Depression:* 50–200 mg/d PO *PTSD:* 25 mg PO qd × 1 wk, then 50 mg PO qd, 200 mg/d max *Peds 6–12 y.* 25 mg qd *13–17 y.* 50 mg PO qd **W/P:** [C, ?/–] Serotonin synd: ↑ risk w/ concomitant use of serotonin antags (haloperidol, etc), hepatic impair **CI:** MAOI use w/in 14 d; concomitant pimozide **Disp:** Tabs 25, 50, 100 mg; 20 mg/mL oral **SE:** Activate manic/hypomanic state, ↑/↓ Wt, insomnia, somnolence, fatigue, tremor, xerostomia, N/D, dyspepsia, ejaculatory dysfunction, ↓ libido, hepatotox

Sevelamer Carbonate (Renvela) **Uses:** *Control ↑ PO₄³⁻ in ESRD* **Acts:** Intestinal phosphate binder **Dose:** Start 0.8 or 1.6 g PO tid w/ meals; titrate 0.8 g/meal for target PO₄ 3.5–5.5 mg/dL; switch g/g among sevelamer forms, titrate PRN **W/P:** [C, ?] w/ Swallowing disorders, bowel problems, may ↓ absorption of vits D, E, K, ↓ ciprofloxacin & other medicine levels **CI:** Bowel obst **Disp:** Tabs 800 mg; powder 0.8/2.4 g **SE:** N/V/D, dyspepsia, Abd pain, flatulence, constipation **Notes:** Separate other meds 1 h before or 3 h after

Sevelamer Hydrochloride (Renagel) **Uses:** *↓ PO₄³⁻ in ESRD* **Acts:** Binds intestinal PO₄³⁻ **Dose:** *Initial:* PO₄³⁻ > 5.5 and < 7.5 mg/dL: 800 mg PO tid; ≥ 7.5 mg/dL: 1200–1600 mg PO tid *Switching from sevelamer carbonate:* per-g basis; titrate ↑/↓ 1 tab/meal 2-wk intervals PRN; take w/ food 2–4 caps PO tid w/ meals; adjust based on PO₄³⁻; max 4 g/dose **W/P:** [C, ?] May ↓ absorption of vits D, E, K, ↓ ciprofloxacin & other medicine levels **CI:** ↓ PO₄³⁻, bowel obst **Disp:** Tabs 400, 800 mg **SE:** N/V/D, dyspepsia, ↑ Ca²⁺ **Notes:** Do not open/chew caps; separate other meds 1 h before or 3 h after; 800 mg sevelamer = 667 mg Ca acetate

Short Ragweed Pollen Allergen Extract (Ragwitek) **BOX:** Can cause life-threatening allergic Rxn (anaphylaxis, laryngopharyngeal edema); DO NOT use w/ severe unstable/uncontrolled asthma; observe for 30 min after 1st dose; Rx and train to use auto-injectable epi; may not be suitable for pts unresponsive to epi or Inh bronchodilators (pts on β-blockers) or w/ certain conditions that could ↓ ability to respond to severe allergic reaction **Uses:** *Immunotherapy of short ragweed pollen-induced allergic rhinitis w/ or w/o conjunctivitis confirmed by + skin test or pollen-specific IgE Ab* **Acts:** Allergen immunotherapy **Dose:** *Adults.* 1 tab SL/day; do not swallow for 1 min **Peds.** Not approved **W/P:** [C, ?/–] Discuss severe allergic Rxn; if oral lesions, stop Tx, restart after healed **CI:** Severe uncontrolled/unstable asthma; Hx severe systemic/local allergic reaction to SL allergen immunotherapy; eosinophilic esophagitis; component hypersens **Disp:** Tabs 30/90 day blister packs **SE:** Throat irritation, oral/ear/tongue pruritus, mouth edema, oral paraesthesia **Notes:** 1st dose in healthcare setting; start 12 wk before expected onset of Sx; give auto-injectable epi; D/C with ↑ local symptoms and seek care; only for adults 18–65 yrs

Sildenafil (Revatio, Viagra) **Uses:** *Viagra:* *ED*; *Revatio:* *Pulm artery HTN (adults only)* **Acts:** ↓ PDE5 (responsible for cGMP breakdown); ↑ cGMP activity to relaxation of smooth muscles & ↑ flow to corpus cavernosum and pulm vasculature; ? antiproliferative on pulm artery smooth muscle **Dose:** *ED:* 25–100 mg PO 1 h before sexual activity, max 1/d; ↓ if > 65 y *Revatio: Pulm HTN:* 20 mg PO tid or 10 mg IV tid **W/P:** [B, ?/–] w/ CYP3A4 inhib (Table 10, p 356); retinitis pigmentosa; hepatic/severe renal impair; w/ sig hypo-/hypertension *Revatio* approved only in adults, not peds; must consider risk/benefit in each pt **CI:** w/ Nitrates or if sex not advised; w/ protease inhib **Disp:** Tabs *Viagra:* 25, 50, 100 mg, tabs *Revatio:* Tabs 20 mg; Inj 5–10 mg/vial **SE:** HA; flushing; dizziness; blue haze visual change, hearing loss, priapism **Notes:** Cardiac events in absence of nitrates debatable; transient global amnesia reports; avoid fatty food w/ dose

Silodosin (Rapaflo) **Uses:** *BPH* **Acts:** α-Blockers of prostatic α_{1a} **Dose:** 8 mg/d; 4 mg/d w/ CrCl 30–50 mL/min; take w/ food **W/P:** [B, ?] Not for use in females; do not use w/ other α-blockers or glycoprotein inhib (ie, cyclosporine); R/O PCa before use; IFIS possible w/ cataract surgery **CI:** Severe hepatic/renal impair (CrCl < 30 mL/min), w/ CYP3A4 inhib (eg, ketoconazole, clarithromycin, itraconazole, ritonavir) **Disp:** Caps 4, 8 mg **SE:** Retrograde ejaculation, dizziness, D, syncope, somnolence, orthostatic ↓ BP, nasopharyngitis, nasal congestion, IFIS during cataract surgery **Notes:** Not for use as antihypertensive; no effect on QT interval

Silver Nitrate (Generic) **Uses:** *Removal of granulation tissue & warts; prophylaxis in burns* **Acts:** Caustic antiseptic & astringent **Dose:** *Adults & Peds.* Apply to moist surface 2–3 × wk for 2–3 wk or until effect **W/P:** [C, ?] **CI:** Do not use on broken skin **Disp:** Topical impregnated applicator sticks, soln 0.5, 10, 25, 50%; topical ointment 10% **SE:** May stain tissue black, usually resolves; local irritation, methemoglobinemia **Notes:** D/C if redness or irritation develops; no longer used in US for newborn Px of gonococcus conjunctivitis

Silver Sulfadiazine (Silvadene, Thermazene, Generic) **Uses:** *Px & Rx of Infxn in 2nd- & 3rd-degree burns* **Acts:** Bactericidal **Dose:** *Adults & Peds.* Aseptically cover the area w/ 1/16-in coating bid **W/P:** [B unless near term, ?/–] **CI:** Infants < 2 mo, PRG near term **Disp:** Cream 1% **SE:** Itching, rash, skin discoloration, blood dyscrasias, hep, allergy **Notes:** Systemic absorption w/ extensive application

Simeprevir (Olysio) Uses: *Hep C w/ genotype 1 & compensated liver Dz in combo w/ ribavirin & peginterferon alpha or w/ sofosbuvir* Acts: NS3/4A protease inhib Dose: See PI W/P: [C, –] NOTE: Ribavirin & peginterferon alpha are [X, –], BOTH are embryo-fetal toxic; avoid PRG (patient or in partner) before & 6 mo post; use at least 2 birth control methods and monthly PRG test CI: PRG or males w/ PRG partner Disp: Caps 150 mg SE: Photosens, rash, pruritus, N, dyspnea Notes: DO NOT use as monotherapy; use w/ ribavirin & peginterferon alpha; monitor W/P & SE from other meds; screen for NS3 Q80K polymorphism; do not use w/ CYP3A inducers/inhib; monitor HCV RNA levels

Simethicone (Generic [OTC]) Uses: *Flatulence* Acts: Defoaming, alters gas bubble surface tension action Dose: *Adults & Peds > 12 y.* 40–360 mg PO after meals and at bedtime PRN; 500 mg/d max *Peds < 2 y.* 20 mg PO qid PRN *2–12 y.* 40 mg PO qid PRN W/P: [C, ?] CI: GI perf or obst Disp: [OTC] Tabs 80, 125 mg; caps 125 mg; susp 40 mg/0.6 mL; chew tabs 80, 125 mg; caps: 125, 180 mg; ODT strip: 40, 62.5 mg SE: N/D Notes: Available in combo products OTC

Simvastatin (Zocor, Generic) Uses: ↓ Cholesterol Acts: HMG-CoA reductase inhib Dose: *Adults.* 5–40 mg PO q P.M.; w/ meals; ↓ in renal Insuff; w/o grapefruit *Peds 10–17 y.* 10 mg, 40 mg/d max W/P: [X, –] Max 10 mg qd w/ verapamil, diltiazem; max 20 mg qd w/ amlodipine, ranolazine, amiodarone; 80 mg dose restricted to those taking > 12 mo w/o muscle tox; w/ Chinese pt on lipid modifying meds CI: PRG, liver Dz, strong CYP3A4 inhib Disp: Tabs 5, 10, 20, 40, 80 mg SE: HA, GI upset, myalgia, myopathy (pain, tenderness, weakness w/ creatine kinase 10 × ULN) & rhabdomyolysis, hep Notes: Combo w/ ezetimibe/simvastatin; follow LFTs; ↑ blood glu w/ DM

Sipuleucel-T (Provenge) Uses: *Asymptomatic/minimally symptomatic met CRPC* Acts: Autologous (pt-specific) cellular immunotherapy Dose: 3 doses over 1 mo @ 2-wk intervals; premed w/ APAP & diphenhydramine W/P: [N/A, N/A] Confirm identity/expiry date before Inf; acute transfusion Rxn possible; not tested for transmissible Dz CI: Ø Disp: 50 mill units autologous CD54+ cells activated w/ PAP GM-CSF in 250 mL LR SE: Chills, fatigue, fever, back pain, N, jt ache, HA Notes: Pt must undergo leukophoresis, w/ shipping and autologous cell processing at manufacturing facility before each Inf

Sirolimus [Rapamycin] (Rapamune) BOX: Use only by physicians experienced in immunosuppression; immunosuppression associated w/ lymphoma, ↑ Infxn risk; do not use in lung transplant (fatal bronchial anastomotic dehiscence); do not use in liver transplant: ↑ risk hepatic arterythrombosis, graft failure, and mortality (w/ evidence of Infxn) Uses: *Px organ rejection in new renal Tx pts* Acts: ↓ T-lymphocyte activation and proliferation Dose: *Adults > 40 kg.* 6 mg PO on d 1, then 2 mg/d PO *Peds < 40 kg & ≥ 13 y.* 3 mg/m² load, then 1 mg/m²/d (in H₂O/orange juice; no grapefruit juice w/ sirolimus); take 4 h after cyclosporine; ↓ in hepatic impair W/P: [C, ?/–] Impaired wound healing & angioedema; grapefruit juice, ketoconazole CI: Component allergy Disp: Soln 1 mg/mL; tabs 0.5, 1, 2 mg

SE: HTN, edema, CP, fever, HA, insomnia, acne, rash, ↑ cholesterol, GI upset, ↑/↓ K⁺, Infxns, blood dyscrasias, arthralgia, tachycardia, renal impair, graft loss & death in liver transplant (hepatic artery thrombosis), ascites **Notes:** Levels: *Trough:* 4–20 ng/mL; varies w/ assay method and indication

Sitagliptin (Januvia) **Uses:** *Monotherapy or combo for type 2 DM* **Acts:** Dipeptidyl peptidase-4 (DDP-4) inhib, ↑ insulin synth/release **Dose:** 100 mg PO qd; CrCl 30–50: 50 mg PO qd; CrCl < 30 mL/min: 25 mg PO qd **W/P:** [B/?] May cause ↓ blood sugar when used w/ insulin secretagogues such as sulfonylureas; not for type 1 DM or DKA; not studied w/ pancreatitis **CI:** Component hypersens **Disp:** Tabs 25, 50, 100 mg **SE:** URI; peripheral edema, nasopharyngitis, severe joint pain **Notes:** No evidence for ↑ CV risk

Sitagliptin/Metformin (Janumet, Janumet XR) **BOX:** See Metformin, p 210 **Uses:** *Adjunct to diet and exercise in type 2 DM* **Acts:** See individual agents **Dose:** 1 tab PO bid, titrate; 100 mg sitagliptin & 2000 mg metformin/d max; take w/ meals **W/P:** [B, ?/–] Not for type 1 DM or DKA; not studied w/ pancreatitis **CI:** Type 1 DM, DKA, male Cr > 1.5; female Cr > 1.4 mg/dL **Disp:** Tabs 50/500, 50/1000, 100/1000; *XR:* 50/500, 50/1000, 100/1000 mg **SE:** Nasopharyngitis, N/V/D, flatulence, Abd discomfort, dyspepsia, asthenia, HA, severe joint pain **Notes:** Hold w/ contrast study; ✓ Cr, CBC

Sitagliptin/Simvastatin (Juvisync) **Uses:** *DM2 and hyperlipidemia* **Acts:** ↑ Insulin synth/release and ↓ cholesterol, ↓ VLDL, ↓ triglycerides, ↑ HDL; DPP-4 inhib w/ HMG-CoA reductase inhib **Dose:** Start 100/40 mg or maintain simvastatin dose **W/P:** [X, –] ↑ AST/ALT; myopathy (↑ risk of myopathy w/ age > 65 y), female, renal impair, meds (eg, niacin, amiodarone, CCBs, fibrates, colchicine); renal failure, hypoglycemia w/ sulfonylureas, or insulin; pancreatitis, anaphylaxis **CI:** Hx hypersens Rxn; w/ CYP3A4 inhib, gemfibrozil, cyclosporine, danazol, ketoconazole, itraconazole, erythromycin, clarithromycin, HIV protease inhib; liver Dz; PRG or women who may get PRG; nursing **Disp:** Tabs mg sitagliptin/mg simvastatin): 100/10, 100/20, 100/40, 50/10, 50/20, 50/40 **SE:** *Simvastatin:* HA, GI upset, myalgia, myopathy (pain, tenderness, weakness w/ creatine kinase 10× ULN) and rhabdomyolysis, hep; *sitagliptin:* URI, nasopharyngitis, UTI, HA, severe joint pain **Notes:** ↑ Myopathy w/ coadministration of CYP3A4 inhib; risk of myopathy dose related

Smallpox Vaccine (ACAM2000) **BOX:** Acute myocarditis and other infectious complications possible; CI in immunocompromised, eczema or exfoliative skin conditions, infants < 1 y **Uses:** Immunization against smallpox (variola virus) **Acts:** Active immunization (live attenuated cowpox virus) **Dose:** *Primary and revaccination:* 15 punctures w/ bifurcated needle dipped in vaccine into deltoid, ✓ site for Rxn in 6–8 d; if major Rxn, site scabs & heals, leaving scar **W/P:** [D, ?] **CI:** *Nonemergency use:* febrile illness, immunosuppression, Hx eczema & in household contacts. *Emergency:* No absolute CI **Disp:** Vial for reconstitution: 100 mill pock-forming units/mL **SE:** Malaise, fever, regional lymphadenopathy, encephalopathy, rashes, spread of inoculation to other sites; SJS, eczema vaccinatum w/ severe disability **Notes:** Avoid infants for 14 d; intradermal use only; restricted distribution; Dryvax discontinued

Sodium Bicarbonate [NaHCO₃] (Generic) Uses: *Alkalinization of urine, RTA, metabolic acidosis, ↑ K⁺, TCA OD* **Acts:** Alkalinizing agent **Dose:** *Adults.* **ECC 2010.** Cardiac arrest w/ good ventilation, hyperkalemia, OD of TCAs, ASA, cocaine, diphenhydramine: 1 mEq/kg IV bolus; repeat 1/2 dose q10min PRN *Metabolic acidosis:* 2–5 mEq/kg IV over 8 h & PRN based on acid–base status. ↑ K⁺: 50 mEq IV over 5 min *Alkalinize urine:* 4 g (48 mEq) PO, then 12–24 mEq q4h; adjust based on urine pH; 2 amp (100 mEq)/1 L D₅W at 100–250 mL/h IV, monitor urine pH & serum bicarbonate *Chronic renal failure:* 1–3 mEq/kg/d *Distal RTA:* 0.5–2 mEq/kg/d in 4–5 ÷ doses *Peds.* **ECC 2010.** *Severe metabolic acidosis, hyperkalemia:* 1 mEq/kg IV slow bolus; 4.2% conc in infants < 1 mo *Chronic renal failure:* See Adults dosage *Distal RTA:* 2–3 mEq/kg/d PO *Proximal RTA:* 5–10 mEq/kg/d; titrate based on serum bicarbonate *Urine alkalinization:* 84–840 mg/kg/d (1–10 mEq/kg/d) in ÷ doses; adjust based on urine pH **W/P:** [C, ?] **CI:** Alkalosis, ↑ Na⁺, severe pulm edema, ↓ Ca²⁺ **Disp:** Powder, tabs; 325 mg = 3.8 mEq; 650 mg = 7.6 mEq; Inj 1 mEq/1 mL, 4.2% (5 mEq/10 mL), 7.5% (8.92 mEq/10 mL), 8.4% (10 mEq/10 mL) vial or amp **SE:** Belching, edema, flatulence, ↑ Na⁺, metabolic alkalosis **Notes:** 1 g neutralizes 12 mEq of acid; 50 mEq bicarbonate = 50 mEq Na; can make 3 amps in 1 L D₅W = 0.2N5 w/ 150 mEq bicarbonate

Sodium Citrate/Citric Acid (Bicitra, Oracit) Uses: *Chronic metabolic acidosis, alkalinize urine; dissolve uric acid & cysteine stones* **Acts:** Urinary alkalinizer **Dose:** *Adults.* 10–30 mL in 1- to 3- oz H₂O pc & hs. *Peds.* 5–15 mL in 1- to 3- oz H₂O pc & hs; best after meals **W/P:** [?, ?] **CI:** Severe renal impair or Na-restricted diets **Disp:** 15- or 30-mL unit dose: 16 (473 mL) or 4 fl oz **SE:** Tetany, metabolic alkalosis, ↑ K⁺, GI upset; avoid use of multiple 50-mL amps; can cause ↑ Na⁺/hyperosmolality **Notes:** 1 mL = 1 mEq Na & 1 mEq bicarbonate

Sodium Oxybate/Gamma Hydroxybutyrate/GHB (Xyrem) [C-III] BOX: Known drug of abuse even at recommended doses; confusion, depression, resp depression may occur **Uses:** *Narcolepsy-associated cataplexy* **Acts:** Inhibitory neurotransmitter **Dose:** *Adults & Peds > 16 y.* 2.25 g PO qhs, 2nd dose 2.5–4 h later; may ↑ 9 g/d max **W/P:** [C, ?/–] **CI:** Succinic semialdehyde dehydrogenase deficiency; potentiates EtOH & other CNS depressants **Disp:** 500 mg/mL (180-mL) PO soln **SE:** Confusion, depression, ↓ diminished level of consciousness, incontinence, sig V, resp depression, psychological Sxs **Notes:** May lead to dependence; GHB abused as a "date rape" drug; controlled distribution (prescriber & pt registration); must be administered when pt in bed

Sodium Phosphate (Osmoprep, Visicol) BOX: Acute phosphate nephropathy reported w/ permanent renal impair risk; w/ ↑ age, hypovolemia, bowel obst or colitis, baseline kidney Dz, w/ meds that affect renal perf/Fxn (diuretics, ACE inhib, ARB, NSAIDs) **Uses:** *Bowel prep prior to colonoscopy*, short-term constipation **Acts:** Hyperosmotic laxative **Dose:** 3 tabs PO w/ at least 8 oz clear liq q15min for 6 doses; then 2 additional tabs in 15 min, 3–5 h prior to colonoscopy; 3 tabs q15min for 6 doses, then 2 additional tabs in 15 min **W/P:** [C, ?] Renal impair, electrolyte disturbances **CI:** Megacolon, bowel obst **Disp:** Tabs 0.398, 1.102 g (32/bottle) **SE:** ↑ QT, ↑ PO₄⁻, ↓ Ca, D, flatulence, cramps, Abd bloating/pain

Sodium Polystyrene Sulfonate (Kayexalate, Kionex, Generic) Uses: *Rx of ↑ K⁺* **Acts:** Na⁺/K⁺ ion-exchange resin **Dose:** *Adults.* 15–60 g PO or 30–50 g PR q6h based on serum K⁺ *Peds.* 1 g/kg/dose PO or PR q6h based on serum K⁺ **W/P:** [C, ?] **CI:** Obstructive bowel Dz; ↑ Na⁺; neonates w/ ↓ gut motility **Disp:** Powder; susp 15 g/60 mL sorbitol **SE:** ↑ Na⁺, ↓ K⁺, GI upset, fecal impaction **Notes:** Enema acts more quickly than PO; PO most effective, onset action > 2 h

Sofosbuvir (Sovaldi) Uses: *Chronic hep C, genotypes 1, 2, 3, & 4 and co-infection w/ HIV* **Acts:** Nucleotide analog NS5B RNA polymerase inhib **Dose:** 400 mg qd w/ ribavirin (genotype 2 & 3; for 12 and 24 wk) or ribavirin + pegylated interferon (genotype 1 or 4 for 12 wk) **W/P:** [X, –] Embryo-fetal tox; avoid PRG (pt or in partner) before & 6 mo post; use at least 2 birth control methods and monthly PRG test **CI:** PRG or may become PRG; men w/ PRG partner **Disp:** Tabs 400 mg **SE:** (*SE from combo*) HA, fatigue, insomnia, N, anemia, pancytopenia, depression, **Notes:** Avoid w/ P-gp inducers; use in post-liver transplant or w/ CrCl < 30 mL/min not studied

Solifenacin (VESIcare) Uses: *OAB* **Acts:** Antimuscarinic, ↓ detrusor contractions **Dose:** 5 mg PO qd, 10 mg/d max; ↓ w/ renal/hepatic impair **W/P:** [C, ?/–] BOO or GI obst, UC, MyG, renal/hepatic impair, QT prolongation risk **CI:** NAG, urinary/gastric retention **Disp:** Tabs 5, 10 mg **SE:** Constipation, xerostomia, dyspepsia, blurred vision, drowsiness **Notes:** CYP3A4 substrate; azole antifungals ↑ levels; recent concern over cognitive effects

Somatropin (Genotropin, Nutropin AQ, Omnitrope, Saizen, Serostim, Zorbtive) Uses: *HIV-associated wasting/cachexia* **Acts:** Anabolic peptide hormone **Dose:** 0.1 mg/kg SQ hs; max 6 mg/d **W/P:** [B, ?] Lipodystrophy (rotate sites) **CI:** Active neoplasm; acute critical illness postop; benzyl alcohol sensitivity; hypersens **Disp:** Powder for Inj 4, 5, 6 mg **SE:** Arthralgia, edema, ↑ blood glu

Sorafenib (Nexavar) Uses: *Unresectable hepatocellular CA, met RCC, thyroid CA* **Acts:** Tyrosine kinase inhib **Dose:** 400 mg PO on empty stomach **W/P:** [D, –] w/ Irinotecan, doxorubicin, warfarin; avoid conception (male/female); avoid inducers **Disp:** Tabs 200 mg **SE:** Hand–foot synd; Tx-emergent hypertension; bleeding, ↑ INR, cardiac infarction/ischemia; ↑ pancreatic enzymes, hypophosphatemia, lymphopenia, anemia, fatigue, alopecia, pruritus, D, GI upset, HA, neuropathy **Notes:** Monitor BP first 6 wk; may require ↓ dose (daily or q other day); impaired metabolism w/ Asian descent; may affect wound healing, D/C before major surgery

Sorbitol (Generic) Uses: *Constipation* **Acts:** Osmotic laxative **Dose:** 30–150 mL PO of a 20–70% soln PRN **W/P:** [C, ?] **CI:** Anuria **Disp:** Liq 70% **SE:**

Edema, lyte loss, lactic acidosis, GI upset, xerostomia **Notes:** Vehicle for many liq formulations (eg, zinc, Kayexalate)

Sotalol (Betapace, Sorine, Sotylize, Generic) **BOX:** To minimize risk of induced arrhythmia, pts initiated/reinitiated on *Betapace AF* should be placed for a minimum of 3 d (on their maint) in a facility that can provide cardiac resuscitation, cont ECG monitoring, & calculations of CrCl; *Betapace* should not be substituted for *Betapace AF* because of labeling; adjust dose base on CrCl; can cause life-threatening ventricular tachycardia w/ prolonged QT; do not initiate if QT > 450 ms; if QTc > 500 ms during Tx, ↓ dose **Uses:** *Ventricular arrhythmias, AF* **Acts:** β-Adrenergic-blocking agent **Dose:** **Adults.** *CrCl > 60 mL/min:* 80 mg PO bid, may ↑ to 240–320 mg/d; CrCl 30–60 mL/min: 80 mg q24h; CrCl 10–30 mL/min: dose 80 mg q36–48h *ECC 2010. SVT and ventricular arrhythmias:* 1–1.5 mg/kg IV over 5 min **Peds** *< 2 y.* Dosing dependent on age, renal Fxn, heart rate, QT interval ≥ 2 y. 30 mg/m² tid; to max dose of 60 mg/m² tid; ↓ w/ renal impair **W/P:** [B, + (monitor child)] **CI:** Asthma, ↓ HR, ↑ prolonged QT interval, 2nd-/3rd-degree heart block w/o pacemaker, cardiogenic shock, uncontrolled CHF **Disp:** Tabs 80, 120, 160, 240 mg; *Sotylize* 5 mg/mL soln **SE:** ↓ HR, CP, palpitations, fatigue, dizziness, weakness, dyspnea

Sotalol (Betapace AF) **BOX:** See Sotalol (*Betapace*) **Uses:** *Maint sinus rhythm for symptomatic AF/A flutter* **Acts:** β-Adrenergic-blocking agent **Dose:** **Adults.** *CrCl > 60 mL/min:* 80 mg PO q12h, max 320 mg/d *CrCl 40–60 mL/min:* 80 mg PO q24h; ↑ to 120 mg bid during hospitalization; monitor QT interval 2–4 h after each dose, dose reduction or D/C if QT interval ≥ 500 ms **Peds.** *< 2 y.* Dose adjusted based on logarithmic scale (see PI); *> 2 y:* 9 mg/m²/d ÷ tid, may ↑ to 180 mg/m²/d **W/P:** [B, +] When converting from other antiarrhythmic **CI:** Asthma, ↓ HR, ↑ QT interval, 2nd-/3rd-degree heart block w/o pacemaker, cardiogenic shock, K⁺ < 4, SSS, baseline QT > 450 ms uncontrolled CHF, CrCl < 40 mL/min **Disp:** Tabs 80, 120, 160 mg **SE:** ↓ HR, CP, palpitations, fatigue, dizziness, weakness, dyspnea **Notes:** Follow renal Fxn & QT interval; Betapace should not be substituted for Betapace AF because of differences in labeling

Spinosad (Natroba) **Uses:** *Head lice* **Acts:** Neuronal excitation of lice, w/ paralysis & death **Dose:** Cover dry scalp w/ suspension, then apply to dry hair; rinse off in 10 min, may repeat after 7 d; unlabeled to use < 4 y **W/P:** [B, ?/–] **Disp:** 0.9% topical susp **SE:** Scalp/ocular erythema **Notes:** Shake well before use; use w/ overall lice management program; in benzyl alcohol, serious Rxns in neonates, in breast milk, pump and discard milk for 8 h after use

Spironolactone (Aldactone, Generic) **BOX:** Tumorogenic in anmial studies; avoid unnecessary use **Uses:** *Hyperaldosteronism, HTN, class III/IV CHF, ascites from cirrhosis* **Acts:** Aldosterone antag; K⁺-sparing diuretic **Dose:** **Adults.** *CHF* (NYHA class III–IV) 12.5–25 mg/d (w/ ACE and loop diuretic); *HTN* 25–50 mg/d; *Ascites:* 100–400 mg q A.M. w/ 40–160 mg of furosemide, start w/ 100 mg/40 mg, wait at least 3 d before ↑ dose **Peds.** 1–3.3 mg/kg/24 h PO ÷ bid q12–24h, take w/ food **W/P:** [C, + (D/C w/ breast-feeding)] **CI:** ↑ K⁺, acute renal failure, anuria **Disp:** Tabs 25, 50, 100 mg **SE:** ↑ K⁺ & gynecomastia, arrhythmia, sexual dysfunction, confusion, dizziness, D/N/V, abnormal menstruation

Starch, Topical, Rectal (Tucks Suppositories [OTC]) **Uses:** *Temporary relief of anorectal disorders (itching, etc)* **Acts:** Topical protectant **Dose:** *Adults & Peds ≥ 12 y.* Cleanse, rinse, and dry, insert 1 supl rectally 6×/d × 7 d max **W/P:** [?, ?] **CI:** Ø Disp: Supp **SE:** D/C w/ or if rectal bleeding occurs or if condition worsens or does not improve w/in 7 d

Stavudine (Zerit, Generic) **BOX:** Lactic acidosis & severe hepatomegaly w/ steatosis & pancreatitis reported w/ didanosine **Uses:** *HIV in combo w/ other antiretrovirals* **Acts:** NRTI **Dose:** *Adults > 60 kg.* 40 mg bid *< 60 kg.* 30 mg bid *Peds Birth–13 d.* 0.5 mg/kg q12h *> 14 d & < 30 kg.* 1 mg/kg q12h *≥ 30 kg.* Adult dose; ↓ w/ renal Insuff **W/P:** [C, −] **CI:** Allergy **Disp:** Caps 15, 20, 30, 40 mg; soln 1 mg/mL **SE:** Peripheral neuropathy, HA, chills, rash, GI upset, anemias, lactic acidosis, ↑ LFTs, pancreatitis **Notes:** Take w/ plenty of H₂O

Steroids, Systemic (See Table 2, p 335) The following relates only to the commonly used systemic glucocorticoids **Uses:** *Endocrine disorders (adrenal Insuff), rheumatoid disorders, collagen–vascular Dzs, derm Dzs, allergic states, cerebral edema*, nephritis, nephrotic synd, immunosuppression for transplantation, ↑ Ca²⁺, malignancies (breast, lymphomas), preop (pt who has been on steroids in past year, known hypoadrenalism, preop for adrenalectomy); Inj into jts/tissue **Acts:** Glucocorticoid **Dose:** Varies w/ use & institutional protocols.

- *Adrenal Insuff, acute: Adults. Hydrocortisone:* 100 mg IV, then 300 mg/d ÷ q8h for 48 h, then convert to 50 mg PO q8h × 6 doses, taper to 30–50 mg/d ÷ bid. *Peds. Hydrocortisone:* 1–2 mg/kg IV, then 150–250 mg/d ÷ q6h–q8h
- *Adrenal Insuff, chronic (physiologic replacement):* May need mineralocorticoid supl such as Florinef *Adults. Hydrocortisone:* 20 mg PO q A.M., 10 mg PO q P.M.; *cortisone:* 25–35 mg PO qd *Dexamethasone:* 0.03–0.15 mg/kg/d or 0.6–0.75 mg/m²/d ÷ q6–12h PO, IM, IV *Peds. Hydrocortisone:* 8–10 mg/m²/d ÷ q8h; some may require up to 12 mg/m²/d *Hydrocortisone succinate:* 0.25–0.35 mg/kg/d IM
- *Asthma, acute: Adults. Methylprednisolone:* 40–80 mg/d in 1–2 ÷ dose PO/IV or *dexamethasone* 12 mg IV q6h *Peds. Prednisolone* 1–2 mg/kg/d or *prednisone* 1–2 mg/kg/d ÷ qd-bid for up to 5 d; *methylprednisolone* 12 mg/kg/d IV ÷ bid; *dexamethasone* 0.1–0.3 mg/kg/d ÷ q6h
- *Cerebral edema: Dexamethasone:* 10 mg IV; then 4 mg IV q4–6h
- *Congenital adrenal hyperplasia: Peds.* Initial *hydrocortisone* 10–20 mg/m²/d in 3 ÷ doses
- *Extubation/airway edema: Adults. Dexamethasone:* 0.5–2 mg/kg/d IM/IV ÷ q6h (start 24 h prior to extubation; continue × 4 more doses) *Peds. Dexamethasone:* 0.5–2 mg/kg/d ÷ q6h (start 24 h before & continue for 4–6 doses after extubation)
- *Immunosuppressive/anti-inflam: Adults & Older Peds. Hydrocortisone:* 15–240 mg PO, IM, IV q12h *Methylprednisolone:* 2–60 mg/d PO in 1–4 ÷ doses taper to

lowest effective dose *Methylprednisolone Na succinate:* 10–80 mg/d IM or 10–40 mg/d IV *Adults. Prednisone or prednisolone:* 5–60 mg/d PO ÷ qd-qid *Infants & Younger Children.* Hydrocortisone: 2.5–10 mg/kg/d PO ÷ q6–8h; 1–5 mg/kg/d IM/IV ÷ qd-bid.

* *Nephrotic synd:* **Peds**. *Prednisolone or prednisone:* 2 mg/kg/d PO tid-qid until urine is protein-free for 5 d, use up to 28 d; for persistent proteinuria, 4 mg/kg/dose PO q other day max, 120 mg/d for an additional 28 d; maint 2 mg/kg/dose q other day for 28 d; taper over 4–6 wk (max 80 mg/d)
* *Perioperative steroid coverage:* Hydrocortisone: 100 mg IV night before surgery, 1 h preop, intraoperative; & 4, 8, & 12 h postop; postop d 1 100 mg IV q6h; postop d 2 100 mg IV q8h; postop d 3 100 mg IV q12h; postop d 4 50 mg IV q12h; postop d 5 25 mg IV q12h; resume prior PO dosing if chronic use or D/C if only perioperative coverage required
* *Rheumatic Dz:* Intra-articular: *Hydrocortisone acetate:* 25–37.5 mg large jt, 10–25 mg small jt *Methylprednisolone acetate:* 20–80 mg large jt, 4–10 mg small jt *Intrabursal: Hydrocortisone acetate:* 25–37.5 mg. *Intra-ganglial: Hydrocortisone acetate:* 25–37.5 mg *Tendon sheath: Hydrocortisone acetate:* 5–12.5 mg
* *Status asthmaticus:* **Adults & Peds.** Hydrocortisone: 1–2 mg/kg/dose IV q6h for 24h; then ↓ by 0.5–1 mg/kg q6h

W/P: [C/D, ?] **CI:** Active varicella Infxn, serious Infxn except TB, fungal Infxns **Disp:** See Table 2, p 335 **SE:** ↑ Appetite, hyperglycemia, ↓ K⁺, osteoporosis, nervousness, insomnia, "steroid psychosis," adrenal suppression **Notes:** Hydrocortisone succinate for systemic, acetate for intraarticular; never abruptly D/C steroids, taper dose; also used for bacterial and TB meningitis

Steroids, Topical (See Table 3, p 336) **Uses:** *Steroid-responsive dermatoses (seborrheic/atopic dermatitis, neurodermatitis, anogenital pruritus, psoriasis)* **Acts:** Glucocorticoid; ↓ capillary permeability, stabilizes lysosomes to control inflam; controls protein synth; ↓ migration of leukocytes, fibroblasts **Dose:** Use lowest potency product for shortest period for effect (see Table 3, p 336) **W/P:** [C, +] Do not use occlusive dressings; high potency topical products not for rosacea, perioral dermatitis; not for use on face, groin, axillae; none for use in a diapered area **CI:** Component hypersens **Disp:** See Table 3, p 336 **SE:** Skin atrophy w/ chronic use; chronic administration or application over large area may cause adrenal suppression or hyperglycemia

Streptokinase (Generic) **Uses:** *Coronary artery thrombosis, acute massive PE, DVT, & some occluded vascular grafts* **Acts:** Activates plasminogen to plasmin that degrades fibrin **Dose:** *Adults. PE:* Load 250,000 units peripheral IV over 30 min, then 100,000 units/h IV for 24–72 h *Coronary artery thrombosis:* 1.5 mill units IV over 60 min *DVT or arterial embolism:* Load as w/ PE, then 100,000 units/h for 24 h *ECC 2010. AMI:* 1.5 mill units over 1 h *Peds.* 1000–2000 units/kg over 30 min, then 1000 units/kg/h for up to 24 h *Occluded catheter (controversial):*

10,000–25,000 units in NS to final vol of catheter (leave in for 1 h, aspirate & flush w/ NS) **W/P:** [C, +] **CI:** Streptococcal Infxn or streptokinase in last 6 mo, active bleeding, CVA, TIA, spinal surgery/trauma in last mo, vascular anomalies, severe hepatic/renal Dz, severe uncontrolled HTN **Disp:** Powder for Inj 250,000, 750,000, 1,500,000 units **SE:** Bleeding, ↓ BP, fever, bruising, rash, GI upset, hemorrhage, anaphylaxis **Notes:** If Inf inadequate to keep clotting time 2–5 × control, see PI for adjustments; antibodies remain 3–6 mo following dose

Streptomycin (Generic) **BOX:** Neuro/oto/renal tox possible; neuromuscular blockage w/ resp paralysis possible **Uses:** *TB combo Rx therapy*, streptococcal or enterococcal endocarditis **Acts:** Aminoglycoside; ↓ protein synth **Dose:** **Adults.** IM route. *Endocarditis:* 1 g q12h 1–2 wk, then 500 mg q12h 1–4 wk in combo w/ PCN; *TB:* 15 mg/kg/d (up to 1 g), DOT 2 × wk 20–30 mg/kg/dose (max 1.5 g), DOT 3 × wk 25–30 mg/kg/dose (max 1.5 g) **Peds.** 20–40 mg/kg/d, 1 g/d max; DOT 2 × wk 25–30 mg/kg/d (max 1.5 g max 1g); DOT 3× wk 25–30 mg/kg/dose (max 1.5 g/d); ↓ w/ renal Insuff, either IM (preferred) or IV over 30–60 min **W/P:** [D, –] **CI:** PRG **Disp:** Inj 400 mg/mL (1-g vial) **SE:** ↑ Incidence of vestibular & auditory tox, ↑ neurotox risk in pts w/ impaired renal Fxn **Notes:** Monitor levels: *Peak:* 20–30 mcg/mL; *Trough:* < 5 mcg/mL; *Toxic peak:* > 50 mcg/mL; *Trough:* > 10 mcg/mL

Streptozocin (Zanosar) **BOX:** Administer under the supervision of a physician experienced in the use of chemotherapy; renal tox dose-related/cumulative and may be severe or fatal; other major tox: N/V, may be Tx-limiting; liver dysfunction, D, hematologic changes possible; streptozocin is mutagenic **Uses:** *Pancreatic islet cell tumors*, carcinoid tumors **Acts:** DNA–DNA (intrastrand) cross-linking; DNA, RNA, & protein synth inhib **Dose:** Per protocol; ↓ in renal failure **W/P:** w/ Renal failure [D, –] **CI:** w/ PRG **Disp:** Inj 1 g **SE:** N/V/D, duodenal ulcers, depression, ↓ BM rare (20%) & mild; nephrotox (proteinuria & azotemia dose related), ↑ LFT hypophosphatemia dose limiting; hypoglycemia; Inj site Rxns **Notes:** ✓ SCr

Succimer (Chemet) **Uses:** *Lead poisoning (levels > 50 mcg/dL w/ sig Sxs)* **Acts:** Heavy metal-chelating agent **Dose:** **Adults & Peds.** 10 mg/kg/dose q8h × 5 d, then 10 mg/kg/dose q12h for 14 d **W/P:** [C, ?] w/ Hepatic/renal Insuff **CI:** Allergy **Disp:** Caps 100 mg **SE:** Rash, fever, GI upset, hemorrhoids, metallic taste, drowsiness, ↑ LFTs **Notes:** Monitor lead levels, maintain hydration, may open caps

Succinylcholine (Anectine, Quelicin, Generic) **BOX:** Acute rhabdomyolysis w/ hyperkalemia followed by ventricular dysrhythmias, cardiac arrest, and death; seen in children w/ skeletal muscle myopathy (Duchenne muscular dystrophy) **Uses:** *Adjunct to general anesthesia, facilitates ET intubation; induce skeletal muscle relaxation during surgery or mechanical ventilation* **Acts:** Depolarizing neuromuscular blocker; rapid onset, short duration (3–5 min) **Dose:** **Adults.** Rapid sequence intubation 1–1.5 mg/kg IV over 10–30 s or 3–4 mg/kg IM (up to 150 mg) **(ECC 2010).** **Peds.** 1–2 mg/kg/dose IV, then by 0.3–0.6 mg/kg/dose q5min; ↓ w/ severe renal/hepatic impair **W/P:** See PI [C, ?] **CI:** w/ Malignant hyperthermia risk, myopathy, recent major burn, multiple trauma, extensive skeletal muscle denervation **Disp:** Inj 20, 100 mg/mL **SE:** Fasciculations, ↑ IOP, ↑ ICP, intragastric pressure, salivation, myoglobinuria, malignant hyperthermia, resp depression, prolonged apnea; multiple drugs potentiate CV effects (arrhythmias, ↓ BP, brady/tachycardia) **Notes:** May be given IV push/Inf/IM deltoid

Sucralfate (Carafate, Generic) **Uses:** *Duodenal ulcers*, gastric ulcers, stomatitis, GERD, Px stress ulcers, esophagitis **Acts:** Forms ulcer-adherent complex that protects against acid, pepsin, & bile acid **Dose:** *Adults.* 1 g PO qid, 1 h prior to meals & hs **Peds.** 40–80 mg/kg/d ÷ q6h; continue 4–8 wk unless healing demonstrated by x-ray or endoscopy; separate from other drugs by 2 h; take on empty stomach ac **W/P:** [B, ?] **CI:** Component allergy **Disp:** Tabs 1 g; susp 1 g/10 mL **SE:** Constipation, D, dizziness, xerostomia **Notes:** Al may accumulate in renal failure; do not give w/ tube feeds

Sucroferric Oxyhydroxide (Velphoro) **Uses:** *↓ Phosphate in ESRD/CKD* **Acts:** Binds phosphate **Dose:** Chew 500 mg tid w/ meals; may ↑ dose weekly to target phosphate < 5.5 mg/dL; max dose studied 3000 mg/d **W/P:** [B, +] ✓ Fe^{+2} w/ peritonitis in dialysis; hepatic or GI disorders, post-GI surgery or Dz resulting in Fe^{+2} accumulation **CI:** Ø **Disp:** Tabs 500 mg SE: D, discolored feces **Notes:** DO NOT prescribe with levothyroxine or vit D; take alendronate or doxycycline 1 h before

Sulfacetamide, Ophthalmic (Bleph-10, Cetamide, Klaron, Generic) **Uses:** *Conjunctival Infxns*, topical acne, seborrheic dermatitis **Acts:** Sulfonamide Abx **Dose:** Ophthal soln: 1–2 gtt q2–3 h while awake for 7–10 d; 10% oint apply qid & hs; soln for keratitis apply q2–3h based on severity **W/P:** [C, M] **CI:** Sulfonamide sensitivity; age < 2 mo **Disp:** Opthal: Oint soln 10%; topical cream 10%; foam, gel, lotion, pad all 10% **SE:** Irritation, burning, blurred vision, brow ache, SJS, photosens

Sulfacetamide/Prednisolone (Blephamide, Others) **Uses:** *Steroid-responsive inflam ocular conds w/ Infxn or a risk of Infxn* **Acts:** Abx & anti-inflam **Dose:** *Adults & Peds > 2 y.* Apply oint lower conjunctival sac qd-qid; soln 1–3 gtt q4h while awake **W/P:** [C, ?/–] Sulfonamide sensitivity; age < 2 mo **Disp:** *Oint:* sulfacetamide 10%/prednisolone 0.2%; *Susp:* sulfacetamide 10%/prednisolone 0.2% **SE:** Irritation, burning, blurred vision, brow ache, SJS, photosens **Notes:** OK ophthal susp use as otic agent

Sulfasalazine (Azulfidine, Azulfidine EN, Generic) **Uses:** *UC, RA, juvenile RA* **Acts:** Sulfonamide; actions unclear **Dose:** *Adults. UC:* Initial, 1 g PO tid-qid; ↑ to a max of 4–6 g/d in 4 ÷ doses; maint 500 mg PO qid *RA:* (EC tab) 0.5–1 g/d, ↑ weekly to max 2 g ÷ bid **Peds.** *UC:* Initial: 40–60 mg/kg/24 h PO ÷ q4–6h; maint: 30 mg/kg/24 h PO ÷ q6h *RA > 6 y.* 30–50 mg/kg/24 h in 2 doses, start w/ 1/4–1/3 maint dose, ↑ weekly until dose reached at 1 mo, 2 g/d max **W/P:** [B, M] Not rec w/ renal or hepatic impair **CI:** Sulfonamide or salicylate sensitivity, porphyria, GI or GU obst **Disp:** Tabs 500 mg; EC DR tabs 500 mg **SE:** GI upset; discolors urine; dizziness,

HA, photosens, oligospermia, anemias, SJS **Notes:** May cause yellow-orange skin/contact lens discoloration; avoid sunlight exposure

Sulindac (Clinoril, Generic) BOX: May ↑ risk MI/CVA & GI bleeding; do not use for post-CABG pain control Uses: *Arthritis & pain* Acts: NSAID; ↓ prostaglandins **Dose:** 150–200 mg bid, 400 mg/d max; w/ food W/P: [B (D if 3rd tri or near term), ?] Not rec w/ severe renal impair CI: Allergy to component, ASA or any NSAID, postop pain in CABG Disp: Tabs 150, 200 mg SE: Dizziness, rash, GI upset, pruritus, edema, ↓ renal blood flow, renal failure (? fewer renal effects than other NSAIDs), peptic ulcer, GI bleeding

Sumatriptan (Alsuma, Imitrex, Imitrex Nasal Spray, Imitrex Statdose, Sumavel DosePro, Generic) Uses: *Rx acute migraine and cluster HA* Acts: Vascular serotonin receptor agonist **Dose:** *Adults.* SQ: 6 mg SQ as a single dose PRN; repeat PRN in 1 h to a max of 12 mg/24 h PO: 25–100 mg, repeat in 2 h, PRN, 200 mg/d max Nasal spray: 1 spray into 1 nostril, repeat in 2 h to 40 mg/24 h max *Peds.* Nasal spray: *6–9 y.* 5–20 mg/d. *10–17 y.* 5–20 mg, up to 40 mg/d W/P: [C, ?] CI: IV use, angina, ischemic heart Dz, CV syndromes, PUD, cerebrovascular Dz, uncontrolled HTN, severe hepatic impair, ergot use, MAOI use w/in 14 d, hemiplegic or basilar migraine Disp: Imitrex Oral: OD tabs 25, 50, 100 mg; Imitrex Injection: 4, 6 mg/0.5 mL; ODTs 25, 50, 100 mg; Imitrex Nasal Spray: 5, 20 mg/spray; Alsuma Auto-Injector: 6 mg/0.5 mL SE: Pain & bruising at Inj site; dizziness, hot flashes, paresthesias, CP, weakness, numbness, coronary vasospasm, HTN

Sumatriptan Needleless System (Sumavel DosePro) Uses: *Rx acute migraine and cluster HA* Acts: Vascular serotonin receptor agonist **Dose:** 6 mg SQ as a single dose PRN; repeat PRN in 1 h to a max of 12 mg/24 h; administer in abdomen/thigh W/P: [C, M] CI: See Sumatriptan Disp: Needle-free SQ injector 6 mg/0.5 mL SE: Inj site Rxn, tingling, warm/hot/burning sensation, feeling of heaviness/pressure/tightness/numbness, feeling strange, lightheadedness, flushing, tightness in chest, discomfort in nasal cavity/sinuses/jaw, dizziness/vertigo, drowsiness/sedation, HA

Sumatriptan/Naproxen Sodium (Treximet) BOX: ↑ Risk of serious CVA (MI, stroke) serious GI events (bleeding, ulceration, perforation) of the stomach or intestines Uses: *Px migraines* Acts: Anti-inflam NSAID w/ 5-HT₁ receptor agonist, constricts CNS vessels **Dose:** 1 tab PO; repeat PRN after 2 h; max 2 tabs/24 h, w/ or w/o food W/P: [C, −] CI: CV Dz, severe hepatic impair, severe ↑ BP Disp: Tabs (mg naproxen/mg sumatriptan) 500/85 SE: Dizziness, somnolence, paresthesia, N, dyspepsia, dry mouth, chest/neck/throat/jaw pain, tightness, pressure Notes: Do not split/crush/chew

Sunitinib (Sutent) BOX: Hepatotox that may be severe and/or result in fatal liver failure Uses: *Advanced GIST refractory/intolerant of imatinib; advanced RCC; well-differentiated pancreatic neuroendocrine tumors unresectable, locally advanced, met* Acts: TKI; VEGF inhib **Dose:** *Adults.* 50 mg PO qd × 4 wk, followed by 2 wk holiday = 1 cycle; ↓ to 37.5 mg w/ CYP3A4 inhib (Table 10, p 356), to ↑ 87.5 mg or

62.5 mg/d w/ CYP3A4 inducers **CI:** Ø **W/P:** [D, –] Multiple interactions require dose modification (eg, St. John's wort) **Disp:** Caps 12.5, 25, 50 mg **SE:** ↓ WBC & plt, bleeding, ↑ BP, ↓ ejection fraction, DVT, Szs, adrenal insufficiency, N/V/D, skin discoloration, oral ulcers, taste perversion, hypothyroidism **Notes:** Monitor left ventricular ejection fraction, ECG, CBC/plts, chemistries (K⁺/Mg²⁺/phosphate), TFT & LFTs periodically; ↓ dose in 12.5-mg increments if not tolerated

Suvorexant (Belsomra) **Uses:** *Insomnia* **Acts:** Orexin receptor antag **Dose:** Lowest effective; start 10 mg qhs × 1 30 min before bed w/ at least 7 h before planned awakening; if 10 mg tolerated and ineffective, may ↑ dose **W/P:** [C, M] Daytime somnolence, ↓ alertness, ↓ motor coordination, driving risk; nighttime sleep-driving; ↑ depression/suicidal thoughts; ↓ resp Fxn; sleep paralysis, hallucinations, cataplexy-like Sxs **CI:** Narcolepsy **Disp:** Tabs 5,10, 15, 20 mg **SE:** Somnolence **Notes:** Re-evaluate for comorbid cond if insomnia persists > 7–10 d; w/ concomitant CYP3A inhib, use 5-mg dose; CYP3A inducers may ↓ efficacy; do NOT use w/ severe hepatic impair

Sweet Vernal, Orchard, Perennial Rye, Timothy and Kentucky Blue Grass Mixed Pollens Allergenic Extract (Oralair) **BOX:** Can cause life-threatening allergic Rxn (anaphylaxis, laryngopharyngeal edema); DO NOT use w/ severe uncontrolled/unstable asthma; observe for 30 min after 1st dose; Rx and train to use auto-injectable epi; may not be suitable for pts unresponsive to epi or Inh bronchodilators (pts on β-blockers) or w/ certain conditions that could ↓ ability to respond to severe allergic reaction **Uses:** *Immunotherapy of grass pollen-induced allergic rhinitis w/ or w/o conjunctivitis confirmed by + skin test or pollen-specific IgE Ab* **Acts:** Allergen immunotherapy **Dose:** *Adults.* 300 IR SL × 1/d daily **Peds.** 100 IR SL d 1, 2 × 100 IR SL d 2, and then 300 IR SL qd starting d 3 (NOT approved age < 10 y) **W/P:** [B, ?/–] Discuss severe allergic Rxn; if oral lesions, stop Tx, restart after healed **CI:** Severe uncontrolled/unstable asthma; Hx of severe systemic allergic reaction or severe local reaction to SL allergen immunotherapy; hypersens **Disp:** IR tabs 100, 300 **SE:** Pruritus of mouth, tongue, or ear; mouth/lip edema, throat irritation, oropharyngeal pain, cough **Notes:** 1st dose in healthcare setting; do not eat w/in 5 mins of admin; start Tx 4 mo before expected onset of Sxs; have auto-injectable epi available

Tacrolimus, Extended Release (Astagraf XL) **BOX:** Only physicians experienced in immunosuppression should prescribe; ↑ risk of malignancy; use in liver transplant not rec due to ↑ mortality in female patients **Uses:** *Px kidney transplant rejection w/ MMF and steroids, w/ or w/o basiliximab induction* **Acts:** Calcineurin inhib/immunosuppressant **Dose:** *w/ Basiliximab induction:* 0.15 mg/kg/d (target level d 1–60: 5–17 ng/mL; mo 3–12: 4–12 ng/mL; *w/o induction: Preop:* 0.1 mg/kg/d; *Postop:* 0.2 mg/kg/d (target level: d 1–60: 6–20 ng/mL; mo 3–12: 6–14 ng/mL; take daily q A.M.; empty stomach; do not take w/ alcohol or grapefruit juice; take w/eve food **W/P:** [C, –] Not interchangeable w/ IR; follow glu, Cr,

K+, can ↑ BP, can ↑ QT interval; do not use w/ sirolimus, CYP3A inhib/inducers; avoid live vaccines, monitor for red cell aplasia w/ Cyclosporine; avoid topical if < 2 y; neuro & nephrotox, ↑ risk opportunistic Infxns; avoid grapefruit juice **CI:** Component allergy, castor oil allergy w/ IV form **Disp:** ER caps 0.5, 1, 5 mg **SE:** N/D, constipation, edema, tremor, anemia **Notes:** Monitor levels; African Americans may need ↑ dose; see *Tacrolimus, Immediate Release*

Tacrolimus, Immediate Release (Prograf, Generic) BOX: ↑ Risk of Infxn and lymphoma; only physicians experienced in immunosuppression should prescribe Uses: *Px organ rejection (kidney/liver/heart)* **Acts:** Calcineurin inhib/immunosuppressant **Dose:** *Adults. IV:* 0.03–0.05 mg/kg/d in kidney and liver, 0.01 mg/kg/d in heart IV Inf *Peds. IV:* 0.03–0.05 mg/kg/d as cont Inf *PO:* 0.15–0.2 mg/kg/d PO ÷ q12h *Adults & Peds. Eczema:* Take on empty stomach; ↓ w/ hepatic/renal impair **W/P:** [C, –] w/ Cyclosporine; avoid topical if < 2 y; Neuro & nephrotox, ↑ risk opportunistic Infxns; avoid grapefruit juice **CI:** Component allergy, castor oil allergy w/ IV form **Disp:** Caps 0.5, 1, 5 mg; Inj 5 mg/mL **SE:** HTN, edema, HA, insomnia, fever, pruritus, ↑/↓ K+, hyperglycemia, GI upset, anemia, leukocytosis, tremors, paresthesias, pleural effusion, Szs, lymphoma, PRES, BK nephropathy, PML **Notes:** Monitor levels; *Trough:* 5–12 ng/mL based on indication and time since transplant; see *Tacrolimus, Extended Release*

Tacrolimus, Ointment (Protopic) BOX: Long-term safety of topical calcineurin inhibs not established; avoid long-term use; ↑ risk of Infxn and lymphoma; not for peds < 2yr Uses: *2nd line mod–severe atopic dermatitis* **Acts:** Topical calcineurin inhib/immunosuppressant **Dose:** *Adult & Peds > 15 y.* Apply thin layer (0.03–0.1%) bid; D/C when S/Sxs clear *Peds 2–15 y.* Apply thin layer (0.03%) bid, D/C when S/Sxs clear **W/P:** [C, –] Reevaluate if no response in 6 wk; not for < 2 y; avoid cont long-term use, ↑ risk opportunistic Infxns **CI:** Component allergy **Disp:** Oint 0.03, 0.1% **SE:** Local irritation **Notes:** Avoid occlusive dressing; only use 0.03% in peds

Tadalafil (Adcirca) Uses: *Pulm artery hypertension* **Acts:** PDE5 inhib, ↑ cyclic guanosine monophosphate & NO levels; relaxes pulm artery smooth muscles **Dose:** 40 mg qd w/o regard to meals; ↓ w/ renal/hepatic Insuff **W/P:** [B, –] w/ CV Dz, impaired autonomic control of BP, aortic stenosis α-blockers (except tamsulosin); use w/ CYP3A4 inhib/inducers (eg, ritonavir, ketoconazole); monitor for sudden ↓/loss of hearing or vision (NAION), priapism **CI:** w/ Nitrates, component hypersens **Disp:** Tabs 20 mg **SE:** HA **Notes:** See Tadalafil (*Cialis*) for ED

Tadalafil (Cialis) Uses: *ED, BPH* **Acts:** PDE5 inhib, ↑ cyclic guanosine monophosphate & NO levels; relaxes smooth muscles, dilates cavernosal arteries **Dose:** *Adults. PRN:* 10 mg PO before sexual activity (5–20 mg max based on response), 1 dose/24 h *Daily dosing:* 2.5 mg qd, may ↑ to 5 mg qd *BPH:* 5 mg PO qd; w/o regard to meals; ↓ w/ renal/hepatic Insuff **W/P:** [B, –] w/ α-Blockers (except tamsulosin); use w/ CYP3A4 inhib (Table 10, p 356) (eg, ritonavir, ketoconazole, itraconazole) 2.5 mg qd or 5 mg PRN; CrCl < 30 mL/min, hemodialysis/severe hepatic impair, do not use daily dosing **CI:** CI w/Nitrates & guanylate cyclase stimulators (eg, riociguat) (risk [down arrow] BP) **Disp:** Tabs 2.5, 5, 10, 20 mg **SE:** HA, flushing, dyspepsia, back/limb pain, myalgia, nasal congestion, urticaria, SJS, dermatitis, visual field defect, NAION, sudden ↓/loss of hearing, tinnitus **Notes:** Longest acting of class (36 h); daily dosing may ↑ drug interactions; excessive EtOH may ↑ orthostasis; transient global amnesia reports

Tafluprost (Zioptan) Uses: *Open-angle glaucoma* **Acts:** ↓ IOP by ↑ uveoscleral outflow; prostaglandin analog **Dose:** 1 gtt evening **W/P:** [C, ?/–] **CI:** Ø **Disp:** Soln 0.0015% **SE:** Periorbital/iris pigmentation, eyelash darkening/thickening; ↑ eye redness blurred vision, HA, Cold, Cough, UTI **Notes:** Pigmentation maybe permanent

Talc [Sterile Talc Powder] (Sclerosol, Generic) Uses: *↓ Recurrence of malignant pleural effusions (pleurodesis)* **Acts:** Sclerosing agent **Dose:** Mix slurry: 50 mL NS w/ 5-g vial, mix, distribute 25 mL into two 60-mL syringes, vol to 50 mL/syringe w/ NS. Infuse each into chest tube, flush w/ 25 mL NS. Keep tube clamped; have pt change positions q15min for 2 h, unclamp tube; aerosol 4–8 g intrapleurally **W/P:** [B, ?] **CI:** Planned further surgery on site **Disp:** 5-g powder; (*Sclerosol*) 400 mg/spray **SE:** Pain, Infxn **Notes:** May add 10–20 mL 1% lidocaine/syringe; must have chest tube placed, monitor closely while tube clamped (tension pneumothorax), not antineoplastic

Taliglucerase Alfa (Elelyso) Uses: *Long-term enzyme replacement for type 1 Gaucher Dz* **Acts:** Catalyzes hydrolysis of glucocerebroside to glu & ceramide **Dose:** 60 units/kg IV every other wk; Inf over 1–2 h **W/P:** [B, ?/–] **CI:** Ø **Disp:** Inj 200 units/vial **SE:** Inf Rxns (allergic, HA, CP, asthenia, fatigue, urticaria, erythema, ↑ BP, back pain, arthralgia, flushing), anaphylaxis, URI, pharyngitis, influenza, UTI, extremity pain **Notes:** For Rxns: ↓ Inf rate, give antihistamines/antipyretics or D/C

Tamoxifen (Generic) **BOX:** CA of the uterus or endometrium; stroke, and blood clots can occur Uses: *Breast CA [postmenopausal, estrogen receptor(+)], ↓ risk of breast CA in high-risk, met male breast CA*, ovulation induction **Acts:** Nonsteroidal antiestrogen; mixed agonist–antag effect **Dose:** 20–40 mg/d; doses > 20 mg ÷ bid **Px:** 20 mg PO qd × 5 y **W/P:** [D, –] w/ ↓ WBC, ↓ plts, hyperlipidemia **CI:** PRG, w/ warfarin, Hx thromboembolism **Disp:** Tabs 10, 20 mg **SE:** Uterine malignancy & thrombosis events seen in breast CA prevention trials; menopausal Sxs (hot flashes, N/V) in premenopausal pts; Vag bleeding & menstrual irregularities; skin rash, pruritus vulvae, dizziness, HA, peripheral edema; acute flare of bone met pain & ↑ Ca^{2+}; retinopathy reported (high dose)

Tamsulosin (Flomax, Generic) Uses: *BPH* **Acts:** Prostatic α-receptor antag **Dose:** 0.4 mg/d, may ↑ to 0.8 mg PO qd **W/P:** [B, ?] IFIS w/ cataract surgery **Disp:** Caps 0.4 mg **SE:** HA, dizziness, syncope, somnolence, ↓ libido, GI upset, retrograde ejaculation, rhinitis, rash, angioedema, IFIS **Notes:** Not for use as antihypertensive; do not open/crush/chew; approved for use w/ dutasteride for BPH

Tapentadol (Nucynta) [C-II] **BOX:** Provider should be alert to problems of abuse, misuse, & diversion; avoid use w/ alcohol **Uses:** *Mod–severe acute pain* **Acts:** Mu-opioid agonist and norepinephrine reuptake inhib **Dose:** 50–100 mg PO q4–6h PRN (max 600 mg/d); w/ mod hepatic impair: 50 mg q8h PRN (max 3 doses/24 h) ER dosing: initial 50 mg PO bid (max daily dose 500 mg) **W/P:** [C, –] Hx of Szs, CNS depression; ↑ ICP, severe renal impair, biliary tract Dz, elderly, serotonin synd w/ concomitant serotonergic agents **CI:** ↓ Pulm Fxn, use w/ or w/in 14 d of MAOI, Ileus **Disp:** Tabs 50, 75, 100 mg; tabs ER 50, 100, 150, 200, 250 mg **SE:** N/V, dizziness, somnolence, HA, constipation **Notes:** Taper dose w/ D/C

Tasimelteon (Hetlioz) **Uses:** *Non–24 h sleep–wake disorder* **Acts:** Melatonin agonist at MT_1 & MT_2 receptors **Dose:** 20 mg **W/P:** [C, ?] May cause somnolence and impair performance **CI:** Ø **Disp:** Caps 20 mg **SE:** Somnolence, ↓ attention to task, HA, unusual dreams or nightmares, URI, UTI, ↑ alt **Notes:** Avoid use w/ strong CYP3A4 inhib or inducers; no dose adjustment w/ ESRD or mild to mod hepatic impairment (class sleep aid, insomnia, melatonin-like)

Tavaborole (Kerydin) **Uses:** *Onychomycosis* **Acts:** Oxaborole antifungal *Spectrum: Trichophyton rubrum, Trichophyton mentagrophytes* **Dose:** Apply to affected toenail(s) entire surface and under tip qd × 48 wk **W/P:** [C, ?/–] Local irritation **CI:** Ø **Disp:** Topical soln 5% **SE:** Dermatitis, erythema, exfoliation at application site; ingrown toenails

Tazarotene (Avage, Fabior, Tazorac) **Uses:** *Facial acne vulgaris; stable plaque psoriasis up to 20% BSA* **Acts:** Keratolytic **Dose:** *Adults & Peds > 12 y. Acne:* Cleanse face, dry, apply thin film qhs lesions *Psoriasis:* Apply qhs **W/P:** [X, ?/–] **CI:** Retinoid sensitivity, PRG, use in women of childbearing age unable to comply w/ birth control requirements **Disp:** Gel 0.05, 0.1%; cream 0.05, 0.1%; foam 0.1% **SE:** Burning, erythema, irritation, rash, photosens, desquamation, bleeding, skin discoloration **Notes:** D/C w/ excessive pruritus, burning, skin redness, or peeling until Sxs resolve; external use only, not for broken or sunburned skin

Tedizolid (Sivextro) **Uses:** *ABSSSI; use only in confirmed Infxn to ↓ resistance* **Acts:** Oxazolidinone; bacteriostatic; *Spectrum: S. aureus* (MRSA/MSSA), *S. pyogenes & others, E. faecalis* **Dose:** 200 mg qd PO or IV over 1 h × 6 d **W/P:** [C, +/–] w/ Neutropenia (neutrophils < 1000 cells/mm³); CDAD reported **CI:** Ø **Disp:** Tabs 200 mg; powder for INJ **SE:** N/V/D, HA, dizziness **Notes:** Not approved in peds

Teduglutide [rDNA Origin] (Gattex) **Uses:** *Short bowel synd dependent on parenteral support* **Acts:** GLP-2 analog ↑ intest & portal blood flow & ↓ gastric acid secretion **Dose:** 0.05 mg/kg SQ qd; ↓ 50% w/ mod–severe renal impair; alternate INJ site between Abd, thighs, arms **W/P:** [B, ?/–] Acceleration neoplastic growth (colonoscopy baseline, 1 y, & q5y); D/C w/ intestinal obst; biliary/pancreatic Dz (baseline & q6mo bili, alk phos, lipase, amylase); may ↑ absorption of oral meds **CI:** Ø **Disp:** Inj vial 5 mg **SE:** N/V, Abd pain, Abd distention, Inj site Rxn, HA, URI, fluid overload

Telaprevir (Incivek) Uses: *HCV, genotype 1, w/ compensated liver Dz including naïve to Tx, nonresponders, partial responders, relapsers; w/ peginterferon and ribavirin* Acts: Hep C antiviral; NS3/4A protease inhib Dose: 750 mg tid, w/ food, must be used w/ peginterferon and ribavirin × 12 wk, then peginterferon and ribavirin × 12 wk (if hep C undetectable at 4 and 12 wk) or 36 wk (if hep C detectable at 4 and/or 12 wk) W/P: [X, −] CI: All CIs to peginterferon and ribavirin; men if PRG female partner; w/ CYP3A metabolized drugs (eg, alfuzosin, sildenafil, tadalafil, lovastatin, simvastatin, ergotamines, cisapride, midazolam, rifampin, St. John's wort) Disp: Tabs 375 mg SE: Rash > 50% of pts, include SJS, DRESS; pruritus, anemia, N/V, fatigue, anorectal pain, dysgeusia, hemorrhoids Notes: Must not be used as monotherapy

Telavancin (Vibativ) BOX: Fetal risk; must have PRG test prior to use in childbearing age Uses: *Comp skin/skin structure Infxns d/t susceptible Gram(+) bacteria* Acts: Lipoglycopeptide antibacterial; *Spectrum:* Good gram(+) aerobic and anaerobic include MRSA, MSSA, some VRE; poor gram(−) Dose: 10 mg/kg IV q24h; 7.5 mg/kg q24h w/CrCl 30–50 mL/min; 10 mg/kg q48h w/CrCl 10–30 mL/min W/P: [C, ?] Nephrotox, CDAD, insomnia, HA Dz, ↑ QTc, interferes w/ some coagulation tests CI: Ø Disp: Inj 250, 750 mg SE: Insomnia, psychiatric disorder, taste disturbance, HA, N/V, foamy urine Notes: Contains cyclodextrin, which can accumulate in renal dysfunction

Telbivudine (Tyzeka) BOX: May cause lactic acidosis and severe hepatomegaly w/ steatosis when used alone or w/ antiretrovirals; D/C may lead to exacerbations of hep B; monitor LFTs Uses: *Rx chronic hep B* Acts: Nucleoside RT inhib Dose: *CrCl > 50 mL/min:* 600 mg PO qd; *CrCl 30–49 mL/min:* 600 mg q48h; *CrCl < 30 mL/min:* 600 mg q72h; *ESRD:* 600 mg q96h; dose after hemodialysis W/P: [B, ?/−] May cause myopathy; follow closely w/ other myopathy-causing drugs Disp: Tabs 600 mg SE: Fatigue, Abd pain, N/V/D, HA, URI, nasopharyngitis, ↑ LFTs, CPK, myalgia/myopathy, flu-like Sxs, dizziness, insomnia, dyspepsia Notes: Use w/ PEG-interferon may ↑ peripheral neuropathy risk

Telithromycin (Ketek) BOX: CI in MyG; life-threatening RF occured in PF w/ MyG Uses: *Mild–mod CAP* Acts: Unique macrolide; blocks ↓ protein synth; bactericidal. *Spectrum:* S. aureus, S. pneumoniae, H. influenzae, M. catarrhalis, C pneumoniae, M. pneumoniae Dose: *CAP:* 800 mg (2 tabs) PO qd × 7–10 d W/P: [C, ?] Pseudomembranous colitis, ↑ QTc interval, visual disturbances, hepatic dysfunction; dosing in renal impair unknown CI: Macrolide allergy; w/ pimozide or cisapride, Hx of hep or jaundice; w/ macrolide abx, w/ MyG Disp: Tabs 300, 400 mg SE: N/V/D, dizziness, blurred vision Notes: A CYP450 inhib; multiple drug interactions; hold statins d/t ↑ risk of myopathy

Telmisartan (Micardis, Generic) BOX: Use of renin-angiotensin agents in PRG can cause fetal injury and death, D/C immediately when PRG detected Uses: *HTN, CHF* Acts: Angiotensin II receptor antag Dose: 40–80 mg/d W/P: [C (1st tri, D 2nd & 3rd tri), ?/−] ↑ K⁺ CI: Angiotensin II receptor antag sensitivity Disp: Tabs 20, 40, 80 mg SE: Edema, GI upset, HA, angioedema, renal impair, orthostatic ↓ BP

Telmisartan/Amlodipine (Twynsta) **BOX:** Use of renin-angiotensin agents in PRG can cause fetal injury and death, D/C immediately when PRG detected **Uses:** *Hypertension* **Acts:** CCB; relaxes coronary vascular smooth muscle & angiotensin II receptor antag **Dose:** Start 40/5 mg telmisartan/amlodipine; max 80/10 mg PO/d; ↑ dose after 2 wk **W/P:** [C 1st tri; D 2nd, 3rd; ?/–] ↑ K+ **CI:** PRG **Disp:** Tabs (mg telmisartan/mg amlodipine) 40/5, 40/10, 80/5, 80/10 **SE:** HA, edema, dizziness, N, ↓ BP **Notes:** Titrate w/ hepatic/renal impair; avoid w/ ACE/other ARBs; correct hypovolemia before; w/ CHF monitor

Temazepam (Restoril, Generic) [C-IV] **Uses:** *Insomnia*, anxiety, depression, panic attacks **Acts:** Benzodiazepine **Dose:** 15–30 mg PO hs PRN; ↓ in elderly **W/P:** [X, ?/–] Potentiates CNS depressive effects of opioids, barbs, EtOH, antihistamines, MAOIs, TCAs **CI:** NAG, PRG **Disp:** Caps 7.5, 15, 22.5, 30 mg **SE:** Confusion, dizziness, drowsiness, hangover **Notes:** Abrupt D/C after > 10 d use may cause withdrawal

Temozolomide (Temodar, Generic) **Uses:** *GBM, refractory anaplastic astrocytoma* **Acts:** Alkylating agent **Dose:** *GBM, new:* 75 mg/m^2 PO/IV/d × 42 d w/ RT, maint 150 mg/m^2/d 1–5 of 28-d cycle × 6 cycles; may ↑ to 200 mg/m^2/d × 5 d every 28 d in cycle 2; *Refractory astrocytoma:* 150 mg/m^2 PO/IV/d × 5 d per 28-d cycle; Adjust dose based on ANC and plt count (per PI and local protocols) **W/P:** [D, ?/–] w/ Severe renal/hepatic impair, myelosuppression (monitor ANC & plt), myelodysplastic synd, secondary malignancies, PCP pneumonia (PCP prophylaxis required) **CI:** Hypersens to components or dacarbazine **Disp:** Caps 5, 20, 100, 140, 180, & 250 mg; powder for Inj 100 mg **SE:** N/V/D, fatigue, HA, asthenia, Sz, hemiparesis, fever, dizziness, coordination abnormality, alopecia, rash, constipation, anorexia, amnesia, insomnia, hepatotox viral Infxn, ↓ WBC, ↓ plt **Notes:** Infuse over 90 min; swallow caps whole; if caps open avoid Inh and contact w/ skin/mucous membranes

Temsirolimus (Torisel) **Uses:** *Advanced RCC* **Acts:** Multikinase inhib, ↓ mTOR, ↓ hypoxic-induced factors, ↓ VEGF **Dose:** 25 mg IV over 30–60 min 1×/wk. Hold w/ ANC < 1000/mm^3 plt < 75,000/mm^3 or NCI grade 3 tox. Resume when tox grade 2 or less, restart w/ dose ↓ 5 mg/wk not < 15 mg/wk. w/ CYP3A4 inhib: ↓ 12.5 mg/wk. w/ CYP3A4 inducers: ↑ 50 mg/wk **W/P:** [D, –] Avoid live vaccines, ↓ wound healing, avoid periop, hypersens Rxn **CI:** Bili > 1.5 × ULN **Disp:** Inj 25 mg/mL w/ 250 mL diluent **SE:** Rash, asthenia, mucositis, N, bowel perf, angioedema, impaired wound healing; interstitial lung Dz anorexia, edema, ↑ lipids, ↑ glu, ↑ triglycerides, ↑ LFTs, ↑ Cr, ↓ WBC, ↓ HCT, ↓ plt, ↓ PO$_4$ **Notes:** Premedicate w/ antihistamine; ✓ lipids, CBC, plt, Cr, glu; w/ sunitinib dose-limiting tox likely; females use w/ contraception

Tenecteplase (TNKase) **Uses:** *Restore perfusion & ↓ mortality w/ AMI* **Acts:** Thrombolytic; TPA **Dose:** 30–50 mg; see table below **W/P:** [C, ?], ↑ Bleeding w/ NSAIDs, ticlopidine, clopidogrel, GPIIb/IIIa antags **CI:** Bleeding, AVM aneurysm, CVA, CNS neoplasm, uncontrolled ↑ BP, major surgery (intracranial, intraspinal) or trauma w/in 2 mo **Disp:** Inj 50 mg, reconstitute w/ 10 mL sterile H_2O only **SE:** Bleeding, allergy **Notes:** Do not shake w/ reconstitution; start ASA ASAP, IV heparin ASAP w/ aPTT 1.5–2 × UL of control

Tenecteplase Dosing (From 1 vial of reconstituted TNKase)

Weight (kg)	TNKase (mg)	TNKase Volume (mL)
< 60	30	6
60–69	35	7
70–79	40	8
80–89	45	9
≥ 90	50	10

Tenofovir (Viread) **BOX:** Lactic acidosis/hepatomegaly w/ steatosis (some fatal) reported w/ use of NRTIs; exacerbations of hep reported w/ HBV pts who D/C hep B Rx, including Viread; ✓ LFTs in these pts, may need to resume hep B Rx **Uses:** *HIV & chronic hep B Infxn* **Acts:** NRTI & HBV RT inhib **Dose:** *Adults & Peds > 12 y, > 35 kg*. 300 mg PO qd w/ or w/o food *Adults w/ renal impair*. CrCl 30–49 mL/min: 300 mg q48h; CrCl 10–29 mL/min q72–96h; hemodialysis: 300 mg q7d *Peds 2–12 y, > 17 kg, can swallow tabs*. 150, 200, 250, or 300 mg based on BW PO qd; powder: 8 mg/kg PO qd w/food (max 300 mg) **W/P:** [B, –] May ↓ renal Fxn; do not give w/ other tenofovir products; caution w/ didanosine; HIV test before HBV Rx; ↓ BMD; redistribution of body fat, immune reconstitution synd **CI:** Ø **Disp:** Tabs 150, 200, 250, 300 mg; oral powder 40 mg/g **SE:** Rash, N/D, HA, pain, depression, asthenia **Notes:** Combo product w/ emtricitabine is *Truvada*

Tenofovir/Emtricitabine (Truvada) **BOX:** Lactic acidosis/hepatomegaly w/ steatosis (some fatal) reported w/ the use of NRTI; not approved for chronic hep B; exacerbations of hepatitis reported w/ HBV pts who D/C *Truvada*; may need to resume hep B Rx; if used for PrEP, confirm (–) HIV before and q3mo; drug-resistant HIV-1 variants have been identified **Uses:** *HIV Infxn PrEP for HIV-1* **Acts:** Dual nucleotide RT inhib **Dose:** 1 tab PO qd w/ or w/o a meal; adjust w/ renal impair **W/P:** [B, ?/–] w/ Known risk factors for liver Dz **CI:** Ø **Disp:** Tabs: 200 mg emtricitabine/300 mg tenofovir **SE:** GI upset, rash, metabolic synd, hepatotox; Fanconi synd; OK in peds > 12 y

Terazosin (Generic) **Uses:** *BPH & HTN* **Acts:** α_1-Blocker (blood vessel & bladder neck/prostate) **Dose:** Initial, 1 mg PO hs; ↑ 20 mg/d max; may ↓ w/ diuretic or other BP medicine **W/P:** [C, ?] w/ β-Blocker, CCB, ACE inhib; use w/ PDE5 inhib (eg, sildenafil) can cause ↓ BP, IFIS w/ cataract surgery **CI:** α-Antag sensitivity **Disp:** Tabs 1, 2, 5, 10 mg; caps 1, 2, 5, 10 mg **SE:** Angina, ↓ BP, syncope following 1st dose or w/ PDE5 inhib; dizziness, weakness, nasal congestion, peripheral edema, palpitations, GI upset **Notes:** Caution w/ 1st dose syncope; if for HTN, combine w/ thiazide diuretic

Terbinafine (Lamisil, Lamisil AT, Generic) [OTC] Uses: *Onychomycosis, athlete's foot, jock itch, ringworm*, cutaneous candidiasis, pityriasis versicolor **Acts:** ↓ Squalene epoxidase resulting in fungal death **Dose:** *PO:* 250 mg/d PO for 6–12 wk *Topical:* Apply to area tinea pedis bid, tinea cruris & corporus qd-bid, tinea versicolor soln bid; ↓ PO in renal/hepatic impair **W/P:** [B, –] PO ↑ effects of drug metabolism by CYP2D6, w/ liver/renal impair **CI:** CrCl < 50 mL/min, WBC < 1000/mm³, severe liver Dz **Disp:** Tabs 250 mg; oral granules 125 mg/pkt, 187.5 mg/pkt *Lamisil AT* [OTC] cream, gel, soln 1% **SE:** HA, N/V/D, dizziness, rash, pruritus, alopecia, GI upset, taste perversion, neutropenia, retinal damage, SJS, ↑ LFTs **Notes:** Effect may take months d/t need for new nail growth; topical not for nails; do not use occlusive dressings; PO follow CBC/LFTs; give granules w/ non-acidic food

Terbutaline (Generic)   BOX: Not approved and should not be used > 48–72h for tocolysis; serious adverse Rxns possible, including death **Uses:** *Reversible bronchospasm (asthma, COPD); inhib labor* **Acts:** Sympathomimetic; tocolytic **Dose:** *Adults. Bronchodilator:* 2.5–5 mg PO qid or 0.25 mg SQ; repeat in 15 min PRN; max 0.5 mg SQ in 4 h; max 15 mg/24 h PO *Premature labor:* 0.25 mg SQ every 1–4 h × 24 h, 5 mg max/24 h; 2.5–5 mcg/min IV, ↑ 5 mcg/min q10min as tolerated, 25 mcg/min max; when controlled ↓ to lowest effective dose; SQ pump: basal 0.05–0.10 mg/h, bolus over 25 mg PRN *Peds. PO:* 0.05–0.15 mg/kg/ dose PO tid; max 5 mg/24 h; ↓ in renal failure **W/P:** [B, +] ↑ Tox w/ MAOIs, TCAs; DM, HTN, hyperthyroidism, CV Dz, convulsive disorders, K⁺ **CI:** Component allergy, prolonged tocolysis **Disp:** Tabs 2.5, 5 mg; Inj 1 mg/mL **SE:** HTN, hyperthyroidism, β₁-adrenergic effects w/ high dose, nervousness, trembling, tachycardia, arrhythmia, HTN, dizziness, ↑ glu **Notes:** Tocolysis requires close monitoring of mother and fetus

Terconazole (Terazol 3, Terazol 7, Zazole, Generic) Uses: *Vulvo-Vag candidiasis* **Acts:** Topical triazole antifungal **Dose:** 1 applicatorful or 1 supp intravag hs × 3 d **W/P:** [C, ?] **CI:** Component allergy **Disp:** Vag cream (*Terzsol 7*) 0.4%, (*Terzsol 3, Zazole*) 0.8%; Vag supp (*Terzsol 3*) 80 mg **SE:** Vulvar/Vag burning **Notes:** Insert high into Vag

Teriflunomide (Aubagio)   BOX: Hepatotox; ✓ LFT baseline & ALT qmo × 6 mo; D/C w/ liver injury & begin accelerated elimination procedure; CI in PRG & women of childbearing potential w/o reliable contraception Uses: *Relapsing MS* **Acts:** Pyrimidine synth inhib **Dose:** 7 or 14 mg PO qd **W/P:** [X, –] w/ CYP2C8, CYP1A2 metabolizing drugs, warfarin, ethinylestradiol, levonorgestrel; ↑ elimination w/ cholestyramine or activated charcoal × 11 d; **CI:** PRG; severe hepatic impair; w/leflunomide **Disp:** Tabs 7, 14 mg **SE:** ↑ ALT, alopecia, N/D, influenza, paresthesia, ↓ WBC, neuropathy, ↑ BP, SJS, TEN, ARF, ↑ K⁺ **Notes:** ✓ CBC & TB screen prior to Rx; ✓ BP, S/Sxs of Infxn; do not give w/ live vaccines

Teriparatide (Forteo) **BOX:** ↑ Osteosarcoma risk in animals; use only where potential benefits outweigh risks **Uses:** *Severe/refractory osteoporosis* **Acts:** PTH (recombinant) **Dose:** 20 mcg SQ qd in thigh or Abd **W/P:** [C, –]; Caution in urolithiasis **Disp:** 250 mcg/mL in 2.4-mL prefilled syringe **SE:** Orthostatic ↓ BP on administration, N/D, ↑ Ca²⁺; leg cramps, ↑ uric acid **Notes:** 2 y max use

Tesamorelin (Egrifta) **Uses:** *↑↓ Excess Abd fat in HIV-infected pts w/ lipodystrophy* **Acts:** Binds/stimulates growth hormone-releasing factor receptors **Dose:** 2 mg SQ/d **W/P:** [X; HIV-infected mothers should not breast-feed] **CI:** Hypothalamic-pituitary axis disorders; hypersen to tesamorelin, mannitol, or any component, head radiation/trauma; malignancy; PRG; child w/ open epiphyses **Disp:** Vial 1 mg **SE:** Arthralgias, Inj site Rxn, edema, myalgia, ↑ glu, N/V **Notes:** ✓ Glu, ? ↑ mortality w/ acute critical illness; ↑ IGF

Testosterone, Implant (Testopel) [C-III] **Uses:** *Male hypogonadism (congenital/acquired)* **Acts:** Testosterone replacement **Dose:** 150–450 mg (2–6 pellets) SQ implant q3–6mo (implant two 75-mg pellets for each 25 mg testosterone required weekly; eg: for 75 mg/wk, implant 450 mg or 6 pellets) **W/P:** [X, –] May cause polycythemia, worsening of BPH Sxs, PCa, edema may worsen CHF; may ↓ blood glu and insulin requirements; venous thrombosis risk **CI:** PCa, male breast CA, PRG women **Disp:** 75 mg/implant (3.2 mm × 9 mm) **SE:** Pain/inflam at site, gynecomastia, excessive erections, oligospermia, hirsutism, male pattern baldness, acne, retention of sodium and electrolytes, suppression of clotting factors, polycythemia, N, jaundice, ↑ LFT/cholesterol, rare hepatocellular neoplasms and peliosis hepatitis, ↑/↓ libido, sleep apnea, ↑ PSA, may ↑ CV risk **Notes:** ✓ Levels and adjust PRN (300–1000 ng/dL testosterone range); follow periodic LFT and CBC; typical site upper outer posterior gluteal region using sterile technique, local anesthesia, 4-mm stab wound and provided 16-gauge insertion trocar

Testosterone, Nasal Gel (Natesto) [C-III] **BOX:** Virilization reported in children exposed to topical testosterone products; children to avoid contact w/ unwashed or unclothed application sites **Uses:** *Adult male hypogonadism (congenital/ acquired)* **Acts:** Testosterone replacement **Dose:** 11 mg (2 pumps) in 1 nostril tid (total 33 mg/d); blow nose before use; avoid blowing for 1 h after **W/P:** [X, –] Avoid with nasal pathology; monitor BPH Sxs and for DVT; may cause azoospermia, edema, sleep apnea; not rec if < 18 y; venous thrombosis risk, may ↑ CV risk **CI:** PCa, male breast cancer, women **Disp:** Metered-dose pump; one pump = 5.5 mg of testosterone **SE:** ↑ PSA, HA, rhinorrhea, epistaxis, nasal discomfort, nasopharyngitis, bronchitis, URI, sinusitis, nasal scab **Notes:** Previously known as *CompleoTRT*; may minimize exposure of testosterone to women or children; ✓ testosterone, PSA, Hgb, LFTs, and lipids periodically

Testosterone, Topical (Androderm, AndroGel 1%, AndroGel 1.62%, Axiron, Fortesta, Striant, Testim, Vogelxo, Generic) [C-III] **BOX:** Virilization reported in children exposed to topical testosterone products; children to avoid contact w/ unwashed or unclothed application sites **Uses:** *Male hypogonadism (congenital/acquired)* **Acts:** Testosterone replacement; ↑ lean body mass, libido **Dose:** All daily applications: *AndroGel 1%:* 50 mg (4 pumps); *AndroGel 1.62%:* 40.5 mg (2 pumps), apply to clean skin on upper body only; *Androderm:* 2- or 4-mg patch qhs; *Axiron:* 60 mg (1 pump = 30 mg each axilla) qA.M.; *Fortesta:* 40 mg (4 pumps) on clean, dry thighs; adjust from 1–7 pumps based on blood test 2 h after (d 14 and 35); *Striant:* 30-mg buccal tabs bid; *Testim:* 50-mg gel; *Vogelxo:* 50 mg (one tube or packet or 4 pump actuations) qd at same time **W/P:** [X, –] May cause polycythemia, worsening of BPH Sx, edema, azoospermia, sleep apnea, DVT, may ↑ CV risk **CI:** PCa, male breast CA, women, venous thrombosis risk **Disp:** *AndroGel 1%:* 12.5-mg/pump; *AndroGel 1.62%:* 20.25-mg/pump; *Androderm:* 2, 4 mg patches; *Axiron:* Metered-dose pump 30-mg/pump; *Fortesta:* Metered-dose gel pump 10-mg/pump; *Striant:* 30-mg buccal tab; *Vogelxo:* 50-mg tube or packet, 12.5-mg/pump **SE:** Site Rxns, acne, edema, Wt gain, gynecomastia, HTN, ↑ sleep apnea, prostate enlargement, ↑ PSA **Notes:** PO agents (*methyltestosterone & oxandrolone*) associated w/ hepatic tumors; transdermal/mucosal/implant forms preferred; wash hands immediately after topical applications; *AndroGel* formulations not equivalent; ✓ T levels and adjust PRN (300–1000 ng/dL testosterone range)

Testosterone Undecanoate, Inj (Aveed) [C-III] **BOX:** POME Rxns (urge to cough, dyspnea, throat tightening, chest pain, dizziness, syncope) and episodes of anaphylaxis, including life-threatening Rxns, have been reported after administration; observe pts for 30 min after dosing **Uses:** *Male hypogonadism (congenital/ acquired)* **Acts:** Testosterone replacement; ↑ lean body mass, libido **Dose:** 3 mL (750 mg) IM (gluteal) initially, at 4 wk, every 10 wk thereafter; observe for 30 min for POME or anaphylaxis **W/P:** [X, –] May worsen BPH Sx, azoospermia possible, edema w/ pre-existing cardiac/renal/hepatic Dz, sleep apnea w/ other risk factors, monitor PSA, Hgb/Hct, lipids periodically; may reduce insulin requirements, monitor INR if on warfarin; w/ steriods may ↑ fluid retention; venous thrombosis risk may ↑ CV risk **CI:** PCa, male breast cancer, women, component sens **Disp:** 3-mL (750 mg) in castor oil and benzyl benzoate **SE:** Acne, Inj site pain, ↑ PSA and estradiol, hypogonadism, fatigue, irritability, ↑ hemoglobin, insomnia, mood swings **Notes:** Available only through a restricted program (Aveed REMS); other IM forms not commonly used: testosterone enanthate (*Delatestryl; Testro-L.A.*) & cypionate (*Depo-Testosterone*) dosed q14–28d w/ variable serum levels

Tetanus Immune Globulin (HyperTET S/D, Generic) **Uses:** Prophylaxis *passive tetanus immunization* (suspected contaminated wound w/ unknown immunization status, see Table 7, p 352), or Tx of tetanus **Acts:** Passive immunization **Dose:** *Adults & Peds.* Prophylaxis: 250 mg units IM × 1; *Tx:* 500–6000 (30–300 units/kg) units IM **W/P:** [C, ?] Anaphylaxis Rxn **CI:** Thimerosal sensitivity **Disp:** Inj 250-unit vial/syringe **SE:** Pain, tenderness, erythema at site; fever, angioedema **Notes:** May begin active immunization series at different Inj site if required

Tetanus Toxoid (TT) (Generic) Uses: *Tetanus prophylaxis* Acts: Active immunization Dose: Based on previous immunization, Table 7, p 352 W/P: [C, ?/–] CI: Thimersal hypersens neurologic Sxs w/ previous use, active Infxn w/ routine primary immunization Disp: Inj TT fluid, 5 Lf units/0.5 mL; TT adsorbed, 5 units/0.5 mL SE: Inj site erythema, induration, sterile abscess; arthralgias, fever, malaise, neurologic disturbances Notes: DTaP rather than TT for all adults 19–64 y who have not previously received 1 dose of DTaP (protection adult pertussis); also use DT or Td instead of TT to maintain diphtheria immunity; if IM, use only preservative-free Inj; do not confuse TD (for adults) w/ DT (for children)

Tetrabenazine (Xenazine) BOX: ↑ Risk of depression, suicide w/ Huntington Dz Uses: *Rx chorea in Huntington Dz* Acts: Monoamine depleter Dose: 25–100 mg/d ÷ doses; 12.5 mg PO qd × 1 wk, ↑ to 12.5 mg bid, may ↑ to 12.5 mg tid if > 37.5 mg/d tid after 1 wk; if > 50 mg needed, ✓ for CYP2D6 gene; if poor metabolizer, 25 mg/dose, 50 mg/d max; extensive/indeterminate metabolizer 37.5 mg dose max, 100 mg/d max W/P: [C, ?/–] 1/2 dose w/ strong CYP2D6 inhib 50 mg/d max (paroxetine, fluoxetine) CI: Want 20 d after reserpine D/C before use, suicidality, untreated or inadequately treated depression; hepatic impair; w/ MOAI or reserpine Disp: Tabs 12.5, 25 mg SE: Sedation, insomnia, depression, anxiety, irritability, akathisia, Parkinsonism, balance difficulties, NMS, fatigue, N/V, dysphagia, ↑ QT, EPS Szs, falls

Tetracycline (Generic) Uses: *Broad-spectrum Abx* Acts: Bacteriostatic; ↓ protein synth. *Spectrum:* Gram(+): *Staphylococcus, Streptococcus.* Gram(–): *H. pylori.* Atypicals: *Chlamydia, Rickettsia,* & *Mycoplasma* Dose: **Adults.** 250–500 mg PO bid-qid *Peds > 8 y.* 25–50 mg/kg/24 h PO ÷ q6–12h; ↓ w/ renal/hepatic impair, w/o food preferred W/P: [D, –] CI: PRG, children < 8 y Disp: Caps 250, 500 mg; SE: Photosens, GI upset, renal failure, pseudotumor cerebri, hepatic impair Notes: Can stain tooth enamel & depress bone formation in children; do not administer w/ antacids or milk products

Thalidomide (Thalomid) BOX: Restricted use; use associated w/ severe birth defects and ↑ risk of venous thromboembolism Uses: *Erythema nodosum leprosum ENL, multiple myeloma, GVHD, aphthous ulceration in HIV(+)* Acts: ↓ Neutrophil chemotaxis, ↓ monocyte phagocytosis Dose: *GVHD:* 50–100 tid, max 600–1200 mg/d *Multiple myeloma:* 200 mg qhs w/ dexamethasone *Stomatitis:* 200 mg bid for 5 d, then 200 mg qd up to 8 wk *Erythema nodosum leprosum:* 100–300 mg PO qhs W/P: [X, –] May ↑ HIV viral load; Hx Szs CI: PRG or females not using 2 forms of contraception Disp: 50, 100, 150, 200 mg Caps SE: Dizziness, drowsiness, rash, fever, orthostasis, SJS, thrombosis, fatigue, peripheral neuropathy, Szs Notes: MD must register w/ STEPS risk-management program; informed consent necessary; immediately D/C if rash develops

Theophylline (Elixophylline, Theo-24, Theolair, Uniphyl, Generic) Uses: *Asthma, bronchospasm* Acts: Bronchodilator & suppression of airways to stimuli Dose: For IV administration, see PI for dose based on age, smoking status, & serum levels *Adults.* 300–600 mg/d PO ÷ q6–8h IR; ER products ÷ qd-bid *Peds.* 12–20 mg/kg/24 h PO ÷ q6h; ER products ÷ qd-bid; ↓ in hepatic failure **W/P:** [C, +] Multiple interactions (eg, caffeine, smoking, carbamazepine, barbiturates, β-blockers, ciprofloxacin, E-mycin, INH, loop diuretics), arrhythmia, hyperthyroidism, uncontrolled Szs **CI:** Component hypersens **Disp:** Elixir 80 mg/15 mL; soln 80 mg/15 mL; ER 12-h caps 300 mg; ER 12-h tabs 100, 200, 300, 480 mg; ER 24-h caps 100, 200, 300, 400 mg; ER 24-h tabs 400, 600 mg; IV soln **SE:** N/V, tachycardia, Szs, nervousness, arrhythmias **Notes:** IV levels: ✓ IV levels 12–24 h after Inf started; *Therapeutic:* 5–15 mcg/mL; *Toxic:* > 20 mcg/mL; PO levels: *Trough:* just before next dose; *Therapeutic:* 5–15 mcg/mL

Thiamine [Vitamin B₁] (Generic) **Uses:** *Thiamine deficiency (beriberi), alcoholic neuritis, Wernicke encephalopathy* **Acts:** Dietary supl **Dose:** *Adults. Deficiency:* 5–30 mg IM or IV TID, then 5–30 mg/d PO for 1 mo *Wernicke encephalopathy:* 100 mg IV single dose, then 100 mg/d IM for 2 wk *Peds.* 10–25 mg/d IM for 2 wk, then 5–10 mg/24 h PO for 1 mo **W/P:** [A, +] **CI:** Component allergy **Disp:** Tabs 50, 100, 250, 500 mg; Inj 100 mg/mL **SE:** Angioedema, paresthesias, rash, anaphylaxis w/ rapid IV **Notes:** IV use associated w/ anaphylactic Rxn; give IV slowly

Thioguanine (Tabloid) **Uses:** *AML, ALL, CML* **Acts:** Purine-based antimetabolite (substitutes for natural purines interfering w/ nucleotide synth) **Dose:** *Adults.* 2–3 mg/kg/d *Peds.* 60 mg/m²/d for 14 d; no renal adjustment in peds; D/C if pt develops jaundice, VOD, portal hypertension; ↓ in severe renal/hepatic impair **W/P:** [D, –] **CI:** Resistance to mercaptopurine **Disp:** Tabs 40 mg **SE:** ↓ BM (leukopenia/thrombocytopenia), N/V/D, anorexia, stomatitis, rash, hyperuricemia, rare hepatotox

Thioridazine (Generic) **BOX:** Dose-related QTc prolongation; elderly pts w/ dementia-related psychosis & pts treated w/ antipsychotics are at an ↑ risk of death **Uses:** *Schizophrenia*, psychosis **Acts:** Phenothiazine antipsychotic **Dose:** *Adults.* Initial, 50–100 mg PO tid; maint 200–800 mg/24 h PO in 2–4 ÷ doses *Peds > 2 y.* 0.5–3 mg/kg/24 h PO in 2–3 ÷ doses **W/P:** [C, ?] Phenothiazines, QTc-prolonging agents, AI **CI:** Phenothiazine sensitivity, severe CNS depression, severe ↑/↓ BP, heart DZ, coma, combo w/ drugs that prolong QTc or CYPZD6 inhib; pt w/ congenital prolonged QTc or Hx cardiac arrhythmia **Disp:** Tabs 10, 15, 25, 50, 100 mg **SE:** Low incidence of EPS; ventricular arrhythmias; ↓ Szs, dizziness, drowsiness, NMS, Szs, skin discoloration, photosens, constipation, sexual dysfunction, blood dyscrasias, pigmentary retinopathy, hepatic impair **Notes:** Avoid EtOH

Thiothixene (Generic) **BOX:** Not for dementia-related psychosis; increased mortality risk in elderly pts on antipsychotics **Uses:** *Psychosis* **Acts:** ? May antagonize DA receptors **Dose:** *Adults & Peds > 12 y. Mild–mod psychosis:* 2 mg PO tid, up to 20–30 mg/d *Rapid tranquilization for agitated pts:* 5–10 mg q30–60 min; avg: 15–30 mg total *Severe psychosis:* 5 mg PO bid; ↑ to max of 60 mg/24 h PRN. *Peds < 12 y.* 0.25 mg/kg/24 h PO ÷ q6–12h **W/P:** [C, ?] Avoid w/ ↑ QT interval or meds that can ↑ QT **CI:** Severe CNS depression; circulatory collapse; blood dyscrasias, phenothiazine sensitivity **Disp:** Caps 1, 2, 5, 10 mg **SE:** Drowsiness, EPS most common; ↓ BP, dizziness, drowsiness, NMS, Szs, skin discoloration, photosens, constipation, sexual dysfunction, leukopenia, neutropenia and agranulocytosis, pigmented retinopathy, hepatic impair

Tiagabine (Gabitril, Generic) Uses: *Adjunct in partial Szs*, bipolar disorder **Acts:** Antiepileptic, enhances activity of GABA **Dose:** *Adults & Peds ≥ 12 y.* (*Dose if already on enzyme-inducing AED; use lower dose if not on AED*) Initial 4 mg/d PO, ↑ by 4 mg during 2nd wk; ↑ PRN by 4–8 mg/d based on response, 56 mg/d max; take w/ food **W/P:** [C, −] May ↑ suicidal risk **CI:** Component allergy **Disp:** Tabs 2, 4, 12, 16 mg **SE:** Dizziness, HA, somnolence, memory impair, tremors, N **Notes:** Use gradual withdrawal; used in combo w/ other anticonvulsants

Ticagrelor (Brilinta) BOX: ↑ Bleeding risk; can be fatal; daily aspirin > 100 mg may ↓ effectiveness; do not start w/ active bleeding, Hx intracranial bleeding, planned CABG; if hypotensive and recent procedure, suspect bleeding; manage any bleeding w/o D/C of ticagrelor Uses: *↓ CV death and heart attack in ACS* **Acts:** Oral antiplatelet; reversibly binding ADP receptor antag inhib **Dose:** Initial 180 mg PO w/ ASA 325 mg, then 90 mg bid w/ ASA 75–100 mg/d **W/P:** [C, −]w/ Mod hepatic impair; w/ strong CYP3A inhib or CYP3A inducers **CI:** Hx intracranial bleeding, active pathologic bleeding, severe hepatic impair **Disp:** Tabs 90 mg **SE:** Bleeding, SOB **Notes:** REMS program in place; D/C 5 days preop

Tigecycline (Tygacil, Generic) BOX: Mortality ↑ in pts treated w/ Tygacil; reserve use when alternatives not suitable Uses: *Rx complicated skin & soft-tissue Infxns & complicated intra-Abd Infxns* **Acts:** A glycycline; binds 30 S ribosomal subunits, ↓ protein synthesis; *Spectrum:* Broad gram(+), gram(−), anaerobic, some mycobacterial; *E. coli, E. faecalis* (vancomycin-susceptible isolates), *S. aureus* (methicillin-susceptible/resistant), *Streptococcus* (*agalactiae, anginosus* grp, *pyogenes*), *Citrobacter freundii, Enterobacter cloacae, B. fragilis* group, *C. perfringens, Peptostreptococcus* **Dose:** 100 mg × 1, then 50 mg q12h IV over 30–60 min **W/P:** [D, ?] Hepatic impair, monotherapy w/ intestinal perf, not OK in peds; w/ tetracycline allergy **CI:** Component sens **Disp:** Inj 50-mg vial **SE:** N/V, Inj site Rxn, anaphylaxis **Notes:** Not indicated for HAP, VAP (↑ mortality for VAP), bacteremia

Timolol (Generic) BOX: Exacerbation of ischemic heart Dz w/ abrupt D/C Uses: *HTN & MI* **Acts:** β-Adrenergic receptor blocker, β₁, β₂ **Dose:** *HTN:* 10–20 mg bid, up to 60 mg/d *MI:* 10 mg bid **W/P:** [C (1st tri; D if 2nd or 3rd tri), +] **CI:** CHF, cardiogenic shock, ↓ HR, heart block, COPD, asthma **Disp:** Tabs 5, 10, 20 mg **SE:** Sexual dysfunction, arrhythmia, dizziness, fatigue, CHF

Timolol, Ophthalmic (Betimol, Istalol, Timoptic, Timoptic XE, Generic) Uses: *Glaucoma* **Acts:** β-Blocker **Dose:** 0.25% 1 gtt bid; ↓ to qd when controlled; use 0.5% if needed; 1-gtt/d gel **W/P:** [C, ?/+] **Disp:** Soln 0.25/0.5%; *Timoptic XE* (0.25, 0.5%) gel-forming soln; *Istalol* 05% soln **SE:** Local irritation

Timothy Grass Pollen Allergen Extract (Grastek) BOX: Can cause life-threatening allergic Rxn (anaphylaxis, laryngopharyngeal edema); DO NOT use w/ severe unstable/uncontrolled asthma; observe for 30 min after 1st dose; Rx and train to use auto-injectable epi; may not be suitable for pts unresponsive to epi or Inh bronchodilators (pts on β-blockers) or w/ certain conds that could ↓ ability to respond to severe allergic reaction Uses: *Immunotherapy of grass pollen–induced allergic rhinitis w/ or w/o conjunctivitis confirmed by + skin test or pollen-specific IgE Ab* Acts: Allergen immunotherapy Dose: *Adults & Peds. 5–17 y:* 1 tab SL/d; do not swallow for 1 min; for sustained effect for one pollen season after D/C may take qd × 3 consecutive y W/P: [B, ?/–] Discuss severe allergic Rxn; if oral lesions, stop Tx, restart after healed CI: Severe uncontrolled/unstable asthma; Hx severe systemic/local allergic reaction to SL allergen immunotherapy; component hypersens Disp: Tabs 30-d blister pack SE: Ear/oral/tongue pruritus, mouth edema, throat irritation Notes: 1st dose in healthcare setting; start 12 wk before expected onset of Sx; give auto-injectable epi; peds give only w/ adult supervision; D/C with ↑ local symptoms and seek care

Tinidazole (Tindamax, Generic) BOX: Carcinogenicity has been seen in mice and rats treated chronically with metronidazole, another nitroimidazole agent Uses: *Trichomoniasis, giardiasis, and amebiasis: in pts age 3 and older; bacterial vaginosis: in non-PRG, adult women* Acts: Nitroimidazole antimicrobial Dose: *Adults. Trichomoniasis, giardiasis:* 2 g PO w/ food × 1. For trichomoniasis treat sexual partners *Bacterial vaginosis:* Non-PRG, adult women: 2 g qd for 2 d w/ food, or 1 g once daily for 5 days w/food *Peds > 3 y:* Giardiasis: 50 mg/kg (up to 2 g) × 1 w/ food Amebiasis: 50 mg/kg/d (up to 2 g per d) × 3 d w/ food *Amebic liver abscess:* same up to 5 d Amebiasis: 2 g/d × 3–5 d W/P: [C, ?] Szs/nephropathy reported; vaginal candidiasis CI: Component allergy; 1st tri PRG, breast-feeding Disp: Tabs 250, 500 mg SE: Metallic/ bitter taste, N, anorexia, dyspepsia, weakness/fatigue, HA, dizziness

Tioconazole (Vagistat-1, Generic [OTC]) Uses: *Vag fungal Infxns* Acts: Topical antifungal Dose: 1 applicator-full intravag hs (single dose) W/P: [C, ?] CI: Component allergy Disp: Vag oint 6.5% SE: Local burning, itching, soreness, polyuria Notes: Insert high into vagina; may damage condom or diaphragm

Tiotropium (Spiriva HandiHaler, Spiriva Respimat) Uses: *Bronchospasm w/ COPD, bronchitis, emphysema* Acts: Synthetic anticholinergic-like atropine Dose: *HandiHaler:* 1 cap/d Inh × 2, DO NOT use w/ spacer; *Respimat:* 2 Inh × 1 qd W/P: [C, ?/–] Hypersens Rxn, w/ BPH, NAG, MyG, renal impair CI: Acute bronchospasm Disp: *HandiHaler:* Inh caps 18 mcg; *Respimat:* Metered-dose inhaler 2.5 mcg/Inh SE: Pharyngitis, cough, dry mouth, sinusitis, dysuria, urinary retention Notes: Monitor FEV1 or peak flow

Tirofiban (Aggrastat) Uses: *ACS* Acts: Glycoprotein IIB/IIIa inhib Dose: 25 mcg/kg w/in 5 min, then 0.15 mcg/kg/min up to 18 h; w/CrCl ≤ 60 mL/min, 25 mcg/kg w/in 5 min, then 0.075 mcg/kg/min *ECC 2010. ACS or PCI:*

0.4 mcg/kg/min IV for 30 min, then 0.1 mcg/kg/min for 18–24 h post-PCI; ↓ in renal Insuff **W/P:** [B, ?/–] **CI:** Component hypersens, internal bleeding, bleeding diathesis, stroke/surgery/trauma w/in last 30 d **Disp:** Inj 50 mcg/mL as 5 mg/100mL and 12.5 mg/250 mL **SE:** Bleeding

Tizanidine (Zanaflex, Generic) Uses: *Rx spasticity* Acts: α$_2$-Adrenergic agonist **Dose: Adults.** 2–4 mg q6–8h, ↑ 2–4 mg PRN, max 12 mg/dose or 36 mg/d; ↓ w/ CrCl < 25 mL/min **Peds.** Not rec **W/P:** [C, ?/–] Do not use w/ potent CYP1A2 inhib or other α$_2$-adrenergic agonists **CI:** w/ Fluvoxamine, ciprofloxacin; hypersens **Disp:** Caps 2, 4, 6 mg; tabs 2, 4 mg **SE:** ↓ BP, ↓ HR, somnolence, hepatotox **Notes:** ✓ LFT & BP; do not abruptly D/C, taper dose; take consistently w/ or w/o food

Tobramycin (Generic) **BOX:** Potential for ototox, neurotox, & nephrotox; monitor levels; avoid w/ other neuro/nephrotox meds; do not give w/ potent diuretics; fetal harm if PRG Uses: *Serious gram(–) Infxns* Acts: Aminoglycoside; ↓ protein synth. *Spectrum:* Gram(–) bacteria (including *Pseudomonas*) **Dose: Adults.** Conventional dosing: 1–2.5 mg/kg/dose IV q8–12h *Once-daily dosing:* 5–7 mg/kg/ dose q24h **Peds.** 2.5 mg/kg/dose IV q8h; ↓ w/ renal Insuff **W/P:** [D, –] **CI:** PRGlt; aminoglycoside sensitivity **Disp:** Inj 10, 40 mg/mL **SE:** Nephro/ototox **Notes:** Follow CrCl & levels. Levels: *Peak:* 30 min after Inf; *Trough:* < 0.5 h before next dose; *Therapeutic Conventional: Peak:* 5–10 mcg/mL, *Trough:* < 2 mcg/mL

Tobramycin, Inh (Bethkis, Kitabis Pak, TOBI, TOBI Podhaler) Uses: *CF pts w/ P. aeruginosa* Acts: Aminoglycoside; ↓ protein synth. *Spectrum:* Gram (–) bacteria **Dose: Adults/Peds > 6 y.** 300 mg Inh q12h by nebulizer; *TOBI Podhaler:* 112 mg (4 × 28-mg caps) Inh q12h; cycle 28 d on, 28 d off **W/P:** [D, –] w/ Renal/auditory/vestibular/neuromusc dysfunction; avoid w/ other neuro/nephro/ ototoxic drugs **CI:** Aminoglycoside sensitivity **Disp:** 300-mg vials for nebulizer; *TOBI Podhaler:* 4-wk supply (56 blister caps w/ Inh device plus reserve); *Kitabis Pak:* single-use ampule 300 mg/5 mL w/ reusable nebulizer (must connect to Pulmo-Aide compressor **SE:** Cough, productive cough, lung disorders, dyspnea, pyrexia, oropharyngeal pain, dysphonia, hemoptysis, ↓ hearing **Notes:** Do not mix w/ dornase alfa in nebulizer; safety not established in peds < 6 y, or w/ FEV1 < 25% or > 80%, or if colonized w/ *Burkholderia cepacia*

Tobramycin, Ophthalmic (Tobradex ST, Tobrex, Generic) Uses: *Ocular bacterial Infxns* Acts: Aminoglycoside **Dose:** 1–2 gtt q2-4h; if bid-tid; if severe, use oint q3–4h, or 2 gtt q60 min, then less frequently **W/P:** [B, –] **CI:** Aminoglycoside sensitivity **Disp:** Oint & soln tobramycin 0.3% **SE:** Ocular irritation

Tobramycin/Dexamethasone, Ophthalmic (TobraDex) Uses: *Ocular bacterial Infxns associated w/ sig inflam* Acts: Abx w/ anti-inflam **Dose:** 0.3% oint apply q6–8h or soln 0.3% apply 1–2 gtt q4–6h (↑ to q2h for first 24–48 h) **W/P:** [C, M] **CI:** Aminoglycoside sensitivity viral, fungal, or mycobacterium Infxn of eye **Disp:** *Tobradex:* Tobramycin 0.3%/dexamethasone 0.1%; oint (3.5 g) & susp 2.5, 5, 10 mL; *Tobradex ST:* Tobramycin 0.3%/dexamethasone 0.05% **SE:** Local irritation/ edema **Notes:** Use under ophthalmologist's direction

Tocilizumab (Actemra) **BOX:** May cause serious Infxn (TB, bacterial, invasive fungal, viral, opportunistic); w/ serious Infxn, stop tocilizumab until Infxn controlled **Uses:** *Mod–severe RA .w/ inadequate response to DMARDs, PJIA, SJIA* **Acts:** IL-6 receptor inhib **Dose:** *Adults. RA:* 4 mg/kg IV q4wk, ↑ 8 mg/kg q4wk PRN, or SQ dosing: < 100 kg, 162 mg q other wk; > 100 kg, 162 mg weekly *Adults & Peds > 2 y. PJIA:* < 30 kg, 10 mg/kg q4wk; > 30 kg, 8 mg/kg q4wk; *SJIA* < 30 kg, 12 mg/kg q2wk; > 30 kg, 8 mg/kg q2wk **W/P:** [C, ?/–] Do not use w/ANC < 2000/mm³, plt ct < 100,000, AST/ALT > 1.5 ULN; serious Infxn; high-risk bowel perf **CI:** Component hypersens **Disp:** Inj 20 mg/mL (4-, 10-, 20-mL vials); prefilled syringe 162 mg/0.9 mL **SE:** URI, nasopharyngitis, HA, ↑ BP, ↑ ALT, Inj site Rxn **Notes:** Do not give live vaccines; ✓ CBC/plt counts, LFTs, lipids; PPD: if (+) treat before starting, w/ prior Hx retreat unless adequate Tx confirmed, monitor for TB even if PPD(–); ↓ mRNA expression of several CYP450 isoenzymes (CYP3A4).

Tofacitinib (Xeljanz) **BOX:** Serious Infxns (bacterial, viral, fungal, TB, opportunistic) possible. D/C w/ severe Infxn until controlled; test for TB w/ Tx; lymphoma/other CA possible; possible EBV-associated renal transplant lymphoproliferative disorder **Uses:** *Mod–severe RA w/ inadequate response/ intolerance to MTX* **Acts:** Janus kinase inhib **Dose:** 5 mg PO bid; ↓ 5 mg qd w/ mod–severe renal & mod hepatic impair, w/ potent inhib CYP3A4, w/ meds w/ both mod inhib CYP3A4 & potent inhib CYP2C19 **W/P:** [C, –] Do not use w/ active Infxn, w/ severe hepatic impair, w/ biologic DMARDs, immunosuppressants, live vaccines; w/ risk of GI perforation **CI:** Ø **Disp:** Tabs 5 mg **SE:** D, HA, URI, nasopharyngitis, ↑ LFTs, HTN, anemia **Notes:** OK w/ MTX or other nonbiologic DMARDs; ✓CBC, LFTs, lipids

Tolazamide (Generic) **Uses:** *Type 2 DM* **Acts:** Sulfonylurea; ↑ pancreatic insulin release; ↑ peripheral insulin sensitivity; ↓ hepatic glu output **Dose:** 100–500 mg/d (no benefit > 1 g/d) **W/P:** [C, ?/–] Elderly, hepatic or renal impair; G6PD deficiency = ↑ risk for hemolytic anemia **CI:** Component hypersens, DM type 1, DKA **Disp:** Tabs 250, 500 mg **SE:** HA, dizziness, GI upset, rash, hyperglycemia, photosens, blood dyscrasias

Tolbutamide (Generic) **Uses:** *Type 2 DM* **Acts:** Sulfonylurea; ↑ pancreatic insulin release; ↑ peripheral insulin sensitivity; ↓ hepatic glu output **Dose:** 500–1000 mg bid; 3 g/d max; ↓ in hepatic failure **W/P:** [C, –] G6PD deficiency = ↑ risk hemolytic anemia **CI:** Sulfonylurea sensitivity **Disp:** Tabs 500 mg **SE:** HA, dizziness, GI upset, rash, photosens, blood dyscrasias, hypoglycemia, heartburn

Tolcapone (Tasmar) **BOX:** Cases of fulminant liver failure resulting in death have occurred **Uses:** *Adjunct to carbidopa/levodopa in Parkinson Dz* **Acts:** Catechol-*O*-methyltransferase inhib slows levodopa metabolism **Dose:** 100 mg PO tid w/ 1st daily levodopa/carbidopa dose, then dose 6 & 12 h later; ↓ /w/ renal Insuff **W/P:** [C, ?] **CI:** Hepatic impair; w/ nonselective MAOI; nontraumatic rhabdomyolysis or hyperpynexia **Disp:** Tabs 100 mg **SE:** Constipation, xerostomia, vivid dreams, hallucinations, anorexia, N/D, orthostasis, liver failure, rhabdomyolysis **Notes:** Do not abruptly D/C or ↓ dose; monitor LFTs

Tolmetin (Generic) BOX: May ↑ risk of MI/CVA & GI bleeding **Uses:** *Arthritis & pain* **Acts:** NSAID; ↓ prostaglandins **Dose:** 400 mg PO tid, titrate up to 1.8 g/d max **W/P:** [C, −] **CI:** NSAID or ASA sensitivity; use for pain; CABG **Disp:** Tabs 200, 600 mg; caps 400 mg **SE:** Dizziness, rash, GI upset, edema, GI bleeding, renal failure

Tolnaftate (Tinactin, Generic) [OTC]) **Uses:** *Tinea pedis, cruris, corporis, manus, versicolor* **Acts:** Topical antifungal **Dose:** Apply to area bid for 2–4 wk **W/P:** [C, ?] **CI:** Nail & scalp Infxns **Disp:** OTC 1% liq; powder; topical cream; oint, spray soln **SE:** Local irritation **Notes:** Avoid ocular contact, Infxn should improve in 7–10 d

Tolterodine (Detrol, Detrol LA, Generic) **Uses:** *OAB (frequency, urgency, incontinence)* **Acts:** Anticholinergic **Dose:** *Detrol:* 1–2 mg PO bid; *Detrol LA:* 2–4 mg/d **W/P:** [C, −] w/ CYP2D6 & 3A3/4 inhib (Table 10, p 356); w/ QT prolongation **CI:** Urinary retention, gastric retention, or uncontrolled NAG **Disp:** Tabs 1, 2 mg; *Detrol LA* tabs 2, 4 mg **SE:** Xerostomia, blurred vision, HA, constipation **Notes:** LA form; patient may see "intact" pill in stool

Tolvaptan (Samsca) BOX: Hospital use only w/ close monitoring of Na⁺; too rapid Na⁺ correction can cause severe neurologic Sxs; correct slowly w/ ↑ risk (malnutrition, alcoholism, liver Dz) **Uses:** *Hypervolemic or euvolemic ↓ Na⁺* **Acts:** Vasopressin V_2-receptor antag **Dose:** 15 mg PO qd; after ≥ 24 h, may ↑ to 30 mg × 1 qd; max 60 mg qd; titrate at 24-h intervals to Na⁺ goal **W/P:** [C, −] Monitor Na⁺, volume, neurologic status; GI bleeding risk w/ cirrhosis, avoid w/ CYP3A inducers and moderate inhib, ↓ dose w/ P-gp inhib, ↑ K⁺; limit Rx to 30 d; avoid w/ liver Dz; can ↑ ALT and injure liver **CI:** Hypovolemic hyponatremia; urgent need to raise Na⁺; in pts incapable of sensing/reacting to thirst; anuria; w/ strong CYP3A inhib **Disp:** Tabs 15, 30 mg **SE:** N, xerostomia, pollakiuria, polyuria, thirst, weakness, constipation, hyperglycemia **Notes:** Monitor K⁺

Topiramate (Qudexy XR, Topamax, Topamax Sprinkle, Trokendi XR, Generic) **Uses:** *Initial monotherapy or adjunctive for complex partial Szs & tonic–clonic Szs; adjunct for Lennox-Gastaut synd, bipolar disorder, neuropathic pain, migraine prophylaxis* **Acts:** Anticonvulsant **Dose:** *Adults. Szs:* Total dose 400 mg/d; see PI for 8-wk schedule *Migraine Px:* titrate 100 m/d total dose *Peds 2–9.* See PI; ↓ w/ renal impair **W/P:** [D, ?/−] Visual field defects unrelated to ↑ ocular pressure, nystagmus, acute glaucoma requires D/C; memory impair, psychomotor slowing, suicidal ideation/ behavior, metabolic acidosis, kidney stones, hyperthermia, ↓ sweating, embryo-fetal tox, ↑ ammonia w/encephalopathy **CI:** Component allergy; for ER recent EtOH use or w/ metabolic acidosis **Disp:** Tabs 25, 50, 100, 200 mg; caps sprinkles 15, 25 mg; ER Caps 25, 50, 100, 150, 200 mg **SE:** Somnolence, fatigue, paresthesias, Wt loss, GI upset, tremor, ↓ serum HCO_3^-, **Notes:** If metabolic acidosis, ↓ dose or D/C or give alkali Tx; ✓ bicarbonate; when

D/C must taper; ↓ efficacy of OCPs; use w/ phenytoin or carbamazepine ↓ topiramate levels; monitor HCO_3^- if on carbonic anhydrase inhib; Li levels ↑, ask if taking both; avoid other CNS depressants

Topotecan (Hycamtin, Generic) **BOX:** Chemotherapy precautions, for use by physicians familiar w/ chemotherapeutic agents, BM suppression possible **Uses:** *Ovarian CA (cisplatin-refractory), cervical CA, SCLC*, sarcoma, ped NSCLC **Acts:** Topoisomerase I inhib; ↓ DNA synth **Dose:** 1.5 mg/m²/d as a 1-h IV Inf × 5 d, repeat q3wk; ↓ w/ renal impair **W/P:** [D, –] **CI:** PRG, breast-feeding; severe bone marrow suppression **Disp:** Inj 4-mg vials; caps 0.25, 1 mg **SE:** ↑ BM, N/V/D, drug fever, skin rash, interstitial lung Dz

Torsemide (Demadex, Generic) **Uses:** *Edema, HTN, CHF, & hepatic cirrhosis* **Acts:** Loop diuretic; ↓ reabsorption of Na⁺ & Cl⁻ in ascending loop of Henle & distal tubule **Dose:** 5–20 mg/d PO or IV; 200 mg/d max **W/P:** [B, ?] **CI:** Sulfonylurea sensitivity, anuria **Disp:** Tabs 5, 10, 20, 100 mg; Inj 10 mg/mL **SE:** Orthostatic ↓ BP, HA, dizziness, photosens, electrolyte imbalance, blurred vision, renal impair **Notes:** 10–20 mg torsemide = 40 mg furosemide = 1 mg bumetanide

Tramadol (ConZip, Ultram, Ultram ER, Generic) [C-IV] **Uses:** *Mod–severe pain* **Acts:** Centrally acting synthetic opioid analgesic **Dose:** *Adults.* 50–100 mg PO q4–6h PRN, start 25 mg PO q A.M., ↑ q3d to 25 mg PO qid; ↑ 50 mg q3d, 400 mg/d max (300 mg if > 75 y); *ER:* 100–300 mg PO qd *Peds.* (ER form not rec) 1–2 mg/kg q4–6h (max single dose 100 mg); max 400 mg/d or 8 mg/kg/d (whichever is less); ↓ w/ renal Insuff **W/P:** [C, –] Suicide risk in addiction prone, w/ tranquilizers or antidepressants; ↑ Szs risk w/ MAOI; serotonin syndrome **CI:** Opioid dependency; w/ MAOIs; sensitivity to opioids, acute alcohol intoxication, hypnotics, centrally acting analgesics, or w/ psychotropic drugs **Disp:** Tabs 50 mg; ER tabs 100, 200, 300 mg; ER caps: 100, 150, 200, 300 mg; susp 10 mg/mL **SE:** Dizziness, HA, somnolence, GI upset, resp depression, anaphylaxis **Notes:** ↓ Sz threshold; tolerance/dependence may develop; abuse potential d/t μ-opioid agonist activity; avoid EtOH; do not cut, chew ODT tabs

Tramadol/Acetaminophen (Ultracet) [C-IV] **BOX:** Acetaminophen hepatotox (acute liver failure, liver transplant, death) reported; often d/t acetaminophen > 4000 mg/d or more than one acetaminophen product **Uses:** *Short-term Rx acute pain (< 5 d)* **Acts:** Centrally acting opioid analgesic w/ APAP **Dose:** 2 tabs PO q4–6h PRN; 8 tabs/d max *Elderly/renal impair:* Lowest possible dose; 2 tabs q12h max if CrCl < 30 mL/min **W/P:** [C, –] Szs, hepatic/renal impair, suicide risk in addiction prone, w/ tranquilizers or antidepressants **CI:** Acute intoxication, w/ EtOH, hypnotics, centrally acting analgesics or psychotropic drugs, hepatic dysfunction **Disp:** Tab 37.5 mg tramadol/325 mg APAP **SE:** SSRIs, TCAs, opioids, MAOIs ↑ risk of Szs; dizziness, somnolence, tremor, HA, N/V/D, constipation, xerostomia, liver tox, rash, pruritus, ↑ sweating, physical dependence **Notes:** Avoid EtOH; abuse potential μ-opioid agonist activity (tramadol); see Acetaminophen note, p 40

Trametinib (Mekinist) Uses: *Met melanoma w/ BRAF V600E or V600K mutations; single drug or combo w/ dabrafenib* **Acts:** TKI **Dose:** 2 mg qd; may need to reduce dose or hold or D/C for SEs or tox **W/P:** [D, –] w/ Dabrafenib new cutaneous and non-cutaneous Ca can occur, bleeding, DVT/PE, cardiomyopathy; ocular tox, retinal vein thrombosis; ILD, serious skin Rxns; ↑ glu; embryofetal tox **CI:** Ø **Disp:** Tabs 0.5, 1, 2 mg **SE:** Fever, chills, night sweats, N/V/D, constipation, Abd pain, anorexia, fatigue, HA, arthralgias/myalgias, cough; rash; lymphedema; hemolytic anemia w/ G6PD def; ↑ glu; ↑ AST, ↑ ALT, ↑ alk phos, ↓ albumin, ↓ WBC, plt **Notes:** Not a single agent if prior BRAF-inhib Tx; ✓ LV function before, 1 mo after start, and q 2–3 mo; hold w/ pulm Sx; ✓ glu and monitor w/ DM or ↑ glu; D/C w/ retinal vein thrombosis, ILD, pneumonitis, or rash (grade, 2, 3, or 4) not improved after off 3 wk; w/ dabrafenib avoid inhib or inducers of CYP3A4/CYP2C8 ; use contraception during and 4 mo post-Tx; w/dabrafenib, must use non-hormonal contraception (class kinase inhibitor)

Trandolapril (Mavik, Generic) **BOX:** Use in PRG in 2nd/3rd tri can result in fetal death Uses: *HTN, heart failure, LVD, post-AMI* **Acts:** ACE inhib **Dose:** *HTN:* 1–4 mg/d, max 8 mg/d. *Heart failure/LVD:* Start 1 mg/d, titrate to 4 mg/d; ↓ w/ severe renal/hepatic impair **W/P:** [C first, D in 2nd + 3rd, –] ACE inhib sensitivity, angioedema w/ ACE inhib **Disp:** Tabs 1, 2, 4 mg **SE:** ↓ BP, ↓ HR, dizziness, ↑ K⁺, GI upset, renal impair, cough, angioedema **Notes:** African Americans: minimum dose is 2 mg vs 1 mg in caucasians

Tranexamic Acid (Cyklokapron, Lysteda, Generic) Uses: *↓ Cyclic heavy menstrual bleeding* **Acts:** ↓ Dissolution of hemostatic fibrin by plasmin **Dose:** 2 tabs tid (3900 mg/d), 5 d max, during monthly menstruation; ↓ w/ renal impair (see PI) **W/P:** [B, +/–] ↑ thrombosis risk **CI:** Component sens; active or ↑ thrombosis risk **Disp:** Tabs 650 mg; Inj 100 mg/mL **SE:** HA, sinus and nasal symptoms, Abd pain, back/musculoskeletal/jt pain, cramps, migraine, anemia, fatigue, retinal/ocular occlusion; allergic Rxns **Notes:** Inj used off label trauma associated hemorrhage

Tranylcypromine (Parnate, Generic) **BOX:** Antidepressants ↑ risk of suicidal thinking and behavior in children and adolescents w/ MDD and other psychiatric disorders Uses: *Depression* **Acts:** MAOI **Dose:** 30 mg/d PO ÷ doses, may ↑ 10 mg/d over 1–3 wk to max 60 mg/d **W/P:** [C, +/–] Minimize foods w/ tyramine **CI:** CV Dz, cerebrovascular defects, Pheo, w/ MAOIs, TCAs, SSRIs, SNRIs, sympathomimetics, bupropion, meperidine, dextromethorphan, buspirone **Disp:** Tabs 10 mg **SE:** Orthostatic hypotension, ↑ HR, sex dysfunction, xerostomia **Notes:** False(+) amphetamine drug test

Trastuzumab (Herceptin) **BOX:** Can cause cardiomyopathy and ventricular dysfunction; Inf Rxns and pulm tox reported; use during PRG can lead to pulm hypoplasia, skeletal malformations, & neonatal death Uses: *Met breast CA that overexpresses the HER2/neu protein*, breast CA adjuvant, w/ doxorubicin, cyclophosphamide, and paclitaxel if pt HER2/neu(+) **Acts:** MoAb; binds HER2 protein;

mediates cellular cytotox **Dose:** Per protocol, typical 2 mg/kg/IV/wk **W/P:** [D, –] CV dysfunction, allergy/Inf Rxns **CI:** Ø **Disp:** Inf 440 mg **SE:** Anemia, cardiomyopathy, nephrotic synd, pneumonitis, N/V/D, rash, pain, fever, HA, insomnia **Notes:** Inf-related Rxns minimized w/ acetaminophen, diphenhydramine, & meperidine

Trazodone (Oleptro, Generic) **BOX:** Closely monitor for worsening depression or emergence of suicidality, particularly in pts < 24 y; Oleptro not approved in peds **Uses:** *Depression*, hypnotic, augment other antidepressants **Acts:** Antidepressant; ↓ reuptake of serotonin & norepinephrine **Dose:** *Adults & Adolescents.* 50–150 mg PO qd–tid; max 600 mg/d (div) *Sleep:* 25–50 mg PO, qhs, PRN *Adults. Oleptro:* Start 150 mg PO daily, may ↑ by 75 mg q3d, max 375 mg/d; take qhs on empty stomach **W/P:** [C, ?/–] Serotonin/neuroleptic malignant syndromes reported; ↑ QTc; may activate manic states; syncope reported; may ↑ bleeding risk; avoid w/in 14 d of MAOI **CI:** Component allergy **Disp:** Tabs 50, 100, 150, 300 mg; *Oleptro:* Scored ER tabs 150, 300 mg **SE:** Dizziness, HA, sedation, N, xerostomia, syncope, confusion, ↓ libido, ejaculation dysfunction, tremor, hep, EPS **Notes:** Takes 1–2 wk for Sx improvement; may interact w/ CYP3A4 inhib to ↑ trazodone concentrations, carbamazepine ↓ trazodone concentrations

Treprostinil, Extended Release (Orenitram) **Uses:** *Pulm arterial HTN to improve exercise capacity* **Acts:** Vasodilator **Dose:** *Adults.* Start 0.25 mg bid; ↑ by 0.25 or 0.5 mg bid or 0.125 mg tid q 3–4 d; max dose based on tolerance **W/P:** [C, ?/–] ↑ Risk of bleeding; do not take with EtOH; do not abruptly D/C; tabs may lodge in colonic diverticulum **CI:** Severe hepatic Dz **Disp:** ER Tabs 0.125, 0.25, 1, 2.5 mg **SE:** HA, N/D, Abd pain, flushing, pain in jaw or ext, ↓ K+ **Notes:** Risk of ↓ BP with antihypertensive drugs; if co-admin w/ strong CYP2C8 inhib starting dose 0.125 mg bid; pitch Abd aggregation; see also Treprostinil Sodium

Treprostinil Sodium (Remodulin, Tyvaso) **Uses:** *NYHA class II–IV pulm arterial HTN* **Acts:** Vasodilation, ↓ plt aggregation **Dose:** *Remodulin:* 0.625–1.25 ng/kg/min cont Inf/SQ (preferred), titrate to effect; *Tyvaso:* Initial: 18 mcg (3 Inh) qid; if not tolerated, ↓ to 1–2 Inh, then ↑ to 3 Inh; Maint: ↑ additional 3 Inh 1–2 wk intervals; 54 mcg (or 9 Inh) qid max **W/P:** [B, ?/–] **CI:** Component allergy **Disp:** *Remodulin:* Inj 1, 2.5, 5, 10 mg/mL; *Tyvaso:* 0.6 mg/mL (2.9 mL) ~6 mcg/Inh **SE:** Additive effects w/ anticoagulants, antihypertensives; Inf site Rxns; N/D, HA, ↓ BP **Notes:** Initiate in monitored setting; do not D/C or ↓ dose, abruptly, will cause rebound pulm HTN; see also Treprostinil, Extended Release

Tretinoin, Topical [Retinoic Acid] (Atralin, Avita, ReFissa, Renova, Retin-A, Retin-A Micro) **Uses:** *Acne vulgaris, sun-damaged skin, wrinkles* (photo aging), some skin CAs **Acts:** Exfoliant retinoic acid derivative **Dose:** *Adults & Peds > 12 y.* Apply qd hs (w/ irritation, ↓ frequency) *Photoaging:* Start w/ 0.025%, ↑ to 0.1% over several mo (apply only q3d if on neck area; dark skin may require bid use) **W/P:** [C, ?] **CI:** Retinoid sensitivity **Disp:** Cream 0.02, 0.025, 0.05, 0.0375, 0.1%; gel 0.01, 0.025, 0.05%; micro formulation gel 0.1, 0.04, 0.08%

SE: Avoid sunlight; edema; skin dryness, erythema, scaling, changes in pigmentation, stinging, photosens

Triamcinolone/Nystatin (Mycolog-II, Generic) Uses: *Cutaneous candidiasis* **Acts:** Antifungal & anti-inflam **Dose:** Apply lightly to area bid **W/P:** [C, ?] **CI:** Varicella; systemic fungal Infxns **Disp:** Cream & oint: triamcinolone 1 mg/g and 100,000 units nystatin/g **SE:** Local irritation, hypertrichosis, pigmentation changes **Notes:** For short-term use (< 7 d)

Triamterene (Dyrenium) BOX: Hyperkalemia can occur **Uses:** *Edema associated w/ CHF, cirrhosis* **Acts:** K⁺-sparing diuretic **Dose:** *Adults.* 100–300 mg/24 h PO ÷ daily-bid *Peds.* HTN: 2–4 mg/kg/d in 1–2 ÷ doses; ↓ w/ renal/hepatic impair **W/P:** [C (Expert opinion), ?] **CI:** ↑ K⁺, renal impair; caution w/ other K⁺-sparing diuretics **Disp:** Caps 50, 100 mg **SE:** ↓ K⁺, ↓ BP, bradycadia, cough, HA

Triazolam (Halcion, Generic) [C-IV] Uses: *Short-term management of insomnia* **Acts:** Benzodiazepine **Dose:** 0.125–0.25 mg/d PO hs PRN; ↓ in elderly **W/P:** [X, ?/–] **CI:** Concurrent fosamprenavir, ritonavir, nelfinavir, itraconazole, ketoconazole, nefazodone or other moderate/strong CYP3A4 inhib; PRG **Disp:** Tabs 0.125, 0.25 mg **SE:** Tachycardia, CP, drowsiness, fatigue, memory impair, GI upset **Notes:** Additive CNS depression w/ EtOH & other CNS depressants, avoid abrupt D/C

Triethylenethiophosphoramide (Tespa, Thioplex, Thiotepa, TSPA) Uses: *Breast & ovarian CAs, lymphomas (infrequently used), preparative regimens for allogeneic & ABMT w/ high doses, intravesical for bladder CA, intracavitary effusion control* **Acts:** Polyfunctional alkylating agent **Dose:** Per protocol typical 0.3–0.4 mg/kg IV q1–4 wk *Effusions:* Intracavitary 0.6-0.8 mg/kg; *Bladder CA* 60 mg into the bladder & retained 2 h q1–4wk; 900–125 mg/m² in ABMT regimens (highest dose w/o ABMT is 180 mg/m²); ↓ in renal failure **W/P:** [D, –] w/ BM suppression, renal and hepatic impair **CI:** Component allergy **Disp:** Inj 15 mg/vial **SE:** ↓ BM, N/V, dizziness, HA, allergy, paresthesias, alopecia **Notes:** Intravesical use in bladder CA infrequent today

Trifluoperazine (Generic) BOX: ↑ Mortality in elderly patients w/ dementia-related psychosis **Uses:** *Psychotic disorders* **Acts:** Phenothiazine; blocks postsynaptic CNS dopaminergic receptors **Dose:** *Adults.* *Schizophrenia/psychosis:* initial 1–2 mg PO bid (outpatient) or 2–5 mg PO bid (inpatient); typical 15–20 mg/d, max 40 mg/d *Nonpsychotic anxiety:* 1–2 mg PO/d, 6 mg/d max *Peds 6–12 y.* 1 mg PO qd-bid initial, gradually ↑ to 15 mg/d; ↓ in elderly/debilitated pts **W/P:** [C, ?/ –] **CI:** Hx blood dyscrasias; phenothiazine sens, severe hepatic Dz **Disp:** Tabs 1, 2, 5, 10 mg **SE:** Orthostatic ↓ BP, EPS, dizziness, NMS, skin discoloration, lowered Sz threshold, photosens, blood dyscrasias **Notes:** Several weeks for onset of effects

Trifluridine, Ophthalmic (Viroptic) Uses: *Herpes simplex keratitis & conjunctivitis* **Acts:** Antiviral **Dose:** 1 gtt q2h, max 9 gtt/d, then 1 gtt q4h × 7 d after healing begins; Rx up to 21 d **W/P:** [C, ?] **CI:** Component allergy **Disp:** Soln 1% **SE:** Local burning, stinging

Trihexyphenidyl (Generic) Uses: *Parkinson Dz, drug-induced EPS* **Acts:** Blocks excess acetylcholine at cerebral synapses **Dose:** *Parkinson:* 1 mg PO qd, ↑ by 2 mg q3–5d to usual dose 6–10 mg/d in 3–4 ÷ doses **CI:** *EPS:* 1 mg PO qd, ↑ to 5–15 mg/d in 3–4 ÷ doses **W/P:** [C, –] NAG, GI obst, MyG, BOO **CI: Disp:** Tabs 2, 5 mg; elixir 2 mg/5 mL **SE:** Dry skin, constipation, xerostomia, photosens, tachycardia, arrhythmias

Trimethobenzamide (Tigan, Generic) Uses: *N/V* **Acts:** ↓ Medullary chemoreceptor trigger zone **Dose:** 300 mg PO or 200 mg IM tid-qid PRN. **W/P:** [C, ?] **CI:** Benzocaine sensitivity; children < 40 kg **Disp:** Caps 300 mg; Inj 100 mg/mL **SE:** Drowsiness, ↓ BP, dizziness; hepatic impair, blood dyscrasias, Szs, Parkinsonian-like synd **Notes:** In the presence of viral Infxns, may mask emesis or mimic CNS effects of Reye synd

Trimethoprim (Primsol, Generic) Uses: *UTI d/t susceptible gram(+) & gram(–) organisms, Rx PCP w/ dapsone* suppression of UTI **Acts:** ↓ Dihydrofolate reductase. *Spectrum:* Many gram(+) & (–) except *Bacteroides, Branhamella, Brucella, Chlamydia, Clostridium, Mycobacterium, Mycoplasma, Nocardia, Neisseria, Pseudomonas,* & *Treponema* **Dose:** *Adults.* 100 mg PO bid or 200 mg PO qd; *PCP:* 15 mg/kg/d ÷ in 3 doses w/ dapsone *Peds ≥ 2 mo.* 4–6 mg/kg/d in 2 ÷ doses; *otitis media* (> or equal to 6 mo): 10 mg/kg/d in 2 ÷ doses × 10 d; ↓ w/ renal failure **W/P:** [C, +] **CI:** Megaloblastic anemia d/t folate deficiency **Disp:** Tabs 100 mg; (*Primsol*) PO soln 50 mg/5 mL **SE:** Rash, pruritus, megaloblastic anemia, hepatic impair, blood dyscrasias **Notes:** Take w/ plenty of H_2O

Trimethoprim [TMP]/sulfamethoxazole [SMX] [Co-Trimoxazole, TMP-SMX] (Bactrim, Bactrim DS, Septra DS, Sulfatrim, Generic) Uses: *UTI Rx & prophylaxis, otitis media, sinusitis, bronchitis, Px PCP pneumonia (HIV w/ CD4 count < 200 cells/mm³)* **Acts:** SMX ↓ synth of dihydrofolic acid, TMP ↓ dihydrofolate reductase to impair protein synth. *Spectrum:* Includes *Shigella,* PCP, & *Nocardia* Infxns, *Mycoplasma, Enterobacter* sp, *Staphylococcus, Streptococcus,* & more **Dose:** All doses based on TMP *Adults.* 1 DS tab PO bid or 8–20 mg TMP/kg/d IV ÷ q6–12h. *PCP:* 15–20 mg TMP/kg/d IV or PO (TMP) in 4 ÷ doses *Nocardia:* 10–15 mg/kg/d IV or PO (TMP) in 4 ÷ doses *PCP prophylaxis:* 1 regular tab qd or DS tab 3 × wk *UTI prophylaxis:* 1 PO bid *Peds.* 8–10 mg TMP/kg/d PO ÷ in 2 doses or 3–4 doses IV; do not use in < 2 mo; ↓ in renal failure; maintain hydration **W/P:** [C (D if near term), –] **CI:** Sulfonamide sensitivity, porphyria, megaloblastic anemia w/ folate deficiency, PRG, breastfeeding Inf < 2 mo, sig hepatic impair **Disp:** Regular tabs 80 mg TMP/400 mg SMX; DS tabs 160 mg TMP/800 mg SMX; PO susp 40 mg TMP/200 mg SMX/5 mL; Inj 80 mg TMP/400 mg SMX/5 mL **SE:** Allergic skin Rxns, photosens, GI upset, SJS, blood dyscrasias, hep **Notes:** Synergistic combo, interacts w/ warfarin

Triptorelin (Trelstar) Uses: *Palliation of advanced PCa* **Acts:** LHRH analog; ↓ GNRH w/ cont dosing; transient ↑ in LH, FSH, testosterone, & estradiol 7–10 d after 1st dose; w/ chronic use (usually 2–4 wk), sustained ↓ LH & FSH w/ ↓ testicular &

ovarian steroidogenesis similar to surgical castration **Dose:** 3.75 mg IM q4wk or 11.25 mg IM q12wk or 22.5 mg q24wk **W/P:** [X, N/A] **CI:** Component hypersens, ♀ **Disp:** Inj depot 3.75, 11.25, 22.5 mg, MixJect system **SE:** Dizziness, emotional lability, fatigue, HA, insomnia, HTN, V/D, ED, retention, UTI, pruritus, anemia, Inj site pain, musculoskeletal pain, osteoporosis, allergic Rxns **Notes:** ✓ periodic testosterone levels & PSA

Trospium (Generic) **Uses:** *OAB w/ Sx of urge incontinence, urgency, frequency* **Acts:** Muscarinic antag, ↓ bladder smooth muscle tone **Dose:** 20 mg PO bid; 60 mg ER PO daily A.M., 1 h ac or on empty stomach; ↓ w/ CrCl < 30 mL/min and elderly **W/P:** [C, +/–] w/ EtOH use, in hot environments, UC, MyG, renal/hepatic impair **CI:** Urinary/gastric retention, NAG **Disp:** Tabs 20 mg; caps ER 60 mg **SE:** Dry mouth, constipation, HA, rash

Ulipristal Acetate (Ella) **Uses:** *Emergency contraceptive for PRG Px (unprotected sex/contraceptive failure)* **Acts:** Progesterone agonist/antag, delays ovulation **Dose:** 30 mg PO ASAP w/in 5 d of unprotected sex or contraceptive failure **W/P:** [X, –] CYP3A4 inducers ↓ effect **CI:** PRG **Disp:** Tabs 30 mg **SE:** HA, N, Abd pain, dysmenorrhea **Notes:** NOT for routine contraception; fertility after use unchanged, maintain routine contraception; use any day of menstrual cycle

Umeclidinium (Incruse Ellipta) **Uses:** *COPD* **Acts:** Anticholinergic **Dose:** 1 Inh qd **W/P:** [C, ?/–] Not for acute Sxs; may worsen NAG, BPH/BOO; paradoxical bronchospasm **CI:** Milk protein hypersens **Disp:** Powder 62.5 mcg/Inh **SE:** Cough, URI, nasopharyngitis, arthralgia, ↑ HR **Notes:** Do not open the inhaler cover until ready to use; do not close cover until dose is inh; discard 6 wk after opening

Umeclidinium/Vilanterol (Anoro Ellipta) **BOX:** LABA, such as vilanterol, ↑ risk of asthma-related death; safety and efficacy in asthma has not been established **Uses:** *Maint COPD* **Acts:** Combo antimuscarinic (anticholinergic) and LABA (B$_2$) **Dose:** 1 inh/d **W/P:** [C, ?/–] May cause asthma-related deaths; NOT for acute exacerbations or deteriorations; do NOT use w/ other LABA; paradoxical bronchospasm; caution w/ CV Dz, seizure Hx, thyrotoxicosis, DM, ketoacidosis, NAG, and Hx of urinary retention or BPH **CI:** Hypersens to milk proteins **Disp:** Inhaler w/ double-foil blister strips of powder, 62.5 mcg umeclidinium & 25 mcg vilanterol **SE:** Sinusitis, pharyngitis, resp Infxn, D, constipation, pain (chest, neck, ext); ↓ K$^+$, ↑ glu **Notes:** DO NOT use to Tx asthma; caution w/ MAOIs, TCA, β-blockers (may block bronchodilator effect); diuretics (may potentiate ↓ K$^+$); other anticholinergic meds; strong P450 3A4 inhib

Ustekinumab (Stelara) **Uses:** *Mod–severe plaque psoriasis, psoriatic arthritis* **Acts:** Human IL-12 & 23 antag **Dose:** *Psoriasis:* Wt < 100 kg, 45 mg SQ initially & 4 wk later, then 45 mg q12wk; Wt > 100 kg, 90 mg SQ initially & 4 wk later, then 90 mg q12wk; *Psoriatic arthritis:* 45 mg SQ initially & 4 wk later, then 45 mg q12wk **W/P:** [B/?] Serious Infxns, TB may ↑ risk of malignancy **CI:** Component hypersens **Disp:** Prefilled syringe & single-dose vial 45 mg/0.5 mL, 90 mg/1 mL **SE:** Nasopharyngitis, URI, HA, fatigue **Notes:** Do not use w/ live vaccines

Valacyclovir (Valtrex, Generic) Uses: *Herpes zoster; genital herpes; herpes labialis* **Acts:** Prodrug of acyclovir; ↓ viral DNA replication. **Spectrum:** Herpes simplex I & II **Dose:** *Zoster:* 1 g PO tid × 7 d *Genital herpes (initial episode):* 1 g bid × 7–10 d, *(recurrent)* 500 mg PO bid × 3 d *Herpes prophylaxis:* 500–1000 mg/d *Herpes labialis:* 2 g PO q12h × 1 d; ↓ w/ renal failure **W/P:** [B, +] ↑ CNS effects in elderly **Disp:** Tabs 500, 1000 mg **SE:** HA, GI upset, ↑ LFTs, dizziness, pruritus, photophobia

Valganciclovir (Valcyte) **BOX:** Granulocytopenia, anemia, and thrombocytopenia reported; carcinogenic, teratogenic, and may cause aspermatogenesis Uses: *CMV retinitis and CMV prophylaxis in solid-organ transplantation* **Acts:** Ganciclovir prodrug; ↓ viral DNA synth **Dose:** *CMV Retinitis induction:* 900 mg PO bid w/ food × 21 d, then 900 mg PO qd; *CMV Px:* 900 mg PO qd × 100 d posttransplant, ↓ w/ renal dysfunction **W/P:** [C, ?/–] Use w/ imipenem/cilastatin, nephrotox drugs; ANC < 500 cells/mcL; plt < 25,000 cells/mcL; Hgb < 8 g/dL **CI:** Allergy to acyclovir, ganciclovir, valganciclovir **Disp:** Tabs 450 mg; oral soln: 50 mg/mL **SE:** BM suppression, HA, GI upset **Notes:** Monitor CBC & Cr

Valproic Acid (Depakene, Depakote, Stavzor, Generic) **BOX:** Fatal hepatic failure (usually during first 6 mo of Tx, peds < 2 y high risk, monitor LFTs at baseline and at frequent intervals), teratogenic effects, and life-threatening pancreatitis reported Uses: *Rx epilepsy, mania; Px migraines*, Alzheimer behavior disorder **Acts:** Anticonvulsant; ↑ availability of GABA **Dose:** *Adults & Peds. Szs:* 10–15 mg/kg/24 h PO ÷ tid (after initiation, ↑ by 5–10 mg/kg/d weekly until therapeutic level) *Mania:* 750 mg in 3 ÷ doses, ↑ 60 mg/kg/d max *Migraines:* 250 mg bid, ↑ 1000 mg/d max; ↓ w/ hepatic impair **W/P:** [X, –] Many drug interactions, DRESS, hepatotoxic, pancreatitis, fetal neural tube defects **CI:** Severe hepatic impair, urea cycle disorder **Disp:** Caps 250 mg; caps w/ coated particles 125 mg; tabs DR 125, 250, 500 mg; tabs ER 250, 500 mg; caps DR (*Stavzor*) 125, 250, 500 mg; syrup 250 mg/5 mL; Inj 100 mg/mL **SE:** Somnolence, dizziness, GI upset, diplopia, ataxia, rash, ↓ plt, hep, pancreatitis, ↑ bleeding times, sperm abnormalities, alopecia, ↑ Wt, hyperammonemic encephalopathy in pts w/ urea cycle disorders; if taken during PRG may ↓ childs IQ test **Notes:** Monitor LFTs & levels: *Trough:* Just before next dose; *Therapeutic: Trough:* 50–100 mcg/mL; *Toxic trough:* > 100 mcg/mL. *Half-life:* 9–16 h; phenobarbital & phenytoin may alter levels

Valsartan (Diovan) **BOX:** Use during 2nd/3rd tri of PRG can cause fetal harm Uses: *HTN, CHF (NYHA class II-IV); ↓ mortality after MI*, DN **Acts:** Angiotensin II receptor antag **Dose:** *Adults. HTN:* 80–160 mg/d, max 320 mg/d; *CHF:* 40 mg PO bid, target 160 mg bid; *Post-MI:* 20 mg PO bid, target 160 mg BID *Peds 6–16 y.* 1.3 mg/kg qd (up to 40 mg; total range up to 40–160 mg total) **W/P:** [D, ?/-] w/ K⁺-sparing diuretics or K⁺ supls **W/P:** Severe hepatic impair, biliary cirrhosis/obst, primary hyperaldosteronism, bilateral RAS **CI:** Component hypersens; use in DM w/ aliskiren **Disp:** Tabs 40 (scored), 80, 160, 320 mg **SE:** HA, dizziness, viral Infxn, fatigue, Abd pain, ↓ BP, D, arthralgia, ↑ K+, back pain, cough, ↑ Cr

Vancomycin (Vancocin, Generic)   Uses: *Serious MRSA Infxns; enterococcal Infxns; PO Rx of *S. aureus* & *C. difficile* pseudomembranous colitis* Acts: ↓ Cell wall synth. *Spectrum:* Gram(+) bacteria & some anaerobes (includes MRSA, *Staphylococcus, Enterococcus, Streptococcus* sp, *C. difficile*) Dose: *Adults.* 15–20 mg/kg/dose IV q8–48h based on CrCl; *C. difficile:* 125–500 mg PO q6h × 10 d. *Peds.* 40–60 mg/kg/d IV in ÷ doses q6–12 h; *C. difficile:* 40 mg/kg/d PO in ÷ 3–4 doses × 7–10 d W/P: [B oral + C Inj, –] CI: Component allergy; avoid in Hx hearing loss Disp: Caps 125, 250 mg; oral soln 25, 50 mg/mL, powder for Inj SE: Oto-/nephrotox, GI upset (PO) Notes: Not absorbed PO, effect in gut only; give IV slowly (over 1–3 h) to Px "red-man synd" (flushing of head/neck/upper torso); IV product used PO for colitis. *Levels: Trough:* < 0.5 h before next dose; *Therapeutic: Trough:* 10–20 mcg/mL; *Trough:* 15–20 mcg/mL. *Half-life:* 6–8 h; peak monitoring is not useful (tox > 80 mcg/mL)

Vandetanib (Caprelsa)   BOX: Can ↑ QT interval, Torsades de pointes, sudden death; do not use in pts w/ ↓ K⁺, ↓ Ca²⁺, ↓ Mg²⁺, prolonged QT, avoid drugs that prolong QT, monitor QT baseline, 2–4 wk, 8–12 wk, then q3mo Uses: *Advanced medullary thyroid CA* Acts: Multi-TKI inhib Dose: 300 mg/d; ↓ dose w/ ↓ renal Fxn W/P: [D, –] Can ↑ QT; avoid w/ CYP3A inducers or drugs that ↑ QT (eg, amiodarone, sotalol, clarithromycin); avoid w/ mod–severe liver impair CI: Prolonged QT synd Disp: Tabs 100, 300 mg SE: Anorexia, Abd pain, N/V, HA, ↑ BP, PRES, fatigue, rash (eg, acne), ↑ QT interval, ILD Notes: Half-life 19 d; restricted distribution, providers and pharmacies must be certified; may need ↑ thyroid replacement

Vardenafil (Levitra, Staxyn, Generic)   Uses: *ED* Acts: PDE5 inhib, increases cGMP and NO levels; relaxes smooth muscles, dilates cavernosal arteries Dose: *Levitra:* 10 mg PO 60 min before sexual activity; titrate; max × 1 = 20 mg; 2.5 mg w/ CYP3A4 inhib (Table 10, p 356); *Staxyn:* 1 10-mg ODT 60 min before sex, max 1×/d W/P: [B, –] w/ CV, hepatic, or renal Dz or if sex activity not advisable; potentiates the hypotensive effects of nitrates, alpha-blockers, and antihypertensives CI: w/nitrates, guanylate cyclase stim (eg, riociguat) Disp: *Levitra:* Tabs 2.5, 5, 10, 20 mg; *Staxyn:* 10-mg ODT (contains phenylalanine) SE: ↑ QT interval, ↓ BP, HA, dyspepsia, priapism, flushing, rhinitis, sinusitis, flu synd, sudden ↓/loss of hearing, tinnitus, NIAON Notes: Concomitant alpha-blockers may cause ↓ BP; transient global amnesia reports; place Staxyn on tongue to disintegrate w/o liquids; ODT not interchangeable w/ oral pill, reaches higher levels

Varenicline (Chantix)   BOX: Serious neuropsychiatric events (depression, suicidal ideation/attempt) reported Uses: *Smoking cessation* Acts: Nicotine receptor partial agonist Dose: 0.5 mg PO qd × 3 d, 0.5 mg bid × 4 d, then 1 mg PO bid for 12 wk total; after meal w/ glass of water W/P: [C, ?/–] ↓ Dose w/ renal impair, may increase risk of CV events in pts w/ CV Dz Disp: Tabs 0.5, 1 mg SE: Serious psychological disturbances, N/V, insomnia, flatulence, constipation, unusual dreams Notes: Slowly ↑ dose to ↓ N; initiate 1 wk before desired smoking cessation date; monitor for changes in behavior

Varicella Zoster Immune Globulin (VariZIG) BOX: Prepared from pools of human plasma, which may contain causative agents of hep & other viral Dz; may cause rare hypersens w/ shock; (Investigational, call (800)843-7477) Uses: Postexposure prophylaxis for persons w/o immunity, exposure likely to result in Infxn (household contact > 5 min) and ↑ risk for severe Dz (immunosuppression, PRG)* Acts: Passive immunization Dose: 125 Int units/10 kg up to 625 Int units IV or IM (deltoid or proximal thigh); give w/in 4–5 d (best < 72 h) of exposure W/P: [?, –] Indicated for PRG women exposed to varicella zoster CI: IgA deficiency, Hx, anaphylaxis to immunoglobulins; known immunity to varicella zoster Disp: 125–Int-unit unit vials SE: Inj site Rxn, dizziness, fever, HA, N; ARF, thrombosis rare Notes: Wait 5 mo before varicella vaccination after varicella immune globulin; may ↓ vaccine effectiveness; observe for varicella for 28 d; if VariZIG administration not possible w/in 96 h of exposure, consider administration of IGIV (400 mg/kg)

Varicella Virus Vaccine (Varivax) Uses: *Px varicella (chickenpox)* Acts: Active immunization w/ live attenuated virus Dose: Adults. 0.5 mL SQ, repeat 4–8 wk Peds 12 mo–12 y. 0.5 mL SQ; repeat ≥ 3 mo later W/P: [C, M] CI: Immunosuppression; PRG, fever, untreated TB, neomycin-anaphylaxic Rxn, febrile Rxn; Disp: Inj 1350 plaque-forming units/0.5 mL SE: Varicella rash, generalized or at Inj site, arthralgias/myalgias, fatigue, fever, HA, irritability, GI upset Notes: OK for all children & adults who have not had chickenpox; avoid PRG for 3 mo after; do not give w/in 3 mo of IgG and no IgG w/in 2 mo of vaccination; avoid ASA for 6 wk in peds; avoid high-risk people for 6 wk after vaccination

Vasopressin [Antidiuretic Hormone, ADH] (Vasostrict, Generic) Uses: *DI; Rx postop Abd distention*; adjunct Rx of GI bleeding & esophageal varices; asystole, PEA, pulseless VT & VF, adjunct systemic vasopressor (IV drip) Acts: Posterior pituitary hormone, potent GI, and peripheral vasoconstrictor Dose: Adults & Peds. DI: 5–10 units SQ or IM bid-tid GI hemorrhage: 0.2–0.4 units/min; ↓ in cirrhosis; caution in vascular Dz VT/VF: 40 units IV push × 1 Vasopressor: 0.01–0.03 units/min Peds. (ECC 2010). Cardiac arrest: 0.4–1 unit/kg IV/IO bolus; max dose 40 units Hypotension: 0.2–2 mill units/kg/min cont Inf W/P: [C, +] w/ Vascular Dz CI: Allergy Disp: Inj 20 units/mL SE: HTN, arrhythmias, fever, vertigo, GI upset, tremor Notes: Addition of vasopressor to concurrent norepinephrine or epi Infs

Vecuronium (Generic) BOX: To be administered only by appropriately trained individuals Uses: *Skeletal muscle relaxation* Acts: Nondepolarizing neuromuscular blocker; onset 2–3 min Dose: Adults & Peds. 0.1–0.2 mg/kg IV bolus (also rapid intubation) (ECC 2010); maint 0.010–0.015 mg/kg after 25–40 min; additional doses q12–15min PRN; ↓ w/ severe renal/hepatic impair W/P: [C, ?] Drug interactions cause ↑ effect (eg, aminoglycosides, tetracycline, succinylcholine) CI: Component hypenses Disp: Powder for Inj 10, 20 mg SE: ↓ HR, ↓ BP, itching, rash, tachycardia, CV collapse, muscle weakness Notes: Fewer cardiac effects than succinylcholine

Vedolizumab (Entyvio) Uses: *Adult UC or Crohn Dz w/ inadequate response to TNF blocker, immunomodulators, or steroids* Acts: Integrin receptor antag Dose: 300 mg IV over 30 min wk 0, 2, 6, then q8wk; D/C w/o benefit at wk 14; give w/in 4 h of reconstitution W/P: [B, M] Not rec w/ active Infxn; PML CI: Hypersens Rxn Disp: Single-use vial 300 mg/20 mL SE: N, HA, fever, pain (back, extremity, joints, oropharyngeal), fatigue, pruritus, URI, nasopharyngitis, sinusitis, cough, bronchitis, influenza Notes: Update all immunizations before start; ✓ neurologic S/Sxs

Vemurafenib (Zelboraf) Uses: *Unresectable met melanoma w/ BRAF mutation* Acts: BRAF serine-threonine kinase inhib Dose: Adults. 960 mg bid W/P: [D, –] If on warfarin, monitor closely CI: Ø Disp: Tabs 240 mg SE: Rash including SJS; anaphylaxis, pruritus, alopecia, photosens, arthralgias, skin SCC (> 20%), ↑ QT Notes: ✓ Derm exams q2mo for SCC; monitor ECG 15 d and qmo × 3; if QTc > 500 ms, D/C temporarily; ✓ LFT and bili baseline and qmo; mod CYP1A2 inhib, weak CYP2D6 inhib and CYP3A4 inducer

Venlafaxine (Effexor XR, Generic) BOX: Monitor for worsening depression or emergence of suicidality, particularly in ped pts Uses: *Depression, generalized anxiety, social anxiety disorder; panic disorder*, OCD, chronic fatigue synd, ADHD, autism Acts: Potentiation of CNS neurotransmitter activity Dose: 75–225 mg/d ÷ in 2–3 equal doses (IR) or qd (ER); 375 mg IR or 225 mg ER max/d; ↓ w/ renal/hepatic impair W/P: [C, ?/–] CI: MAOIs Disp: Tabs IR 25, 37.5, 50, 75, 100 mg; ER caps 37.5, 75, 150 mg; ER tabs 37.5, 75, 150, 225 mg SE: HTN, ↑ HR, HA, somnolence, xerostomia, insomnia, GI upset, sexual dysfunction; actuates mania or Szs Notes: Avoid EtOH; taper on D/C to avoid withdral Sxs

Verapamil (Calan, Calan SR, Isoptin SR, Verelan, Verelan PM, Generic) Uses: *Angina, HTN, PSVT, AF/A flutter*, migraine prophylaxis, hypertrophic cardiomyopathy, bipolar Dz Acts: CCB Dose: Adults. Arrhythmias: 2nd line for PSVT w/ narrow QRS complex & adequate BP 2.5–10 mg IV over 1–2 min; repeat 5–10 mg in 15–30 min PRN (30 mg max) Angina: 80–120 mg PO tid, ↑ 480 mg/24 h max HTN: 80–180 mg PO tid or SR tabs 120–240 mg PO qd to 240 mg bid ECC 2010: Reentry SVT w/ narrow QRS: 2.5–5 mg IV over 2 min (slower in older pts); repeat 5–10 mg, in 15–30 min, PRN max of 20 mg; or 5-mg bolus q15min (max 30 mg) Peds < 1 y. 0.1–0.2 mg/kg IV over 2 min (may repeat in 30 min) 1–16 y. 0.1–0.3 mg/kg IV over 2 min (may repeat in 30 min); 5mg max PO: 3–4 mg/kg/d PO ÷ in 3 doses, max 8 mg/kg/d up to 480 mg/d > 5 y. 80 mg q6–8h; ↓ in renal/hepatic impair W/P: [C, +] Amiodarone/β-blockers/flecainide can cause ↓ HR; statins, midazolam, tacrolimus, theophylline levels may be ↑; use w/ clonidine may cause severe ↓ HR w/ elderly pts CI: EF < 30%, severe LV dysfunction, BP < 90 mm Hg, SSS, 2nd-, 3rd-AV block AF/A flutter w/ bypass tract Disp: Calan SR: Tabs 120, 180, 240 mg; Verelan: Caps 120, 180, 240, 360 mg; Verelan PM: Caps (ER) 100, 200, 300 mg; Calan: Tabs 80, 120 mg; Isoptin SR: 24-h tabs 120, 180, 240 mg; Inj 2.5 mg/mL SE: Gingival hyperplasia, constipation,

↓ BP, bronchospasm, HR or conduction disturbances; edema; ↓ BP and bradyarrhythmias taken w/ telithromycin

Vigabatrin (Sabril) **BOX:** Vision loss reported; assess vision periodically; D/C w/in 2–4 wk if no effects seen **Uses:** *Refractory complex partial Sz disorder, infantile spasms* **Acts:** ↓ GABA-T to ↑ levels of brain GABA **Dose:** *Adults.* Initially 500 mg bid, then ↑ daily dose by 500 mg at weekly intervals based on response and tolerability; 1500 mg bid max **Peds.** *Seizures:* 10–15 kg: 0.5–1 g/d ÷ bid; 16–30 kg: 1–1.5 g/d ÷ bid; 31–50 kg: 1.5–3 g/d ÷ bid; > 50 kg: 2–3 g/d ÷ bid; *Infantile spasms:* Initially 50 mg/kg/d ÷ bid, ↑ 25–50 mg/kg/d q3d to 150 mg/kg/d max **W/P:** [C, +/–] ↓ Dose by 25% w/ CrCl 50–80 mL/min, ↓ dose 50% w/ CrCl 30–50 mL/min, ↓ dose 75% w/ CrCl 10–30 mL/min; MRI signal changes reported in some infants **Disp:** Tabs 500 mg; powder/oral soln 500 mg/packet **SE:** Vision loss/blurring, anemia, peripheral neuropathy, fatigue, somnolence, nystagmus, tremor, memory impair, ↑ Wt, arthralgia, abn coordination, confusion **Notes:** ↓ Phenytoin levels reported; taper slowly to avoid withdrawal Szs; restricted distribution; see PI for powder dosing in peds

Vilazodone (Viibryd) **BOX:** ↑ Suicide risk in children/adolescents/young adults on antidepressants for MDD and other psychiatric disorders **Uses:** *MDD* **Acts:** SSRI and 5HT1A receptor partial agonist **Dose:** 40 mg/d; start 10 mg PO/d × 7 d, then 20 mg/d × 7 d, then 40 mg/d; ↓ to 20 mg w/ CYP3A4 inhib **W/P:** [C, ?/–] **CI:** MOAI, < 14 d between D/C MAOI and start **Disp:** Tabs 10, 20, 40 mg **SE:** Serotonin syndrome, NMS, N/V/D, dry mouth, dizziness, insomnia, restlessness, abnormal dreams, sexual dysfunction **Notes:** NOT approved for peds; w/ D/C, ↓ dose gradually

Vinblastine (Generic) **BOX:** Chemotherapeutic agent; handle w/ caution; only individuals experienced in use of vinblastine should administer; IV only; tissue damage w/ extrav **Uses:** *Hodgkin Dz & NHLs, mycosis fungoides, CAs (testis, renal cell, breast, NSCLC), AIDS-related Kaposi sarcoma*, choriocarcinoma, histiocytosis **Acts:** ↓ Microtubule assembly **Dose:** Based on specific protocol; ↓ in hepatic failure **W/P:** [D, ?] **CI:** Granulocytopenia, bacterial Infxn **Disp:** Inj 1 mg/mL in 10-mg vial **SE:** ↓ BM (especially leukopenia), N/V, constipation, neurotox, alopecia, rash, myalgia, tumor pain **Notes:** Its use can be fatal

Vincristine [Vincristine PFS] (Marquibo, Generic) **BOX:** Chemotherapeutic agent; handle w/ caution; fatal if administered IT; IV only; administration by individuals experienced in use of vincristine only; severe tissue damage w/ extrav **Uses:** *ALL, breast CA, SCLC, sarcoma (eg, Ewing tumor, rhabdomyosarcoma), Wilms tumor, Hodgkin Dz & NHLs, neuroblastoma, multiple myeloma* **Acts:** Promotes disassembly of mitotic spindle, causing metaphase arrest, vinca alkaloid **Dose:** Per protocols; 0.4–1.4 mg/m² (single doses 2 mg/max); ↓ in hepatic failure **W/P:** [D, –] **CI:** Charcot-Marie-Tooth synd **Disp:** Inj 1 mg/mL **SE:** Neurotox commonly dose limiting jaw pain, (trigeminal neuralgia), fever, fatigue, anorexia, constipation & paralytic ileus, bladder atony; no sig ↓ BM w/ standard doses; tissue necrosis w/ extrav; myelosuppression

Vinorelbine (Navelbine, Generic) BOX: Chemotherapeutic agent; administration by physician experienced in CA chemotharapy only; severe granulocytopenia possible; extra may cause tissue irritation and necrosis; IV only **Uses:** *Breast CA & NSCLC* (alone or w/ cisplatin) **Acts:** ↓ Polymerization of microtubules, impairing mitotic spindle formation; semisynthetic vinca alkaloid **Dose:** Per protocols; 30 mg/m^3/wk; ↓ in hepatic failure **W/P:** [D, –] **CI:** Intrathecal IT use, granulocytopenia (< 1000/mm^3) **Disp:** Inj 10 mg/mL **SE:** ↓ BM (leukopenia), mild GI, neurotox (6–29%); constipation/paresthesias (rare); tissue damage from extrav, alopecia

Vismodegib (Erivedge) BOX: Embryo-fetal death and severe birth defects; verify PRG status before start; advise female and male pts to these risks; advise females on need for contraception and males of potential risk of exposure through semen **Uses:** *Met basal cell carcinoma, postsurgery local recurrence, not surgical candidate* **Acts:** Binds/inhibs transmembrane protein involved in hedgehog signal transduction **Dose:** 150 mg PO daily **W/P:** [D, –] **CI:** Ø **Disp:** Caps 150 mg **SE:** N/V/D, constipation, ↓ Wt, anorexia, dysgeusia, ageusia, arthralgias, muscle spasms, fatigue, alopecia, ↓ Na$^+$, ↑ K$^+$, azotemia; ↑ SE if coadministered w/ P-gp inhib **Notes:** w/ Missed dose DO NOT make up missed dose, resume w/ next scheduled dose; DO NOT donate blood while on Tx and for 7 mo after last Tx; immediately report exposure if PRG

Vitamin B$_1$ (See Thiamine, p 302)
Vitamin B$_6$ (See Pyridoxine, p 267)
Vitamin B$_{12}$ (See Cyanocobalamin, p 103)
Vitamin K (See Phytonadione, p 257)
Vitamin, Multi (See Multivitamins, Oral & Table 12, p 359)
Vorapaxar (Zontivity) BOX: Do not use w/ stroke, TIA, intracranial hemorrhage, active bleeding; anti-plt agents ↑ bleeding risk **Uses:** *↓ Thrombotic events w/ MI or peripheral artery Dz* **Acts:** PAR1 antag **Dose:** 1 tab PO qd w/ ASA or clopidogrl **W/P:** [C, –] ↑ Bleeding risk; avoid w/ strong CYP3A inhib/ inducers **CI:** see PI **Disp:** Tabs 2.08 mg **SE:** Bleeding possibly fatal

Voriconazole (VFEND, Generic) **Uses:** *Invasive aspergillosis, candidemia, serious fungal Infxns* **Acts:** ↓ Ergosterol synth. *Spectrum: Candida, Aspergillus, Scedosporium, Fusarium* sp **Dose:** *Adults & Peds > 12 y.* IV: 6 mg/kg q12h × 2 doses, then 4 mg/kg bid PO; < 40 kg: 100 mg q12h, up to 150 mg; > 40 kg: 200 mg q12h, up to 300 mg; w/ mild–mod hepatic impair; IV not rec d/t accumulation of IV diluent; w/ CYP3A4 substrates (Table 10, p 356); do not use w/ clopidogrel (↓ effect) **W/P:** [D, ?/–] SJS, electrolyte disturbances **CI:** w/ Terfenadine, astemizole, cisapride, pimozide, quinidine, sirolimus, rifampin, carbamazepine, long-acting barbiturates, ritonavir, rifabutin, ergot alkaloids, St. John's wort; in pt w/ galactose intol; skeletal events w/ long term use; w/ proarrhythmic cond **Disp:** Tabs 50, 200 mg; susp 200 mg/5 mL; Inj 200 mg **SE:** Visual changes, fever, rash, GI upset, ↑ LFTs, edema **Notes:** ✓ for multiple drug interactions (eg, ↓ dose w/ phenytoin); ✓ LFT before and during; ✓ vision w/ use 28 d

Vorinostat (Zolinza) **Uses:** *Rx cutaneous manifestations in cutaneous T-cell lymphoma* **Acts:** Histone deacetylase inhib **Dose:** 400 mg PO qd w/ food; if intolerant, 300 mg PO qd × 5 consecutive d each wk; ↓ w/ mild–mod hepatic impair **W/P:** [D, ?/ –] w/ Warfarin (↑ INR) **CI:** Severe hepatic impair **Disp:** Caps 100 mg **SE:** N/V/D, dehydration, fatigue, anorexia, dysgeusia, DVT, PE, ↓ plt, anemia, ↑ SCr, hyperglycemia, ↑ QTc, edema, muscle spasms **Notes:** Monitor CBC, lytes (K+, Mg2+, Ca2+), glu, & SCr q2wk × 2 mo then monthly; baseline & periodic ECGs; drink 2 L fluid/d

Vortioxetine (Brintellix): **BOX:** ↑ Risk of suicidal behavior/thinking in children, adolescents, and young adults; monitor for ↑ suicidal behaviors or thought; has not been evaluated in peds **Uses:** *MDD* **Acts:** Inhib serotonin reuptake **Dose:** *Adults.* 10 mg qd, ↑ to 20 mg as tolerated; consider 5 mg/d if intol to higher doses **W/P:** [C, –] Serotonin syndrome risk ↑ w/ other serotonergic drugs (TCA, tramadol, lithium, triptans, buspirone, St. John's Wort); ↑ bleeding risk; may induce mania or hypomania; SIADH w/ ↓ Na+ **CI:** w/ MAOIs, linezolid, or methylene blue (IV); stop MAOIs 14 d before; stop 21 d before starting MAOIs **Disp:** Tabs 5, 10, 15, 20 mg **SE:** N/V, constipation, sexual dysfunction **Notes:** w/ strong CYP2D6 inhib, ↓ dose by ½; w/ strong CYP2D6 inducers for > 2 wk, consider ↑ dose, NOT to exceed 3 × original dose

Warfarin (Coumadin, Jantoven, Generic) **BOX:** Can cause major/fatal bleeding; monitor INR; drugs, dietary changes, other factors affect INR; instruct pts about bleeding risk **Uses:** *Prophylaxis & Rx of PE & DVT, AF w/ embolization* **Acts:** ↓ Vit K-dependent clotting factors in this order: VII-IX-X-II **Dose:** *Adults.* Titrate, INR 2.0–3.0 for most; mechanical valves INR is 2.5–3.5. *American College of Chest Physicians guidelines:* 5 mg initial, may use 7.5–10 mg; ↓ if pt elderly or w/ other bleeding risk factors; maint 2–10 mg/d PO, follow daily INR initial to adjust dosage (Table 8, p 353). *Peds.* 0.05–0.34 mg/kg/24 h PO or IV; follow PT/INR to adjust dosage; monitor vit K intake; ↓ w/ hepatic impair/ elderly **W/P:** [X, +] **CI:** Bleeding, peptic ulcer, PRG **Disp:** Tabs 1, 2, 2.5, 3, 4, 5, 6, 7.5, 10 mg **SE:** Bleeding d/t overanticoagulation or injury & therapeutic INR; bleeding, alopecia, skin necrosis, purple toe synd **Notes:** Monitor vit K intake (↓ effect); INR preferred test; to rapidly correct overanticoagulation: vit K, fresh-frozen plasma, or both. Caution pt on taking w/ other meds that can ↑ risk of bleed. *Common warfarin interactions: Potentiated by:* APAP, EtOH (w/ liver Dz), amiodarone, cimetidine, ciprofloxacin, cotrimoxazole, erythromycin, fluconazole, flu vaccine, isoniazid, itraconazole, metronidazole, omeprazole, phenytoin, propranolol, quinidine, tetracycline. *Inhibited by:* barbiturates, carbamazepine, chlordiazepoxide, cholestyramine, dicloxacillin, nafcillin, rifampin, sucralfate, high–vit K foods. Consider genotyping for VKORC1 & CYP2C9

Witch Hazel (Tucks Pads, Others) [OTC] **Uses:** After BM, cleansing to decrease local irritation or relieve hemorrhoids; after anorectal surgery, episiotomy, Vag hygiene **Acts:** Astringent; shrinks blood vessels locally **Dose:** Apply PRN

W/P: [?, ?] External use only **CI:** Ø **Supplied:** Presoaked pads **SE:** Mild itching or burning

Zafirlukast (Accolate, Generic) Uses: *Adjunctive Rx of asthma* Acts: Selective & competitive inhib of leukotrienes **Dose: *Adults & Peds > 12 y.*** 20 mg bid *Peds 5–11 y.* 10 mg PO bid (on empty stomach) **W/P:** [B, –] Interacts w/ warfarin, ↑ INR **CI:** Component allergy, hepatic impair **Disp:** Tabs 10, 20 mg **SE:** Hepatic dysfunction, usually reversible on D/C; HA, dizziness, GI upset; Churg-Strauss synd, neuropsych events (agitation, restlessness, suicidal ideation) **Notes:** Not for acute asthma

Zaleplon (Sonata, Generic) [C-IV] Uses: *Insomnia* Acts: Nonbenzodiazepine sedative/hypnotic, pyrazolopyrimidine **Dose:** 5–20 mg hs PRN; not w/ high-fat meal; ↓ w/ hepatic Insuff, elderly **W/P:** [C, ?/–] Angioedema, anaphylaxis; w/ mental/psychological conditions **CI:** Component allergy **Disp:** Caps 5, 10 mg **SE:** HA, edema, amnesia, somnolence, photosens **Notes:** Take immediately before desired onset

Zanamivir (Relenza) Uses: *Influenza A & B w/ Sxs < 2 d; prophylaxis for influenza* Acts: ↓ Viral neuraminidase **Dose: *Adults & Peds > 7 y.*** 2 Inh (10 mg) bid × 5d, initiate w/in 48 h of Sxs *Prophylaxis household:* 10 mg qd × 10 d *Prophylaxis community:* 10 mg qd × 28 d **W/P:** [C, ?] Not OK for pt w/ airway Dz, reports of severe bronchospasms **CI:** Component or milk allergy **Disp:** Powder for Inh 5 mg **SE:** Bronchospasm, HA, GI upset, allergic Rxn, abn behavior, ear, nose, throat Sx **Notes:** Uses a Diskhaler for administration; dose same time each d

Ziconotide (Prialt) **BOX:** Psychological, cognitive, neurologic impair may develop over several wk; monitor frequently; may necessitate D/C Uses: *IT Rx of severe, refractory, chronic pain* Acts: N-type CCB in spinal cord **Dose:** Max initial dose 2.4 mcg/d IT at 0.1 mcg/h; may ↑ 2.4 mcg/d 2–3×/wk to max 19.2 mcg/d (0.8 mcg/h) by d 21 **W/P:** [C, ?/–] w/ Neuro-/psychological impair **Disp:** Inj (mcg/mL): 100/1, 500/5, 500/20 **SE:** Dizziness, N/V, confusion, psych disturbances, abn vision, edema, ↑ SCF, amnesia, ataxia, meningitis; may require dosage adjustment **Notes:** May D/C abruptly; uses specific pumps (eg, Medtronic SynchroMed systems); do not ↑ more frequently than 2–3×/wk

Zidovudine (Retrovir, Generic) **BOX:** Neutropenia, anemia, lactic acidosis, myopathy, & hepatomegaly w/ steatosis Uses: *HIV Infxn, Px maternal HIV transmission* Acts: NRTI **Dose: *Adults.*** 200 mg PO tid or 300 mg PO bid or 1 mg/kg/dose IV q4h *PRG:* 100 mg PO 5×/d until labor; during labor 2 mg/kg IV over 1 h, then 1 mg/kg/h until cord clamped *Peds 4 wk–18 y.* 160 mg/m²/dose tid or see table below; ↓ in renal failure **W/P:** [C, ?/–] w/ Ganciclovir, interferon alpha, ribavirin; may alter many other meds (see PI) **CI:** Allergy **Disp:** Caps 100 mg; tabs 300 mg; syrup 50 mg/5 mL; Inj 10 mg/mL **SE:** Hematologic tox, HA, fever, rash, GI upset, malaise, myopathy, fat redistribution **Notes:** w/ Severe anemia/neutropenia dosage interruption may be needed

Recommended Pediatric Dosage of Retrovir

Body Weight (kg)	Total Daily Dose	Dosage Regimen and Dose	
		bid	tid
4 to < 9	24 mg/kg/d	12 mg/kg	8 mg/kg
≥ 9 to < 30	18 mg/kg/d	9 mg/kg	6 mg/kg
≥ 30	600 mg/d	300 mg	200 mg

Zidovudine/Lamivudine (Combivir, Generic) BOX: Neutropenia, anemia, lactic acidosis, myopathy & hepatomegaly w/ steatosis **Uses:** *HIV Infxn* **Acts:** Combo of RT inhib **Dose:** *Adults & Peds > 12 y.* 1 tab PO bid; ↓ in renal failure **W/P:** [C, ?/–] **CI:** Component allergy **Disp:** Tabs zidovudine 300 mg/lamivudine 150 mg **SE:** Hematologic tox, HA, fever, rash, GI upset, malaise, pancreatitis **Notes:** Combo product ↓ daily pill burden; refer to individual component listings

Zileuton (Zyflo, Zyflo CR) **Uses:** *Chronic Rx asthma* **Acts:** Leukotriene inhib (↓ 5-lipoxygenase) **Dose:** *Adults & Peds > 12 y.* 600 mg PO qid; CR 1200 mg bid 1 h after A.M./P.M. meal **W/P:** [C, ?/–] **CI:** Hepatic impair **Disp:** Tabs 600 mg; CR tabs 600 mg **SE:** Hepatic damage, HA, N/D, upper Abd pain, leukopenia, neuropsych events (agitation, restlessness, suicidal ideation) **Notes:** Monitor LFTs qmo × 3, then q2–3mo; take regularly; not for acute asthma; do not chew/crush CR

Ziprasidone (Geodon, Generic) BOX: ↑ Mortality in elderly w/ dementia-related psychosis **Uses:** *Schizophrenia, acute agitation bipolar disorder* **Acts:** Atypical antipsychotic **Dose:** 20 mg PO bid, may ↑ in 2-d intervals up to 80 mg bid; *agitation:* 10–20 mg IM PRN up to 40 mg/d; separate 10-mg doses by 2 h & 20-mg doses by 4 h (w/ food) **W/P:** [C, –] w/ ↓ Mg²⁺, ↓ K⁺ **CI:** QT prolongation, recent MI, uncompensated heart failure, meds that ↑ QT interval **Disp:** Caps 20, 40, 60, 80 mg; Inj 20 mg/mL **SE:** ↓ HR; rash, somnolence, resp disorder, EPS, Wt gain, orthostatic ↓ BP **Notes:** ✓ lytes

Ziv-Aflibercept (Zaltrap) BOX: Severe/fatal hemorrhage possible, including GI hemorrhage; D/C w/ GI perf; D/C w/ compromised wound healing, suspend Tx 4 wk prior to & after surgery & until surgical wound is fully healed **Uses:** *Met colorectal CA (PI/institution protocol)* **Acts:** Binds VEGF-A & PIGF w/ ↓ neovascularization & ↓ vascular permeability **Dose:** 4 mg/kg IV Inf over 1 h q2wk **W/P:** [C, –] Severe D w/ dehydration; D/C w/ fistula, ATE, hypertensive crisis, RPLS; ✓ urine protein, suspend Tx if proteinuria ≥ 2 g/24 h, D/C w/ nephrotic synd or thrombotic microangiopathy; ✓ neutrophils, delay until ≥ 1.5 × 10⁹/L **CI:** Ø **Disp:** Inj vial 25 mg/mL (100 mg/4 mL, 200 mg/8 mL) **SE:** D, ↓ WBC, ↓ plts, stomatitis, proteinuria, ↑ ALT/AST, fatigue, epistaxis, Abd pain, ↓ appetite, ↓ Wt, dysphonia, ↑ SCr, HA **Notes:** Males/females: use contraception during Tx & for 3 mo after last dose

Zoledronic Acid (Reclast, Zometa, Generic) Uses: *HCM, ↓ skeletal-related events in PCa multiple myeloma, & met bone lesions (*Zometa*)*; *Px/Rx of postmenopausal osteoporosis, Paget Dz, ↑ bone mass in men w/ osteoporosis, steroid-induced osteoporosis (*Reclast*)* Acts: Bisphosphonate; ↓ osteoclastic bone resorption Dose: *Zometa HCM:* 4 mg IV over ≥ 15 min; may retreat in 7 d w/ adequate renal Fxn *Zometa bone lesions/myeloma:* 4 mg IV over > 15 min, repeat q3–4wk PRN; extend w/ ↑ Cr. *Reclast Rx osteoporosis:* 5 mg IV annually *Reclast:* Px postmenopausal osteoporosis 5 mg IV q2y *Paget:* 5 mg IV × 1 W/P: [D, ?/–] w/ Diuretics, aminoglycosides; ASA-sensitive asthmatics; avoid invasive dental procedures CI: Bisphosphonate allergy; hypocalcemia, angioedema, CrCl < 35 Disp: Vial 4 mg, 5 mg SE: Fever, flu-like synd, GI upset, insomnia, anemia; electrolyte abnormalities, bone/jt/muscle pain, AF, ONJ, atyp femur Fx Notes: Requires vigorous prehydration; do not exceed rec doses/Inf duration to ↓ renal dysfunction; follow Cr; effect prolonged w/ Cr ↑; avoid oral surgery; dental exam recommended prior to Rx; ↓ dose w/ renal dysfunction; give Ca²⁺ and vit D supls; may ↑ atypical subtrochanteric femur fractures

Zolmitriptan (Zomig, Zomig Nasal, Zomig ZMT) Uses: *Acute Rx migraine* Acts: Selective serotonin agonist; causes vasoconstriction Dose: Initial 2.5 mg PO, may repeat after 2 h, 10 mg max in 24 h; nasal 2.5–5 mg; if HA returns, repeat after 2 h, 10 mg max 24 h W/P: [C, ?/–] CI: Ischemic heart Dz, Prinzmetal angina, uncontrolled HTN, accessory conduction pathway disorders, ergots, MAOIs Disp: Tabs 2.5, 5 mg; rapid tabs (*Zomig ZMT*) 2.5, 5 mg; nasal 2.5, 5 mg, SE: Dizziness, hot flashes, paresthesias, chest tightness, myalgia, diaphoresis, unusual taste, coronary artery spasm

Zolpidem (Ambien CR, Ambien IR, Edluar, Intermezzo, ZolpiMist, Generic) [C-IV] Uses: *Short-term Tx of insomnia; *Ambien and Edluar* w/ difficulty of sleep onset; *Ambien CR* w/ difficulty of sleep onset and/or sleep maint* Acts: Hypnotic agent Dose: *Adults, Men. Ambien:* 5–10 mg or 12.5 mg *CR* PO qhs; *Edluar:* 10 mg SL qhs; *Intermezzo:* 3.5 mg qhs; *Zolpimist:* 10 mg spray qhs *Women.* 5 mg for IR (*Ambien, Edluar, and Zolpimist*); 6.25 mg for ER (*Ambien CR*); *Intermezzo:* 1.75 mg qhs; ↓ dose in elderly, debilitated, & hepatic impair (5 mg or 6.25 mg CR) W/P: [C, M] May cause anaphylaxis, angioedema, abn thinking, CNS depression, withdrawal; evaluate for other comorbid conditions; next-day psychomotor impairment/impaired driving when Ambien is taken w/ less than a full night of sleep remaining (7–8 h) CI: Ø Disp: *Ambien IR:* Tabs 5, 10 mg; *Ambien CR* 6.25, 12.5 mg; *Edluar:* SL tabs 5, 10 mg; *Intermezzo:* SL tabs 1.75, 3.5 mg; *Zolpimist:* Oral soln 5 mg/spray (60 actuations/unit) SE: Drowsiness, dizziness, D, drugged feeling, HA, dry mouth, depression Notes: Take tabs on empty stomach; be able to sleep 7–8 h; *Zolpimist:* Prime w/ 5 sprays initially, and w/ 1 spray if not used in 14 d; store upright

Zonisamide (Zonegran, Generic) Uses: *Adjunct Rx complex partial Szs* Acts: Anticonvulsant Dose: Initial 100 mg/d PO; may ↑ by 100 mg/d q2wk to

400 mg/d **W/P:** [C, −] ↑ q2wk w/ CYP3A4 inhib; ↓ levels w/ carbamazepine, phenytoin, phenobarbital, valproic acid **CI:** Allergy to sulfonamides **Disp:** Caps 25, 50, 100 mg **SE:** Metabolic acidosis, dizziness, drowsiness, confusion, ataxia, memory impair, paresthesias, psychosis, nystagmus, diplopia, tremor, anemia, leukopenia; GI upset, nephrolithiasis (? d/t metabolic acidosis), SJS; monitor for ↓ sweating & ↑ body temperature **Notes:** Swallow caps whole

Zoster Vaccine, Live (Zostavax) **Uses:** *Px varicella zoster in adults > 50 y* **Acts:** Active immunization (live attenuated varicella) virus **Dose:** 0.65 mL SQ × 1 **CI:** Gelatin, neomycin anaphylaxis; fever, untreated TB, immunosuppression, PRG **W/P:** [C, ?/−] **Disp:** Single-dose vial **SE:** Inj site Rxn, HA **Notes:** May be used if previous Hx of zoster; do not use in place of varicella virus vaccine in children; contact precautions not necessary; antivirals and immune globulins may ↓ effectiveness

NATURAL AND HERBAL AGENTS

The following is a guide to some common herbal products. These may be sold separately or in combination with other products. According to the FDA, "Manufacturers of dietary supplements can make claims about how their products affect the structure or function of the body, but they may not claim to prevent, treat, cure, mitigate, or diagnose a disease without prior FDA approval." The table on p 331 summarizes some of the common dangerous aspects of natural and herbal agents.

Black Cohosh Uses: Sx of menopause (eg, hot flashes), PMS, hypercholesterolemia, peripheral arterial Dz; has anti-inflam & sedative effects Efficacy: May have short-term benefit on menopausal Sx Dose: 20–40 mg bid W/P: May further ↓ lipids &/or BP w/ prescription meds CI: PRG (miscarriage, prematurity reports); lactation SE: w/ OD, N/V, dizziness, nervous system & visual changes, ↓ HR, & (possibly) Szs, liver damage/failure

Chamomile Uses: Antispasmodic, sedative, anti-inflam, astringent, antibacterial Dose: 10–15 g PO qd (3 g dried flower heads tid–qid between meals; can steep in 250 mL hot H_2O) W/P: w/ Allergy to chrysanthemums, ragweed, asters (family *Compositae*) SE: Contact dermatitis; allergy, anaphylaxis Interactions: w/ Anticoagulants, additive w/ sedatives (benzodiazepines); delayed ↓ gastric absorption of meds if taken together (↓ GI motility)

Cranberry (*Vaccinium macrocarpon*) Uses: Px & Rx UTI Efficacy: Possibly effective Dose: 300–400 mg bid, in 6-oz juice qid; tincture 1/2–1 tsp up to tid, tea 2–3 tsp of dried flowers/cup; creams apply topically bid-tid PO W/P: May ↑ kidney stones in some susceptible individuals, V SE: None known Interactions: May potentiate warfarin

Dong Quai (*Angelica polymorpha, sinensis*) Uses: Uterine stimulant; anemia, menstrual cramps, irregular menses, & menopausal Sx; anti-inflam, vasodilator, CNS stimulant, immunosuppressant, analgesic, antipyretic, antiasthmatic Efficacy: Possibly effective for menopausal Sx Dose: 3–15 g qd, 9–12 g PO tab bid W/P: Avoid in PRG & lactation SE: D, photosens, skin CA Interactions: Anticoagulants (↑ INR w/ warfarin)

Echinacea (*Echinacea purpurea*) Uses: Immune system stimulant; Px/Rx URI of colds, flu; supportive care in chronic Infxns of the resp/lower urinary tract Efficacy: Not established; may ↓ severity & duration of URI Dose: Caps 500 mg, 6–9 mL expressed juice or 2–5 g dried root PO W/P: Do not use w/progressive systemic or immune Dzs (eg, TB, collagen–vascular disorders, MS); may interfere w/ immunosuppressive Rx, not OK w/ PRG; do not use > 8 consecutive wk; possible immunosuppression; 3 different commercial forms **SE:** N; rash **Interactions:** Anabolic steroids, amiodarone, MTX, corticosteroids, cyclosporine

Evening Primrose Oil **Uses:** PMS, diabetic neuropathy, ADHD **Efficacy:** Possibly for PMS, not for menopausal Sx **Dose:** 2–4 g/d PO **SE:** Indigestion, N, soft stools, HA **Interactions:** ↑ Phenobarbital metabolism, ↓ Sz threshold

Feverfew (*Tanacetum parthenium*) **Uses:** Px/Rx migraine; fever; menstrual disorders; arthritis; toothache; insect bites **Efficacy:** Weak for migraine prevention **Dose:** 125 mg PO of dried leaf (standardized to 0.2% of parthenolide) PO **W/P:** Do not use in PRG **SE:** Oral ulcers, gastric disturbance, swollen lips, Abd pain; long-term SE unknown **Interactions:** ASA, warfarin

Fish Oil Supplements (Omega-3 Polyunsaturated Fatty Acid) **Uses:** CAD, hypercholesterolemia, hypertriglyceridemia, type 2 DM, arthritis **Efficacy:** No definitive data on ↓ cardiac risk in general population; may ↓ lipids & help w/ secondary MI prevention **Dose:** One FDA approved (see Lovaza, p 238) OTC 1500–3000 mg/d; AHA rec: 1 g/d **W/P:** Mercury contamination possible; some studies suggest ↑ cardiac events **SE:** ↑ Bleeding risk, dyspepsia, belching, aftertaste **Interactions:** Anticoagulants

Garlic (*Allium sativum*) **Uses:** Antioxidant; hyperlipidemia; HTN; antiinfective (antibacterial, antifungal); tick repellent (oral) **Efficacy:** ↓ Cholesterol by 4–6%; soln ↓ BP; possible ↓ GI/CAP risk **Dose:** 2–5 g, fresh garlic; 0.4–1.2 g of dried powder; 2–5 mg oil; 300–1000 mg extract or other formulations = 2–5 mg of allicin daily, 400–1200 mg powder (2–5 mg allicin) PO **W/P:** Do not use in PRG (abortifacient); D/C 7 d preop (bleeding risk) **SE:** ↑ Insulin/lipid/cholesterol levels, anemia, oral burning sensation, N/V/D **Interactions:** Warfarin & ASA (↓ plt aggregation), additive w/ DM agents (↑ hypoglycemia), CYP3A4 inducer (may ↑ cyclosporine, HIV antivirals, oral contraceptives)

Ginger (*Zingiber officinale*) **Uses:** Px motion sickness; N/V d/t anesthesia **Efficacy:** Benefit in ↓ N/V w/ motion or PRG; weak for postop or chemotherapy **Dose:** 1–4 g rhizome or 0.5–2 g powder PO qd **W/P:** Pt w/ gallstones; excessive dose (↑ depression, & may interfere w/ cardiac Fxn or anticoagulants) **SE:** Heartburn **Interactions:** Excessive consumption may interfere w/ cardiac, DM, or anticoagulant meds (↓ plt aggregation)

Ginkgo Biloba **Uses:** Memory deficits, dementia, anxiety, improvement Sx peripheral vascular Dz, vertigo, tinnitus, asthma/bronchospasm, antioxidant, premenstrual Sx (especially breast tenderness), impotence, SSRI-induced sexual dysfunction **Dose:** 60–80 mg standardized dry extract PO bid–tid **Efficacy:** Small cognition benefit w/ dementia; no other demonstrated benefit in healthy adults **W/P:** ↑ Bleeding risk (plt-activating factor antag), concerning w/ anti-plt agents (D/C 3 d preop); reports of ↑ Sz risk **SE:** GI upset, HA, dizziness, heart palpitations, rash **Interactions:** ASA, salicylates, warfarin, antidepressants

Ginseng **Uses:** "Energy booster" general; also for pt undergoing chemotherapy, stress reduction, enhance brain activity & physical endurance (adaptogenic)

antioxidant, aid to control type 2 DM; Panax ginseng being studied for ED **Efficacy:** Not established **Dose:** 1–2 g of root or 100–300 mg of extract (7% ginsenosides) PO tid **W/P:** w/ Cardiac Dz, DM, ↓ BP, HTN, mania, schizophrenia, w/ corticosteroids; avoid in PRG; D/C 7 d preop (bleeding risk) **SE:** Controversial "ginseng abuse synd" w/ high dose (nervousness, excitation, HA, insomnia); palpitations, Vag bleeding, breast nodules, hypoglycemia **Interactions:** Warfarin, antidepressants, & caffeine (↑ stimulant effect), DM meds (↑ hypoglycemia)

Glucosamine Sulfate (Chitosamine) and Chondroitin Sulfate

Uses: Osteoarthritis (*Glucosamine:* rate-limiting step in glycosaminoglycan synth), ↑ cartilage rebuilding; *Chondroitin:* biological polymer, flexible matrix between protein filaments in cartilage; draws fluids/nutrients into joint, "shock absorption") **Efficacy:** Controversial **Dose:** *Glucosamine:* 500 PO tid, chondroitin 400 mg PO tid **W/P:** Many forms come from shellfish, so avoid if have shellfish allergy **SE:** ↑ Insulin resistance in DM; concentrated in cartilage, theoretically unlikely to cause tox/teratogenic effects **Interactions:** *Glucosamine:* None. *Chondroitin:* Monitor anticoagulant Rx

Kava Kava (Kava Kava Root Extract, *Piper methysticum*) Uses:

Anxiety, stress, restlessness, insomnia **Efficacy:** Possible mild anxiolytic **Dose:** Standardized extract (70% kavalactones) 100 mg PO bid–tid **W/P:** Hepatotox risk, banned in Europe/Canada; not OK in PRG, lactation; D/C 24 h preop (may ↑ sedative effect of anesthetics) **SE:** Mild GI disturbances; rare allergic skin/rash Rxns, may ↑ cholesterol; ↑ LFTs/jaundice; vision changes, red eyes, puffy face, muscle weakness **Interactions:** Avoid w/ sedatives, alcohol, stimulants, barbiturates (may potentiate CNS effect)

Melatonin Uses:

Insomnia, jet lag, antioxidant, immunostimulant **Efficacy:** Sedation most pronounced w/ elderly pts w/ ↓ endogenous melatonin levels; some evidence for jet lag **Dose:** 1–3 mg 20 min before hs (w/ CR 2 h before hs) **W/P:** Use synthetic rather than animal pineal gland **SE:** "Heavy head", HA, depression, daytime sedation, dizziness **Interactions:** β-Blockers, steroids, NSAIDs, benzodiazepines

Milk Thistle (*Silybum marianum*) Uses:

Px/Rx liver damage (eg, from alcohol, toxins, cirrhosis, chronic hep); preventive w/ chronic toxin exposure (painters, chemical workers, etc) **Efficacy:** Use before exposure more effective than use after damage has occurred **Dose:** 80–200 mg PO tid **SE:** GI intolerance **Interactions:** Ø

Red Yeast Rice Uses:

Hyperlipidemia **Efficacy:** HMG-CoA reductase activity, naturally occurring lovastatin; ↓ LDL, ↓ triglycerides, ↑ HDL; ↓ secondary CAD events **Dose:** 1200–1800 mg bid **W/P:** CI w/ PRG, lactation; do not use w/ liver Dz, recent surgery, serious Infxn; may contain a mycotoxin, citrinin, can cause renal failure **Disp:** Caps 600–1200 mg **SE:** N/V, Abd pain, hep, myopathy, rhabdomyolysis **Interactions:** Possible interactions many drugs, avoid w/ CYP3A4 inhib or EtOH **Notes:** Use only in adults; generic lovastatin cheaper

Resveratrol Uses:

Cardioprotective, Px aging; ? antioxidant **Efficacy:** Limited human research **W/P:** Avoid w/ Hx of estrogen-responsive CA or w/

CYP3A4-metabolized drugs **Disp:** Caps, tabs 20–500 mg, skins of red grapes, plums, blueberries, cranberries, red wine **SE:** N/D, anorexia, insomnia, anxiety, jt pain, anti-plt aggregation **Interactions:** Avoid w/ other antiplatelet drugs or anticoagulants; CYP3A4 inhib

Saw Palmetto (*Serenoa repens*) Uses: Rx BPH, hair tonic, PCa Px (weak 5α-reductase inhib like finasteride, dutasteride) **Efficacy:** Small, no sig benefit for prostatic Sx **Dose:** 320 mg qd **W/P:** Possible hormonal effects, avoid in PRG, w/ women of childbearing years **SE:** Mild GI upset, mild HA, D w/ large amounts **Interactions:** ↑ Iron absorption; ↓ estrogen replacement effects

St. John's Wort (*Hypericum perforatum*) Uses: Mild–mod depression, anxiety, gastritis, insomnia, vitiligo; anti-inflam; immune stimulant/anti-HIV/antiviral **Efficacy:** Variable; benefit w/ mild–mod depression in several trials, but not always seen in clinical practice **Dose:** 2–4 g of herb or 0.2–1 mg of total hypericin (standardized extract) qd; also 300 mg PO tid (0.3% hypericin) **W/P:** Excess doses may potentiate MAOI, cause allergic Rxn, not OK in PRG **SE:** Photosens, xerostomia, dizziness, constipation, confusion, fluctuating mood w/ chronic use **Interactions:** CYP3A enzyme inducer; do not use w/ Rx antidepressants (especially MAOI); ↓ cyclosporine efficacy (may cause rejection), digoxin (may ↑ CHF), protease inhib, theophylline, OCP; potency varies between products/batches

Valerian (*Valeriana officinalis*) Uses: Anxiolytic, sedative, restlessness, dysmenorrhea **Efficacy:** Probably effective sedative (reduces sleep latency) **Dose:** 2–3 g in extract PO qd-bid added to 2/3 cup boiling H_2O, tincture 15–20 drops in H_2O, oral 400–900 mg hs (combined w/ OTC sleep product Alluna) **W/P:** Hepatotox w/ long-term use **SE:** Sedation, hangover effect, HA, cardiac disturbances, GI upset **Interactions:** Caution w/ other sedating agents (eg, alcohol or prescription sedatives): may cause drowsiness w/ impaired Fxn

Yohimbine (*Pausinystalia Yohimbe*) (*Yocon, Yohimex*) Uses: Improve sexual vigor, Rx ED **Efficacy:** Variable **Dose:** 1 tab = 5.4 mg PO tid (use w/ physician supervision) **W/P:** Do not use w/ renal/hepatic Dz; may exacerbate schizophrenia/mania (if pt predisposed); $α_2$-adrenergic antag (↓ BP, Abd distress, weakness w/ high doses), OD can be fatal; salivation, dilated pupils, arrhythmias **SE:** Anxiety, tremors, dizziness, ↑ BP, ↑ HR **Interactions:** Do not use w/ antidepressants (eg, MAOIs or similar agents)

(Adapted from Haist SA and Robbins JB. *Internal Medicine on Call*. 4th ed. New York, NY: McGraw-Hill; 2005; and the FDA. http://dietarysupplements.nlm.nih.gov/dietary/index.jsp. Accessed July 2014.)

Unsafe Herbs With Known Toxicity

Agent	Toxicities
Aconite	Salivation, N/V, blurred vision, cardiac arrhythmias
Aristolochic acid	Nephrotox
Calamus	Possible carcinogenicity
Chaparral	Hepatotox, possible carcinogenicity, nephrotox
"Chinese herbal mixtures"	May contain ma huang or other dangerous herbs
Coltsfoot	Hepatotox, possibly carcinogenic
Comfrey	Hepatotox, carcinogenic
Ephedra/ma huang	Adverse cardiac events, stroke, Sz
Juniper	High allergy potential, D, Sz, nephrotox
Kava kava	Hepatotox
Licorice	Chronic daily amounts (> 30 g/mo) can result in increased K^+, Na/fluid retention w/ HTN, myoglobinuria, hyporeflexia
Life root	Hepatotox, liver CA
Pokeweed	GI cramping, N/V/D, labored breathing, increased BP, Sz
Sassafras	V, stupor, hallucinations, dermatitis, abortion, hypothermia, liver CA
Usnic acid	Hepatotox
Yohimbine	Hypotension, Abd distress, CNS stimulation (mania/psychosis in predisposed individuals)

Source: Haist SA, Robbins JB. *Internal Medicine on Call.* 4th ed. New York, NY: McGraw-Hill; 2005.

Tables

TABLE 1
Local Anesthetic Comparison Chart for Commonly Used Injectable Agents

Agent	Proprietary Names	Onset	Duration	Maximum Dose mg/kg	Maximum Dose Volume in 70-kg Adult[a]
Bupivacaine	Marcaine	7–30 min	5–7 h	3	70 mL of 0.25% solution
Lidocaine	Xylocaine, Anestacon	5–30 min	2 h	4	28 mL of 1% solution
Lidocaine with epinephrine (1:200,000)		5–30 min	2–3 h	7	50 mL of 1% solution
Mepivacaine	Carbocaine	5–30 min	2–3 h	7	50 mL of 1% solution
Procaine	Novocaine	Rapid	30 min–1 h	10–15	70–105 mL of 1% solution

[a] To calculate the maximum dose if not a 70-kg adult, use the fact that a 1% solution has 10 mg/mL drug.

TABLE 2
Comparison of Systemic Steroids (See also p 287)

Drug	Relative Equivalent Dose (mg)	Relative Mineralocorticoid Activity	Duration (h)	Route
Betamethasone	0.75	0	36–72	PO, IM
Cortisone	25	2	8–12	PO, IM
Dexamethasone	0.75	0	36–72	PO, IV
Hydrocortisone (Solu-Cortef, Hydrocortone)	20	2	8–12	PO, IM, IV
Methylprednisolone acetate (Depo-Medrol)	4	0	36–72	PO, IM, IV
Methylprednisolone succinate (Solu-Medrol)	4	0	8–12	PO, IM, IV
Prednisone	5	1	12–36	PO
Prednisolone	5	1	12–36	PO, IM, IV

TABLE 3
Topical Steroid Preparations (See also p 288)

Agent	Common Trade Names Dosage/Strength	Potency	Apply
Alclometasone dipropionate	Aclovate, cream, oint 0.05%	Low	bid/tid
Amcinonide	Cream, lotion, oint 0.1%	High	bid/tid
Betamethasone			
Betamethasone valerate	Cream, lotion, oint 0.1%	Low	qd/bid
Betamethasone valerate	Luxiq foam 0.12%	Intermediate	qd/bid
Betamethasone dipropionate	Cream, lotion, oint 0.05%; aerosol 0.1%	High	qd/bid
Betamethasone dipropionate, augmented	Diprolene oint, lotion, gel 0.05%	Ultrahigh	qd/bid
Clobetasol propionate	Diprolene AF cream 0.05%	Ultrahigh	bid (2 wk max)
	Temovate, Clobex, Cormax cream, gel, oint, lotion, foam, aerosol, shampoo, soln, 0.05%, 00.05%, 0.5%	Ultrahigh	bid (2 wk max)
Clocortolone pivalate	Cloderm cream 0.1%	Intermediate	qd-qid
Desonide	DesOwen, cream, oint, lotion 0.05%	Low	bid-qid
Desoximetasone			
Desoximetasone 0.05%	Topicort cream, gel 0.05%	Intermediate	qd-qid
Desoximetasone 0.25%	Topicort cream, gel 0.025%	High	qd/bid
Dexamethasone base	Aerosol 0.01%, cream 0.1%	Low	bid-qid
Diflorasone diacetate	ApexiCon cream, oint 0.05%	Ultrahigh	bid-qid
Fluocinolone			
Fluocinolone acetonide 0.01%	Synalar cream, soln 0.01%	Low	bid/tid
	Capex shampoo 0.01%		

336

Fluocinolone acetonide 0.025%	Synalar oint, cream 0.025%	Intermediate	bid/tid
Fluocinonide 0.1%	Vanos cream 0.1%	High	qd/bid
Flurandrenolide	Cordran cream, oint 0.25%	Intermediate	qd
Fluticasone propionate	Cutivate cream, lotion 0.05%, oint 0.005%	Intermediate	bid
Halobetasol	Ultravate cream, oint 0.05%	Very high	bid
Halcinonide	Halog cream oint 0.1%	High	qd/bid
Hydrocortisone			
Hydrocortisone	Cortizone, Caldecort, Hycort, Hytone, etc—aerosol 1%, cream 0.5, 1, 2.5%, gel 0.5%, oint 0.5, 1, 2.5%, lotion 0.5, 1, 2.5%, paste 0.5%, soln 1%	Low	tid/qid
Hydrocortisone acetate	Cream, oint 0.5, 1%	Low	tid/qid
Hydrocortisone butyrate	Locoid oint, cream, lotion soln 0.1%	Intermediate	bid/tid
Hydrocortisone valerate	Cream, oint 0.2%	Intermediate	bid/tid
Mometasone furoate	Elocon cream, oint, lotion, soln 0.1%	Intermediate	qd
Prednicarbate	Dermatop cream, oint 0.1%	Intermediate	bid
Triamcinolone			
Triamcinolone acetonide 0.025%	Cream, oint, lotion 0.025%	Low	tid/qid
Triamcinolone acetonide 0.1%	Cream, oint, lotion 0.1%	Intermediate	tid/qid
	Kenalog aerosol 0.147 mg/g		
Triamcinolone acetonide 0.5%	Cream, oint 0.5%	High	tid/qid

Table 4
Comparison of Insulins (See also p 177)

Products are classified based on onset and duration of action. Insulin is 100 units per mL unless otherwise noted. Cartridge volume of insulin pens is 3 mL. Approximate performance characteristics of the different insulins are listed. See individual package inserts for specifics.

Type of Insulin			
Ultra Rapid	Onset < 0.25 h	Peak 0.5–1.5 h	3–4 h
Glulisine [rDNA origin] • Apidra, Apidra SoloSTAR pen			
Lispro [rDNA origin] • HumaLOG, HumaLOG KwikPen • HumaPen Luxura HD pen			
Aspart [rDNA origin] • NovoLOG, NovoLOG FlexPen • NovoPen Echo			
Rapid (regular insulin)	Onset 0.5–1 h	Peak 2–3h	Duration 4–6 h
Regular • HumuLIN R, NovoLIN R			

Intermediate	Onset 1–4 h	Peak 6–10 h	Duration 10–16 h

NPH
- HumuLIN N, HumuLIN N Pen
- NovoLIN N

Prolonged	Onset 1–4 h	Peak/No Peak/ max effect 5h	Duration 24 h

Glargine [rDNA origin]
- Lantus, Lantus SoloSTAR pen, Toujeo[a]

Detemir [rDNA origin]
- Levemir, Levemir FlexPen

Combination Insulins	Onset < 0.25 h	Peak Dual based on agent	Duration Up to 10 h

Lispro protamine suspension/Insulin lispro
- HumaLOG Mix 75/25
- HumaLOG Mix 75/25 KwikPen
- HumaLOG Mix 50/50
- HumaLOG Mix 50/50 KwikPen

339

(Continued)

Table 4 (continued)
Comparison of Insulins (See also p 177)

Combination Insulins	Onset < 0.25 h	Peak Dual Based on Agent	Duration Up to 10 h

Aspart protamine suspension/Insulin aspart
- NovoLOG Mix 70/30
- NovoLOG patients on NovoLOG 70/30 FlexPen

	Onset 0.5–1 h	Peak Dual Based on Agent	Duration Up to 10–16 h

NPH/Insulin regular
- HumuLIN 70/30
- HumuLIN 70/30 Pen
- NovoLIN 70/30

340

^aOnset 6h

About insulin pens:

Insulin pens can increase patient acceptance and adherence. Depending on the pen, the insulin cartridges may be prefilled disposable single use OR refillable/reusable. Dosage ranges vary but are typically 1 to 60–80 units, in increments of 1 unit, with **HumPen Luxura HD** and **NovoPen Echo** offering 0.5 unit increments. Features that are helpful for patients with reduced vision are a large or magnified dosing window and audible dosing clicks (end of dose click). Many pens allow for adjusting the dose without wasting insulin and prevent dialing a dose that is larger than the number of units remaining in the pen. **NovoPen Echo** is the first pen to record the dose and time of last injection and can accommodate different types of insulin in the cartridges. The CDC stresses patients not share injection pens.

Do not confuse **HumaLOG, NovoLOG, HumaLOG Mix,** and **NovoLOG Mix** with each other or with other agents, as serious medication errors can occur. Use **"TALL MAN LETTERS" for the "LOGs and the "LINs** per FDA recommendations to avoid prescribing errors.

TABLE 5
Oral Contraceptives (See also p 240)

(Note: 21 = 21 Active pills; 24 = 24 Active pills; Standard for most products is 28 [unless specified] = 21 Active pills + 7 Placebo[a])

Drug	Note	Progestin (mg)	Estrogen (mcg)	Extra
Altavera		Levonorgestrel (0.15)	Ethinyl estradiol (30)	
Alyacen 1/35		Norethindrone (1)	Ethinyl estradiol (35)	
Apri		Desogestrel (0.15)	Ethinyl estradiol (30)	
Aviane		Levonorgestrel (0.1)	Ethinyl estradiol (20)	
Balziva		Norethindrone (0.4)	Ethinyl estradiol (35)	
Beyaz	b, c, e	Drospirenone (3)	Ethinyl estradiol (20)	0.451 mg levomefolate in all including 7 placebo
Monophasics				
Brevicon		Norethindrone (0.5)	Ethinyl estradiol (35)	
Briellyn		Norethindrone (0.4)	Ethinyl estradiol (35)	
Cryselle		Norgestrel (0.3)	Ethinyl estradiol (30)	
Cyclafem 1/35		Norethindrone (1)	Ethinyl estradiol (35)	
Elinest		Norgestrel (0.3)	Ethinyl estradiol (30)	
Emoquette		Desogestrel (0.15)	Ethinyl estradiol (30)	
Enskyce		Desogestrel (0.15)	Ethinyl estradiol (30)	
Estarylla		Norgestimate (0.25)	Ethinyl estradiol (35)	

[Continued]

341

TABLE 5 (continued)
Oral Contraceptives (See also p 240)

(Note: 21 = 21 Active pills; 24 = 24 Active pills; Standard for most products is 28 [unless specified] = 21 Active pills + 7 Placebo[a])

Drug	Note	Progestin (mg)	Estrogen (mcg)	Extra
Monophasics				
Gianvi	c, e	Drospirenone (3)	Ethinyl estradiol (20)	
Gildagia		Norethindrone (0.4)	Ethinyl estradiol (35)	
Falmina		Levonorgestrel (0.1)	Ethinyl estradiol (20)	
Femcon Fe		Norethindrone (0.4)	Ethinyl estradiol (35)	75 mg Fe x 7 d in 28 d
Junel Fe 1/20		Norethindrone acetate (1)	Ethinyl estradiol (20)	75 mg Fe x 7 d in 28 d
Junel Fe 1.5/30		Norethindrone acetate (1.5)	Ethinyl estradiol (30)	75 mg Fe x 7 d in 28 d
Kelnor		Ethynodiol Diacetate (1)	Ethinyl estradiol (35)	
Kurvelo		Levonorgestrel (0.15)	Ethinyl estradiol (30)	
Lessina		Levonorgestrel (0.1)	Ethinyl estradiol (20)	
Levlen		Levonorgestrel (0.15)	Ethinyl estradiol (30)	
Levora		Levonorgestrel (0.15)	Ethinyl estradiol (30)	
Lo Minastrin Fe		Norethindrone (1)	Ethinyl estradiol (10)	2 10 mcg est/2 Fe
Loestrin 24 Fe		Norethindrone (1)	Ethinyl estradiol (20)	75 mg Fe x 4 d
Loestrin Fe 1.5/30		Norethindrone acetate (1.5)	Ethinyl estradiol (30)	75 mg Fe x 7 d in 28 d
Loestrin Fe 1/20		Norethindrone acetate (1)	Ethinyl estradiol (20)	75 mg Fe x 7 d in 28 d
Loestrin 1/20		Norethindrone acetate (1)	Ethinyl estradiol (20)	

342

Loestrin 1.5/20		Norethindrone acetate (1.5)	Ethinyl estradiol (20)	
Lo/Ovral		Norgestrel (0.3)	Ethinyl estradiol (30)	
Loryna	c, e	Drospirenone (3)	Ethinyl estradiol (20)	
Low-Ogestrel	c	Drospirenone (3)	Ethinyl estradiol (30)	
Lutera		Levonorgestrel (0.1)	Ethinyl estradiol (20)	
Marlissa		Levonorgestrel (0.15)	Ethinyl estradiol (30)	
Microgestin 1/20		Norethindrone acetate (1)	Ethinyl estradiol (20)	
Microgestin 1.5/30		Norethindrone acetate (1.5)	Ethinyl estradiol (30)	
Microgestin Fe 1/20		Norethindrone acetate (1)	Ethinyl estradiol (20)	75mg Fe x 7 d in 28 d
Microgestin Fe 1.5/30		Norethindrone acetate (1.5)	Ethinyl estradiol (30)	75mg Fe x 7 d in 28 d
Minastrin 24 Fe (chew)		Norethindrone 1 mg	Ethinyl estradiol (20)	75mg Fe x 4 d
Mircette		Desogestrel (0.15)	Ethinyl estradiol (20, 0, 10)	2 inert, 2 ethinyl estradiol 10 mcg
Modicon		Norethindrone (0.5)	Ethinyl estradiol (35)	
Mono-Linyah		Norgestimate (0.25)	Ethinyl estradiol (35)	
MonoNessa		Norgestimate (0.25)	Ethinyl estradiol (35)	
Necon 0.5/35		Norethindrone (0.5)	Ethinyl estradiol (35)	
Necon 1/50		Norethindrone (1)	Mestranol (35)	
Necon 1/35		Norethindrone (1)	Mestranol (50)	
Nordette		Levonorgestrel (0.15)	Ethinyl estradiol (30)	
Norethin 1/35E		Norethindrone (1)	Ethinyl estradiol (35)	
Norinyl 1/35		Norethindrone (1)	Ethinyl estradiol (35)	
Norinyl 1/50		Norethindrone (1)	Mestranol (50)	

[Continued]

TABLE 5 (continued)
Oral Contraceptives (See also p 240)

(Note: 21 = 21 Active pills; 24 = 24 Active pills; Standard for most products is 28 [unless specified] = 21 Active pills + 7 Placebo[a])

Drug	Note	Progestin (mg)	Estrogen (mcg)	Extra
Nortrel 0.5/35		Norethindrone (0.5)	Ethinyl estradiol (35)	
Nortrel 1/35		Norethindrone (1)	Ethinyl estradiol (35)	
Ocella	c	Drospirenone (3)	Ethinyl estradiol (30)	
Ogestrel 0.5/50		Norgestrel (0.5)	Ethinyl estradiol (50)	
Orsythia		Levonorgestrel (0.1)	Ethinyl estradiol (20)	
Ortho-Cept		Desogestrel (0.15)	Ethinyl estradiol (30)	
Ortho-Cyclen		Norgestimate (0.25)	Ethinyl estradiol (35)	
Ortho-Novum		Norethindrone (1)	Ethinyl estradiol (35)	
Ovcon 35		Norethindrone (0.4)	Ethinyl estradiol (35)	
Ovcon 35 Fe		Norethindrone (0.4)	Ethinyl estradiol (35)	75 mg Fe × 7 d in 28 d
Philith		Norethindrone (0.4)	Ethinyl estradiol (35)	
Pirmella 1/35		Norethindrone (1)	Ethinyl estradiol (35)	
Previfem		Norgestimate (0.25)	Ethinyl estradiol (35)	
Portia		Levonorgestrel (0.15)	Ethinyl estradiol (30)	
Reclipsen		Desogestrel (0.15)	Ethinyl estradiol (30)	
Safyral	b, c	Drospirenone (3)	Ethinyl estradiol (30)	0.451 mg levomefolate in all including 7 placebo

344

Solia	Desogestrel (0.15)	Ethinyl estradiol (30)
Sprintec	Norgestimate (0.25)	Ethinyl estradiol (35)
Sronyx	Levonorgestrel (0.1)	Ethinyl estradiol (20)
Syeda	c	Drospirenone (3)	Ethinyl estradiol (30)
Vestura	c, e	Drospirenone (3)	Ethinyl estradiol (20)
Vyfemla		Norethindrone (0.4)	Ethinyl estradiol (35)
Wera		Norethindrone (0.5)	Ethinyl estradiol (35)
Wymza Fe		Norethindrone (0.4)	Ethinyl estradiol (35) 75 mg Fe x 7 d in 28 d
Yasmin	c, d	Drospirenone (3)	Ethinyl estradiol (30)
Yaz	d, e, f	Drospirenone (3)	Ethinyl estradiol (20) 4 inert in 28 d
Zarah	c	Drospirenone (3)	Ethinyl estradiol (30)
Zenchent		Ethynodiol Diacetate (0.4)	Ethinyl estradiol (35)
Zeosa		Norgestimate (0.25)	Ethinyl estradiol (35)
Zovia 1/35		Ethynodiol Diacetate (1)	Ethinyl estradiol (35)
Zovia 1/50		Ethynodiol Diacetate (1)	Ethinyl estradiol (50)
Multiphasics		
Alyacen 7/7/7		Norethindrone (0.5, 0.75, 1)	Ethinyl estradiol (35, 35, 35)
Aranelle		Norethindrone (0.5, 1, 0.5)	Ethinyl estradiol (35, 35, 35)
Azurette		Desogestrel (0.15, 0, 0)	Ethinyl estradiol (20, 0, 10)
Caziant		Desogestrel (0.1, 0.125, 0.15)	Ethinyl estradiol (25, 25, 25)

345

(Continued)

TABLE 5 (continued)
Oral Contraceptives (See also p 240)

(Note: 21 = 21 Active pills; 24 = 24 Active pills; Standard for most products is 28 [unless specified] = 21 Active pills + 7 Placebo⁹)

Drug	Note	Progestin (mg)	Estrogen (mcg)	Extra
Multiphasics				
Cesia		Desogestrel (0.1, 0.125, 0.15)	Ethinyl estradiol (25, 25, 25)	
Cyclafem 7/7/7		Norethindrone (0.5, 0.75, 1)	Ethinyl estradiol (35, 35, 35)	
Cyclessa		Desogestrel (0.1, 0.125, 0.15)	Ethinyl estradiol (25, 25, 25)	
Dasetta 7/7/7		Norethindrone (0.5, 0.75, 1)	Ethinyl estradiol (35, 35, 35)	
Enpresse		Levonorgestrel (0.05, 0.075, 0.125)	Ethinyl estradiol (30, 40, 30)	
Estrostep Fe	e	Norethindrone acetate (1, 1, 1)	Ethinyl estradiol (20, 30, 35)	75 mg Fe x 7 d in 28 d
Generess Fe	e	Norethindrone acetate (0.8)	Ethinyl estradiol (25)	75 mg Fe x 4 d
Kariva		Desogestrel (0.15, 0, 0)	Ethinyl estradiol (20, 0, 10)	
Leena		Norethindrone (0.5, 1, 0.5)	Ethinyl estradiol (35, 35, 35)	
Lessina		Levonorgestrel (0.1)	Ethinyl estradiol (20)	

346

Levonest		Levonorgestrel (0.05, 0.075, 0.125)	Ethinyl estradiol (30, 40, 30)
Lo Loestrin Fe		Norethindrone acetate (1.0)	Ethinyl estradiol (10, 10)
Lutera		Levonorgestrel (0.1)	Ethinyl estradiol (20)
Mircette		Desogestrel (0.15, 0, 0)	Ethinyl estradiol (20, 0, 10)
Myzilra		Levonorgestrel (0.05, 0.075, 0.125)	Ethinyl estradiol (30, 40, 30)
Natazia	g	Dienogest (0, 2, 3, 0)	Estradiol valerat (3, 2, 2, 1)
Necon 10/11		Norethindrone (0.5, 1)	Ethinyl estradiol (35)
Necon 7/7/7		Norethindrone (0.5, 0.75, 1)	Ethinyl estradiol (35, 35, 35)
Nortrel 7/7/7		Norethindrone (0.5, 0.75, 1)	Ethinyl estradiol (35, 35, 35)
Orsythia		Levonorgestrel (0.1)	Ethinyl estradiol (20)
Ortho-Novum 10/11		Norethindrone (0.5, 1)	Ethinyl estradiol (35)
Ortho-Novum 7/7/7		Norethindrone (0.5, 0.75, 1)	Ethinyl estradiol (35, 35, 35)
Ortho Tri-Cyclen	e	Norgestimate (0.18, 0.215, 0.25)	Ethinyl estradiol (25, 25, 25)
Ortho Tri-Cyclen Lo		Norgestimate (0.18, 0.215, 0.25)	Ethinyl estradiol (35, 35, 35)
Pirmella 7/7/7		Norethindrone (0.5, 0.75, 1)	Ethinyl estradiol (35, 35, 35)
Previfem		Norgestimate (0.25)	Ethinyl estradiol (35)

(Continued)

TABLE 5 (continued)
Oral Contraceptives (See also p 240)

(Note: 21 = 21 Active pills; 24 = 24 Active pills; Standard for most products is 28 [unless specified] = 21 Active pills + 7 Placebo[a])

Drug	Note	Progestin (mg)	Estrogen (mcg)	Extra
Multiphasics				
Tilia Fe		Norethindrone acetate (1, 1, 1)	Ethinyl estradiol (20, 30, 35)	75 mg Fe x 7 d in 28 d
Tri-Estarylla		Norgestimate (0.18, 0.215, 0.25)	Ethinyl estradiol (25, 25, 25)	
Tri-Legest		Norethindrone acetate (1, 1, 1)	Ethinyl estradiol (20, 30, 35)	
Tri-Legest Fe		Norethindrone acetate (1, 1, 1)	Ethinyl estradiol (20, 30, 35)	75 mg Fe x 7 d in 28 d
Tri-Levlen		Levonorgestrel (0.05, 0.075, 0.125)	Ethinyl estradiol (30, 40, 30)	
Tri-Linyah		Norgestimate (0.18, 0.215, 0.25)	Ethinyl estradiol (25, 25, 25)	
Tri-Nessa		Desogestrel (0.1, 0.125, 0.15)	Ethinyl estradiol (25, 25, 25)	
Tri-Norinyl		Norethindrone (0.5, 1, 0.5)	Ethinyl estradiol (35, 35, 35)	
Tri-Previfem		Desogestrel (0.1, 0.125, 0.15)	Ethinyl estradiol (25, 25, 25)	

Tri-Sprintec	Desogestrel (0.1, 0.125, 0.15)	Ethinyl estradiol (25, 25, 25)	
Trivora	Levonorgestrel (0.05, 0.075, 0.125)	Ethinyl estradiol (30, 40, 30)	
Velivet	Desogestrel (0.1, 0.125, 0.15)	Ethinyl estradiol (25, 25, 25)	
Viorele	Desogestrel (0.15, 0, 0)	Ethinyl estradiol (20, 0, 10)	

Progestin Only (aka "mini-pills")

Camila	Norethindrone (0.35)	None	
Errin	Norethindrone (0.35)	None	
Heather	Norethindrone (0.35)	None	
Jencycla	Norethindrone (0.35)	None	
Jolivette	Norethindrone (0.35)	None	
Micronor	Norethindrone (0.35)	None	
Nor-QD	Norethindrone (0.35)	None	
Nora-BE	Norethindrone (0.35)	None	

Extended-Cycle Combination (aka COCP [combined oral contraceptive pills]) 91 d

Daysee	Levonorgestrel (0.15)	Ethinyl estradiol (30)	7 (0 mg/10 mcg)
Introvale	Levonorgestrel (0.15)	Ethinyl estradiol (30)	7 inert
Jolessa	Levonorgestrel (0.15)	Ethinyl estradiol (30)	7 inert
LoSeasonique	Levonorgestrel (0.1)	Ethinyl estradiol (20, 10)	7 (0 mg/10 mcg)

349

(Continued)

TABLE 5 (continued)
Oral Contraceptives (See also p 240)

(Note: 21 = 21 Active pills; 24 = 24 Active pills; Standard for most products is 28 [unless specified] = 21 Active pills + 7 Placebo[a])

Drug	Note	Progestin (mg)	Estrogen (mcg)	Extra
Extended-Cycle Combination (aka COCP [combined oral contraceptive pills]) 91 d				
Quasense		Levonorgestrel (0.15)	Ethinyl estradiol (30)	7 inert
Seasonale		Levonorgestrel (0.15)	Ethinyl estradiol (30)	7 inert
Seasonique		Levonorgestrel (0.15)	Ethinyl estradiol (30)	7 (0 mg/10 mcg)
Extended-Cycle Combination, ascending dose				
Quartette 91 d		Ethinyl estradiol	Levonorgestrel	
		0.02 mg (42 d)	0.15 mg (42 d)	
		0.025 mg (21 d)	0.15 mg (21 d)	
		0.03 mg (21 d)	0.15 mg (21 d)	
		0.01 mg (7 d)		

[a] The designations 21 and 28 refer to number of days in regimen available; if not listed, assume 28.

[b] Raises folate levels to help decrease neural tube defect risk with eventual pregnancy.

[c] Drospirenone-containing pills have increased risk for blood clots compared to other progestins.

[d] Avoid in patients with hyperkalemia risk.

[e] Also approved for acne.

[f] Approved for PMDD in women who use contraception for birth control.

[g] First "four-phasic" OCP.

TABLE 6
Oral Potassium Supplements (See also p 261)

Brand Name	Salt	Form	mEq Potassium/Dosing Unit
Glu-K	Gluconate	Tablet	2 mEq/tablet
Kaon elixir	Gluconate	Liquid	20 mEq/15 mL
Kaon-Cl 10	KCl	Tablet, SR	10 mEq/tablet
Kaon-Cl 20%	KCl	Liquid	40 mEq/15 mL
K-Dur 20	KCl	Tablet, SR	20 mEq/tablet
KayCiel	KCl	Liquid	20 mEq/15 mL
K-Lor	KCl	Powder	20 mEq/packet
K-lyte/Cl	KCl/bicarbonate	Effervescent tablet	25 mEq/tablet
Klorvess	KCl/bicarbonate	Effervescent tablet	20 mEq/tablet
Klotrix	KCl	Tablet, SR	10 mEq/tablet
K-Lyte	Bicarbonate/citrate	Effervescent tablet	25 mEq/tablet
Klor-Con/EF	Bicarbonate/citrate	Effervescent tablet	25 mEq/tablet
K-Tab	KCl	Tablet, SR	10 mEq/tablet
Micro-K	KCl	Capsule, SR	8 mEq/capsule
Potassium Chloride 10%	KCl	Liquid	20 mEq/15 mL
Potassium Chloride 20%	KCl	Liquid	40 mEq/15 mL
Slow-K	KCl	Tablet, SR	8 mEq/tablet
Tri-K	Acetate/bicarbonate and citrate	Liquid	45 mEq/15 mL
Twin-K	Citrate/gluconate	Liquid	20 mEq/5 mL

SR = sustained release.

Note: Alcohol and sugar content vary between preparations.

TABLE 7
Tetanus Prophylaxis (See also p 301)

History of Absorbed Tetanus Toxoid Immunization	Clean, Minor Wounds		All Other Wounds[a]	
	Td[b]	TIG[c]	Td[d]	TIG[c]
Unknown or < 3 doses	Yes	No	Yes	Yes
= 3 doses	No[e]	No	No[f]	No

[a] Such as, but not limited to, wounds contaminated with dirt, feces, soil, saliva, etc; puncture wounds; avulsions; and wounds resulting from missiles, crushing, burns, and frostbite.

[b] Td = tetanus-diphtheria toxoid (adult type), 0.5 mL IM.
  • For children < 7 y, DPT (DT, if pertussis vaccine is contraindicated) is preferred to tetanus toxoid alone.
  • For persons > 7 y, Td is preferred to tetanus toxoid alone.
  • DT = diphtheria-tetanus toxoid (pediatric), used for those who cannot receive pertussis.

[c] TIG = tetanus immune globulin, 250 units IM.

[d] If only 3 doses of fluid toxoid have been received, then a fourth dose of toxoid, preferably an adsorbed toxoid, should be given.

[e] Yes, if > 10 y since last dose.

[f] Yes, if > 5 y since last dose.

Data from Guidelines from the Centers for Disease Control and Prevention and reported in *MMWR* (*MMWR*, December 1, 2006; 55(RR-15):1-48).

TABLE 8
Oral Anticoagulant Standards of Practice (See also Warfarin, p 321)

Thromboembolic Disorder	INR	Duration
Deep Venous Thrombosis & Pulmonary Embolism		
Treatment of single episode		
Transient risk factor	2–3	3 mo
Idiopathic[a]	2–3	long-term
Recurrent systemic embolism	2–3	long-term
Prevention of Systemic Embolism		
Atrial fibrillation (AF)[b]	2–3	long-term
AF: cardioversion	2–3	3 wk prior; 4 wk post sinus rhythm
Mitral valvular heart dx[c]	2–3	long-term
Cardiomyopathy (usually ASA)[d]	2–3	long-term
Acute Myocardial Infarction		
High risk[e]	2–3 + low-dose aspirin	long-term
All other infarcts (usually ASA)[f]		

TABLE 8
Oral Anticoagulant Standards of Practice (See also Warfarin, p 321) (continued)

Thromboembolic Disorder	INR	Duration
Prosthetic Valves		
Bioprosthetic heart valves		
Mitral position	2–3	3 mo
Aortic position[g]	2–3	3 mo
Bileaflet mechanical valves in aortic position[h]	2–3	long-term
Other mechanical prosthetic valves[i]	2.5–3.5	long-term

[a] 3 mo if mod or high risk of bleeding or distal DVT; if low risk of bleeding, then long-term for proximal DVT/PE.

[b] Paroxysmal AF or ≥ 2 risk factors (age > 75, Hx, BP, DM, mod–severe LV dysfunction or CHF), then warfarin; 1 risk factor warfarin or 75–325 mg ASA; 0 risk factors ASA.

[c] Mitral valve Dz: rheumatic if Hx systemic embolism, or AF or LA thrombus or LA > 55 mm; MVP: only if AF, systemic embolism or TIAs on ASA; mitral valve calcification: warfarin if AF or recurrent embolism on ASA; aortic valve w/ calcification: warfarin not recommended.

[d] In adults only ASA; only indication for anticoagulation cardiomyopathy in children, to begin no later than their activation on transplant list.

[e] High risk = large anterior MI, significant CHF, intracardiac thrombus visible on TE, AF, and Hx of a thromboembolic event.

[f] If meticulous INR monitoring and highly skilled dose titration are expected and widely accessible, then INR 3.5 (3.0–4.0) w/o ASA or 2.5 (2.0–3.0) w/ ASA long-term (4 years).

[g] Usually ASA 50–100 mg; warfarin if Hx embolism, LA thrombus, AF, low EF, hypercoagulable state, 3 mo, or until thrombus resolves.

[h] Target INR 2.5–3.5 if AF, large anterior MI, LA enlargement, hypercoagulable state, or low EF.

[i] Add ASA 50–100 mg if high risk (AF, hypercoagulable state, low EF, or Hx of ASCVD).

Data from ACCP guidelines-Antithrombotic Therapy and Prevention of Thrombosis: American College of Chest Physicians Evidence-Based Clinical Practice Guidelines (9th Ed.) CHEST. 2012;141 (suppl 2) 1s-801s.

TABLE 9
Antiarrhythmics: Vaughn Williams Classification

Class I: Sodium Channel Blockade

A. **Class Ia:** Lengthens duration of action potential (↑ the refractory period in atrial and ventricular muscle, in SA and AV conduction systems, and Purkinje fibers)
   1. Amiodarone (also classes II, III, IV)
   2. Disopyramide (Norpace)
   3. Imipramine (MAO inhibitor)
   4. Procainamide (Pronestyl)
   5. Quinidine
B. **Class Ib:** No effect on action potential
   1. Lidocaine (Xylocaine)
   2. Mexiletine (Mexitil)
   3. Phenytoin (Dilantin)
   4. Tocainide (Tonocard)
C. **Class Ic:** Greater sodium current depression (blocks the fast inward Na^+ current in heart muscle and Purkinje fibers, and slows the rate of ↑ of phase 0 of the action potential)
   1. Flecainide (Tambocor)
   2. Propafenone

Class II: β-Blocker

D. Amiodarone (also classes Ia, III, IV)
E. Esmolol (Brevibloc)
F. Sotalol (also class III)

Class III: Prolong Refractory Period via Action Potential

G. Amiodarone (also classes Ia, II, IV)
H. Sotalol

Class IV: Calcium Channel Blocker

I. Amiodarone (also classes Ia, II, III)
J. Diltiazem (Cardizem)
K. Verapamil (Calan)

TABLE 10
Cytochrome P450 Isoenzymes and Common Drugs
They Metabolize, Inhibit, and Induce

Increased or decreased (primarily hepatic cytochrome P450) metabolism of medications may influence the effectiveness of drugs or result in significant drug–drug interactions. Understanding the common cytochrome P450 isoforms (eg, CYP2C9, CYP2D9, CYP2C19, CYP3A4) and common drugs that are metabolized by (aka "substrates"), inhibit, or induce activity of the isoform helps identify and minimize significant drug interactions.

CYP1A2	
Substrates:	Acetaminophen, caffeine, cyclobenzaprine, clozapine, imipramine, mexiletine, naproxen, propranolol, theophylline
Inhibitors:	Amiodarone, cimetidine, most fluoroquinolone antibiotics, fluvoxamine, verapamil
Inducers:	Carbamazepine, charcoal-broiled foods, cruciferous vegetables, omeprazole, modafinil, tobacco smoking
CYP2C9	
Substrates:	Most NSAIDs (including COX-2), glipizide, irbesartan, losartan, phenytoin, tamoxifen, warfarin
Inhibitors:	Amiodarone, fluconazole, isoniazid (INH), ketoconazole, metronidazole
Inducers:	Aprepitant, Barbiturates, rifampin
CYP2C19	
Substrates:	Amitriptyline, clopidogrel, cyclophosphamide, diazepam, lansoprazole, omeprazole, pantoprazole, phenytoin, rabeprazole
Inhibitors:	Fluoxetine, fluvoxamine, isoniazid, ketoconazole, lansoprazole, omeprazole, ticlopidine
Inducers:	Barbiturates, carbamazepine, prednisone, rifampin
CYP2D6	
Substrates:	**Antidepressants:** Most tricyclic antidepressants, clomipramine, fluoxetine, paroxetine, venlafaxine **Antipsychotics:** Aripiprazole, clozapine, haloperidol, risperidone, thioridazine **Beta-blockers:** Carvedilol, metoprolol, propranolol, timolol

(Continued)

TABLE 10
Cytochrome P450 Isoenzymes and Common Drugs
They Metabolize, Inhibit, and Induce (*continued*)

CYP2D6 (continued)

Opioids: Codeine, hydrocodone, oxycodone, tramadol
Others: Amphetamine, dextromethorphan, duloxetine, encainide, flecainide, mexiletine, ondansetron, propafenone, selegiline, tamoxifen

Inhibitors: Amiodarone, bupropion, cimetidine, clomipramine, doxepin, duloxetine, fluoxetine, haloperidol, methadone, paroxetine, quinidine, ritonavir

Inducers: Dexamethasone, rifampin

CYP3A
(involved in the metabolism of > 50% of drugs metabolized by the liver)

Substrates: **Anticholinergics:** Darifenacin, oxybutynin, solifenacin, tolterodine
Benzodiazepines: Alprazolam, diazepam, midazolam, triazolam
Calcium channel blockers: Amlodipine, diltiazem, felodipine, nifedipine, nimodipine, nisoldipine, verapamil
Chemotherapy: Cyclophosphamide, erlotinib, ifosfamide, paclitaxel, tamoxifen, vinblastine, vincristine
HIV protease inhibitors: Atazanavir, indinavir, nelfinavir, ritonavir, saquinavir
HMG-CoA reductase inhibitors: Atorvastatin, lovastatin, simvastatin
Immunosuppressive agents: Cyclosporine, tacrolimus
Macrolide-type antibiotics: Clarithromycin, erythromycin, telithromycin, troleandomycin
Opioids: Alfentanil, cocaine, fentanyl, methadone, sufentanil
Steroids: Budesonide, cortisol, 17-β-estradiol, progesterone
Others: Acetaminophen, amiodarone, carbamazepine, delavirdine, efavirenz, nevirapine, quinidine, repaglinide, sildenafil, tadalafil, trazodone, vardenafil

Inhibitors: Amiodarone, amprenavir, aprepitant, atazanavir, ciprofloxacin, cisapride, clarithromycin, diltiazem, erythromycin, fluconazole, fluvoxamine, grapefruit juice (in high ingestion), indinavir, itraconazole, ketoconazole, nefazodone, nelfinavir, norfloxacin, ritonavir, saquinavir, telithromycin, troleandomycin, verapamil, voriconazole

(Continued)

TABLE 10
Cytochrome P450 Isoenzymes and Common Drugs
They Metabolize, Inhibit, and Induce (*continued*)

CYP3A (continued)

Inducers:	Carbamazepine, efavirenz, glucocorticoids, modafinil, nevirapine, phenytoin, phenobarbital, rifabutin, rifapentine, rifampin, St. John's wort

Data from Katzung B, ed. *Basic and Clinical Pharmacology*. 12th ed. New York, NY: McGraw-Hill; 2012 *The Medical Letter*. July 4, 2004; 47; 1 *N Engl J Med*. 2005;352:2211–2221. Flockhart DA. Drug Interactions Cytochrome P450 Drug Interaction Table. Indiana University School of Medicine. http://medicine.iupui.edu/clinpharm/ddis/table.aspx. Accessed August 31, 2013.

TABLE 11
SSRIs/SNRIs/Triptans and Serotonin Syndrome

A life-threatening condition, when selective serotonin reuptake inhibitors (SSRIs) and 5-hydroxytryptamine receptor agonists (triptans) are used together. However, many other drugs have been implicated (see below). Signs and symptoms of serotonin syndrome include the following:

Restlessness, coma, N/V/D, hallucinations, loss of coordination, overactive reflexes, hypertension, mydriasis, rapid changes in BP, increased body temperature

Class	Drugs
Antidepressants	MAOIs, TCAs, SSRIs, SNRIs, mirtazapine, venlafaxine
CNS stimulants	Amphetamines, phentermine, methylphenidate, sibutramine
5-HT$_1$ agonists	Triptans
Illicit drugs	Cocaine, methylenedioxymethamphetamine (ecstasy), lysergic acid diethylamide (LSD)
Opioids	Tramadol, oxycodone, morphine, meperidine
Others	Buspirone, chlorpheniramine, dextromethorphan, linezolid, lithium, selegiline, tryptophan, St. John's wort

Management includes removal of the precipitating drugs and supportive care. To control agitation, the serotonin antagonist cyproheptadine can be used. When symptoms are mild, discontinuation of the medication or medications and the control of agitation with benzodiazepines may be needed. Critically ill patients may require sedation and mechanical ventilation as well as control of hyperthermia. (Ables AZ, Nagubilli R. Prevention, recognition, and management of serotonin syndrome. *Am Fam Physician*. May 1, 2010;81(9):1139–1142.
MAOI = monoamine oxidase inhibitor.
TCA = tricyclic antidepressant.
SNRI = serotonin–norepinephrine reuptake inhibitors.

TABLE 12

Selected Multivitamin Supplements

This table lists common multivitamins available without a prescription, and most chains have generic versions. Many specialty vitamin combinations are available and are not included in this table. (Examples are B vitamins plus C; disease-specific supplements; pediatric and infant formulations; prenatal vitamins, etc.) A check (✓) indicates the component is found in the formulation; NA indicates it is not in the formulation. Details of the specific composition of these multivitamins can be found at www.eDrugbook.com or on the product site.

Brand	Fat-Soluble Vitamins		Water-Soluble Vitamins[a]		Minerals[b]								Trace Elements[b]				Other
	A, D, E	K	C, B₁, B₂, B₃, B₅, B₆, B₁₂, Folate	Biotin	Ca	P	Mg	Fe	Zn	I	Se	K	Mn	Cu	Cr	Mo	
Centrum	✓	✓	✓	✓	✓	✓	✓	✓	✓	✓	✓	✓	✓	✓	✓	✓	
Centrum Performance	✓	✓	✓	✓	✓	✓	✓	✓	✓	✓	✓	✓	✓	✓	✓	✓	Lycopene Ginseng Ginkgo
Centrum Silver	✓	✓	✓	✓	✓	✓	✓	NA	✓	✓	✓	✓	✓	✓	✓	✓	
NatureMade Multi Complete	✓	✓	✓	✓	✓	NA	✓	✓	✓	✓	✓	✓	✓	✓	✓	✓	
NatureMade Multi Daily	✓	NA	✓	NA	✓	NA	NA	✓	✓	NA	NA	NA	NA	NA	NA	NA	Lycopene
NatureMade Multi Max	✓	✓	✓	✓	✓	✓	✓	✓	✓	✓	✓	NA	✓	✓	✓	NA	Lutein

(Continued)

TABLE 12 (continued)
Selected Multivitamin Supplements

This table lists common multivitamins available without a prescription, and most chains have generic versions. Many specially vitamin combinations are available and are not included in this table. (Examples are B vitamins plus C; disease-specific supplements; pediatric and infant formulations; prenatal vitamins; etc.) A check (✓) indicates the component is found in the formulation; NA indicates it is not in the formulation. Details of the specific composition of these multivitamins can be found at www.eDrugbook.com or on the product site.

Brand	Fat-Soluble Vitamins		Water-Soluble Vitamins[a]		Minerals[b]								Trace Elements[b]				Other
	A, D, E	K	C, B₁, B₂, B₃, B₅, B₆, B₁₂, Folate	Biotin	Ca	P	Mg	Fe	Zn	I	Se	K	Mn	Cu	Cr	Mo	
NatureMade Multi 50+	✓	✓	✓	✓	✓	✓	✓	✓	✓	✓	✓	✓	✓	✓	✓	✓	
One-A-Day 50 Plus	✓	✓	✓	✓	✓	NA	✓	NA	✓	✓	✓	✓	✓	✓	✓	✓	Lutein
One-A-Day Essential	✓	NA	✓	NA	✓	NA	NA	✓	✓	NA	NA	NA	NA	NA	NA	NA	
One-A-Day Maximum	✓	✓	✓	✓	✓	✓	✓	✓	✓	✓	✓	✓	✓	✓	✓	✓	
Therapeutic Vitamin	✓	NA	✓	✓	✓	NA	NA	✓	NA	NA	NA	NA	NA	NA	NA	NA	

Product																			
Theragran-M Advanced Formula High Potency	✓		✓		✓		✓	✓	✓	✓		✓	✓	✓	✓		✓	✓	✓
Theragran-M Premier High Potency	✓		✓		✓		✓	✓	✓	✓		✓	✓	✓	✓		✓	✓	✓ Lutein
Theragran-M Premier 50 Plus High Potency	✓		✓		✓		NA	✓	✓	✓		✓	✓	✓	✓		✓	✓	✓ Lutein
Therapeutic Vitamin + Minerals Enhanced	NA		NA		NA		✓	✓	✓	✓	low	✓	✓	✓	✓		✓	✓	✓
Unicap M	NA		NA		NA		NA	✓	✓	✓	NA low	✓	✓	✓	✓		NA NA		
Unicap Senior	✓		NA		✓		✓	✓	✓	✓	NA low	✓	✓	✓	✓		NA NA		
Unicap T	✓		NA		NA		NA NA	NA	NA	✓	✓ low	✓	✓	✓	✓		NA NA		

361

a Vitamin B₁ = thiamine; B₂ = riboflavin; B₃ = niacin; B₅ = pantothenic acid; B₆ = pyridoxine; B₁₂ = cyanocobalamin.

b Ca = calcium; Cr = chromium; Cu = copper; Fe = iron; Fl = fluoride; I = iodine; K = potassium; Mg = magnesium; Mn = manganese; Mo = molybdenum; P = phosphorus; Se = selenium; Zn = zinc.

TABLE 13
Influenza Vaccine Strains for 2015–2016 (See also pp 176–177)

The 2015–2016 trivalent influenza vaccine is made from the following three viruses:

- A/California/7/2009 (H1N1)-like virus
- A/Switzerland/9715293/2013 (H3N2)-like virus
- B/Phuket/3073/2013-like virus

This represents changes in the influenza A (H3N2) virus and the influenza B virus as compared with the 2014–15 season. Quadrivalent influenza vaccines will contain these vaccine viruses, and a B/Brisbane/60/2008-like (Victoria lineage) virus, which is the same Victoria lineage virus recommended for quadrivalent formulations in 2013–14 and 2014–15 .(http://www.cdc.gov/flu/about/season/flu-season-2015-2016.htm. Accessed September 20, 2015)

Age	Brand Name Product	Dosage Form/Strength
6–35 mo	Fluzone	0.25 ml; 5 ml multi-dose vial
	Fluzone Quadrivalent	0.25 ml prefilled syringe
2–49 y	FluMist Quadrivalent	0.2 ml prefilled intranasal sprayer
≥36 mo	FluLaval	5 ml multi-dose vial
	Fluzone	0.5 ml; 5 ml multi-dose vial
	Fluarix Quadrivalent	0.5 ml prefilled syringe
	Fluzone Quadrivalent	0.5 ml prefilled syringe, single-dose via, & multi-dose vial
≥4 y	Fluvirin	0.5 ml prefilled syringe & 5 ml multi-dose vial
≥ 5 ya	Afluria	0.5 ml prefilled syringe & 5 ml multi-dose vial
≥ 18 y	Flucelvax	0.5 ml prefilled syringe
	Flublok[b]	0.5 ml single-dose vial
18–64 y	Fluzone Intradermal	0.1 ml prefilled microinjection system
≥ 65 y	Fluzone High-Dose	0.5 ml prefilled syringe

[a]Age indication per package labeling is ≥ 5 y; ACIP (http://www.cdc.gov/vaccines/hcp/acip-recs/vacc-specific/flu.html) recommends Afluria not be used in children 6–8 y due to increased risk of febrile Rxn.

[b]Adolescents of age 18 yrs and older with egg allergy of any severity can receive the recombinant influenza vaccine (RIV) (Flublok). RIV does not contain any egg protein.

Index

Note: Page numbers are followed by a "t" indicate tables.